9R

# Eye Movements in Reading

PERCEPTUAL AND LANGUAGE PROCESSES

PERSPECTIVES IN
NEUROLINGUISTICS, NEUROPSYCHOLOGY, AND
PSYCHOLINGUISTICS: A Series of Monographs and Treatises

**Harry A. Whitaker, Series Editor**
DEPARTMENT OF HEARING AND SPEECH SCIENCES
UNIVERSITY OF MARYLAND
COLLEGE PARK, MARYLAND 20742

The list of titles in this series continues on the last page of this volume.

# Eye Movements in Reading

## PERCEPTUAL AND LANGUAGE PROCESSES

Edited by

## KEITH RAYNER

*Department of Psychology*
*University of Massachusetts*
*Amherst, Massachusetts*

1983

**ACADEMIC PRESS**

A Subsidiary of Harcourt Brace Jovanovich, Publishers

New York    London
Paris   San Diego   San Francisco   São Paulo   Sydney   Tokyo   Toronto

ACADEMIC PRESS, INC.
111 Fifth Avenue, New York, New York 10003

*United Kingdom Edition published by*
ACADEMIC PRESS, INC. (LONDON) LTD.
24/28 Oval Road, London NW1 7DX

Library of Congress Cataloging in Publication Data
Main entry under title:

Eye movements in reading.

(Perspectives in neurolinguistics, neuropsychology,
and psycholinguistics)
Based on a conference sponsored by the Sloan Foundation
and held at the University of Massachusetts in June of
1981.
Includes index.
1. Eye--Movements--Congresses. 2. Reading--Physiologi-
cal aspects--Congresses. 3. Visual perception--Congresses.
I. Rayner, Keith. II. Alfred P. Sloan Foundation.
III. Series.
QP477.5.E953 1983      152.1'4      82-11565
ISBN 0-12-583680-5

PRINTED IN THE UNITED STATES OF AMERICA

83 84 85 86      9 8 7 6 5 4 3 2 1

# Contents

## I

## Eye Movements and Psychophysical Processes

## 1

### Sensory Masking, Persistence, and Enhancement in Visual Exploration and Reading

BRUNO G. BREITMEYER

# 2
## Retinal Image Size and the Perceptual Span in Reading
### ROBERT E. MORRISON

# 3
## The Temporal Characteristics of Visual Information Extraction during Reading
### GARY S. WOLVERTON and DAVID ZOLA

# 4
## Locations and Contents
### PAUL A. KOLERS

# II
## Eye Movements and Perceptual Processes

# 5
## Eye Movements and Perception during Reading

GEORGE W. McCONKIE

# 6
## The Perceptual Span and Eye Movement Control during Reading

KEITH RAYNER

# 7
## Elementary Perceptual and Eye Movement Control Processes in Reading

J. KEVIN O'REGAN

# 8
## Perceptual Factors in Reading

ARNOLD D. WELL

# III

# Eye Movements and Context Effects

## 9

### Eye Movements and Context Effects during Reading of Extended Discourse

WAYNE L. SHEBILSKE and DENNIS F. FISHER

## 10

### Attentional Strategies during the Reading of Short Stories

ALBRECHT WERNER INHOFF

## 11

### Contextual Influences on Eye Movements in Reading

SUSAN F. EHRLICH

# 12
## Context, Form, and Interaction

### PHILIP B. GOUGH

# IV
## Eye Movements and Language Processes I

# 13
## Processing Sentence Structure

### LYN FRAZIER

# 14
## On Looking into Space

### ALAN KENNEDY

# 15
## Eye Movements in Pronoun Assignment: A Study of Sentence Integration

### KATE EHRLICH

# 16
## Psycholinguistic Factors Reflected in the Eye
### CHARLES CLIFTON, JR.

# V
# Eye Movements and Language Processes II

# 17
## What Your Eyes Do while Your Mind Is Reading
### PATRICIA A. CARPENTER and MARCEL ADAM JUST

# 18
## Reading Patterns in Eye Movement Data
### THOMAS W. HOGABOAM

# 19
## On Problems of Unconfounding Perceptual and Language Processes

REINHOLD, KLIEGL, RICHARD K. OLSON, and BRIAN J. DAVIDSON

# 20
## What Does the Mind Do While the Eyes Are Gazing?

MARIA L. SLOWIACZEK

# VI
## Eye Movements in Picture Processing and Visual Search

# 21
## Eye Fixations on Text and Scenes

GEOFFREY R. LOFTUS

# 22
## A Spatial-Relational Logic behind Visual Differentiation: Gibosonian Constructivism?
### CALVIN F. NODINE

# 23
## Saccadic Reaction Time in Visual Search
### JONATHAN VAUGHAN

# 24
## Representational Buffers: The Eye–Mind Hypothesis in Picture Perception, Reading, and Visual Search
### MARY C. POTTER

# VII
## Eye Movements and Dyslexia

## 25
### The "Dyslexia Syndrome" and Its Objective Diagnosis by Erratic Eye Movements

#### GEORGE Th. PAVLIDIS

## 26
### Eye Movements in Reading Disability

#### RICHARD K. OLSON, REINHOLD KLIEGL, and BRIAN J. DAVIDSON

## 27
### Abnormal Patterns of Normal Eye Movements in Specific Dyslexia

#### ASHBY JONES and LAWRENCE STARK

# 28
## Eye Movements and Reading Disability

### FRANCIS J. PIROZZOLO

# 29
## What Can Eye Movements Tell Us about Dyslexia?

### ALEXANDER POLLATSEK

# Contributors

*Numbers in parentheses indicate the pages on which the authors' contributions begin.*

**BRUNO G. BREITMEYER** (3), *Department of Psychology, University of Houston, Houston, Texas 77004*

**PATRICIA A. CARPENTER** (275), *Department of Psychology, Carnegie-Mellon University, Pittsburgh, Pennsylvania 15231*

**CHARLES CLIFTON, JR.** (269), *Department of Psychology, University of Massachusetts, Amherst, Massachusetts 01003*

**BRIAN J. DAVIDSON** (333, 467), *Department of Psychology, University of Colorado, Boulder, Colorado 80309*

**KATE EHRLICH**[1] (253), *Department of Psychology, University of Massachusetts, Amherst, Massachusetts 01003*

**SUSAN F. EHRLICH**[2] (193), *Department of Psychology and Social Relations, Harvard University, Cambridge, Massachusetts 02173*

**DENNIS F. FISHER** (153), *Behavioral Research Directorate, U.S. Army Human Engineering Laboratory, Aberdeen Proving Ground, Aberdeen, Maryland 21005*

**LYN FRAZIER** (215), *Department of Linguistics, University of Massachusetts, Amherst, Massachusetts 01003*

**PHILIP B. GOUGH** (203), *Department of Psychology, University of Texas, Austin, Texas 78712*

[1]Present address: Department of Computer Science, Yale University, New Haven, Connecticut 06520

[2]Present address: Advanced Systems Laboratory, Wang Laboratories, Lowell, Massachusetts 01851

THOMAS W. HOGABOAM[3] (309), *Center for the Study of Reading, University of Illinois at Urbana–Champaign, Champaign, Illinois 61820*

ALBRECHT WERNER INHOFF (181), *Department of Psychology, University of Massachusetts, Amherst, Massachusetts 01003*

ASHBY JONES (481), *Physiological Optics, School of Optometry, University of California at Berkeley, Berkeley, California 94720*

MARCEL ADAM JUST (275), *Department of Psychology, Carnegie-Mellon University, Pittsburgh, Pennsylvania 15231*

ALAN KENNEDY (237), *Department of Psychology, University of Dundee, Dundee, Scotland*

REINHOLD KLIEGL (333, 467), *Department of Psychology, University of Colorado, Boulder, Colorado 80309*

PAUL A. KOLERS (53), *Department of Psychology, University of Toronto, Toronto, Ontario M5S 1A1, Canada*

GEOFFREY R. LOFTUS (359), *Department of Psychology, University of Washington, Seattle, Washington 98195*

GEORGE W. McCONKIE (65), *Center for the Study of Reading and Department of Educational Psychology, University of Illinois at Urbana–Champaign, Champaign, Illinois 61802*

ROBERT E. MORRISON (31), *Department of Psychology, University of Massachusetts, Amherst, Massachusetts 01003*

CALVIN F. NODINE (377), *Department of Educational Psychology, Temple University, Philadelphia, Pennsylvania 19122*

J. KEVIN O'REGAN (121), *Laboratoire de Psychologie Experimentale, Paris, France*

RICHARD K. OLSON (333, 467), *Department of Psychology, University of Colorado, Boulder, Colorado 80309*

GEORGE Th. PAVLIDIS (441), *Reading Disabilities Research Institute, Department of Psychiatry, Rutgers Medical School, Piscataway, New Jersey 08854*

FRANCIS J. PIROZZOLO (499), *Department of Neurology, Baylor College of Medicine, Houston, Texas 77030*

ALEXANDER POLLATSEK (511), *Department of Psychology, University of Massachusetts, Amherst, Massachusetts 01003*

MARY C. POTTER (413), *Department of Psychology, Massachusetts Institute of Technology, Cambridge, Massachusetts 02139*

KEITH RAYNER (97), *Department of Psychology, University of Massachusetts, Amherst, Massachusetts 01003*

WAYNE L. SHEBILSKE (153), *Department of Psychology, University of Virginia, Charlottesville, Virginia 22901*

MARIA L. SLOWIACZEK[4] (345), *Bell Laboratories, Murray Hill, New Jersey 07974*

LAWRENCE STARK (481), *Department of Engineering Sciences and of Physiological Optics and Department of Neurology, University of California, Berkeley, California 94720*

---

[3]Present address: Bell Laboratories, 6 Corporate Place, Piscataway, New Jersey 08854
[4]Present address: Department of Psychology, University of Texas, Austin, Texas 78712

JONATHAN VAUGHAN *(397), Department of Psychology, Hamilton College, Clinton, New York 13323*

ARNOLD D. WELL *(141), Department of Psychology, University of Massachusetts, Amherst, Massachusetts 01003*

GARY S. WOLVERTON *(41), Center for the Study of Reading, University of Illinois, Champaign, Illinois 61820*

DAVID ZOLA *(41), Center for the Study of Reading, University of Illinois, Champaign, Illinois 61820*

# Preface

This volume originated with my observation that an increasing number of researchers were beginning to use eye movement data as a way to study the reading process. Although there are articles reviewing the use of eye movements to study reading, the material has not been treated in great depth, and so I decided to ask a number of colleagues to prepare chapters describing their research and how they use eye movements to reveal aspects of the reading process, including underlying cognitive processes. It is my hope that this volume will be useful to various researchers interested in the reading process.

Other recent books concerning eye movements and cognitive processes have emerged, but none of them has been solely directed to the reading process. The strength of the current volume lies in the fact that all the chapters illustrate interesting and informative ways that eye movements can be used to study reading; the volume is unique in this respect. Neither I nor any of the chapter authors in this volume would want to argue that the only way to study reading is via eye movement data. However, we would all argue that it is a good way, and our enthusiasm should be clear in the chapters contained herein.

This volume presents a comprehensive and up-to-date treatment of current research on the topic. It is divided into a number of major sections with three (or four) chapters followed by a commentary concerning that section. Each section begins with a comprehensive summary chapter on the topic under consideration and is followed by chapters dealing with more specific research.

The first two sections of the volume deal with psychophysical and perceptual factors relevant to eye movements during reading. The first section deals with how various psychophysical factors, such as masking and type size, affect reading performance. Breitmeyer considers the role of sustained and transient cells and their potential effects on reading. He relates his widely known views to the reading process and draws implications from work in physiology to what is known about reading. Morrison discusses work done a number of years ago by Tinker and then analyzes the role of type size on eye movements. Wolverton and Zola then describe some recent research they have done concerning masking during eye fixations and the implications for the time course of information extraction during fixations. The second section deals with perceptual factors during reading. McConkie, O'Regan, and I discuss the work that we have completed concerning the size of the perceptual span in reading, the control of eye movements in reading, and integration of information across eye movements. The first chapter by McConkie provides an excellent overview of this area of research, and he presents some thoughts concerning unanswered questions. O'Regan and I present more focused discussions concerning our most recent research in the area.

The next three sections deal with language processes during reading. The third section deals with contextual effects on reading and on eye movements. The effects of context on various perceptual and language processes has been widely studied recently, and the chapters in this section reflect this widespread interest. Shebilske and Fisher begin with a summary of various types of contextual effects in reading and specifically review how context might affect eye movements and reading comprehension processes. S. Ehrlich and Inhoff then describe recent research they have undertaken demonstrating how eye movement data can be used to reveal the effects of context on reading behavior. The fourth and fifth sections of the volume deal with language processes and eye movements. Many past attempts to study language processes during reading via eye movements have been notably unsuccessful. More recently, however, there have been a number of highly successful research programs that have used fixation duration and fixation location as indices of psycholinguistic processes. These successful programs are well documented in the present volume. Frazier describes work that she and I have collaborated on concerning syntactic effects on reading behavior that can be revealed by tracing the time course of the eye movements. Kennedy and K. Ehrlich then provide demonstrations that language processing influences regressions and that pronoun assignment directly affects fixation duration. Carpenter and Just next present a comprehensive summary of the work that they have completed concerning higher-level language processing during reading as reflected in eye movement data. The next chapters by Hogaboam and by Kliegl, Olson, and Davidson discuss the relationship between language processing and perceptual processing, which is clearly an issue of much debate among researchers interested in eye movements and reading.

The sixth section deals with the relationship between eye movements in reading and in picture perception and visual search. Loftus explicitly describes the similarities and the differences that exist between reading and looking at pictures and then summarizes how eye movements are likewise similar and different in the two tasks. Nodine examines how children discriminate letters when they are learning to read and how this is related to drawing. Vaughan then compares the control of fixation durations in reading and search via some recent experiments.

The final section deals with eye movements and reading disability. Reading disability is an emotionally laden research area where there are often widely divergent viewpoints concerning the nature of the deficit. The chapters in this final section reflect these divergent views. The chapters by Pavlidis, by Olson, Kliegl, and Davidson, by Jones and Stark, and by Pirozzolo all reflect different approaches to using eye movement behavior to investigate reading disability.

Each section is followed by a commentary or discussion of the topic relevant to that particular section. These commentaries by Kolers, Well, Gough, Clifton, Slowiaczek, Potter, and Pollatsek serve to place the research in proper perspective and to consider the strength and weaknesses of various positions. It is clear that some of the commentators do not agree with statements made by various authors and the points of disagreement provide interesting and valuable points of discussion.

Finally, I would like to thank my friends and colleagues at the University of Massachusetts for their assistance in putting this volume together. Particularly, I thank Chuck Clifton, Lyn Frazier, Sandy Pollatsek, and Arnie Well. I also appreciate the advice of Harry Whitaker, the series editor, and the editorial staff at Academic Press. My final appreciation goes to Susan Rayner for her continued support and assistance.

# Eye Movements in Reading

PERCEPTUAL AND LANGUAGE PROCESSES

# I
# Eye Movements
# and Psychophysical Processes

# 1

# Sensory Masking, Persistence, and Enhancement in Visual Exploration and Reading

## I.   Introduction

By way of introduction, there are at least three points of departure for what follows in subsequent sections of the present chapter. For one, like several other perceptual psychologists, among them Hochberg (1978), Neisser (1976), and Rayner (1978a), one can regard reading as a particular variant of a more general class of visual exploratory behavior characterized by directed saccade–fixation sequences. The directedness of visual exploratory behavior and, in particular, of reading deserves emphasis since such behavior seems to be under the control of anticipatory plans or schemata (Hochberg, 1970, 1976, 1978; Neisser, 1976). The schemata presumably are composed of such contents and processes as general knowledge of the world, more restricted task relevant knowledge, intention and attention, as well as sensory–perceptual data.

Moreover, based on these contents and processes, the role of schemata is threefold: (1) to guide saccade amplitude and direction to potentially informative locations in the visual field; (2) to anticipate the sensory–cognitive information to be garnered there during the subsequent fixation interval, and, thus, (3) to integrate information across saccades from a prior to a following fixation. The control and guidance of saccades, in turn, is affected by cognitive and by peripheral sensory processes. Specifically regarding visual search and reading, the sequential direction of gaze via saccades is believed to be to varying degrees under cognitive or linguistic as well as extrafoveal, sensory control (Bouma & de Voogd, 1974; Haber, 1976; Hochberg, 1970, 1976, 1978; Malt & Seamon, 1978; Moffitt, 1980; O'Regan, 1979; O'Regan & Levy-Schoen, 1978; Rayner, 1978a). For instance, the existences of global features such as word length and shape (Rayner & Bertera, 1979; Rayner & McConkie, 1977; Schiepers, 1976a, 1976b) and of lateral masking

3

EYE MOVEMENTS IN READING:
PERCEPTUAL AND LANGUAGE PROCESSES

(Bouma, 1973; Loomis, 1978; Wanatabe, 1977) can affect in positive and adverse manners, respectively, the extrafoveal preprocessing of text or pictorial material (Ikeda & Saida, 1978; Saida & Ikeda, 1979), which, in turn, can facilitate its subsequent, more detailed foveal analysis.

However, the main concern of the present chapter is not with these cognitive and extrafoveal sensory components of the momentary and continually updated schemata employed in visual search or reading. Rather, the focus is placed on several sensory factors involving the following three phenomena in reading and visual exploration: (1) the role of early visual persistence as a mechanism of forward masking; (2) the role of early, peripheral sensory consequences of saccadic image displacements; and (3) the role of central corollary discharges accompanying saccades in effecting changes in visual sensitivity and visual coding.

The first two phenomena define the second point of departure of the introductory remarks. This point assumes that the reader is relatively familiar with recent theories of visual information processing based (*a*) on the existence of sustained and transient channels in human vision, such as those theories proposed by Breitmeyer and Ganz (1976), Matin (1975), and Weisstein, Ozog, and Szoc (1975); and (*b*) on the functional utility of these channels in the sequential analysis of an extended visual scene as proposed by Breitmeyer (1980, in press-a, in press-b). Here, it may be important to note as a third point of departure that theories, such as those cited above, that rely heavily on extant neurophysiological and neuroanatomical findings are meant neither to supplant nor reduce more cognitively oriented theories of visual perception but rather to complement them. Although the danger exists in the former theoretical enterprises, as noted by Uttal (1971), of slipping facilely from neurophysiological fact to psychological theory, one can argue that such enterprises, when carefully considered, also can offer a more comprehensive conceptual scheme or scientific language framework within which to integrate and explain a wide range of seemingly disparate experimental phenomena, be they derived by use of physiological, anatomical, psychophysical, or other behavioral methods. With this in mind, the following section serves as a selective summary for the benefit of readers who are unfamiliar with these recent theoretical developments.

## II.    Sustained and Transient Channels: Their Roles in Visual Masking, Persistence, and Saccadic Suppression

### A.    Masking Mechanisms

Let us briefly outline the main features of a masking model based on transient–sustained channel interactions proposed by Breitmeyer and Ganz (1976). The main assumptions of the model are: (*a*) a brief stimulus elicits a short-latency transient response that persists for a relatively short duration and a longer latency sustained response that persists for a relatively long duration (Cleland, Levick, & Sanderson, 1973); (*b*) the latency (Breitmeyer, 1975; Brietmeyer, Levi, & Harwerth, 1981; Jones & Keck, 1978; Lupp, Hauske, & Wolf, 1976; Parker & Salzen, 1977a, 1977b; Vassilev & Mitov, 1976; Vassilev & Strashimirov, 1979) as well as duration of persistence of sustained channels (Breitmeyer & Ganz, 1976, fig. 9, p. 16; Breitmeyer *et al.* 1981; Corfield, Frosdick, & Campbell, 1978; Meyer & Maguire, 1977) increases as the spatial frequency increases; and (*c*) the transient and sustained channels can reciprocally inhibit each other (Breitmeyer, Rudd, & Dunn, 1981; Singer & Bedworth, 1973; von Grünau, 1978). An ancillary assumption (*d*) is that whereas transient channels can signal the location or change of location, that is, motion, of a stimulus, sustained channels process its figural or spatial properties (see Breitmeyer & Ganz, 1976).

These basic features of the model are illustrated in Figure 1.1. To the left are shown hypothetical activation sequences when a target (Stimulus 1, disk) and a flanking mask (Stimulus 2, annulus), typically employed in metacontrast masking, are flashed synchronously. Both stimuli activate brief, short-latency transient responses and more persistent, long-latency sustained responses. Due to the latency difference between transient and sustained channels, the transient response generated by either stimulus cannot inhibit the sustained response generated by the other stimulus. However, the interchannel inhibition can occur optimally, as shown in the right half of Figure 1.1, when the mask is delayed so that the latency of the mask's faster transient response is synchronous with that of the target's slower sustained response. This transient-on-sustained inhibition is shown by the downward negatively signed arrow. The oppositely directed negative arrow denotes sustained-on-transient channel inhibition which, though irrelevant here, is relevant in the context of the following section. One can see that at either lower or

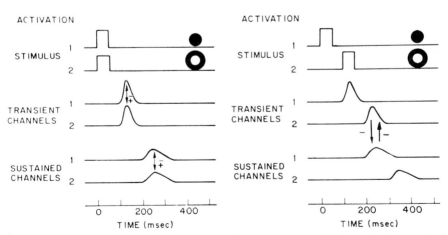

**FIGURE 1.1.** *Hypothetical activation and interactions of transient and sustained channels when two stimuli (target and mask) are presented simultaneously (left panel) and when onset of the first stimulus (target) precedes that of the second stimulus (mask) by 100 msec, which is assumed to be the latency difference between sustained and transient channel responses. See text for further explanations. (From B. G. Breitmeyer [1980]. Unmasking visual masking: A look at the "why" behind the veil of the "how." Psychological Review, 87, 52–69. Copyright 1980 by the American Psychological Association. Reprinted by permission of the publisher and author.)*

higher target-mask onset asynchronies the transient-on-sustained inhibition and hence the suppression of the target's sustained pattern information is less than optimal, hence, a characteristic U-shaped, type B (Kolers, 1962) backward meta-contrast masking function should be generated.

To illustrate another type of masking effect, let us assume that the target and mask overlap spatially. Here the pattern or luminance information of the target can additionally be masked by its being integrated with the pattern information of the mask at the level of common afferent sustained channels (or even as early as the retinal receptors). Such common integration of sustained pattern information, as shown in Figure 1.1, would be optimal at target-mask synchrony and, due to less than optimal temporal superposition, would decrease monotonically at progressively larger asynchronies, thus yielding a type A masking function (Kolers, 1962). In fact, as shown by several investigators (Bachmann & Allik, 1976; Hellige, Walsh, Lawrence, & Cox, 1977; Hellige, Walsh, Lawrence, & Prasse, 1979; Kolers, 1962; Merikle, 1977; Michaels & Turvey, 1979; Turvey, 1973; Weisstein, 1972), by proper arrangements of target-to-mask energy ratios, both type B and type A masking effects can be revealed with spatially adjacent as well as overlapping target and mask stimuli. Moreover, as Breitmeyer and Halpern (1978; see also Breitmeyer, 1980) have shown, masking by common integration is stronger and persists longer in the fovea than in extrafoveal regions of visual space.

Both the U-shaped metacontrast masking and the monotonic masking by integration are fairly local phenomena in that target and mask must occupy either the same or adjacent retinal locations. Recently, however, long-range masking effects, dubbed *jerk-effects*, also have been investigated by Breitmeyer, Valberg, Kurtenbach, and Neumeyer (1980) and Valberg and Breitmeyer (1980). Presumably, these effects index the neurophysiologically identified periphery (McIlwain, 1964) or shift effects (Fischer & Krüger, 1974; Krüger, 1977; Krüger & Fischer, 1973; Krüger, Fischer, & Barth, 1975) and they, like the short-range metacontrast effect, are due to transient-on-sustained inhibition, as indicated by Valberg and Breitmeyer (1980).

Consequential for visual search and reading are two specific properties of the jerk-effect: (1) The sudden, saccadelike displacement of remote, peripheral contours has the effect of (a) reducing the sensitivity of sustained channels but (b) concomitantly increasing the range of contrast and luminance to which they respond (Valberg & Breitmeyer, 1980); (2) as shown in Figure 1.2, this inhibition or reduction of sustained channel response is to be found only in the fovea. Figure 1.2a shows the position of fixation crosses relative to a central incremental test flash surrounded by a remote, jerking grating. Figure 1.2b shows that as an incremental test spot's eccentricity increases, the inhibitory effect on its threshold visibility decreases dramatically; in fact beyond an eccentricity of 1.5°, hardly any reduction in threshold visibility is obtained. This result indicates that the excitation produced in peripheral transient channels by remote contour shifts concenters, via centripetal pathways, at the fovea and inhibits sustained channels only there.

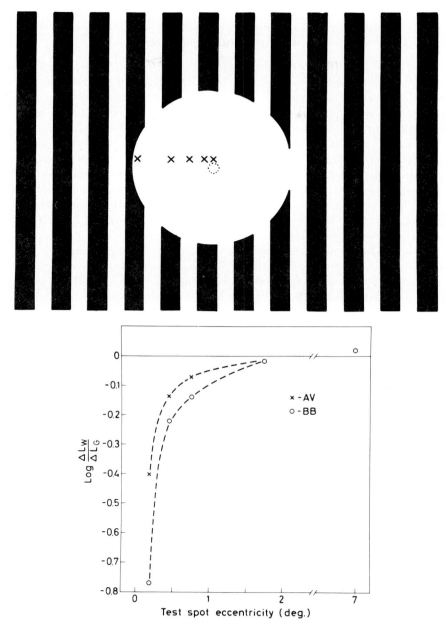

FIGURE 1.2. (a) A representation of the stimulus display used to measure the jerk-effect. The display size was 24 × 19.5°; bar width was .94°; diameter of white background disk was 7.0°; central test spot diameter was .38°. A fixation point could be located at any one of the positions indicated by the X's. (b) The change in increment threshold △ $L_G$ produced by a peripheral, jerking grating relative to the threshold △ $L_W$ obtained in the presence of a uniform outer surround as a function of test spot eccentricity. Negative values of log ($△L_W/△L_G$) indicate that the jerking grating had an inhibitory effect on incremental threshold visibility. (From B. G. Breitmeyer and A. Valberg [1979]. Local foveal inhibitory effects of global peripheral excitation. Science, 203, 463–464. Copyright 1979 by the American Association for the Advancement of Science.)

## B.  Functional Significance

How, one may ask, do the above masking effects relate to visual search and specifically to reading? The answer lies in the fact that both behaviors are characterized by saccade–fixation sequences. For instance, Antes (1974) has demonstrated that visual search of pictorial displays is characterized initially by many high amplitude saccades and short fixation intervals whereas at later search stages the saccades become fewer and smaller in amplitude and the fixation intervals correspondingly become longer. Based on Valberg and Breitmeyer's (1980) findings discussed above, visual search can be characterized by a transition within sustained channels from low sensitivity but high range of contrast effected by the initial high frequency, large amplitude saccades, and short fixation intervals to high sensitivity but low range of contrast effected by the terminal low frequency, low amplitude saccades, and long fixations. This may be a useful characteristic since in the initial phases of target search one is scanning the entire display for global, coarse features based on a larger range of discriminable contrasts that when located allow one to focus on the figural and spatial detail of the target. The latter, detailed inspection is effected by few, small amplitude saccades and longer fixations that optimize spatial sensitivity of sustained channels at the expense of contrast range. For reading the implications seem to be at least two-fold: (1) the finer the print, that is, the higher its spatial frequency components, the greater the need for figural and spatial sensitivity, hence fewer saccades and longer fixations; and (2) as a corollary, for optimal reading performance, size and minimal allowable contrast of print required to read efficiently should vary inversely; that is, the smaller the print, the higher its minimal allowable contrast.

Let us now turn to metacontrast and the foveally restricted inhibitory action of the jerk-effect, and let us for the moment assume that the sole function of saccades is to abruptly change the locus of fixation during visual inspection or reading. The second panel of Figure 1.3, illustrates what happens under this assumption when three 250-msec fixations separated by two 25-msec saccades, as illustrated in the top panel, are performed. Recall that sustained channel response persistence is especially strong and long in the fovea. Hence, especially in the fovea, the sustained pattern activity generated in the afferent channels during a preceding fixation interval should persist and integrate with the sustained channel activity generated in the succeeding fixation interval. That is to say, since afferent, retino-geniculo-striate pathways are retinotopically organized (Brindley & Lewin, 1968; Daniel & Whitteridge, 1961; Hubel & Wiesel, 1977; Malpeli & Baker, 1975; Rolls & Cowey, 1970; Talbot & Marshall, 1941; Whitteridge, 1973), one would generate successive forward masking effects by integration of discordant pattern information within common sustained channels. The net result of such forward masking effects proceeding from one fixation interval to another, is illustrated in Figure 1.4, when one, two, or three fixations are required to read: NORMAL VISION IS ICONOCLASTIC. If we take visual persistence in retinotopically organized afferent sustained channels (or even receptors; Adelson, 1978, 1979; Banks & Barber, 1977, 1980; Sakitt, 1975, 1976) as one possible

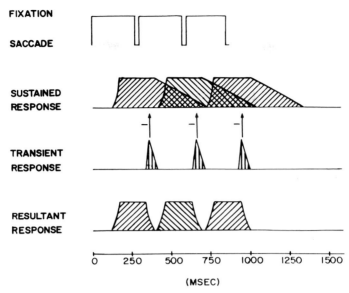

**FIGURE 1.3.** *Panel 1: A hypothetical response sequence of sustained and transient channels during three 250-msec fixation intervals separated by two 25-msec saccades. Panel 2: Response persistence of sustained channels acting as a forward mask from preceding to succeeding fixation interval. Panel 3: Activation of transient channels, shortly after each saccade, which exert inhibition (arrows with minus signs) on the trailing, persisting sustained activity generated in prior fixation intervals. Panel 4: Resultant sustained channel response after the effects of transient-on-sustained inhibition have been taken into account. (From B. G. Breitmeyer [1980]. Unmasking visual masking: A look at the "why" behind the veil of the "how." Psychological Review, 87, 52–69. Copyright 1980 by the American Psychological Association. Reprinted by permission of the publisher and author.)*

definition of the visual icon, we see, as noted also by Hochberg (1978), that normal vision, characterized by multiple saccade–fixation sequences, must eliminate iconic persistence and integration from one fixation to another, that is, it must be iconoclastic.

Fortunately, due to the consequent sudden retinal contour shifts, a saccade not

Normal Vi**NoonaesVINoonaesYicoonclas**iconoclastic        (THREE FIXATIONS)

Normal Vision **NerhaonUceaonics** Iconoclastic        (TWO FIXATIONS)

Normal Vision is Iconoclastic        (ONE FIXATION)

**FIGURE 1.4.** *The perceptual masking effects of temporal integration of persisting sustained activity from preceding fixation intervals with sustained activity generated in succeeding ones when reading a sentence requiring one, two, or three fixations. Here, as in Panel 2 of Figure 1.3, the effects of transient-on-sustained inhibition produced by saccades is not taken into account. (From B. G. Breitmeyer [1980]. Unmasking visual masking: A look at the "why" behind the veil of the "how." Psychological Review, 87, 52–69. Copyright 1980 by the American Psychological Association. Reprinted by permission of the publisher and author.)*

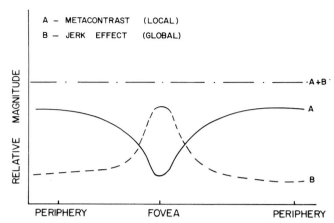

**FIGURE 1.5.** *The relative strength of metacontrast (A) as a short-range, local mechanism of saccadic suppression and (B) the jerk effect as a long-range, global mechanism of saccadic suppression as a function of retinal locus. (From B. G. Breitmeyer [1980]. Unmasking visual masking. A look at the "why" behind the veil of the "how." Psychological Review, 87, 52–69. Copyright 1980 by the American Psychological Association. Reprinted by permission of the publisher and author.)*

only serves to change fixations but also, as shown in the third panel of Figure 1.3, activates and abets the fleeting "hit-and-run" iconoclast—in this case, the transient channel responses that inhibit the otherwise persisting sustained channel responses from the just prior fixation interval. The result, as shown in the lowest panel of Figure 1.3, is to eliminate retinotopic, type A forward masking effects and to ensure that in afferent sustained channels each fixation interval produces its own unmasked pattern activity. The iconoclastic, transient-on-sustained inhibition referred to earlier is only the short-range metacontrast and the long range jerk-effects that comprise the afferent mechanisms of saccadic suppression (Breitmeyer, 1980; Breitmeyer & Ganz, 1976; Matin, 1974; Singer & Bedworth, 1973; Volkman, Riggs, Moore, & White, 1978).[1]

One may ask why both a short-range and a long-range mechanism of saccadic suppression are necessary. The answer lies in considering the peculiar function and structure of the fovea. Without the fovea, reading, as shown by Rayner and Bertera (1979), and, by extension, visual search would be significantly impaired. The fovea contains the highest relative number and activity of sustained channels whereas transient channel activity is relatively more pronounced in the retinal periphery (Breitmeyer & Valberg, 1979; Cleland & Levick, 1974). Both of these inhomogeneities are related to the fact that foveal metacontrast is generally weaker (Alpern, 1953; Bridgeman & Leff, 1979; Lyon, Matteson, & Maras, 1981; Saunders, 1977; Stewart & Purcell, 1970) and of shorter range (Kolers & Rosner, 1960) that extrafoveal metacontrast. Consequently, in view of the stronger and longer response persistence of foveal sustained channels noted earlier, foveal

---

[1]Evidence supporting the existence of additional, efferent, central mechanisms of saccadic suppression has been reported by Riggs, Merton, and Morton (1974).

metacontrast, as a short-range mechanism of saccadic suppression, is too weak. Hence, as shown in Figure 1.5, the long-range jerk-effect, which produces local, foveal inhibition of sustained channels when global, peripheral excitation of transient channels occurs, amplifies and compensates for the weak foveal metacontrast mechanism (see MacLeod, 1978, for similar views).

## III.   Saccades and Extraretinal Signals

The preceding summary review of mechanisms of visual masking, persistence, and suppression and their functional role in visual search and reading restricted itself to a discussion of the afferent sensory consequences of fixations and saccades. However, efferent activity in the form of central processes corollary to the programming and generation of saccades may also play an important role in visual search and reading. Several cortical and subcortical sites have been identified as important in programming and generating saccades. Among those relevant to the present discussion of visual search and reading are the superior colliculus–pulvinar complex, the midbrain reticular areas, and the frontal eye fields (see also Breitmeyer, in press-a).

### A.   Superior Colliculus–Pulvinar Complex

Both the superior colliculus and the pulvinar are involved in the generation and control of saccades (Crommelinck, Roucoux, & Meulders, 1977; Schiller, True, & Conway, 1979). The superior colliculus is composed of three general subdivisions: the superficial, intermediate, and deep layers. Cells in the superficial layers are visually responsive and are characterized by response enhancement beginning about 200 msec before a *goal-directed* saccade is made to a stimulus falling in their receptive field *but not elsewhere* (Goldberg & Wurtz, 1972; Schiller & Koerner, 1971; Wurtz, 1976; Wurtz & Mohler, 1974, 1976a), that is, only if the stimulus is behaviorally relevant. This may be a neurophysiological event corresponding to the psychological phenomenon of selective attention or target selection (Goldberg & Wurtz, 1972) which precedes a saccade or change of fixation. However, after completion of a saccade, the response of superficial-layer cells is suppressed (Goldberg & Robinson, 1978). This would inhibit directing attention to extrafoveal regions while the currently fixated area is being attended to.

The superficial layers of the superior colliculus receive direct retinal input and indirect input from the ipsilateral visual cortex. The foveal and parafoveal representations of the visual field by and large depend on cortical input; peripheral representations depend on direct as well as indirect cortical inputs (Frost & Pöppel, 1976; Wilson & Toyne, 1970). A major portion of each of these inputs is composed of short latency, high velocity transient fibers (Hoffmann, 1973; Leventhal & Hirsch, 1978; Palmer & Rosenquist, 1974) which are particularly sensitive to onset, offset, or rapid displacement of stimuli (Moors & Vendrick, 1979). Moreover the mapping of these transient fibers onto the superficial layers is retinotopically organized (McIlwain, 1973a, 1973b, 1975, 1977; Peck,

Schlag–Rey, and Schlag, 1980). Since reading or visual search usually is characterized by scanning a stationary, nonchanging stimulus array, these onset–offset
or "sudden event" detectors would not be relevant to the reading process, other
than possibly distracting from it when a sudden stimulus change does occur in the
visual field. However, recently, Peck *et al.* (1980) found that in unanesthetized
cat a substantial proportion of cells in the superficial layers of the superior colliculus respond tonically to stationary stimuli. Moreover, their mapping onto the
colliculus is spatiotopically organized in that their response is determined jointly
by the retinal coordinates of a stationary stimulus and the orbital position of the
eyes.[2] For two cogent reasons, the activity of such cells may be involved in the
visual search or reading process: (1) in these processes the direction of saccades is
determined by stationary extrafoveal stimuli; (2) as Mays and Sparks (1980) recently showed, saccades are *spatiotopically* rather than retinotopically organized.

Since the superficial collicular cells project to the pulvinar, which in turn
projects to primary visual cortex (area 17) and secondary visual association areas
(areas 18, 19, and 21 or inferotemporal cortex), the aforementioned collicular
response enhancement accompanying a saccade to a stimulus at a given *spatial*
location in the visual field could render that location more salient to the pulvinar
and, thus, to primary and secondary visual cortex (Chalupa, Anchel, & Lindsley,
1973; Chalupa, Coyle, & Lindsley, 1976; Goldberg & Robinson, 1978; Gross,
1973; Gross, Bender, & Roch–Miranda, 1974; Rezak & Benevento, 1979). This
may be of particular relevance to visual search and reading since the pulvinar is
unresponsive to unpatterned stimuli but, rather, requires a *visual pattern* to yield
an effective response (Perryman & Lindsley, 1977). Consequently, the pulvinar
may be intimately involved in visual pattern analysis (Chalupa *et al.*, 1976).

In the deeper layers of the superior colliculus, cells are not visually responsive.
Rather, they respond prior to eye movements and via ascending fibers may provide
the response-enhancing influence to superficial cells (Goldberg & Robinson, 1978;
Mohler & Wurtz, 1976; Wurtz & Mohler, 1976b). In fact, on physiological and
histological grounds Edwards (1977; Edwards, Ginsberg, Henkel, & Stein, 1979)
argues that the deeper cells are more appropriately classified as reticular rather
than as collicular. In the intermediate layers, many cells combine the properties of
superficial- and deep-layer cells. They seem to integrate information from these
layers and, thus, may constitute an important source of sensory–motor efference
from the superior colliculus (Wurtz & Mohler, 1976b).

## B.   Midbrain Reticular Formation

Electrical stimulation of the midbrain reticular formation (MRF) is known to
produce saccadic eye movements (Büttner, Büttner–Ennever, & Henn, 1977;
Peterson, in press; Singer & Bedworth, 1974). Moreover, it also is known that

---

[2]It is not clear what constitutes the exact source of information about the eye's orbital position. L.
Matin (1976) argues that the source may be an efferent signal, or an afferent proprioceptive signal
originating from extraocular muscles, or both. As such it may be better to use the neutral term
*extraretinal signal* or *corollary signal* (E. Matin, 1976) rather than *efference copy* or *proprioceptive feedback*.

corollary MRF activation occurring with eye movements modulates cortical and lateral geniculate (LGN) excitability (Cohen, Feldman, & Diamond, 1969; McIlwain, 1972; Ogawa, 1963; Pecci–Saacedra, Wilson, & Doty, 1966; Singer, 1973a, 1973b; Singer, 1977; Singer & Bedworth, 1974; Singer, Tretter, & Cynader, 1976; Tatton & Crapper, 1972). According to Singer's findings (Singer, 1977, 1979; Singer & Bedworth, 1974; Singer et al., 1976), the excitability of LGN and cortical sustained neurons generally is globally enhanced whereas the transient channels are generally inhibited (Singer, 1973b).

The latency of the enhancement effect in sustained neurons produced by MRF stimulation is on the order of 60 to 100 msec (Ogawa, 1963; Singer et al., 1976; Singer and Bedworth, 1974). Since electrical stimulation of the MRF also produces saccades (Büttner et al., 1977; Peterson, in press, Singer & Bedworth, 1974), one would expect similar results when saccades are executed. In fact, Singer and Bedworth (1974) obtained the facilitatory effect when MRF stimulation produced saccades. Moreover, Cohen et al. (1969) have shown that the magnitude and time course of such facilitation are equal when MRF stimulation is used and when saccades are performed.

The enhancement of excitability in the geniculo-cortical pathway is thought to occur in one of several ways (Singer, 1977). Inhibition of LGN relay cells can occur either due to activity of intrinsic interneurons or else due to an extrinsic source of activity generated in the adjacent perigeniculate nucleus that comprises part of the "nonspecific" thalamic reticular nucleus. It is believed that whereas the intrinsic inhibitory loops are highly local in nature, the extrinsic ones are involved in more global modifications of LGN excitability (Dubin & Cleland, 1977) and are probably related to changes in an organism's state of alertness or to orienting behavior associated with eye movements (Singer, 1977). MRF stimulation is known also to have a particularly strong excitatory effect on pyramidal cells of lower layers in the striate cortex (Singer, et al., 1976) which, in turn, project corticofugally in a retinotopic manner to LGN. This corticofugal activity could produce local disinhibition of LGN relay cells; however, besides this indirect pathway, disinhibition could also be due to direct global connections between MRF and the intrinsic circuits of the LGN (Singer, 1977, 1979). Stimulation of the MRF also is known to directly inhibit the neurons of the thalamic reticular nucleus, thus increasing the excitability of LGN neurons by eliminating or attenuating extrinsic sources of inhibition (Singer, 1977, 1979). Although there is a gain of contrast or luminance response in sustained channels when the MRF is activated, this gain occurs at the expense of a coarser spatial band-pass selectivity; for example, geniculate sustained neurons respond to a significantly larger stimulus under MRF influence than they do otherwise (Singer, 1973b, 1977). Frizzi (1979) recently reported psychophysical findings on rhesus monkey that showed that MRF stimulation lowers the threshold for luminance increments. This may be one perceptual correlate of the enhanced LGN and cortical excitability produced by MRF stimulation. Another one (though not yet established) may be a steeper attenuation of the response to high spatial frequencies or a greater sensitivity at low spatial frequencies. This trade off of a gain of contrast or luminance response and a loss of spatial sensitivity produced in sustained channels by saccades may very well be a neural correlate of similar psychophysically measured relationships (see discussion of Antes's 1974 and Valberg & Breitmeyer's 1980 findings in Section IIB.)

## C.  Frontal Eye Fields

We know that the generation (Robinson & Fuchs, 1969) as well as the control (Schiller, *et al.*, 1979) of saccades involves activity in the frontal eye fields (area 8). The responses of many visual neurons in the frontal eye fields, like many of those in the superficial layers of the superior colliculus, are *selectively* enhanced when a *goal-directed* saccade is made to stimuli falling in their receptive fields *but not elsewhere* (Goldberg & Robinson, 1977; Mohler, Goldberg, & Wurtz, 1973; Wurtz & Mohler, 1976a). However, in frontal eye field neurons the enhancement occurs *after* saccades, whereas in superficial layers of the superior colliculus it occurs up to 200 msec before and maximally at the time of the saccade.

Moreover, electrical stimulation of the frontal eye fields has been shown to have a facilitatory effect, independent of activation of MRF, on sustained neurons in dorsal LGN and visual cortex (Tsumoto & Suzuki, 1976). The latency of this effect is on the order of 50 to 100 msec, which, by the way, is the same facilitatory latency found after MRF stimulation (Ogawa, 1963; Singer *et al.*, 1976; Singer & Bedworth, 1974). Since mutual inhibition exists between transient and sustained channels, such sustained-response facilitation may consequently result in an attenuation of transient responses in the retino-geniculo-striate pathway shortly after a saccade is completed similar to the postsaccadic suppression of transient neurons in the superficial collicular layers (Goldberg & Robinson, 1978), which presumably are associated with spatial changes of gaze and attention (see Section IIIA.)

## IV.   Consequences for Visual Search and Reading

Let us now turn to some relevant perceptual correlates of the corollary activity generated by the aforementioned sites involved in the generation and direction of saccades. We shall focus particularly on (*a*) postsaccadic enhancement; (*b*) presaccadic enhancement; and (*c*) their respective roles in visual integration across saccades of a spatiotopically organized representation of the visual field.

### A.   Postsaccadic Enhancement

Although corollary discharges exist that may enhance saccadic suppression (Duffy & Burchfiel, 1975), there is also substantial evidence, as noted earlier, that corollary discharges accompanying saccades may enhance visibility by counteracting afferent mechanisms of saccadic suppression. To illustrate this point, let us consider relevant findings reported by Adey and Noda (1973). These investigators showed that single units in LGN and striate cortex can be inhibited by the sudden and rapid displacement of a large global grating when no eye movements occur. In particular a 30-msec saccadelike displacement produced substantial response suppression that reached a maximum at 50 msec after the displacement and then decreased gradually for the following 150 msec. In other words, the entire suppression interval was about 200 msec and presumably was produced by the local and global transient-on-sustained inhibition (metacontrast and jerk-effect) discussed in Sections IIA and IIB.

However, this prolonged afferent inhibition poses a problem. Since an actual saccade is on the order of 20 to 50 msec long, one can see that the suppression would extend appreciably from the saccade into the following fixation interval and thus inhibit sustained activity there. In the context of efficient, rapid pattern processing this problem is overcome by the central corollary discharges discussed in the Section III. To illustrate this fact, Adey and Noda (1973) also recorded responses in visual cells while the organism made saccades in one of three viewing conditions: (1) complete darkness; (2) a Ganzfeld; and (3) a patterned field. In the dark and in the Ganzfeld condition, both of which are characterized by a lack of retinal contour displacement, Adey and Noda (1973) found a *facilitation* of response after the onset of the saccade. Presumably, this would be due to facilitatory signals, converging on sustained cells, from MRF (Singer, 1977) or from frontal cortex (Tsumoto & Suzuki, 1976) after the saccade is executed. With the patterned field, however, one obtains a biphasic response characterized by an initial 50 to 75 msec suppression followed by about 150 msec of facilitation. In a patterned field it is as though the total response produced by the saccade is a summation of afferent neural (transient-on-sustained) inhibition produced by image displacement and a sustained response facilitation produced by central corollary discharges. Thus, due to corollary discharges, there is an effective curtailment of transient-on-sustained inhibition such that it occurs during the saccade but not appreciably after it when, in contrast, one obtains facilitation presumably synchronized with the start of a new fixation interval.

Psychophysical studies, using grating contrast thresholds, conducted by Volkmann, Riggs, Moore, and White (1978) and Volkmann, Riggs, White and Moore (1978) also point to the existence of such a biphasic response characterized by initial saccadic suppression followed by facilitation of visibility. In these studies, the effect of a saccade was characterized by an initial decrease in visibility (suppression) followed by an increase and enhancement of visibility after the saccade was terminated. In the context of Adey and Noda's (1973) results we can take this as tentative evidence that both afferent transient-on-sustained inhibition and central, corollary facilitatory activity play a role in determining visual sensitivity in humans during and after saccades, although more research must be done to clarify this point.

Another form of postsaccadic enhancement involves the effect of viewing a presaccadic stimulus on postsaccadic sensitivity. Wolf, Hauske, and Lupp (1978, 1980), studied how a stationary, extrafoveal presaccadic grating of variable spatial frequency affected foveal contrast sensitivity after a foveating saccade was made to the spatial location of the presaccadic grating (which was extinguished just prior to the saccade). They found that at an eccentricity of 4 to 8°, postsaccadic facilitation of foveal contrast sensitivity was maximal when (a) the spatial frequency of the post- and presaccadic gratings were roughly three cycles per degree; and (b) the gratings were spatially in phase (Wolf et al., 1980).

These highly pattern- and phase-specific effects were taken as evidence that saccades, besides effecting a change of fixation, also are instrumental in integrating spatiotopically coded presaccadic information with the same spatiotopically coded postsaccadic information. Such a process, which may be thought of as a template matching or as cross-correlation or pre- and postsaccadic information, would moreover be instrumental in maintaining visual stability across saccades (Wolf et al., 1980).

In earlier works, Rayner (1975), McConkie and Rayner (1976) and, similarly, Haber (1978) proposed the existence of an *integrative visual buffer* which presumably would serve this function of cross-saccadic integration in reading. By incorporating information about (a) spatial phase or how far the eye had moved and (b) the commonality and specificity of the visual patterns from the pre- and postsaccadic fixations, such a visual buffer could also preserve visual stability in reading. Although Rayner (1978b) reported some evidence consistent with the existence of an *integrative* visual buffer, the results of several subsequent investigations (see McConkie & Zola, 1979; Rayner, 1978a, 1978b, 1979; Rayner, McConkie, & Ehrlich, 1978; Rayner, McConkie, & Zola, 1980) have militated against its existence or its necessity in reading. For instance, although presaccadic parafoveal information was found to facilitate the identification response to the same postsaccadic foveal information, the same facilitation was obtained under a simulated saccade, in which the observer with eyes fixated was presented first a parafoveal stimulus followed by a foveal one (Rayner, 1978b; Rayner et al., 1978; Rayner et al. 1980). Thus, it was concluded that the saccade *per se* does not seem to be necessary for *such* integration. In line with this interpretation, McConkie and Zola (1979) found that changing the visual shapes of letters and words, for example, by substituting uppercase for lowercase letters and vice versa from one fixation to the next, did not affect reading efficiency. Based on this finding, McConkie and Zola (1979) concluded "that such *visual data are not integrated across saccades* [p. 224, italics added]." Rather, the results of this study and also that of Rayner et al. (1980) were taken to show that the cross-saccadic carryover of information of individual or seriate letters occurred in a postvisual, more abstract and deeply encoded form.

Although these results and the associated explanatory hypothesis may hold specifically for the reading process, particularly for that of an experienced and efficient reader, in a broader context in which reading, from a purely visual standpoint, can be considered as merely a particular variant of exploratory behavior, as it might be in the fledgling reader, these results do not disconfirm nor does this hypothesis stand opposed to the integrative visual buffer hypothesis. Moreover, whenever a saccade occurs, either in reading or in visual search, cross-saccadic integration of visual information ought to occur. Unfortunately, some of my own prior theoretical work (Breitmeyer, 1980; Breitmeyer & Ganz, 1976), as illustrated in Figure 1.3 above, seems to run counter to a cross-saccadic visual integration hypothesis (see also Rayner, 1978a) although Footnote 5 of the 1980 article (Breitmeyer, 1980) anticipated some of what shall be discussed next.

What are the bases for these claims? Among other things, cross-saccadic visual integration realized in the spatiotopic, rather than retinotopic, domain as indicated by Wolf et al. (1978, 1980) would (1) be instrumental in and consistent with the maintenance of the visually perceived stability of the world during and across saccades, as recently shown by White, Post, and Leibowitz (1980) and (2) be consistent with (a) Peck et al.'s (1980) finding of spatiotopically organized receptive fields of tonic units found in superficial layers of the superior colliculus; (b) the execution of spatiotopically rather than retinotopically programmed saccades as demonstrated by Mays and Sparks (1980); and (c) Ritter's (1976) study showing that a spatiotopic icon, preserving position constancy, persists during saccades.

## B.  Presaccadic Enhancement and Cross-Saccadic Visual Integration

Facilitation of the visual response also may occur presaccadically. Robinson, Baizer, and Dow (1980) report that the visual response of a significant number of prestriate cortical cells to a visual stimulus is enhanced up to 200 msec prior to onset of a saccade, similar to the presaccadic enhancement found among superficial cells of the superior colliculus. However, whereas the collicular cell responses are specifically enhanced during only goal-directed saccades, the enhancement of prestriate cell responses occurs for any saccade. The function of this more general enhancement is not clear; however, one possibility is that this enhancement is associated with a mapping of cortical retinotopic representations of a visual field changing from one fixation to another onto a stable, nonchanging cortical spatiotopic representation of the world.[3]

A consequence of this hypothesis is that a central, cortical spatiotopically organized representation of a prior fixation persists cross-saccadically and integrates with the cortical spatiotopically organized representation of the succeeding fixation. Ritter (1976) and Wolf et al. (1980) investigated post-saccadic enhancement of contrast sensitivity; the current focus is on presaccadic facilitation and its role in cross-saccadic integration.

[3]Wurtz (1976) suggests that the nonspecific, general enhancement found at cortical levels is an index of general arousal produced, for instance, by signals arriving from the midbrain reticular areas (Singer, 1977). However, this suggestion is flawed since the general arousal produced by reticular input (Singer, 1977) or frontal eye field input (Tsumoto & Suzuki, 1976) to visual cortex occurs after a saccade rather than up to 200 msec before its onset.

To determine the existence and role of presaccadic facilitation on cross-saccadic integration, Breitmeyer, Kropfl, and Julesz (in press) took advantage of the well-known fact that visual persistence under static viewing is curtailed as stimulus duration increases (Bowen, Pola, & Matin, 1974; Bowling and Lovegrove, 1980; Haber & Standing, 1970). Using an integration method of measuring visual persistence (DiLollo, 1977; Eriksen & Collins, 1967, 1968; Hogben & DiLollo, 1974; Ikeda & Uchikawa, 1978; see also Coltheart, 1980, for a review of methods of measuring visual persistence), DiLollo (1980) and DiLollo and Wilson (1978) demonstrated that as the duration of the first stimulus, separated from the second one by an interstimulus interval or ISI of 10 msec, increased beyond about 80 msec, persistence of the first stimulus and thus integration across this mere 10-msec ISI was dramatically curtailed.

Breitmeyer et al., (in press) exploited and further explored this finding in the following manner. The stimuli and method were similar to those employed by DiLollo (1980) and Hogben and DiLollo (1974). A schematic example of the stimulus displays used by Breitmeyer et al. (in press) is shown in Figure 1.6. However, whereas Figure 1.6, for illustrative purposes, uses capitalized O's as elements to form the stimulus displays, the Breitmeyer et al., 1982 study actually employed 25' × 25' filled squares as elements. The square elements were painted on a Hewlett–Packard cathode ray tube with rise and fall times less than 1 msec. The stimulus display consisted of a 4 × 4 array of elements. On any trial 8 of the 16 possible positions were randomly filled by the first flash as shown in Figure 1.6a; and with a probability of .5 either seven, as shown in Figure 1.6b, or eight of the remaining positions were filled by the second flash. In the former case, the integrated composite filled all but one randomly determined element position as shown in Figure 1.6c; in the latter case all interior positions of the composite were filled. The two observers simply indicated whether or not any of the element positions were vacant. The duration of the leading flash was 200 msec; that of the second flash was 20 msec; and their ISI was 40 msec. Since DiLollo (1980) and DiLollo and Wilson (1978) reported poor performance for the same leading stim-

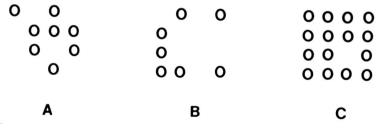

**A**                                  **B**                                  **C**

**FIGURE 1.6.** *Schematic examples of stimuli used to study visual persistence by using the temporal integration paradigm. (A) First stimulus consists of eight randomly filled locations of a 4 × 4 matrix. (B) Second stimulus consists of either seven filled locations as shown or eight filled locations of the remaining and complementary ones. (C) Composite appearance of the first and second stimulus when visually integrated. Here either a random location is left blank as shown or the entire array is filled, depending on whether the second stimulus contains seven or eight filled, complementary locations.*

ulus duration of 200 msec and an ISI of only 10 msec, one would expect that in the present study, employing a larger ISI of 40 msec, performance under static viewing would also be poor, possibly yielding a correct response rate of 50% predicted on the basis of chance guessing.

Three static viewing conditions were employed in the first experiment. In Condition 1a, the two stimuli were flashed foveally; in Condition 1b both stimuli were flashed 6.6° to the right of fixation, and in Condition 1c, the first stimulus was flashed foveally or 6.6° to the right of fixation whereas the second stimulus was flashed 6.6° extrafoveally or foveally, respectively. As expected, in all three conditions the correct response rates ranged between .48 and .52—values of which none differed significantly from the a priori guessing probability of .5. In particular, Condition 1c showed that under static viewing there was no visual integration between a foveal and 6.6° extrafoveal flash.

In a second set of experiments visual integration was measured under dynamic viewing using a method similar to that employed by Ritter (1976) and, more recently, by Jonides, Irwin & Yantis (1982). In Condition 2a, the first flash was viewed foveally. Its onset signalled the observer to saccade to a fixation point 6.6° to the right of the fovea. Since the duration of Flash 1 was 200 msec and the ISI was 40 msec, the observer was allowed 240 msec to initiate and execute the saccade—a value closely approximating the average saccade latency and execution time (Ditchburn, 1973; Fuchs, 1976)—before the second stimulus was flashed at the same spatial location. Hence, although eye movements were not strictly monitored, it is highly likely that on most trials the saccade intervened between the first and second stimulus,[4] thus assuring that they registered at the same spatiotopic, but at 6.6° disparate, retinotopic locations. In Condition 2b, the first stimulus was flashed 6.6° to the right of fixation and also served as a signal to saccade to that extrafoveal location. As in Condition 2a the second stimulus subsequently fell at the same spatiotopic, but at 6.6° disparate retinotopic, locations. In Condition 2c, the first stimulus was flashed in the fovea and the second was also flashed there but only after the saccade intervened and moved the fovea from its prior location to one 6.6° to the right. Consequently, in Conditions 2a and 2b the interesting possibility exists that if visual information persists and is integrated across saccades, the persistence must reside at a spatiotopically rather than retinotopically organized stimulus representation. Moreover, if that were the case

[4]Even if the saccade latency were shorter than 200 msec by several tens of milliseconds, for example, if it were 160 msec, the sustained pattern information in the remaining 40 msec (and even earlier) would be subject to saccadic suppression and therefore would not contribute to the observed, persistence phenomena but rather, by effectively extending the integration interval to 80 msec, reduce the probability of integration. Moreover if the saccadic latency were longer, for example, if it were 240 or 250 msec, the onset of the second 20-msec stimulus could be synchronized with the saccade onset. Hence one would expect to obtain saccadic suppression and second stimulus pattern and consequently no visible integration of the first and second stimulus pattern. The fact that cross-saccadic pattern integration was obtained suggests both of these two eventualities played a minor role in generating the obtained results. Moreover, Jonides et al.'s (1982) recent study, in which saccade latencies were more precisely measured, obtained clearer evidence for such cross-saccadic integration.

20

Bruno G. Breitmeyer

one would not expect cross-saccadic pattern persistence and integration in Condition 2c, since here the two stimuli fell on the same retinal location (i.e., the fovea) but disparate spatiotopic locations. For Conditions 2a and 2b the correct response rate ranged from 0.65 to 0.77—values that were all significantly above the a priori chance guessing probability of .5, whereas in Condition 2c the correct response rates did not differ significantly from .5. This indicates that cross-saccadic visual pattern persistence and integration indeed occurs at the spatiotopically rather than retinotopically coded level of processing, despite the fact that, as in static-viewing Condition 1c, which yielded chance performance, the two stimuli fell on disparate retinotopic locations.

What additional pertinent inferences can one draw from these findings? First, since no visible integration occurred under static viewing, it is highly likely that the corollary or extraretinal signal (E. Matin, 1976) accompanying saccades not only serves to map earlier, changing retinotopic representations into later, stable spatiotopic representations, but also produces a spatiotopically coded visible persistence that otherwise is absent. That is to say, the spatiotopic iconic persistence is merely occasioned by afferent visual input but is in fact produced or enhanced by a stimulus–autonomous extraretinal signal. Second, one can claim, contrary to Sakitt (1975, 1976) and Turvey (1977), that a cortical visible iconic persistence not tied to retinal coordinates exists. Third, cross-saccadic integration seems to occur at a more literal, visual rather than schematic level, as suggested by Neisser (1976) and Hochberg (1978). Moreover, whereas the later spatiotopically organized form of visual persistence constitutes, or contributes to, a visible icon, the earlier retinotopically organized form of visual persistence is previsible. This is due to the following considerations. The effect of a saccade on the spatiotopic icon is to enhance its persistence across saccades whereas earlier retinotopic forms of persistence, as noted in Section IIB above, are suppressed by the saccade. Now, since saccadic suppression presumably partakes of the same transient-on-sustained inhibition as metacontrast and since metacontrast prevents previsible sustained pattern information from ever being transferred to the visible level (see Breitmeyer, 1980, Footnote 5; Michaels & Turvey, 1979), the retinotopically coded form of visual persistence, prevented by saccadic suppression from being transferred to the spatiotopic level, must be previsible. Another reason, supported by phenomenal reports, is that *one normally never sees* retinotopic integration across saccades as illustrated in Figure 1.4 above, except perhaps when abnormally intense stimuli produce retinal afterimages that can persist and mask patterns, falling at the same retinal location, over several saccades.

Thus insofar as the previsible, retinotopic form of visual persistence is suppressed by saccades, *normal vision,* as noted in Section IIB, indeed *is iconoclastic.* However, insofar as the visible, spatiotopic form of visual persistence is produced and prolonged by corollary or extraretinal signals attending saccades, *normal vision* also *is iconoplastic.* To facilitate understanding of this important distinction, consider Figure 1.7, an extension of Figure 1.3. The top four panels replicate Figure 1.3, and show how the retinotopic and previsible sustained pattern information

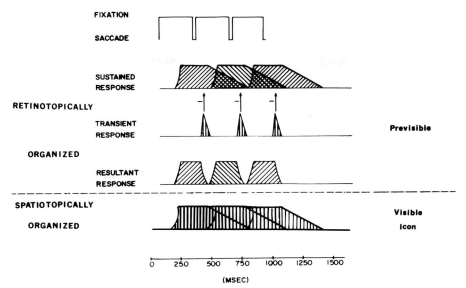

FIGURE 1.7. *Panels 1–4 are the same as in Figure 1.3. The processes depicted in Panels 2–4 are retinotopically organized and occur at previsible levels. Panel 5: Cross-saccadic persistence and integration of spatiotopically coded pattern information occurring at visible level. Transition from processes shown in Panel 4 to those shown in Panel 5 require mapping of pattern information from retinotopic onto spatiotopic representation.*

that otherwise would persist from one fixation to another is suppressed by saccades to form temporally segregated windows of such information which then, as shown in the bottom panel, provides input to the visible, spatiotopic level of analysis where cross-saccadic persistence and integration, the latter analogous to a cross-correlation or template matching, are produced by a corollary or extraretinal signal. In short, saccades, on the one hand, suppress previsible, retinotopic sustained channel persistence and, on the other hand, produce and enhance visible, spatiotopic pattern persistence from one fixation to the next. In this way phenomenal continuity and stability of the visually perceived world is maintained across saccades. Such a process, moreover, would be indifferent to the specific task involved, be it visual search or reading. In both cases cross-saccadic integration of visible, spatiotopically coded pattern information occurs.

## V.    A Brief Look at Application

Recently Lovegrove and Heddle (1980) showed that visual persistence not only increases with spatial frequency (Bowling, Lovegrove, & Mapperson, 1979; Corfield, *et al.*, 1978; Meyer & Maguire, 1977) but also decreases with age. For instance, over spatial frequencies ranging from 1 to 16 c/deg, persistence increased from about 130 to 320 msec for 7-year-old children and from only about 70 to 250 msec for 13-year-old children, with the range of persistence values obtained by 10-year-old children falling between those of the younger and older children. On the assumption that under static viewing, lacking the saccade-produced and - enhanced persistence at the spatiotopic level of processing, retinotopically organized sustained activity fairly early in visual processing primarily contributes to these persistence phenomena, one would expect a more prolonged forward pattern masking effect from one fixation onto the next for younger children (see the second panel of Figures 1.3 and 1.7). On that basis alone one might expect worse performance in visual search or reading in younger than in older children. However, as the results of a recent study conducted by Lawrence, Kee, and Hellige (1980) indicate, the magnitude of U-shaped metacontrast pattern masking also decreases with age. One likely interpretation of these results is that the transient-on-sustained inhibition responsible for metacontrast and, by extension, saccadic suppression, is stronger in younger than in older children. Such a stronger saccadic suppression in younger children would thus more effectively terminate the correlated stronger or longer persistence of retinotopic sustained activity when a saccade is executed. Consequently from a purely visuo—sensory standpoint, visual search or reading ability should not be hampered at younger ages by stronger or longer retinotopic persistence phenomena. Of course, this explanation is highly speculative, and may prove wrong; but it is hoped to define a problem for future research.

Among additional findings reported by Lovegrove, Heddle, and Slaghuis (1980) and Badcock and Lovegrove (1981) is that at any fixed age, specific reading disabled (SRD) children seem to show longer visual persistence particularly at spatial frequencies ranging from about 1 to 10 c/deg and for stimulus durations approximating fixation durations in reading (Badcock & Lovegrove, 1981).[5] The possible implications of this finding depend on whether or not the strength of saccadic suppression (transient-on-sustained inhibition) is more or less equal in reading disabled and normal children. Should it be equal, one might expect longer and stronger forward masking of retinotopic sustained patterns as reading (or visual search) proceeds from one fixation to another. To compensate for this relative deficit produced by forward masking of the early portion of a fixation, reading disabled children may require longer fixation durations (see Rayner, 1978a, for a recent review) to obtain a clarity of visual input equivalent to that of normal readers. On the other hand, in reading disabled children saccadic suppression may be weaker, in which case the aforementioned problem is aggravated, or it

---

[5] Using a variety of methods (for reviews see Coltheart, 1980; Long, 1980) several additional investigators, among them, Lovegrove, Billing, and Slaghuis (1978), Lovegrove and Brown (1978), and Stanley and Hall (1973a, 1973b) have reported longer durations of visible persistence in SRDs, although others such as Arnett and DiLollo (1978), Fisher and Frankfurter (1977), and Morrison, Giordani, and Nagy (1977) have failed to replicate these findings. As noted by Badcock and Lovegrove (1981), these conflicting reports on visual persistence of SRD and control subjects may reflect the fact that different experimental techniques measure different components of visual persistence.

may be stronger, in which case the problem is eliminated or attenuated. Again, these speculations serve only to define problems for further research.

Moreover, they have implications for the development or use of therapeutic techniques. By eliminating or pinpointing the possibility of visuo–sensory or visuo–motor defects one can institute appropriate remediation methods. For instance, Ciuffreda, Bahill, Kenyon, and Stark (1976) report that congenital jerk nystagmus results in reading difficulty. The source of the problem may be at least two-fold. For one, when these jerklike nystagmic movements of the eye occur during fixations, they activate transient channels, and thus, via the local and global mechanisms of transient-on-sustained inhibition, produce suppression of pattern information in sustained channels. Second, insofar as these eye movements, unlike goal-directed saccades, are not voluntary, they may lack an appropriate accompanying corollary discharge, which would, on the basis of the discussion in the prior section, result in visual instability as well as a faulty mapping of pattern information from retinotopic onto spatiotopic coordinates, thus producing masking by mutual integration of spatially discordant pattern information at the level of the central, visible icon (Michaels & Turvey, 1979). Similar explanations may apply to reading defects encountered by functional amblyopes, since latent nystagmus is not uncommon in these patients (Burian, 1969; Hess, Campbell & Greenhalgh, 1978). In these cases, remediation producing acquired control over eyemovements, for example, via biofeedback training (Flom, Kirschen, & Bedell, 1980), may improve the efficiency of reading or visual search. An extensive review of specific reading disabilities may suggest other examples of visuo–sensory and visuo–motor deficiencies that correlate with them. However, that is not the task of this paper. Nonetheless, as a final general implication for the study and diagnosis of reading disabilities and in line with the conclusion reached by Badcock and Lovegrove (1981), one could note that "reading disability without perceptual deficit" by and large may be an empty diagnostic category.

## References

Adelson, E. H. (1978). Iconic storage: The role of rods. *Science, 201,* 544–546.

Adelson, E. H. (1979). Visual persistence without rods. *Perception & Psychophysics, 26,* 245–256.

Adey, W. R., & Noda, H. (1973). Influence of eye movements on geniculo-striate excitability in the cat. *Journal of Physiology (London,)* 235, 805–821.

Alpern, M. (1953). Metacontrast. *Journal of the Optical Society of America, 43,* 648–657.

Antes, J. R. (1974). The time course of picture viewing. *Journal of Experimental Psychology, 103,* 62–70.

Arnett, J. L., & DiLollo, V. (1979). Visual information processing in relation to age and to reading ability. *Journal of Experimental Child Psychology, 27,* 143–152.

Bachman, T., & Allik, J. (1976). Integration and interruption in the masking of form by form. *Perception, 5,* 79–97.

Badcock, D., & Lovegrove, W. (1981). The effects of contrast, stimulus duration and spatial frequency on visual persistence in normal and specifically disabled readers. *Journal of Experimental Psychology: Human Perception and Performance, 7,* 495–505.

Banks, W. P., & Barber, G. (1977). Color information in iconic memory. *Psychological Review, 84,* 536–546.

Banks, W. P., & Barber, G. (1980). Normal iconic memory for stimuli invisible to the rods. *Perception & Psychophysics, 27,* 581–584.

Bouma, H. (1973). Visual interference in the parafoveal recognition of initial and final letters of words. *Vision Research, 13,* 767–782.

Bouma, H., & de Voogd, A. H. (1974). On the control of eye saccades in reading. *Vision Research, 14,* 273–284.

Bowen, R. W., Pola, J., & Matin, L. (1974). Visual persistence: Effects of flash luminance, duration and energy. *Vision Research, 14,* 295–303.

Bowling, A., & Lovegrove, W. (1980). The effect of stimulus duration on the persistence of gratings. *Perception & Psychophysics, 27,* 574–578.

Bowling, A., Lovegrove, W., & Mapperson, B. (1979). The effect of spatial frequency and contrast on visual persistence. *Perception, 8,* 529–539.

Breitmeyer, B. G. (1975). Simple reaction time as a measure of the temporal response properties of transient and sustained channels. *Vision Research, 15,* 1411–1412.

Breitmeyer, B. G. (1978). Disinhibition in metacontrast masking of Vernier acuity targets: Sustained channels inhibit transient channels. *Vision Research, 18,* 1401–1405.

Breitmeyer, B. G. (1980). Unmasking visual masking: A look at the "why" behind the veil of the "how." *Psychological Review, 87,* 52–69.

Breitmeyer, B. G. The directive control of sense receptors and the temporal coupling of sensory consequences to the time course of central control mechanisms. In D. E. Sheer (Ed.), *Attention: Theory, brain function and clinical application.* New York: Academic Press, in press. (a)

Breitmeyer, B. G. *Visual Masking: An Integrated Approach.* Oxford: Oxford University Press, in press. (b)

Breitmeyer, B. G., & Ganz, L. (1976). Implications of sustained and transient channels for theories of visual pattern masking, saccadic suppression, and information processing. *Psychological Review, 83,* 1–36.

Breitmeyer, B., & Halpern, M (1978). *Visual persistence depends on spatial frequency and retinal locus.* Paper presented at the annual meeting of the Psychonomic Society, San Antonio, Texas, November.

Breitmeyer, B., Kropfl, W., & Julesz, B. The existence and role of retinotopic and spatiotopic forms of visual persistence. *Acta Psychologica,* in press.

Breitmeyer, B., Levi, D. M., & Harwerth, R. S. (1981). Flicker masking in spatial vision. *Vision Research, 21,* 1385–1391.

Breitmeyer, B. G., Rudd, M., & Dunn, K. (1981). Metacontrast investigations of sustained-transient channel inhibitory interactions. *Journal of Experimental Psychology: Human Perception and Performance, 7,* 770–779.

Breitmeyer, B., & Valberg, A. (1979). Local, foveal, inhibitory effects of global, peripheral excitation. *Science, 203,* 463–465.

Breitmeyer, B., Valberg, A., Kurtenbach, W., & Neumeyer, C. (1980). The lateral effect of oscillation of peripheral luminance gratings on the foveal incremental threshold. *Vision Research, 20,* 799–805.

Bridgeman, B., & Leff, S. (1979). Interaction of stimulus size and retinal eccentricity in metacontrast masking. *Journal of Experimental Psychology: Human Perception and Performance, 5,* 101–109.

Brindley, G. S., & Lewin, W. S. (1968). The sensations produced by electrical stimulation of the visual cortex. *Journal of Physiology (London) 196,* 479–493.

Burian, H. M. (1969). Pathophysiologic basis of amblyopia and of its treatment. *American Journal of Ophthalmology, 67,* 1–12.

Büttner, U., Büttner–Ennever, J. A., & Henn, V. (1977). Vertical eye movement related unit activity in the rostral mesencephalic reticular formation of the alert monkey. *Brain Research, 130,* 329–352.

Chalupa, L. M., Anchel, H., & Lindsley, D. B. (1973). Effects of cryogenic blocking of pulvinar upon visually evoked responses in the cortex of the cat. *Experimental Neurology, 39,* 112–122.

Chalupa, L. M., Coyle, R. S., & Lindsley, D. (1976). Effect of pulvinar lesion on visual discrimination in monkeys. *Journal of Neurophysiology, 39,* 354–369.

Ciuffreda, K. J., Bahill, A. T., Kenyon, R. V. & Stark, L. (1976). Eye movements during reading: Case reports. *American Journal of Optometry and Physiological Optics, 53,* 389–395.

Cleland, B. G., & Levick, W. R. (1974). Brisk and sluggish concentrically organized ganglion cells in the cat's retina. *Journal of Physiology (London), 240,* 421–456.

Cleland, B. G., Levick, W. R., & Sanderson, K. J. (1973). Properties of sustained and transient cells in the cat retina. *Journal of Physiology (London), 228,* 649–680.

Cohen, B., Feldman, M., & Diamond, S. P. (1969). Effects of eye movement, brainstem stimulation, and alertness on transmission through lateral geniculate body of monkey. *Journal of Neurophysiology, 32,* 583–595.

Coltheart, M. (1980). Iconic memory and visible persistence. *Perception & Psychophysics, 27,* 183–228.

Corfield, R., Frosdick, J. P., & Campbell, F. W. (1978). Grey-out elimination: The roles of spatial waveform, frequency and phase. *Vision Research, 18,* 1305–1311.

Crommelinck, M., Roucoux, A., & Meulders, M. (1977). Eye movements evoked by stimulation of lateral posterior nucleus and pulvinar in the cat. *Brain Research, 124,* 361–366.

Daniel, P. M., & Whitteridge, D. (1961). The representation of the visual field on the cerebral cortex in monkeys. *Journal of Physiology (London) 159,* 203–221.

DiLollo, V. (1977). Temporal characteristics of iconic memory. *Nature (London), 267,* 241–243.

DiLollo, V. (1980). Temporal integration in visual memory. *Journal of Experimental Psychology: General, 109,* 75–97.

DiLollo, V., & Wilson, A. E. (1978). Iconic persistence and perceptual moment as determinants of temporal integration in vision. *Vision Research, 18,* 1607–1610.

Ditchburn, R. W. (1973). *Eye-movements and visual perception.* Oxford: Clarendon Press.

Dubin, M. W., & Cleland, B. G. (1977). Organization of visual inputs to interneurons of lateral geniculate nucleus of the cat. *Journal of Neurophysiology, 40,* 410–427.

Duffy, F. H., & Burchfield, J. L. (1975). Eye movement related inhibition of primate visual neurons. *Brain Research, 89,* 121–132.

Edwards, S. B. (1977). The commissural projection of the superior colliculus in the cat. *Journal of Comparative Neurology, 173,* 23–40.

Edwards, S. B., Ginsberg, C. L., Henkel, C. K., & Stein, B. E. (1979). Sources of subcortical projections to the superior colliculus in the cat. *Journal of Comparative Neurology, 184,* 301–330.

Eriksen, C. W., & Collins, J. F. (1967). Some temporal characteristics of visual pattern perception. *Journal of Experimental Psychology, 74,* 476–484.

Eriksen, C. W., & Collins, J. F. (1968). Sensory traces versus the psychological moment in the temporal organization of form. *Journal of Experimental Psychology, 77,* 376–382.

Fischer, B., & Krüger, J. (1974). The shift-effect in the cat's lateral geniculate nucleus. *Experimental Brain Research, 21,* 225–227.

Fisher, D. F., & Frankfurter, A. (1977). Normal and disabled readers can locate and identify letters: Where's the perceptual deficit? *Journal of Reading Behavior, 10,* 31–43.

Flom, M. C., Kirschen, D. G., & Bedell, H. E. (1980). Control of unsteady, eccentric fixation in amblyoptic eyes by auditory feedback of eye position. *Investigative Opthalmology & Visual Science, 19,* 1371–1381.

Frizzi, T. J. (1979). Midbrain reticular stimulation and brightness detection. *Vision Research, 19,* 123–130.

Frost, D., & Pöppel, E. (1977). Different programming modes of human saccadic eye movements as a function of stimulus eccentricity: Indications of a functional subdivision of the visual field. *Biological Cybernetics, 23,* 39–48.

Fuchs, A. F. (1976). The neurophysiology of saccades. In R. A. Monty & J. W. Senders (Eds.), *Eye moevements and pyschological processes.* Hillsdale, New Jersey: Erlbaum, Pp. 39–53.

Goldberg, M. E., & Robinson, D. L. (1977). Visual mechanisms underlying gaze: Function of the cerebral cortex. In R. A. Baker & A. Berthoz (Eds.), *Developments in neuroscience* (Vol. 1: *Control of gaze by brainstem neurons*). Amsterdam: Elsevier/North-Holland Biomedical Press, Pp. 445–451.

Goldberg, M. E., & Robinson, D. L. (1978). Visual system: Superior colliculus. In R. B. Masterson (Ed.), *Handbook of behavioral neurobiology* (Vol. 1). New York: Plenum, Pp. 119–164.

Goldberg, M. E., & Wurtz, R. H. (1972). Activity of superior colliculus in behaving monkey. I. Visual receptive fields of single neuronal responses. *Journal of Neurophysiology, 35,* 542–559.

Gross, C. G. (1973). Inferotemporal cortex in vision. In E. Stellar & J. M. Sprague (Eds.), *Progress in physiological psychology* (Vol. 5). New York: Academic Press, Pp. 77–123.

Gross, C. G., Bender, D. B., & Roch–Miranda, C. E. (1974). Infero-temporal cortex: A single unit analysis. In F. O. Schmitt & F. G. Worden (Eds.), *The neuro-sciences third study program.* Cambridge: MIT Press, Pp. 229–338.

Haber, R. N. (1976). Control of eye movements during reading. In R. A. Monty & J. W. Senders (Eds.), *Eye movements and psychological processes.* Hillsdale, New Jersey: Erlbaum, Pp. 443–452.

Haber, R. N. (1978). Visual perception. In M. R. Rosenzweig & L. W. Porter (Eds.), *Annual review of psychology.* Palo Alto: Annual Reviews, Pp. 31–59.

Haber, R. N., & Standing, L. G. (1970). Direct estimates of the apparent duration of a flash. *Canadian Journal of Psychology, 24,* 216–229.

Hellige, J. B., Walsh, D. A., Lawrence, V. W., & Cox, P. J. (1977). The importance of figural relationships between target and mask. *Perception & Psychophysics, 21,* 285–286.

Hellige, J. B., Walsh, D. A., Lawrence, V. W., & Prasse, M. (1979). Figural relationship effects and mechanisms of visual masking. *Journal of Experimental Psychology: Human Perception and Performance, 5,* 88–100.

Hess, R. F., Campbell, F. W. & Greenhalgh, T. (1978). On the nature of neural abnormality in human amblyopia; neural abberations and visual sensitivity loss. *Pflügers Archiv., 377,* 201–207.

Hochberg, J. (1970). Components of literacy: Speculations and exploratory research. In H. Levin & J. P. Williams (Eds.), *Basic studies in reading.* New York: Basic Books, Pp. 74–89.

Hochberg, J. (1976). Toward a speech-plan eye-movement model of reading. In R. A. Monty & J. W. Senders (Eds.), *Eye movements and psychological processes.* Hillsdale, New Jersey: Erlbaum, Pp. 397–416.

Hochberg, J. E. (1978). *Perception.* Englewood Cliffs, New Jersey: Prentice–Hall.

Hoffman, K.-P. (1973). Conduction velocity in pathways from retina to superior colliculus in the cat: A correlation with receptive field properties. *Journal of Neurophysiology, 36,* 409–424.

Hogben, J. H., & DiLollo, V. (1974). Perceptual integration and perceptual segregation of brief visual stimuli. *Vision Research, 14,* 1059–1069.

Hubel, D. H., & Wiesel, T. N. (1977). Functional architecture of macaque monkey visual cortex. *Proceedings of the Royal Society (London), 198B,* 1–59.

Ikeda, M., & Saida, S. (1978). Span of recognition in reading. *Vision Research, 18,* 83–88.

Ikeda, M., & Uchikawa, K. (1978). Integrating time for visual pattern perception and a comparison with tactile mode. *Vision Research, 18,* 1565–1571.

Jones, R., & Keck, J. M. (1978). Visual evoked response as a function of grating spatial frequency. *Investigative Ophthalmology & Visual Science, 17,* 652–659.

Jonides, J., Irwin, D. E. & Yantis, S. (1982). Integrating visual information from successive saccades. *Science, 215,* 192–194.

Kolers, P. A. (1962). Intensity and contour effects in visual masking. *Vision Research, 2,* 277–294.

Kolers, P. A., & Rosner, B. S. (1960). On visual masking (metacontrast): Dichoptic observations. *American Journal of Psychology, 73,* 2–21.

Krüger, J. (1977). The shift-effect in the lateral geniculate body of the rhesus monkey. *Experimental Brain Research, 29,* 387–392.

Krüger, J., & Fischer, B. (1973). Strong periphery effect in cat retinal ganglion cells. Excitatory responses in ON- and OFF-center neurons to single grid displacements. *Experimental Brain Research, 18,* 316–318.

Krüger, J., Fischer, B., & Barth, G. (1975). The shift-effect in retinal ganglion cells of the rhesus monkey. *Experimental Brain Research, 23,* 443–446.

Lawrence, V. W., Kee, D. W., & Hellige, J. B. (1980). Developmental differences in visual backward masking. *Child Development, 51,* 1081–1089.

Leventhal, A. G., & Hirsch, H. V. B. (1978). Receptive field properties of neurons in different laminae of visual cortex of cat. *Journal of Neurophysiology, 41,* 948–962.

Long, G. M. (1980). Iconic memory: A review and critique of the study of short-term visual storage. *Psychological Bulletin, 88,* 785–820.

Loomis, J. M. (1978). Lateral masking in foveal and eccentric vision. *Vision Research, 18,* 335–338.

Lovegrove, W., Billing, G., & Slaghuis, W. (1978). Processing of visual contour orientation information in normal and disabled reading children. *Cortex, 14,* 268–278.

Lovegrove, W., & Brown, C. (1978). Development of information processing in normal and disabled readers. *Perceptual and Motor Skills, 46,* 1047–1054.

Lovegrove, W., & Heddle, M. (1980). Visual persistence as a function of spatial frequency and age. *Perception, 9,* 529–532.

Lovegrove, W. J., Heddle, M., & Slaghuis, W. (1980). Reading disability: Spatial frequency specific deficits in visual information store. *Neuropsychologia, 18,* 111–115.

Lupp, U., Hauske, G., & Wolf, W. (1976). Perceptual latencies to sinusoidal gratings. *Vision Research, 16,* 969–972.

Lyon, J. E., Matteson, H. H., & Maras, M. S. (1981). Metacontrast in the fovea. *Vision Research, 21,* 217–219.

MacLeod, D. I. A. (1978). Visual sensitivity. In M. R. Rosenzweig & L. W. Porter (Eds.), *Annual review of psychology.* Palo Alto: Annual Reviews, Pp. 613–645.

Malpeli, J. G., & Baker, F. H. (1975). The representation of the visual field in the lateral geniculate nucleus of *macaca mulatta. Journal of Comparative Neurology, 161,* 569–594.

Malt, B. C., & Seamon, J. G. (1978). Peripheral and cognitive components of eye guidance in filled-space reading. *Perception & Psychophysics, 23,* 399–402.

Matin, E. (1974). Saccadic suppression: A review and analysis. *Psychological Bulletin, 81,* 899–917.

Matin, E. (1975). The two-transient (masking) paradigm. *Psychological Review, 82,* 451–461.

Matin, E. (1976). Saccadic suppression and the stable world. In R. A. Monty and J. W. Senders (Eds.), *Eye movements and psychological processes.* Hillsdale, New Jersey: Erlbaum, Pp. 113–119.

Matin, L. (1976). A possible hybrid mechanism for modification of visual direction associated with eye movements—the paralyzed-eye experiment reconsidered. *Perception, 5,* 233–239.

Mays, L. E., & Sparks, D. L. (1980). Saccades are spatially, not retinocentrically, coded. *Science, 208,* 1163–1165.

McConkie, G. W., & Rayner, K. (1976). Identifying the span of the effective stimulus in reading: Literature review and theories of reading. In H. Singer & R. B. Rudell (Eds.), *Theoretical models and processes of reading.* Newark, Delaware: International Reading Association, Pp. 137–162.

McKaukie, G. W. & Zola, D. (1979). Is visual information integrated across successive fixations in reading. *Perception & Psychophysics, 25,* 221–225.

McIlwain, J. T. (1964). Receptive fields of optic tract axons and lateral geniculate cells: Peripheral extent and barbiturate sensitivity. *Journal of Neurophysiology, 27,* 1154–1173.

McIlwain, J. T. (1972). Nonretinal influences on the lateral geniculate nucleus. *Investigative Opthalmology & Visual Science, 11,* 311–322.

McIlwain, J. T. (1973). Topographic relationships in projection from striate cortex to superior colliculus of the cat. *Journal of Neurophysiology, 36,* 690–701. (a)

McIlwain, J. T. (1973). Retinotopic fidelity of striate cortex-superior colliculus interactions in the cat. *Journal of Neurophysiology, 36,* 702–710. (b)

McIlwain, J. T. (1975). Visual receptive fields and their images in superior colliculus of the cat. *Journal of Neurophysiology, 38,* 219–230.

McIlwain, J. T. (1977). Topographic organization and convergence in corticotectal projections from areas 17, 18 and 19 in the cat. *Journal of Neurophysiology, 40,* 189–198.

Merikle, P. M. (1977). On the nature of metacontrast with complex targets and masks. *Journal of Experimental Psychology: Human Perception and Performance, 3,* 607–621.

Meyer, G. E., & Maguire, W. M. (1977). Spatial frequency and the mediation of short-term visual storage. *Science, 198,* 524–534.

Michaels, C. F., & Turvey, M. T. (1979). Central sources of visual masking: Indexing structures supporting seeing at a single, brief glance. *Psychological Research, 41,* 1–61.

Moffitt, K. (1980). Evaluation of the fixation duration in visual search. *Perception & Psychophysics, 27,* 370–372.

Mohler, C. W., Goldberg, M. E., & Wurtz, R. H. (1973). Visual receptive fields of frontal eye field neurons. *Brain Research, 61,* 385–409.

Mohler, C. W., & Wurtz, R. H. (1976). Organization of monkey superior colliculus: Intermediate layers cells discharge before eye movements. *Journal of Neurophysiology, 39,* 722–744.

Moors, J., & Vendrick, A. J. H. (1979). Responses of single units in the monkey superior colliculus to stationary flashing stimuli. *Experimental Brain Research, 35,* 333–347.

Morrison, F. J., Giordani, B., & Nagy, J. (1977). Reading disability: An information processing analysis. *Science, 196,* 77–79.

Neisser, U. (1976). *Cognition and reality.* San Francisco: W. H. Freeman.

Ogawa, T. (1963). Midbrain reticular influences upon single neurons in lateral geniculate nucleus. *Science, 139,* 343–344.

O'Regan, K. (1979). Saccade size control in reading: Evidence for the linguistic control hypothesis. *Perception & Psychophysics, 25,* 501–509.

O'Regan, K., & Levy–Schoen, A. (1978). Les mouvements des yeux au cours de la lecture. *L'Annee Psychologique, 78,* 459–492.

Palmer, L. A., & Rosenquist, A. C. (1974). Visual receptive fields of single striate cortical units projecting to the superior colliculus in the cat. *Brain Research, 67,* 27–42.

Parker, D. M., & Salzen, E. A. (1977). Latency changes in the human visual evoked response to sinusoidal gratings. *Vision Research, 17,* 1201–1204. (a)

Parker, D. M., & Salzen, E. A. (1977). The spatial selectivity of early and late waves within the human visual evoked response. *Perception, 6,* 85–95. (b)

Pecci–Saacedra, J., Wilson, P. D., & Doty, R. W. (1966). Presynaptic inhibition in primate lateral geniculate nucleus. *Nature (London), 210,* 740–742.

Peck, C. K., Schlag–Rey, M., & Schlag, J. (1980). Visuo-oculomotor properties of cells in the superior colliculus of the alert cat. *Journal of Comparative Neurology, 194,* 97–116.

Perryman, K. M., & Lindsley, D. B. (1977). Visual responses in geniculo-striate and pulvino-extrastriate systems to patterned and unpatterned stimuli in squirrel monkeys. *Electroencephalography and Clinical Neurophysiology, 42,* 157–177.

Peterson, B. W. Participation of pontomedullary reticular neurons in specific motor activity. In A. Hobson & M. Brazier (Eds.), *The reticular formation revisited.* New York: Raven Press, in press.

Rayner, K. (1975). The perceptual span and peripheral cues in reading. *Cognitive Psychology, 7,* 65–81.

Rayner, K. (1978). Eye movements in reading and information processing. *Psychological Bulletin, 85,* 618–660. (a)

Rayner, K. (1978). Foveal and parafoveal cues in reading. In J. Requin (Ed.), *Attention and performance* (Vol. 7). Hillsdale, New Jersey: Erlbaum, Pp. 149–162. (b)

Rayner, K. (1979). Eye movements in reading: Eye guidance and integration. In P. A. Kolers, M. Wrolstad, & H. Bouma (Eds.), *Processing of visible language.* New York: Plenum, Pp. 61–76.

Rayner, K., & Bertera, J. H. (1979). Reading without a fovea. *Science, 206,* 468–469.

Rayner, K., & McConkie, G. W. (1977). Perceptual processes in reading: The perceptual spans. In A. Reber & D. Scarborough (Eds.), *Toward a psychology of reading.* Hillsdale, New Jersey: Erlbaum, Pp. 183–206.

Rayner, K., McConkie, G. W., & Ehrlich, S. (1978). Eye movements and integrating information across fixations. *Journal of Experimental Psychology: Human Perception and Performance, 4,* 529–544.

Rayner, K., McConkie, G. W., & Zola, D. (1980). Integrating information across eye movements. *Cognitive Psychology, 12,* 206–226.

Rezak, M., & Benevento, L. A. (1979). A comparison of the organization of the projections of the dorsal lateral geniculate nucleus, the inferior pulvinar and adjacent lateral pulvinar to primary visual cortex (area 17) in the macaque monkey. *Brain Research, 167,* 19–40.

Riggs, L. A., Merton, P. A., & Morton, H. B. (1974). Suppression of visual phosphenes during saccadic eye movements. *Vision Research, 14,* 997–1010.

Ritter, M. (1976). Evidence for visual persistence during saccadic eye movements. *Psychological Research, 39,* 67–85.

Robinson, D. A., & Fuchs, A. (1969). Eye movements evoked by stimulation of frontal eye fields. *Journal of Neurophysiology, 32,* 637–648.

Robinson, D. L., Baizier, J. S., & Dow, B. M. (1980). Behavioral enhancement of visual responses of prestriate neurons of the rhesus monkey. *Investigative Ophthalmology & Visual Science, 19,* 1120–1123.

Rolls, E. T., & Cowey, A. (1970). Topography of the retina and striate cortex and its relationship to visual acuity in rhesus monkeys and squirrel monkeys. *Experimental Brain Research, 10,* 298–310.

Saida, S., & Ikeda, M. (1979). Useful visual field size for pattern perception. *Perception & Psychophysics, 25,* 119–125.

Sakitt, B. (1975). Locus of short-term visual storage. *Science, 190,* 1318–1319.

Sakitt, B. (1976). Iconic memory. *Psychological Review, 83,* 257–276.

Saunders, J. (1977). Foveal and spatial properties of brightness metacontrast. *Vision Research, 17,* 375–378.

Schiepers, C. W. J. (1976). Global attributes in visual word recognition. Part 1: Length perception of letter strings. *Vision Research, 16,* 1343–1349. (a)

Schiepers, C. W. J. (1976). Global attributes in visual word recognition. Part 2: The contribution of word length. *Vision Research, 16,* 1445–1454. (b)

Schiller, P. H., & Koerner, F. (1971). Discharge characteristics of single units in superior colliculus of alert rhesus monkey. *Journal of Neurophysiology, 35,* 920–936.

Schiller, P. H., True, S. D., & Conway, J. L. (1979). Effects of frontal eye field and superior colliculus ablations on eye movements. *Science, 206,* 590–592.

Singer, W. (1973). The effect of mesencephalic reticular stimulation on intracellular potentials of cat lateral geniculate neurons. *Brain Research, 61,* 35–54. (a)

Singer, W. (1973). Brain stem stimulation and the hypothesis of presynaptic inhibition in cat lateral geniculate nucleus. *Brain Research, 61,* 55–68. (b)

Singer, W. (1977). Control of thalamic transmission by corticofugal and ascending reticular pathways in the visual system. *Physiological Review, 57,* 386–420.

Singer, W. (1979). Central-core control of visual cortex function. In F. O. Schmitt & F. G. Worden (Eds.), *The neurosciences fourth study program.* Cambridge, Massachusetts: MIT Press, Pp. 1093–1110.

Singer, W., & Bedworth, N. (1973). Inhibitory interaction between $X$ and $Y$ units in cat lateral geniculate nucleus. *Brain Research, 49,* 291–307.

Singer, W., & Bedworth, N. (1974). Correlation between the effects of brain stem stimulation and saccadic eye movements on transmission in the cat lateral geniculate nucleus. *Brain Research, 72,* 185–202.

Singer, W., Tretter, F., & Cynader, M. (1976). The effect of reticular stimulation on spontaneous and evoked activity in the cat visual cortex. *Brain Research, 102,* 71–90.

Stanley, G., & Hall, R. (1973). A comparison of dyslexics and normals in recalling letter arrays after brief presentation. *British Journal of Educational Psychology, 43,* 301–304. (a)

Stanley, G., & Hall, R. (1973). Short-term visual information processing in dyslexics. *Child Development, 44,* 841–844. (b)

Stewart, A. L., & Purcell, D. G. (1970). U-shaped masking functions in visual backward masking: Effects of target configuration and retinal position. *Perception & Psychophysics, 7,* 253–256.

Talbot, S. A., & Marshall, W. H. (1941). Physiological studies of neural mechanisms of visual localization and discrimination. *American Journal of Opthalmology, 24,* 1255–1264.

Tatton, W. G., & Crapper, D. R. (1972). Central tegmental alteration of cat lateral geniculate activity. *Brain Research, 47,* 371–387.

Tsumoto, T., Suzuki, D. A. (1976). Effects of frontal eye field stimulation upon activities of the lateral geniculate body of the cat. *Experimental Brain Research, 25,* 291–306.

Turvey, M. T. (1973). On peripheral and central processes in vision: Inferences from an information-processing analysis of masking with patterned stimuli. *Psychological Review, 80,* 1–52.

Turvey, M. T. (1977). Contrasting orientations to the theory of visual information processing. *Psychological Review, 84,* 67–88.

Uttal, W. R. (1971). The psychobiologically silly season-or-what happens when neurophysiological data become psychological theories. *Journal of General Psychology, 84,* 151–166.

Valberg, A., & Breitmeyer, B. (1980). The lateral effect of oscillation of peripheral luminance gratings: Test of various hypotheses. *Vision Research, 20,* 789–798.

Vassilev, A., & Mitov, D. (1976). Perception time and spatial frequency. *Vision Research, 16,* 719–730.

Vassilev, A., & Strashimirov, D. (1979). On the latency of human visually evoked response to sinusoidal gratings. *Vision Research, 19,* 843–845.

Volkmann, F. C., Riggs, L. A., Moore, R. K., & White, K. D. (1978). Central and peripheral determinants of saccadic suppression. In J. W. Senders, D. R. Fischer, & R. A. Monty (Eds.), *Eye movements and the higher psychological functions.* Hillsdale, New Jersey: Erlbaum, Pp. 35–54.

Volkmann, F. C., Riggs, L. A., White, K. D., & Moore, R. K. (1978). Contrast sensitivity during saccadic eye movements. *Vision Research, 18,* 1193–1199.

von Grünau, M. E. (1978). Interaction between sustained and transient channels: Form inhibits motion in the human visual system. *Vision Research, 18,* 197–201.

Wanatabe, Y. (1977). Interferences of visual noises with the peripheral matching of letters. *Tohoku Psychologica Folia, 36,* 101–110.

Weisstein, N. (1972). Metacontrast. In D. Jameson & L. M. Hurvich (Eds.), *Handbook of sensory physiology* (Vol. 7/4). New York: Springer, Pp. 233–272.

Weisstein, N., Ozog, G., & Szoc, R. (1975). A comparison and elaboration of two models of metacontrast. *Psychological Review, 82,* 325–343.

White, K. D., Post, R. B., & Leibowitz, H. W. (1980). Saccadic eye movements and body sway. *Science, 208,* 621–623.

Whitteridge, D. (1973). Projection of optic pathways to the visual cortex. In R. Jung (Ed.), *Handbook of sensory physiology* (Vol. 7/3). New York: Springer.

Wilson, M. E., & Toyne, M. J. (1970). Retino-tectal and cortico-tectal projections in *macaca mulatta. Brain Research, 24,* 395–406.

Wolf, W., Hauske, G., & Lupp, U. (1978). How presaccadic gratings modify post-saccadic modulation transfer function. *Vision Research, 18,* 1173–1179.

Wolf, W., Hauske, G., & Lupp, U. (1980). Interaction of pre- and postsaccadic patterns having the same coordinates in space. *Vision Research, 20,* 117–125.

Wurtz, R. H. (1976). Extraretinal influences on the primate visual system. In R. A. Monty & J. W. Senders (Eds.), *Eye movements and psychological processes.* Hillsdale, New Jersey: Erlbaum, pp. 231–244.

Wurtz, R. H., & Mohler, C. W. (1974). Selection of visual targets for the initiation of saccadic eye movements. *Brain Research, 71,* 209–214.

Wurtz, R. H., & Mohler, C. W. (1976). Organization of monkey superior colliculus: Enhanced visual response of superficial layer cells. *Journal of Neurophysiology, 39,* 745–765. (a)

Wurtz, R. H., & Mohler, C. W. (1970). Enhancement of visual responses in monkey striate cortex and frontal eye fields. *Journal of Neurophysiology, 39,* 766–772. (b)

Robert E. Morrison

# 2

# Retinal Image Size and the Perceptual Span in Reading[1]

## I.   Introduction

The issue to be addressed in this chapter is how the perceptual span is affected by changes in the size of the retinal image of the stimulus. The term *perceptual span* refers to the span of the effective stimulus or the amount of textual material that is processed—in some manner—within a fixation.

There are two ways to accomplish identical changes in the retinal image size of the letters in a stimulus text: by changing the physical size of the characters themselves or by changing the distance they are viewed from. With viewing distance held constant larger characters yield a larger retinal image. Decreasing viewing distance will increase the size of the retinal image as well. As retinal image size increases the stimulus presumably becomes more perceptible; however, a given stimulus also extends further into the retinal periphery where acuity is poorer.

The relationship between retinal image size and eccentric acuity is unclear. Is there a trade-off such that the greater perceptibility of larger retinal images compensates for the poorer acuity encountered in the retinal areas subtended? If so, changes in character size or viewing distance (assuming foveal recognition thresholds are not approached) would have a minimal effect on the perceptual span. As type size increased or as distance from stimulus to eye was reduced—both yielding a larger retinal image of the stimulus yet falling into more eccentric

[1]This work was supported by grant HD12727 from the National Institute of Child Health and Human Development.

31

regions of the retina—the poorer acuity might offset any increase in perceptibility of the characters. Conversely, as type size decreased or viewing distance became greater, the resulting smaller retinal image would fall within a more compact region around the fovea and the higher acuity might compensate for any reduction in perceptibility of the stimulus.

Since many psychophysical determinations of acuity show it to be a linearly decreasing function of retinal eccentricity (Anstis, 1974) it has been hypothesized that the trade-off between retinal image size and eccentric acuity is counterbalancing and thus moderate changes in viewing distance may not affect the perceptual span in reading (O'Regan, 1980).

In contrast, it may be that the reader processes text only within some high acuity region of central vision, a critical visual angle, with the perceptual span determined by the amount of text filling this cone of vision. Since psychophysical experiments usually present single stimuli in the visual field those data may not apply to reading situations where the visual field is filled. Here effects of lateral masking may be present to constrain the region of clear vision. Or, even if stimuli are perceptible in more eccentric retinal areas, in an ongoing processing task such as reading different transmission speeds from retina to cortex or attentional factors may induce the reader to adapt a strategy of processing only within a fixed retinal region and then redirecting the eye.

In any event, the question of the relationship between retinal image size and the perceptual span is an interesting one. An answer might tell us three things: (1) whether retinal image size of letters is indeed a determinant of the perceptual span and if so what factors must be controlled in reading research; (2) whether data from the psychophysical literature can lead to accurate inferences about reading behavior; and (3) what the appropriate metric is for discussing the size of the perceptual span and oculomotor variables such as saccade length in reading.

## II.   Tinker's Research

Recent research has used on-line stimulus changes contingent upon eye position to precisely determine the span of the effective stimulus (perceptual span) in reading (e.g., McConkie & Rayner, 1975; Rayner, 1975). In fact we can talk about different perceptual spans for different kinds of information such as specific letter information or word boundary information. However, these studies have not looked at factors such as character size or viewing distance to determine the effects of changes in retinal image size.

A lot of early reading research done in the first half of this century, especially by Miles Tinker and his colleagues, did consider the effects of typographical and psychophysical factors (Tinker, 1963, 1965). Although the technology to make online stimulus changes contingent upon eye position was not available, the early researchers did photograph eye movements and discovered quite a few facts about oculomotor behavior in reading that contemporary research merely replicates.

# physically somewhat longer saccades but these traversed fewer characters. There are two possible explanations for

14-point type, leaded 4 points, 29-pica measure

area in this case. Regression frequency increased only slightly; thus the frequency of forward fixations (total fixation frequency minus regression frequency) increased. This implies by our previous reasoning that mean saccade size decreased, in this case

6-point type, leaded 3 points, 29-pica measure

## noted above, more visual angle may be covered by saccades while reading the text of larger type. But

10-point type, leaded 2 points, 19-pica measure

### picas, which results in a line of approximately

10-point type, leaded 1 point, 9-pica measure

**FIGURE 2.1.** *Examples of typographical variables used by Tinker to investigate the impact on reading behavior of changes in type size, line width, and leading.*[2]

Lacking the on-line methodology, average saccade length or a measure like words per fixation was used as an index of the perceptual span (Paterson & Tinker, 1947). Though saccade length is not equivalent to the perceptual span it will be assumed that mean saccade length bears a monotonic relationship to the average size of the perceptual span and mean saccade length will be used to infer changes in the perceptual span.

---

[2]Type size is traditionally given in units of vertical extent called points. A point is approximately 1/72 in. A pica is a traditional typographical measure of width, approximately equal to 1/6 in. Leading is blank space inserted (vertically) between type set lines of text and is also specified in points. This chapter is set in 10 point type on a 12 point body, that is, 10 point type leaded 2 points.

Tinker (1963, 1965) investigated the effects on reading speed, eye movements, and the perceptual span of manipulations of typographical variables such as type size, line width, and leading (see Figure 2.1). His findings about effects of type size may shed some light on the question of retinal image size.[3]

## A.   Type Size

When type size was varied in a constant-width line of 19 picas the 10- and 11 point type was read most quickly, with fewer fixations and longer saccades on the average. Smaller and larger type sizes were read more slowly, with more fixations and shorter saccades. Tinker concluded that fixation durations were longer on smaller type sizes because the characters were harder to discriminate. The average saccade made on small type traversed fewer characters and a narrower visual angle.

Type sizes larger than 11 point had shorter fixation durations (due to the more easily perceived characters) yet still were read more slowly because there were more fixations. The average saccade traversed fewer characters than on 11 point type. It is interesting to note that these saccades were actually larger physically, covering a wider visual angle than those made on 11 point type.

This experiment shows that saccades traversing fewer characters than those made on an optimal typography can result from saccades of either greater or lesser visual angle. That is, saccade length could increase or decrease in terms of a physical metric like visual angle and still result in fewer characters per saccade, suggesting that an absolute metric is noninformative when discussing the amount of text traversed or similarly when considering the perceptual span. The relative metric of number of characters seems more appropriate.

Tinker's work initially suggests that 10 or 11 point type optimizes some function relating retinal image size and eccentric acuity (and perhaps other factors—e.g., attentional) such that larger or smaller type decreases the perceptual span and saccades traverse fewer characters. However, Tinker realized that the number of characters in a line was confounded with type size in this experiment.

## B.   Line Width

Extensive experiments on line width indeed showed that the width of the line interacted with type size in determining reading speed and eye movement efficiency.

Generally, larger type sizes are read optimally when printed in longer lines (physically, in picas) than smaller type sizes, thus maintaining a similar number of

[3]Tinker's eye movement monitoring apparatus kept a subject's head still by means of a head rest. Thus viewing distance was fixed for any subject having eye movements monitored (not all Tinker's experiments involved eye tracking) although it may have varied between subjects (Morrison & Inhoff, 1981).

characters on a line. Also, for any one type size, Tinker found an intermediate range of line widths that were read equally fast. Lines shorter than these increased fixation durations and decreased saccade length. The fewer characters in a short line make inefficient use of peripheral vision, Tinker believed. Optimal length lines allow the perceptual span to stretch to its fullest, thus increasing saccade length. In addition, mean fixation duration decreases since fixation durations are initially long at the beginning of a line and decrease as portions of the line are fixated that have been successively glimpsed in peripheral vision (Dearborn, 1906; Dodge, 1907). If line lengths are longer than those found optimal this benefit is negated by frequent undershoots on the return sweep and difficulties in fixating the correct line at that point. Increased fixation durations and more fixations there result in a decrease in reading speed with lines longer than optimal.

## C. Leading

Tinker found that leading (space between lines) increases reading speed and saccade length compared with text set solid (no leading). The increased blank space above and below the letters probably reduces lateral masking to increase the perceptual span. Generally 2 points of leading optimized performance on most type sizes investigated. The leading also extended the range of optimal line widths for which a given type size was read equally quickly. Shorter and longer lines were read with no decrement in performance compared with text set solid.

## D. Type Size with Optimal Line Width and Leading

Having established the fact that the various typographical features of a text interact to determine legibility, Tinker investigated type size again while printing each type size in its empirically determined optimal combination of line width and leading. This time no significant differences were found between 9, 10, 11, and 12 point type. Smaller types, 6 and 8 point, were still read slower with increased fixation durations and slightly less characters per saccade. Once above this lower limit, type size seemed to have no effect. Apparently, when type size is not confounded with the number of characters in a line the perceptual span is invariant with changes in retinal image size that result from moderate changes in type size.

It appears that retinal image size (thus perceptability) does trade off evenly with eccentric acuity, within limits. The lower bound of this invariant range is when the stimulus characters become difficult to discriminate. An upper bound would presumably occur when the perceptual span extended out to the 20 or 30° of eccentricity beyond which the decrease in acuity is no longer linear, but accelerates (Anstis, 1974). A practical limit may be reached before this however, at least when successive lines of text requiring return sweeps are read, by causing disruption of the return sweep (perhaps necessitating head movements along with saccades to accomplish such a large redirection of vision). Unfortunately, Tinker did not use type larger than 12 point in this study.

Gilliland (1923) did use larger type sizes of 36, 54, 72, and 90 point (all stimuli had a constant number of characters in a line) and although the study is less carefully controlled than Tinker's and lacks eye movement monitoring, the findings are similar. There seemed to be no difference in reading speed between 9, 12, and 18 point type. Reading speed seemed to decrease for 6 point type or smaller, or 36 point type or larger. Judd (1918) reported equivalence in the span of recognition when 11 point type was doubled or halved in size.

## III.  Viewing Distance

As noted earlier, changes of viewing distance mimic those of type size in producing retinal image size changes.[4] Surprisingly, Tinker did not address the issue of viewing distance. He may have considered it a moot point. Prior to his work Javal (cited in Huey, 1900) and Huey (1900) had reported that the number of fixations on a text does not change with changes in viewing distance. Huey particularly reported that doubling viewing distance had no effect on eye movements. However in the same article Huey reported saccade length data in degrees of visual angle and the perceptual span as millimeters of the stimulus surface. Thus, there seemed to be some confusion about what the appropriate metric was for discussing these measures, which has continued up to the present (Rayner, 1978, p. 624).

The question of viewing distance has been most recently addressed by O'Regan (1980). He claimed that the perceptual span is invariant over moderate changes in viewing distance by the argument set forth earlier that retinal image size (and perceptibility) is offset by the linear decrease in acuity with increasing retinal eccentricity (as found in psychophysical paradigms). Since it is not clear that the psychophysical literature generalizes to reading behavior where a filled visual field exists which may increase lateral masking, or different strategies may be operant for various reasons, it seemed that O'Regan's assertion should be empirically demonstrated.

We (Morrison & Rayner, 1981) monitored the eye movements of subjects who read single sentences on a cathode-ray tube (CRT) at three different viewing distances: 14, 21, and 28 in. (approximately 36, 53, and 71 cm). Eleven sentence triplets were constructed that were matched word by word for word length. One sentence of the three was read at each distance. The letters on the CRT were composed of luminous dots from a 5 × 7 dot matrix approximately equal to a 14 point type size. At the three distances used, the matrix subtended different visual angles which, if caused by type all at a distance of 14 in. (36 cm) would have

---

[4]Of course other limiting factors may come into play such as the ability to focus the eyes in near vision which declines with age (presbyopia).

resulted from sizes of approximately 14, 10, and 7 points. The subjects' task was simply to read the sentences for understanding and press a button when this was done. The experimenter occasionally asked the subject to report or paraphrase the sentence as a check on comprehension. Thirteen triplets of filler sentences were also included.

Two predictions were possible a priori about the eye movements of subjects reading at different distances. One is that the perceptual span and thus the average number of characters traversed by a saccade would be constant. Mean saccade length in character spaces would not differ significantly but it would change drastically in terms of visual angle. Alternatively, if readers process the text only within some critical visual angle, regardless of viewing distance, then the mean saccade length would be a constant visual angle but would differ significantly in terms of character spaces (as would the perceptual span). An intermediate position might be that a certain retinal image size of characters is optimal and deviations in either direction decrease the perceptual span so that the mean characters per saccade data would fit an inverted U-shaped curve. This is still a hypothesis that distance would be a critical variable in determining the perceptual span and is contrasted with the invariant perceptual span hypothesis proposed by O'Regan (1980).

The mean saccade lengths at each viewing distance are plotted in Figure 2.2 both in terms of character spaces and visual angle. The data quite clearly favor the hypothesis of an invariant perceptual span with moderate changes in viewing distance. As can be seen in the lower portion of Figure 2.2, the mean number of characters traversed by saccades did not differ significantly when viewing distance changed by a factor of 2. Of course this means that physically the mean saccade size was quite different when viewing distance was changed. Indeed, the upper portion of Figure 2.2 shows that the visual angle per saccade decreased as distance increased. The data neatly fit the prediction that the number of characters and not the visual angle per saccade would be invariant (solid lines) and strikingly oppose the prediction of constant visual angle, character-space-different saccades (dashed lines).

Mean fixation durations increased somewhat as viewing distance increased—237, 253, and 260 msec at 14, 21, and 28 in., respectively. This was probably due to the stimulus being less discriminable at greater viewing distances.

If moderate changes in retinal image size of the stimulus do not alter or constrain the perceptual span in any way as is claimed and supported by summary data on mean saccade length then eye movement strategies employed by readers should also be unaffected. In other words there should be no systematic difference between the fixation patterns observed when subjects read at different viewing distances. An examination of individual fixation patterns from the experiment shows that this appears to be true. Figure 2.3 gives examples of two fixation sequences made by the same subject on two sentences presented at different viewing distances. Dots below the sentences mark the letter position of individual fixations, with their corresponding durations indicated above the sentence. For

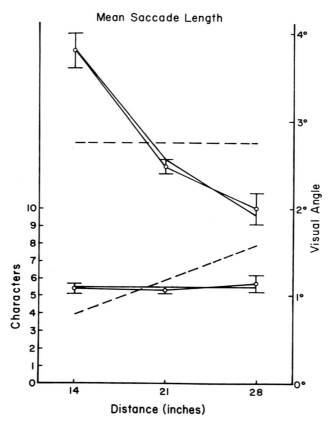

**FIGURE 2.2.** *Mean saccade length data (open circles) as a function of viewing distance plotted in terms of character spaces (lower portion, left ordinate); or the same data plotted as degrees of visual angle (upper portion, right ordinate). Error bars are one standard error. The solid line in the lower portion shows a prediction of constant character space saccades plotted at the data grand mean of 5.47 characters per saccade. When transformed to corresponding values of visual angle the prediction results in the solid line in the upper portion. The dashed line (upper portion) shows a prediction of constant-visual-angle saccades plotted at the data grand mean of 2.75° per saccade. The equivalent in character spaces is shown as the dashed line in the lower portion.*

the example shown, all fixations were forward fixations—there were no regressive eye movements. The sentences are exactly matched for word length which is one variable known to affect fixation behavior (Rayner, 1979). Grammatical class and general gist of meaning is matched as well.

As can be seen in the pattern of individual fixations, "preferred viewing locations within words" as discussed by Rayner (1979) tend to be fixated—primarily the center or first half of words. Also, if two short words occur in succession often only one fixation is needed to process them. The mean saccade lengths in this case mimics the group data—saccade length is quite similar in terms of character spaces but quite different in terms of visual angle traversed.

| Distance (In.) | | Mean saccade length | |
|---|---|---|---|
| | | Characters | Degrees |
| 28 | 182 203 190   183       192   354 419<br>*The crazed boy was locked into a cage.*<br>.    .    .         .        .    . | 5.5 | 1.9 |
| 14 | 191   294 121     269   306     238 534<br>*The unruly guy was heaved into a cell.*<br>.    .   .         .        .       .    . | 5.7 | 4.0 |

**FIGURE 2.3.** *Examples of fixation positions and durations (msec).*

Not all comparisons of individual eye movement records match as well as these do of course, due to random variability. But cases such as those in Figure 2.3 occur frequently enough to sufficiently rule out the possibility that the group data are an artifact caused by real changes in eye movements at different viewing distances canceling out when averaged over subjects.

## IV.   Conclusion

In conclusion it appears that the perceptual span is invariant over changes— within limits—in the retinal image size of the stimulus as caused by moderate changes in viewing distance (as proposed by O'Regan, 1980) or type size (when not confounded by other typographical factors such as number of characters in a line, as shown by Tinker, 1963).

It seems clear that the appropriate metric when discussing saccade lengths in reading is the relative one of character spaces as opposed to an absolute physical metric such as visual angle or distance on the stimulus surface. Both recent results (Morrison & Rayner, 1981; see O'Regan, Chapter 7 of this volume) and Tinker's research show that reading experiments involving independent variables that change the retinal image size of the stimulus can result in changes in the amount of visual angle traversed by the saccades, the direction and magnitude of which is totally uninformative by itself about the effects on the perceptual span. A change in either direction of the visual angle per saccade may be associated with an increase, decrease, or no change at all in the number of characters per saccade.

Furthermore, it seems that viewing distance need not be strictly controlled in reading experiments, at least those reading experiments concerned with using the perceptual span, or saccade length (in characters) as a dependent measure. With-in limits the viewing distance may be varied to accommodate the comfort of the subject or preferences of the experimenter without confounding the data. Type size is also free to vary moderately but since typographical variables interact with type size these must be carefully adjusted. Particularly, line width must be varied along with type size and kept within certain limits. Leading must be controlled as well. Any other typographical variables (type font, etc.) should be controlled.

# References

Anstis, S. M. (1974). A chart demonstrating variations in acuity with retinal position. *Vision Research*, *14*, 589–592.

Dearborn, W. F. (1906). *The psychology of reading*. Columbia University Contribution to Philosophy and Psychology, *14* (1).

Dodge, R. (1907). An experimental study of visual fixation. *Psychological Review Monograph Supplements*, *8* (4).

Gilliland, A. R. (1923). The effect on reading of changes in the size of type. *Elementary School Journal*, *24*, 138–146.

Huey, E. B. (1900). On the psychology and physiology of reading. *American Journal of Psychology*, *11*, 283–302.

Judd, C. H. (1918). Reading: Its nature and development. *Supplementary Educational Monographs*, (10).

McConkie, G. W., & Rayner, K. (1975). The span of the effective stimulus during a fixation in reading. *Perception & Psychophysics*, *17*, 578–586.

Morrison, R. E., & Inhoff, A. W. (1981). Visual factors and eye movements in reading. *Visible Language*, *15*, 129–146.

Morrison, R. E., & Rayner, K. (1981). Saccade size in reading depends upon character spaces and not visual angle. *Perception & Psychophysics*, *30*, 395–396.

O'Regan, K. (1980). The control of saccade size and fixation duration in reading: The limits of linguistic control. *Perception & Psychophysics*, *28*, 112–117.

Paterson, D. G., & Tinker, M. A. (1947). The effect of typography upon the perceptual span in reading. *American Journal of Psychology*, *60*, 388–396.

Rayner, K. (1975). The perceptual span and peripheral cues in reading. *Cognitive Psychology*, *7*, 65–81.

Rayner, K. (1978). Eye movements in reading and information processing. *Psychological Bulletin*, *85*, 618–666.

Rayner, K. (1979). Eye guidance in reading: Fixation locations within words. *Perception*, *8*, 21–30.

Tinker, M. A. (1963). *Legibility of print*. Ames, Iowa: Iowa State University Press.

Tinker, M. A. (1965). *Bases for effective reading*. Minneapolis: University of Minnesota Press.

Gary S. Wolverton and David Zola

# 3

# The Temporal Characteristics of Visual Information Extraction during Reading

## I.   Introduction

We have been studying the nature of the temporal characteristics of silent skilled reading in an attempt to describe the perceptual process of extraction of visual information that is taking place as reading is in progress. This task is difficult because there are few outwardly observable indicators of the cognitive events of the mind that are occurring during reading. Eye movements and electrical activity of the brain are two measurable events that provide indicators of ongoing processing of information during reading with minimal interference on the process. To us, reading is an integrated series of cognitive processes that operate at different levels of abstraction and that occur simultaneously. Eye movement patterns have been shown to reflect this cognitive activity. In this chapter, we consider a series of issues that the eye movement phase of our research has addressed. We present a brief statement from the literature of the current perspective upon each issue and supplement the discussion with our own findings. Since our research activity is in its infancy, our chapter is more of a progress report than a statement of results. We intend to show the critical nature of eye movement research in the investigation of the reading process.

Throughout this chapter we discuss various eye movement events primarily with respect to some contingent display change. To facilitate this discussion, the following conventions are used:

EYE MOVEMENTS IN READING:
PERCEPTUAL AND LANGUAGE PROCESSES

1. In our research, display changes occurred during a specific fixation (F0) or specific saccade (S0).
2. The saccade following the current fixation (F0) is referred to as S1.

A schematic diagram of this nomenclature is presented in Figure 3.1.

All of our research involves an eye movement contingent display manipulation. A computer system has been developed that permits experimental control over a display contingent upon the characteristics of the reader's eye movements. The display can be changed during specific saccades and/or fixations (McConkie, Zola, Wolverton & Burn, 1978). Such rapid display changes are accomplished by programming the computer to detect within a few msec the state of the eyes (i.e., in a saccade or fixation). The parameters supplied to the computer with each individual experimental text line permit the experimental manipulations (i.e., display changes) to be performed in the proper time sequence. By replacing individual letters, words, and text lines, we are able to determine when the reader is sensitive to the visual information provided by the text. The eye position monitoring equipment is a Stanford Research Institute Dual Purkinje Eyetracker. The procedures that are currently in use permit detection of an eye movement of ⅛° of visual angle. Repeatability measures taken before and after the reading of each passage have convinced us that our current optical and mechanical procedures maintain an accuracy well within ¼° of visual angle (approximately one letter position in our current setup). With such high degrees of resolution and accuracy, we are able to make very precise manipulations in the text display being read.

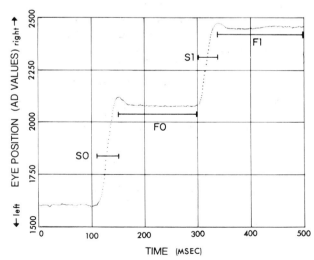

FIGURE 3.1. *Schematic representation of data taken from a typical line of reading showing the sequence of events for a given experimental line.*

## II.  The Extraction of Information during Saccades in Reading

Vision research has demonstrated that the threshold for detecting visual information is raised during saccadic movements (Latour, 1962; Volkmann, 1962; Volkmann, 1976; Volkmann, Schick, & Riggs, 1968). This phenomenon has commonly been referred to as "saccadic suppression." What this line of research has really shown is that the ability to detect a stimulus (usually, a flash of light) is attenuated during saccades. The temporal course of this threshold elevation includes a period of approximately 20 msec prior to and 75 msec after the onset of the saccade (Haber and Hershenson, 1973). This phenomenon raises the interesting question of what visual information is noticed during eye movements in reading. The answer indicates whether or not readers are noticing word information as the eyes are moving, and whether information extraction is occurring only during fixations. Wolverton (1979) investigated this in a representative reading situation. Subjects were asked to read five 30-line passages primarily attempting to understand the meaning of each passage in preparation for a comprehension test. The experimental manipulation caused specified lines of text to be replaced with some alternative line for up to 30 msec during selected saccades and fixations. There were five types of alternative text lines that were used as replacement lines for the original text. These are referred to as the "text substitution" conditions. The replacement line was either the original line of text (as a control condition), a line

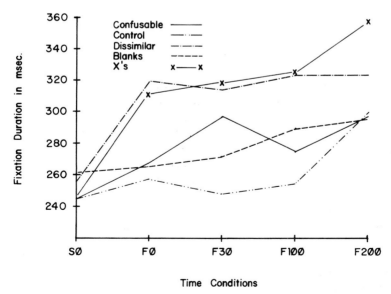

**FIGURE 3.2.** *Mean fixation duration (F0) as a function of experimental conditions.*

of blanks, a line of all capital X's that preserved the spacing of the original line, a line from some totally unrelated passage, or a line of letters that were selected as the letters most visually similar to the original letters in the text (e.g., for example the word *but* was replaced with the letter string *dvr*). By examining the durations of the immediately subsequent two fixations and two saccades, Wolverton was able to determine whether or not there was any disruption in the normal reading pattern (see Fig. 3.2). Overall, the manipulation had no significant effect on reading. Thus, it appears that the extraction of visual information from text occurs only during fixations.

## III.  When during a Fixation Is Visual Information Acquired?

Although we are sure that visual information is extracted during the fixations in reading, we do not know precisely when during individual fixations such perceptual processing takes place. There have been a number of studies investigating the visual processing sequence in identifying words, and this research has led to speculations about perceptual processing in reading. Sperling (1960) suggested that visual input to the cognitive system is very rapid and is accomplished in a parallel fashion. Geyer (1970) argues for a serial input of letters proceeding in a left to right manner across some defined perceptual span that requires approximately 8 msec per letter. However, Geyer further suggests that information can be extracted at any time during the fixation when the reading system is prepared to accept it. Gough (1972) presents a similar argument suggesting a 10–20-msec individual letter-input time. Brown (1970) has hypothesized a precise algorithm for the noticing of information that includes the primacy of first and last letters. Smith (1971) concluded from his word recognition research that the input necessary and sufficient for reading takes place within the first 50 msec of a fixation. Rayner provides support for this position. He and his colleagues (Rayner, Inhoff, Morrison, Słowiaczek, & Bertera, 1981) have reported that the identification of words in short sentences is possible when the text is only available for a limited time. In this study, text was presented for the first 50 msec of each fixation followed by a foveal mask for the remainder of the fixation. Under such conditions, readers were able to verbally report the content of each sentence with a high degree of accuracy. Rayner interprets these and other findings (Rayner, 1975; Rayner & Bertera, 1979; Rayner *et al.*, 1981; Rayner & McConkie, 1976; Rayner, McConkie, & Zola, 1980; Rayner, Well, & Pollatsek, 1980) as evidence that the initial foveal extraction process requires approximately 50 msec and is followed by an extraction of parafoveal then peripheral information which facilitates subsequent processing.

In a study that was described in Section II, Wolverton similarly replaced lines of text with some other line for a 30 msec period at different times during certain fixations (i.e., as soon as the fixation began, or 30, 100, or 200 msec after the fixation began). The X's and the unrelated lines of text had the greatest effect, causing an increase in the duration of the fixation during which the manipulation was made. Blanks and similar-letter lines had less of an effect. However, the main point of interest in this study was that effects were found when an experimental manipulation occurred at each selected time throughout the fixation. (see Figure 3.2) It appears that at no period during a fixation is the visual system insensitive to the textual stimuli because of threshold elevation or because information extraction has been completed. Our results indicate that at all times during the fixation, the stimulus information is being noticed. The finding that only gross changes during the first 30 msecs of the fixation significantly disrupt the process suggests that parafoveal and peripheral information, such as word shape, is being extracted during this initial period. The signification increase in fixation duration for the confusable text condition, which occurs 30 msec after the start of a fixation, suggests that specific foveal information is required during this period. Therefore, although the reader extracts information from the text at various locations during the fixation as needed for processing, specific detailed information from the foveal region need not be processed first.

In a follow-up study, Wolverton (unpublished data) attempted to gain a better understanding of this notion that information is noticed at all times during a fixation. He presented subjects with text where the original stimulus line was replaced with an alternate line in which every letter of the original text was replaced by letters that were most similar to the original letters. Therefore, word

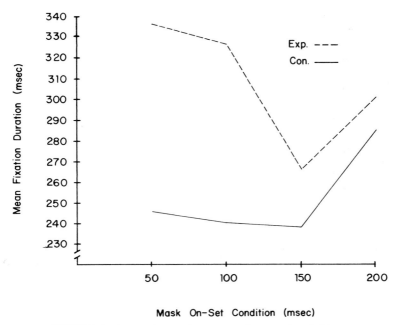

FIGURE 3.3. *Average fixation duration as a function of mask delay.*

shape and spatial information were preserved. The alternate lines were displayed at four different timing conditions: after the first 50, 100, 150, and 200 msec of the fixation, remaining for the rest of the fixation. Figure 3.3 presents mean fixation durations as a function of mask onset condition for the fixation during which the display changed. Significant differences were found for the 50- and 100-msec delay conditions suggesting that information available during the first 100 msec of the current fixation can immediately influence reading behavior. Changes that occur much later than 100 msec apparently have little effect upon the current fixation. An analysis of the following saccade also revealed a significant difference in length; in the 50- and 100-msec delay conditions, the average following saccade was shorter than the control. However, the 150- and 200-msec conditions exhibited no differences. Figures 3.4 and 3.5 present frequency distributions of saccades under both 50- and 100-msec delay conditions. These distributions indicate a dramatic increase in the number of short regressions when changes occur prior to 150 msec into the fixation. This finding supports the previously reported conclusion that information extracted early in the fixation can immediately influence the fixation and the following saccade.

Analysis of the fixation following the fixation where the display change occurred showed that average fixation durations were significantly different from the control in all delay conditions. This finding suggests that the erroneous information was noticed in all conditions, but the system was unable to react during the fixation where the change occurred under the latter two delay conditions. In

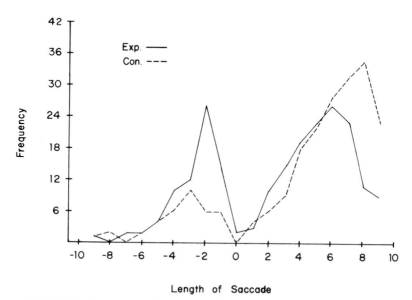

FIGURE 3.4. *Frequency distribution of saccade (S1) for the 50-msec delay condition.*

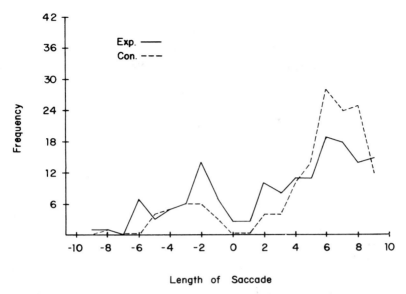

**FIGURE 3.5.** *Frequency distribution of saccade (S1) for the 100-msec delay condition.*

the 150 and 200 msec mask onset conditions, the manipulation did not affect the current fixation or subsequent saccade because the decision of when and where to move the eyes has already been made. However, the new information was noticed and had its effect on the subsequent fixation. We conclude from these results that visual information is noticed throughout the fixation, but that a critical point of movement decision is made around 140 msec prior to the onset of the fixation.

## IV. Is Information Extracted after the Next Movement Has Been Programmed?

The ability to make display changes during fixations dependent upon the precise location of the eyes has led to some intriguing research. In Wolverton's study (1979) an interesting case resulted with the 200-msec mask-on set condition. The data collected under this condition reveal some interesting facts. First, and foremost, the display change occurred too late in the fixation to influence the current fixation (F0) or the subsequent saccade (S1). The disruption caused no effect until the following fixation (F1) which was greatly inflated by the 30-msec mask. In the follow-up study where a mask that lasted until the end of the current fixation (F0) was used, a similar result was observed. Mask presentation time (MPT) is defined as the time from the onset of the mask until the beginning of the following saccade (S1). When the mask presentation time (MPT) was 30 msec or less, only a small elevation in the following fixation (F1) was observed. When the MPT was from 30 to 140, then the following fixation (F1) was significantly inflated (approximately 80 msec). However, when the MPT was greater than 140 msec, only a slight increase in the following fixation (F1) was noted whereas the fixation where the change occurred (F0) was increased. These preliminary results suggest that new information presented late in the fixation (in those cases where the MPT was less than around 150 msec) is noticed but is reflected in the subsequent fixation (F1). Apparently, if the fixation is scheduled for a time sufficient to allow the MPT to be greater than 150 msec, then the influence of the new information is reflected in the current fixation (F0) rather than in the following fixation (F1). In fact, this result was also observed when combining all masking conditions (i.e., 50, 100, 150, and 200 msec).

In a recent pilot study, we used a technique in which a selected word in a line of text is presented for 200 msec. When that word is fixated, an alternative word that differs by only one letter and is syntactically and semantically compatible replaces the original word for the remainder of the fixation. The data indicate that the subject can identify both words in those cases where the alternative word was present for at least 80 msec. This finding suggests that information is extracted late in the fixation (presumably after the movement has been programmed). In most cases the current fixation (F0) and subsequent saccade (S1) are unaffected by this manipulation. The effect is seen in the following fixation (F1). However, there are many instances when the manipulation influences the current fixation (F0). Our data suggest that the decision of when to move the eyes, in most cases, has been made around 140 msec prior to the beginning of the saccade.

## V.  Is Information Extracted within the Initial Portion of the Fixation?

Wolverton (1979) has demonstrated that information present during the first 30 msec of a fixation has an influence on the extraction of information. Other recent data (Rayner et al., 1981) also suggests that the perception of stimulus information is not attenuated or inhibited immediately following a saccade. However, it is rather specious to argue that all necessary and sufficient information is extracted during this period. The metaphor that reading involves discrete periods of information extraction followed by "deadtime" when the visual stimulus is no longer given attention (e.g., Abrams & Zuber, 1972) does not agree with our observations. The reading process, we believe, deals with simultaneous processing. For example, the language processing system furnishes the oculomotor system with a command to move the eyes as it is engaged in semantic and syntactic analysis of the text portion being read. Thus, information is being extracted during the initial portion of the fixation. Furthermore, our observations suggest that information is noticed until just before the onset of the following saccade, and is not limited to the initial portion of the fixation or any specific period in between.

## VI.  Is the Information That Is Extracted on the Current Fixation Immediately Influencing Language Processing?

We want to make two important points regarding this issue. First, during the past several years, eye movement researchers (e.g., Just & Carpenter, 1980; McConkie & Zola, 1979; Rayner, 1975, 1978) have found that text manipulations have an immediate influence on language processing that is reflected in the eye movement data. As we have recently found when new information becomes available it always has some influence. However, if the saccade has already been programmed and insufficient time remains for reprogramming the saccade (approximately 140 msec) then the influence will be evident later.

Second, the question of the immediate influence upon high order language processes is less clear. Introspections about regressions would imply a disruption in higher order processes (e.g., syntactic, semantic). For example, if an ambiguous word is present in the text regressive eye movements from the disambiguating word to the ambiguous word are often seen (Carpenter & Daneman, 1981). These data do not indicate whether the regressions occurred immediately upon encountering the disambiguating word, but if they occurred immediately after this would provide strong support for the notion that information obtained on the current fixation can immediately influence higher order processes. Some of our recent pilot research, involving removing the text during selected fixations, has convinced us that higher order processes continue after removal of the text. In this study, subjects were able to report several words beyond the fixated word when the text was removed. We are convinced that higher order processes lag behind the actual extraction of the visual information due to transmission delays and finite processing times.

## VII.  Do Display Changes during Fixations Cause Disruptions?

In our research we recognize it is possible that display changes during fixations themselves might cause differences in eye movement patterns. Comparisons between data for fixations where no display change occurred and corresponding data for fixations in which the display change consisted of replacing the original line by an identical line showed no differences. This was taken as evidence that the display changes along are not disruptive.

## VIII.  Conclusion

We have dealt with some of the issues involving the temporal characteristics of information extraction during reading. To conceptualize the reading system as involving (*a*) the discrete periods of extraction of visual information; (*b*) periods of language processing; and (c) periods of oculomotor computational processes, portrays a system that is continually waiting for lower order subprocesses to complete a task before a higher order process can start and vice versa. Such a system would be very inefficient. We propose that reading be considered a series of simultaneous integrated processes where information becomes available and is used by the respective processes. Information is noticed throughout fixations and is not restricted to a limited time span. Movement decisions are made contingent upon requirements of several ongoing processes.

# References

Abrams, S. G., & Zuber, B. L. (1972). Some temporal characteristics of information processing during reading. *Reading Research Quarterly, 8*, 46–51.

Brown, R. (1970). Psychology and reading: Commentary on chapters 5 to 10. In H. Levin and J. P. Williams (Eds.), *Basic studies on reading*. New York: Basic Books, Pp. 164–187.

Carpenter, P. A., & Daneman, M. (1981). Lexical retrieval and error recovery in reading: A model based on eye fixations. *Journal of Verbal Learning and Verbal Behavior, 20*, 137–160.

Geyer, J. J. (1970). Models of perceptual processes in reading. In H. Singer and R. B. Ruddell (Eds.), *Theoretical models and processes of reading*. Newark, Deleware: International Reading Association, Pp. 47–94.

Gough, P. B. (1972). One second of reading. In J. F. Kavanagh and I. G. Mattingly (Eds.), *Language by ear and by eye: The relationships between speech and reading*. Cambridge, Massachusetts: M.I.T. Press, Pp. 331–358.

Haber, R. N., & Hershenson, M. (1973). *The psychology of visual perception*. New York: Holt, Rinehart and Winston.

Just, M. A., & Carpenter, P. A. (1980). A theory of reading: From eye fixations to comprehension. *Psychological Review, 4*, 329–354.

Latour, P. (1962). Visual threshold during eye movements. *Vision Research, 2*, 261–262.

McConkie, G. W., & Zola, D. (1979). Is visual information integrated across successive fixations in reading? *Perception & Psychophysics, 25*, 221–224.

McConkie, G. W., Zola, D., Wolverton, G. S., & Burns, D. D. (1978). Eye movement contingent display control in studying reading. *Behavior Research Methods & Instrumentation, 10*, 154–166.

Rayner, K. (1975). The perceptual span and peripheral cues in reading. *Cognitive Psychology, 7*, 68–81.

Rayner, K. (1978). Eye movements in reading and information processing. *Psychological Bulletin, 85*, 618–660.

Rayner, K., & Bertera, J. H. (1979). Reading without a fovea. *Science, 206*, 468–469.

Rayner, K., Inhoff, A. W., Morrison, R. E., Slowiaczek, M. L., & Bertera, J. H. (1981). Masking of foveal and parafoveal vision during eye fixations in reading. *Journal of Experimental Psychology: Human Perception and Performance, 7*, 167–179.

Rayner, K., & McConkie, G. W. (1976). What guides a reader's eye movements? *Vision Research, 16*, 829–837.

Rayner, K., McConkie, G. W., & Zola, D. (1980). Integrating information across eye movements. *Cognitive Psychology, 12*, 206–226.

Rayner, K., Well, A. D., & Pollatsek, A. (1980). Asymmetry of the effective visual field in reading. *Perception & Psychophysics, 27*, 537–544.

Smith, F. (1971). *Understanding reading: A psycholinguistic analysis of reading and learning to read*. New York: Holt, Rinehart and Winston.

Sperling, G. (1960). The information available in brief visual presentations. *Psychological Monographs, 74,* (11).

Volkmann, F. C. (1962). Vision during voluntary saccadic eye movements. *Journal of the Optical Society of America, 1962, 52,* 571–578.

Volkmann, F. C. (1976). Saccadic suppression: A brief review. In R. A. Monty & J. W. Senders (Eds.), *Eye movements and psychological processes.* Hillsdale, New Jersey: Erlbaum, Pp. 73–83.

Volkmann, F. C., Schick, A. M. L., & Riggs, L. A. (1968). Time course of visual inhibition during voluntary saccades. *Journal of the Optical Society of America, 58,* 562–569.

Wolverton, G. S. (1979). *The acquisition of visual information during fixations and saccades in reading.* Paper presented at the annual meeting of the American Educational Research Association in San Francisco, California, April (ERIC Document Reproduction Service No. ED 178 861).

# 4

# Locations and Contents[1]

## I.  Introduction

In the three chapters of Part I. Bruno Breitmeyer tries to establish a neu-rophysiological basis for aspects of eye movement and form perception relevant to reading, Robert Morrison examines the relation between size of display and span of fixation, and Gary Wolverton and David Zola discuss some issues regarding control of fixations and information acquired during them. A melange, indeed, but with correlated components.

## II.  Two Views of Performance

Breitmeyer's tutorial review surveys neurophysiological and psychophysical data to support a theory of perception. The theory proposes that the interaction of transient and sustained detectors performs the greatest part of visual work. The theory is both broad and bold; indeed, reading the papers of the bibliography would by itself provide a distinct education in the psychology and neurophysiology of visual perception. I find the claim to be a little too bold, and the coverage a little too broad to be persuasive, however. I will discuss three aspects of his proposal, relating to neurophysiology, behavior, and the structure of theory.

[1]Preparation of this chapter was aided by Grant A7655 from National Science and Engineering Research Council Canada.

*EYE MOVEMENTS IN READING:*
*PERCEPTUAL AND LANGUAGE PROCESSES*

## A.   Sustained and Transient Cells

What is the sustained–transient contrast? About 30 years ago, Kuffler (1953) identified some kinds of neural organization in the ganglion cells of cat retina. The early electrophysiological tradition that culminated in Kuffler's discoveries had identified types of responses that were called on, off, and on–off: responses to the onset or termination of stimulation, and responses that were maintained during the course of stimulation (Ratliff, 1974). Kuffler showed that these were aspects of organizations such as on-center, off-surround, off-center, and so on. More recently the typology has been refined into a contrast among $X$, $Y$, and sometimes $W$ cells, and their various properties have been explored in detail (Rodieck, 1979).

Two points must be made regarding categorization of cells. One is that the various types of mammalian visual cell are identified principally in terms of their conduction velocity, although sometimes fiber diameter and sometimes cell reactivity are also invoked. That is, the classifications have not been carried out on the basis of visual functions but on the basis of electrical responses, and the latter are at best only loosely identified with the former. Indeed, Rodieck (1979, p. 198) remarks that at present only "vague hints" about function exist even though the claim that "$X$ is for pattern, $Y$ for movement" is very popular. In a word, the functional visual role of the various organizations has still to be worked out. Moreover, it would be erroneous to think that there are only two or three types of cells, for not only are there sustained and transient or $X$ and $Y$ types, Rodieck's (1979) classification identifies at least 12 different types of cell.

A second point is that the greatest part of the research that has been used to identify and classify visual neural organization has been carried out on the cat, a lesser amount on rodents, and still less on monkeys. A great deal of information about the organization of the mammalian retina and its visual pathways has been obtained from this work, as is widely known. It is important to remember, however, that activity shapes structure in the nervous system (Gaze, Keating, Szekeley & Beazley, 1970; Greenough, 1975); and visual organization in these animals differs in important ways not only from that of humans, but among the animals themselves even within species. A well known example is the Siamese cat, whose congenitally crossed eyes lead in time to a different cortical elaboration of visual pathways from that found among other cats (Antonini, Berlucchi, Marzi, & Sprague, 1979). Moreover, the cat's retina contains mainly rods and, in this respect, is very different from the human retina, where the foveal cones are thought to do most of the detailed analysis that reading requires. Indeed, not only do cats not read, they do not even discriminate among forms well nor respond to color in an easily detectable way (Crocker, Ringo, Wolbarsht, & Wagner, 1980).

Psychologists and neurophysiologists have demonstrated repeatedly during the last 25 years that visual exercise is required to maintain normal function, and that visual skills develop out of such exercise (Barlow, 1975; Freeman, 1979; Held & Hein, 1967; Wiesel & Hubel, 1965). It is a plausible conjecture, therefore, that the activity of reading shapes the development of the visual nervous system in literate humans. If true, this claim would set additional limits on the applicability of the analysis of infrahuman visual systems to human function and constitute an occasion for discovery of specialized functions in humans.

## B.   Psychophysical Considerations

Breitmeyer raises a number of points that are interesting to students of cognitive aspects of visual perception. Particularly useful is the effort to declassify the icon from the privileged and important role to which it was assigned in Neisser's (1967) account of acquisition of visual information. There, as in Sperling's (1960) report, the icon was said to be some first detailed mapping of the visual scene onto the retina, from which a language operator saved significant parts by naming them and storing the names away. Breitmeyer instead divides the visual response into two components, high frequency and low frequency, the second associated with motion or location of stimulation (the *on* and *off* cells of the earlier workers), and the first associated with the perception of form (the sustained or *on–off* cells). I will mention a few consequences of rapid presentation of stimuli and comment on a related phenomenon, backward masking, and the issue of "spatiotopic" rather than retinotopic representation.

### 1.   ICONS

Breitmeyer presents an interesting account of the way that the interaction of sustained and transient detectors might serve to limit the problem that long lasting icons would create for perception. As in the proposal of Matin, Clymer, and Matin (1972), masking is put forward as the chief means by which this is accomplished. I believe that the mechanisms, however ingeniously proposed, are too simple for the job, and I will try to show this by appealing to two facts.

In one study (Kolers & Katzman, 1966) letters were presented on the same part of a viewing screen at various rapid rates. The finding was that their correct report increased with a decrease in rate, as might be expected, but that sometimes people got the identity of the letters right and confused their order, or they got the order approximately right and misidentified one or more of the letters. These confusions of order and identity occurred at just about the temporal conditions that characterize the masking effects of interest to Breitmeyer's theory. In a second study using the same general technique (Kolers & Lewis, 1972) it was found that people could *detect* one or a pair of letters in sequence far more accurately than they could *identify* the target and accompanying letters. Since limitations on memory span were not at issue, interaction among sustained and transient cells must provide an account, on Brietmeyer's theory, of the difference between recognition and recall. These two conditions—order of stimulation and the difference between detecting and reporting—yield results that seem to me to be beyond the reach of the theory based on two interacting detectors.

## 2. MASKING

The theory moreover provides a contrast only of the broadest kind, but says nothing about locations or distances of the stimuli presented, their shapes, or other properties. Whether a target can be inhibited by a masking form depends upon the distance separating their borders; the nature of their interaction—whether U-shaped or monotonic—is also so affected (Kolers, 1962). Nothing about distances is apparent in the theory, however. One improvement Breitmeyer has made to the earlier proposal of Breitmeyer and Ganz (1976) accommodates the fact that the two stimuli of a masking experiment actually mask each other (Kolers & Rosner, 1960); but I find there is still no sensitivity in his proposal to the fact that flashes of light to the dark adapted eye and flashes of dark to the light adapted eye do not yield equivalent behavioral or psychophysical results.

Rodieck (1979) points out that two of the 12 retinal organizations that have been identified involve sensitivity to contrast. Perhaps expanding the sustained–transient dichotomy along those lines would be useful. Further expansion might also include chromatic characteristics of the stimuli, for in backward masking experiments the color of the two shapes is important in establishing whether one finds U-shaped or monotonic effects. Shape of the stimuli must also be specified, for their actual geometry is crucial in establishing the nature and extent of their interaction (Werner, 1935). In sum, a collection of fairly basic properties of the stimuli—color, shape, contrast, spatial location, and temporal order—along with whether they are detected or named, seem to be outside the reach of the theory. As I said at the outset, the theory seems to be trying to do too much with too little. A final point along these lines is that forms of backward masking have been found using only semantic relations of target and mask (Jacobson, 1974). With all other important variables controlled, linguistic features of the mask help to establish how much it inhibits perception of a target word.

## 2. TEMPORAL INTEGRATION

Does the visual system have to recompute its world every time the eye moves? Breitmeyer proposes a negative response to this question, asserting the existence of a cross-saccadic buffer or store that maintains object constancy despite movements of the eyes. Part of the argument for this claim involves visual completion experiments where different scenes are flashed in quick succession (illustrated in Breitmeyer's Figure 1.6, Chapter 1 of this volume). The finding important to the argument is that increasing the duration of the first flash in a sequence of two flashes that are separated by a brief interstimulus interval actually decreases persistence (the "icon"). Breitmeyer reviews the work of people claiming this, and I do not question the findings. Rather, I point out that another visual phenomenon whose temporal characteristics are quite similar to those of backward masking actually works oppositely.

The phenomenon is called apparent motion and occurs when two stimuli are presented briefly in sequence in neighboring locations. People see them in movement, a single shape moving between the physical locations of the stimuli. The point of interest is that this is a phenomenon of instability, and the finding is that the greater the duration of the first flash, the greater the likelihood that a movement relation will occur (Kolers, 1964). Hence, "persistence" may be construed as of little significance in discussing the development of form perception, perhaps even irrelevant to the discussion. In apparent motion, increasing the stimulus in a way that decreases its persistence and that might be thought to increase its stability actually increases the likelihood that it will seem to transform. Perhaps the increased duration increases the low frequency (motion detecting) component; but if that is the case here, the result should be the same in the completion experiments. The fact remains that the visible world is stable despite our eye movements, but I find it increasingly difficult to believe that the interaction of sustained and transient cells by themselves creates that stability and so much more for us.

Finally, Brietmeyer proposes that visual locations are coded not in terms of retinal but in terms of phenomenal space—spatiotopic rather than retinotopic representations. The problems of visual direction and spatial localization have been discussed for more than 100 years and seem to be immensely complicated. The modern work begins with Lotze's (1886) claim that the retina is coded with respect to local signs; that is, the retina signals to the brain in absolute terms the retinal location of stimulation. More recent developments have shown that however useful parts of that claim might be, the claim as a whole is excessive (Matin, 1972); indeed, very often the visual system knows where the eye is looking only by virtue of what it is looking at.

Breitmeyer supports the claim that the visual system codes for space, not for retinal location, and adds that successive samples are established in this context. I think this must be right, because successive fixations on a scene do not give us a perception that is organized according to the temporal order of the samples, but give us a scene ordered according to their spatial locations (Kolers, 1976b). Whether the actual order of the samples also is represented in the perceptual outcome of sampling remains to be determined; certainly that claim was implicit in the Noton and Stark (1971) account, although it was not well supported there. Breitmeyer proposes a device to account for the perceptual facts, again in terms of two conponents. I am not sure, whether his account is sufficiently sensitive to the difference between spatial and substantive information, or whether the two run together.

## C.  Aspects of Theory

The notion that Breitmeyer seems to have in mind is that an account in terms of neurophysiology is somehow more informative than an account in terms of behavioral or symbolic variables. How one does science is, of course, largely a matter of taste and interest, but it is easy to show that different descriptions of phenomena, undertaken from the view of different scientific disciplines, do not necessarily map into each other. There is little reason to believe that all of perception psychology can be reduced to neurophysiology or biology any more than there is reason to think that any unformalized universe of discourse can be reduced to another. Neurophysiological descriptors have their reality, and psychological descriptors have theirs.

The sustained–transient dichotomy translates almost too readily, as Rodieck (1979) remarked, into the behavioral correlates of *what* and *where*, of content and location. With respect to form perception at the gross cross-species level that includes cat, monkey, and human, this is a substantial start even though limited: In motion perception, for example, difference in species can make for some substantial differences in behavior (Gruesser & Gruesser–Cornehls, 1973). When we consider a subject as complex, subtle, and elaborate as reading is, I should think that two other contrasts might dominate research: the interpretative functions defined as *how* and *why*. I am solidly among those who believe that the pattern one is analyzing is important to the analysis carried out (Kolers, 1976a), and in this respect vouch for and support Breitmeyer's claim that form perception is important to literacy. But literacy is more than perception of form and location, and its understanding requires that we know something as well about the manipulation of symbols, especially linguistic symbols. Indeed, syntax is not even always visible in the visual display of English; and when it comes to semantic processing, reading surely makes appeal to features that the reader brings to rather than takes from the display.

Breitmeyer tells us of the importance of purpose and adaptation in understanding visual processes. One can only agree and hope that those features, and some of the others mentioned that contribute to the performance of skilled reading, will be taken into consideration in future accounts.

## III.   Skills and Glances

The role of knowledge and skill in shaping performance can be inferred in part from the fixations that people make. As is well known, Tinker (1963) surveyed a large amount of the available literature on the legibility of print; he used the span of apprehension and eye movements to measure the effects of different typographies on reading. Morrison refers to some of that literature and argues that the fixation span is constant over a range of type sizes. He concludes that number of characters per span is probably a better metric than visual angle; if he is right, the metric could provide a reliable base for comparative measurement.

Other factors that interested Tinker also affect performance; the one that interests me most is skill. It is well known that saccadic interval increases with skill in reading (Kolers, 1976b). I should think it might be interesting to study the performance of people reading texts in familiar or unfamiliar typographies. Presumably, amount of text processed per fixation would vary with changes of typography. Many other aspects of skill also modulate performance. One wonders what metric the visual system uses to establish the size of the input that is then found to hold constant across changes in size of type.

## IV.   Segments and Inferences

Two classical issues in the study of perception come together in the study of reading. First, what segments the continuous stimulus flux into discrete perceptible objects? The second is, what is the nature of the control system for eye movements? The two come together in that eye movements have sometimes been proposed as one of the segmenting devices for perception: Wolverton and Zola take a particular position on that and related issues. Their chief claim is that the eye receives stimulation continuously during a fixation. Hence, they argue for a parallel processing model in which the visual system is thought to do simultaneously many things related to acquisition, transformation, and interpretation of visual signals. Information regarding location of a word, its length, its part of speech, its interpretation are run off together, on this view, but at different rates. Movement of the eye itself may then play a role in segmenting or organizing the visual scene.

One must quibble regarding their claim that they find no diminution in sensitivity as a function of an eye's movement. Since the effect of movement on threshold of visibility is not very great in the first place—Volkmann, Schick, and Riggs (1962) measured it at about one-half a log unit, or a factor of only about seven times in luminance—the special procedures of the experiment by Wolverton and Zola may have been inadequate to detect the effect. The postsaccadic influence on perception that Breitmeyer discusses may equally have been missed. In this respect the fact that the details of Wolverton and Zola's experiments are not publicly available for study makes their report less persuasive than it might otherwise be. Moreover, belief that the eye's movement itself acts as a segregator of visible events into objects implicates a particular notion of control of eye motions to which Wolverton and Zola may not actually want to subscribe.

The key question regarding eye movements is whether they are tightly controlled, as McConkie (1979) especially has affirmed, or whether they are loosely controlled, as Kolers (1976b) among others has proposed. The notion of tight control is that each fixation is the sufficient stimulus for computing its content and determining the place the eye is to move next. On this view the eye must acquire immediately intelligible information from each fixation. The fact that the eye regresses sometimes, sometimes skips ahead, sometimes leaves the page altogether, must constitute something of a difficulty for such a view of tight control, for the consequence of the movements would be unintelligible word salads.

The alternative notion of loose control supposes that mind does the intelligent organizing of inputs, the record keeping and place noting, the interpreting and, even, the thinking that sometimes accompanies reading. On this view the eye's job is largely logistic, to acquire the information from the scene, but not necessarily in the order it is on the page. Mind has the capability of ordering misordered inputs, whether they be geometric misorientations of text or temporal misorderings (Kolers & Perkins, 1975). Wolverton and Zola claim that the visual system can compute on the basis of the first 50-msec sample how long to stay where it is and where to go next, but needs at least 140 msec to carry out the actual computation. If they are right, both the notions of loose and of tight control as stated need some refining.

But perhaps nothing needs refining as much as the notion of "information." We all use the term very loosely, discussing the information in the display or the information processing the reader engages in; but lacking is any thought-out description of what the term means, or even what it could mean. It has been taken over a little too readily from the information sciences, but lacks the precision of definition it usually acquires there. One might even ask whether the term has a definition independent of the processing that people engage in.

# References

Antonini, A., Berlucchi, G., Marzi, C. A., & Sprague, J. M. (1979). Behavioral and electrophysiologi-
    cal effects of unilateral optic tract section in ordinary and Siamese cats. *Journal of Comparative
    Neurology, 185,* 183–202.
Barlow, H. B. (1975). Visual experience and cortical development. *Nature, 258,* 199–204.
Breitmeyer, B. G., & Ganz, L. (1976). Implications of sustained and transient channels for theories of
    visual pattern masking, saccadic suppression, and information processing. *Psychological Review,
    53,* 1–36.
Crocker, R. A., Ringo, J., Wolbarsht, M. L., & Wagner, H. G. (1980). Cone contributions to cat
    retinal ganglion receptive fields. *Journal of General Physiology, 76,* 763–785.
Freeman, R. D. (Ed.). (1979). *Developmental neurobiology of vision.* New York: Plenum Press.
Gaze, R. M., Keating, M. J., Szekeley, G., & Beazley, L. (1970). Binocular interaction in the
    formation of specific intertectal neuronal connexions. *Proceedings of the Royal Society (London),
    175B,* 107–147.
Greenough, W. T. (1975). Experiential modification of the developing brain. *American Scientist, 63,*
    37–46.
Gruesser, O. J., & Gruesser–Cornehls, U. (1973). Neuronal mechanisms of visual movement percep-
    tion and some psychophysical and behavioral correlations. In R. Jung (Ed.), *Handbook of sensory
    physiology* (Vol. 7, No. 3A: *Central processing of visual information*). Berlin: Springer–Verlag.
Held, R., & Hein, A. (1967). On the modifiability of form perception. In W. Wathen–Dunn (Ed.),
    *Models for the perception of speech and visual form.* Cambridge, Massachusetts: MIT Press.
Jacobson, J. Z. (1974). Interaction of similarity to words of visual masking and targets. *Journal of
    Experimental Psychology, 102,* 431–434.
Kolers, P. A. (1962). Intensity and contour effects in visual masking. *Vision Research, 2,* 277–294.
Kolers, P. A. (1964). The illusion of movement. *Scientific American, 211* (4), 98–106.
Kolers, P. A. (1976). Reading a year later. *Journal of Experimental Psychology: Human Learning and
    Memory, 2,* 554–565. (a)
Kolers, P. A. (1976). Buswell's discoveries. In R. A. Monty & J. W. Senders (Eds.), *Eye movements and
    psychological processes.* Hillsdale, N.J.: Erlbaum, 1976. (b)
Kolers, P. A., & Katzman, M. T. (1966). Naming sequentially presented letters and words. *Language
    and Speech, 9,* 84–95.
Kolers, P. A., & Lewis, C. L. (1972). Bounding of letter sequences and the integration of visually
    presented words. *Acta Psychologica, 36,* 112–124.

Kolers, P. A., & Perkins, D. N. (1975). Spatial and ordinal components of form perception and literacy. *Cognitive Psychology, 7,* 228–267.

Kolers, P. A., & Rosner, B. S. (1960). On visual masking (metacontrast): dichoptic observation. *American Journal of Psychology, 73,* 2–21.

Kuffler, S. (1953). Discharge patterns and functional organization of mammalian retina. *Journal of Neurophysiology, 16,* 37–68.

Lotze, H. (1886). *Outline of psychology.* G. T. Ladd (Ed. and trans.). Boston: Ginn.

Matin, E., Clymer, A. B., & Matin, L. (1972). Metacontrast and saccadic suppression. *Science, 178,* 179–182.

Matin, L. (1972). Eye movements and perceived visual direction. In D. Jameson & L. M. Hurvich (Eds.), *Handbook of sensory physiology* (Vol. 7, No. 4: *Visual psychophysics*). Berlin: Springer–Verlag.

McConkie, G. W. (1979). On the role and control of eye movements in reading. In P. A. Kolers, M. E. Wrolstad, & H. Bouma (Eds.), *Processing of visible language 1.* New York: Plenum Press.

Neisser, U. (1967). *Cognitive psychology.* New York: Appleton–Century–Crofts.

Noton, D., & Stark, L. (1971). Eye movements and visual perception. *Scientific American, 224,* (6), 34–43.

Ratliff, F. (Ed.). (1974). *Studies on excitation and inhibition in the retina.* New York: Rockefeller University Press.

Rodieck, R. W. (1979). Visual pathways. *Annual Review of Neurosciences, 2,* 193–204.

Sperling, G. (1960). The information available in brief visual presentations. *Psychological Monographs, 74,* (11, Whole No. 498).

Tinker, M. A. (1963). *Legibility of print.* Ames: University of Iowa Press.

Volkmann, F. C., Schick, A. M. L., & Riggs, L. A. (1962). Time course of visual inhibition during voluntary saccades. *Journal of the Optical Society of America, 58,* 362–369.

Werner, H. (1935). Studies on contour: I. Qualitative analyses. *American Journal of Psychology, 47,* 40–64.

Wiesel, T. N., & Hubel, D. H. (1965). Comparison of the effects of unilateral and bilateral eye closure on cortical unit responses in kittens. *Journal of Neurophysiology, 28,* 1029–1040.

# II
# Eye Movements and Perceptual Processes

George W. McConkie

# 5

# Eye Movements and Perception during Reading[1]

## I.  Introduction

The purpose of this chapter is to review some of the issues about perception during reading that have been raised in studies involving eye movement recording, to try to put these issues in perspective, and to evaluate our present knowledge where appropriate. First, however, it is important to recognize that the range of activities that can be called *reading* is very broad, and that the perceptual activities involved in such different tasks are likely to be different enough to lead us astray if we assume that what is occurring during one task is necessarily the same as what is occurring during another (Hochberg, 1976). This chapter will consider the perceptual processes involved in the fairly careful reading of continuous text for the purpose of comprehending and remembering its message.

Since it has been difficult to study the perceptual processes involved in this type of reading, which I will refer to as *careful reading,* most investigations have used other types in which greater information can be obtained about details of the processes involved. This continually raises the question of generality of findings. Are the perceptual processes involved in the task used in a particular experiment similar enough to those involved in careful reading that the results should be accepted as constraining theories of this type of reading?

This issue is of particular concern when dealing with the hundreds of studies employing tachistoscopic presentation. These studies were motivated by a need to

[1]This chapter was prepared with support from Grant MH 32884 from the National Institute of Mental Health to the author, and Contract US-NIE-400-76-0117 from the National Institute of Education to the Center for the Study of Reading.

EYE MOVEMENTS IN READING:
PERCEPTUAL AND LANGUAGE PROCESSES

gain the type of experimental control necessary to investigate perceptual processes in detail. A tachistoscopic presentation was taken as being similar to a single fixation during reading; hence, findings from such studies were assumed to generalize to fixations during reading (Huey, 1908).

There is one way in which a tachistoscopic presentation and a fixation during reading are similar; in both, the visual system is exposed to a relatively stable retinal pattern for a brief period of time. Given our recent history of theoretical behaviorism (as opposed to methodological behaviorism which we still largely abide by), it is understandable that there would be a bias to believe that similar stimulus patterns might evoke similar perceptual processes. However, the growth of cognitive approaches to theorizing has been stimulated by the recognition that, in fact, this is not necessarily true. The organism often processes the same information in different ways, depending on the task being performed.

Even a cursory comparison of a fixation in reading and a tachistoscopic exposure shows significant differences, some inherent in the nature of the tasks appropriately associated with the two types of text presentation, and some more associated with the nature of the stimuli typically used. They typically differ in the complexity of the stimulus pattern (which Bouma, 1978, has demonstrated has substantial effects on perceptibility), in the end toward which the information obtained is used (reporting words and letters or making semantic judgments versus extending one's representation of a message being communicated), in the momentary context within which the exposure is set (having time to become set for a brief exposure and prepared to do identification versus being only a momentary part of a flow of skilled behavior supported by a series of such brief exposures to the text), and in the types of language variables involved (exposure to only one or a few words precludes the influence of most of the language factors involved in normal text).

It seems reasonable for these types of differences to produce substantial differences in the nature of the perceptual processes employed in these two reading tasks. The state of the organism is certainly different at the onset of the exposure to the text, and the nature of the mental activities being carried out during the exposure and the time following must be quite different. To the extent that perceptual processes, especially those involved in selectively attending to available information, are in the service of the mental processes engaged to carry out the task at hand, we would expect quite different activities to result from these situations.

Additional difficulties for generalization are seen when we consider what typically serves as data in studies employing these two different reading tasks and the ways in which those data are analyzed and interpreted. The complexity of the data can be much greater in the careful reading task; in fact, its potential complexity is one force that drives researchers to adopt simpler tasks. Added complexity does not necessarily just add new factors to an additive model; it frequently changes the relation among factors already entered. One reason why the phenomenon of lateral masking has been of such interest is because it produces data patterns different from those expected from simpler displays (Bouma, 1973, points out that letters further into the visual periphery can frequently be identified more readily than letters closer to the fovea.) Introducing a saccadic eye movement into a task changes the degree to which stimulus information at different retinal locations influences performance on the task, due to associated attentional processes (Rayner, McConkie, & Ehrlich, 1978; Remington, 1980). Also, concepts that are useful in accounting for data in the tachistoscopic task, and which are then generalized to discussions of reading, can lead us astray in our theorizing. The usefulness of the concept of the icon for an understanding of careful reading has been challenged (R. N. Haber, 1983) and the notion of a "word superiority effect" seems irrelevant. In studies of reading, the effects of nonwords are not taken as a baseline against which to judge the superiority of words; rather they are taken as indications of the difficulties produced when a letter string does not map nicely onto a known word. These two concepts have, of course, been central to the study of perception from tachistoscopic presentations.

My purpose here is not to argue against conducting research on certain types of reading tasks. All aspects of reading need investigation, and it is often the case that since there is no way to investigate some aspect of the reading processes in one type of task another must be employed. Rather, I wish to emphasize two points. First, we need to take more care to recognize the diversity of tasks involving reading and the differences in perceptual processes that may be involved, thus being more careful not to overgeneralize, than has often been the case in the past. Second, at the same time, we need to be more creative in finding ways of directly studying the types of reading we wish most to understand. In fact, this is one of the primary contributions that recent eye movement research has made to the field of reading. It has provided the means of investigating many perceptual issues by studying people directly engaged in the task of careful reading. It is this literature that is the primary focus of this review.

The issues to be dealt with mainly fall into three areas. First there is a discussion of the control of eye movements, since this determines what visual information will be available to the reader, in what sequence and for how long; second, there is a discussion of perception during a fixation in reading; and third, a discussion of what is involved in maintaining perception across fixations. In each of these, the focus will be on understanding relatively skilled reading, with comments on the development of reading or on reading disabilities where appropriate.

Since there have been two excellent reviews of eye movement studies recently, this review will not try to exhaustively cover the earlier literature (Levy–Schoen & O'Regan, 1979; Rayner, 1978a).

## II.   Control of Eye Movements

During continuous reading and most other real-world visual tasks, the eyes are free to move and they do so at a rapid rate. Where they go and how long they stay at each location is considered to be part of the perceptual process since this determines the degree of clarity of different parts of the display at any given time.

For the present discussion, eye guidance will be considered to involve two factors: a decision of when to launch the eyes to the next location, which will be referred to as the *temporal decision,* and a decision of where the eyes will be sent, which will be referred to as the *spatial decision.* The temporal decision determines the duration of the fixation, and the spatial decision determines the length of the saccade and the location of the next fixation. Other aspects of eye movement will not be considered here.

It is well established that the variability observed in these two aspects of eye behavior is not simply due to error, noise, or inaccuracy; to some extent (and the degree is a matter of dispute) both aspects of eye behavior reflect moment by moment brain state changes induced by interaction of the stimulus pattern and the task of comprehending. Before turning to a discussion of the nature of the control in these decisions, it is important to review timing considerations of when these decisions are made.

## A.  Timing of Decisions Regarding Eye Behavior

McConkie and Underwood (1981) have provided an analysis of the timing of the decisions regarding eye behavior which will be briefly summarized here and which is presented in Figure 5.1. This figure represents a fixation of approximately median duration, 220 msec. Above the line, the times of observable events during the fixation are noted: the termination of one saccade, the onset of the next

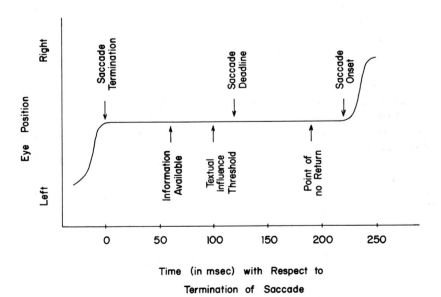

FIGURE 5.1. *Some critical times during the period of a fixation in reading. The line represents relative eye position as in a temporally based eye movement record. [From McConkie and Underwood, 1981.]*

saccade, and the point after which stimulus changes have no effect on the time of onset of the following saccade, here called the *saccade deadline*. The saccade deadline occurs about 100 msec prior to the saccade onset. Nonobservable (by nonneurological means) events are indicated below the line in the figure. The first of these, the time at which the visual information from a new fixation becomes available to the visual centers of the brain, is estimated at 60 msec after the onset of the fixation. The second, the *point of no return*, is the time at which the brain centers actually become committed to the time of onset of the next saccade. This is estimated at 30 msec prior to the saccade onset. Both of these estimates come from the physiological data reviewed by Russo (1978).

One final estimate is of the earliest point at which stable textual information (as opposed to stimulus changes) can influence the present fixation duration. This is estimated at 140 msec, or 40 msec longer than the saccade deadline (McConkie & Underwood, 1981). Thus, it is assumed that language aspects of the text must begin having their influence on processing within about 100 msec after the onset of the fixation. This is labeled as the *textual influence threshold* in Figure 5.1.

From this figure it is possible to estimate the amount of time elapsing between the textual influence threshold and the point of no return—the time during which processing of the visual stimulus encountered on that fixation can influence the duration of that fixation. This varies, of course, with the duration of the fixation, but for a 220 msec fixation this period is only 90 msec. However, for a fixation of the same length, the stimulus is available to the brain for 120 msec after processing can no longer influence the duration of that fixation (assuming a 30-msec saccade). It seems most unlikely, given this timing pattern, that all processing of information obtained on any given fixation has been completed in time to affect the following saccade, or even that all processing that might be capable of affecting the saccade has been completed. This would result in a 120-msec "dead time" (Russo, 1978) which turns out to be over half of the total time for the median fixation–saccade cycle and would seem to be extremely inefficient.

The inevitable conclusion from these considerations is that, contrary to Just and Carpenter's (1980) eye–mind assumption (see also McConkie, Hogaboam, Wolverton, Zola, & Lucas, 1979), processing of the information available during a fixation is not completed by the end of that fixation, and that the onset of the next fixation is not triggered by a completion of processing of information obtained on the present fixation. It appears that most of the time available for processing the information from most fixations, prior to the arrival of information from the next fixation, actually occurs after it is too late to influence the duration of that fixation or probably the length of the next saccade. A second conclusion is that the durations of the shortest fixations (and probably the lengths of the saccades following them) are not being influenced at all by the information perceived from those fixations. This raises many questions, including what processing is typically completed prior to the point of no return, and what processing event triggers the onset of a saccadic eye movement during reading. Some of these issues will be discussed later.

## B.  Some Issues

Saccadic eye movements in reading are typically grouped into three or four categories. These include forward movements, regressions, return sweeps (Levy–Schoen & O'Regan, 1979), and sometimes "corrective movements," regressions frequently seen immediately following return sweeps (Hartje, 1972). This section will deal primarily with forward movements, to some degree with regressions, and the remaining categories will be largely ignored.

### 1.   HOW TO CONCEPTUALIZE EYE MOVEMENT CONTROL

As indicated earlier, the control of eye movements during reading can be considered to involve *temporal* and *spatial* decisions. There is a variety of ways in which one can conceptualize these decisions. For instance, it is possible that they are both the result of a single decision: The eyes are moved at the time the spatial decision is made.

On the other hand, assuming that a separate temporal decision is made, one can think of it as being either a true timing decision or simply as the mind responding to some processing state. In the first case, the mind is seen as a timing device, attempting to make optimal estimates of how long the eyes should pause at each location. Such timing decisions could, of course, be made early in a fixation or even prior to its onset, anticipating the time that will be required to process the information expected at that location. In the second case, the mind is not perceived as making temporal decisions at all, but rather as acting on an interrupt-driven basis, with eye control events occurring as they are called for in support of the mental task at hand, or by external attention capturing events. By this view, the mind does not decide how long the eyes will be left centered at a given location; rather, the eyes are simply left there until some critical mental event occurs that elicits a saccadic movement.

Likewise, there are different ways of thinking of the nature of the spatial decision. Here a primary distinction is between a push versus a pull view: Does the mind decide to send the eyes a certain distance in a certain direction, or are the eyes drawn to a certain location in the text? Either view can take several forms. In the push view, the eyes might be considered to be sent some general distance (perhaps a standard amount modified by some parameter reflecting local text or processing conditions, as with Koler's, 1976, "kicker" plus gain control) or some distance that has been calculated to be likely to be optimal under present information seeking or hypothesis testing conditions. Once again it would be possible for such a decision to be made early in a fixation, or even prior to it. In the pull view, on the other hand, the eyes are considered to be drawn to a certain location. As examples, during a fixation a reader may attend to different regions at different times, with the eyes being drawn to a text region when the level of visual detail needed to support the identification process is not readily available (McConkie, 1979), or the eyes may be drawn to the centers of words (O'Regan, 1981; Rayner, 1979).

A basic distinction that underlies these different ways of conceptualizing eye movement control is whether these mental activities are thought of as being planfully calculated and executed, or as being interrupt driven, responding to certain critical mental events when they occur. I do not believe that present evidence on eye movement guidance during reading is capable of selecting among most of these alternatives. There are some specific issues on which evidence is accumulating, however, and some of these will be briefly reviewed.

## 2.  RELATION OF TEMPORAL AND SPATIAL DECISIONS

It would have seemed reasonable to find that there was a close relationship between the temporal and spatial decisions, such that when processing difficulties occur reading is slowed both by shortening saccades and by extending the fixation periods, resulting in a respectable autocorrelation between successive fixation durations and between successive saccade lengths, and in correlations between the durations of fixations and the lengths of saccades preceding or following them. This pattern has not been found (Andriessen & deVoogd, 1973; Kliegl, Olson, & Davidson, Chapter 19 of this volume; Rayner & McConkie, 1976). This stands as evidence for independent control of fixation durations and saccade extents, and for individual control of each of these measures from fixation to fixation. Certain relationships can be found (regressions are more likely to occur following longer saccades, Andriessen & deVoogd, 1973, and fixations prior to regressions tend to be shorter than normal (Hawley, Stern, & Chen, 1974; Kliegl *et al.* Chapter 19 of this volume, for instance), but the more global relationships appear to be largely absent. This fact has given encouragement to those who suspect that the variability in eye fixation patterns reflect local cognitive and stimulus pattern effects.

## 3.  GLOBAL, LOCAL, OR IMMEDIATE CONTROL

A second issue around which much controversy has centered has to do with the degree of global, local, and immediate control of eye movements. Global influences are those that operate over entire texts or large segments of texts. The tendency of early eye movement research to use mean eye movement measures as data encouraged a focus on global influences of such factors as age, reading ability, passage difficulty, or reading strategy (Woodworth, 1938). Although these studies showed differences in averaged measures, it is not clear whether they resulted from the setting of general parameters in the eye movement system or from the cumulative effects of hundreds of local decisions. A more recent proposal is that prior to reading (in fact, prior to any visual task) the subject establishes a general scanning routine and that although there may be local adjustments these are simply modifications of, or overrides to, the routine initially established (Levy–Schoen, 1981).

The demonstration of local influences on eye movement control has been a primary contribution of the recent wave of eye movement research in the study of reading. Some examples are provided in Table 5.1. Both the durations of fixations and the lengths of saccades have been shown to vary with local stimulus and information processing characteristics. However, this has raised the further issue

### TABLE 5.1
#### Local Influences on Eye Movement Patterns

*Fixation durations are*

| | |
|---|---|
| Longer on low frequency words | Kliegl, Olson, and Davidson, Chapter 19, this volume; Rayner, 1977 |
| Longer on technical words, where readers have a poorer technical vocabulary | Buswell (cited by Kolers, 1976) |
| Longer on shorter words | O'Regan, 1980, 1981 |
| Longer when erroneous letters were in the periphery on the prior fixation | O'Regan, 1980; Rayner, 1975a; Underwood & McConkie, 1981 |
| Longer if foveal letters are replaced by a grating | Rayner and Bertera, 1979 |
| Longer when text is masked for the first part of the fixation, or during the fixation (if not too near the end) | Rayner and Pollatsek, 1981; Wolverton, 1979 |
| Longer on less constrained words | Zola, 1981 |
| Longer on "semantically primed" words | Kennedy, 1980 |
| Longer on words if indirect, rather than direct, inference is required | Just and Carpenter, 1978 |
| Longer on certain grammatical elements | Wanat, 1971; Rayner, 1977 |
| Longer on first fixations on lines | Woodworth, 1938; Rayner, 1977 |
| Longer on words containing spelling errors | Zola, 1981 |
| Longer in regions of text containing more important ideas | Shebilske & Fisher, 1981 |
| Longer on numbers whose names have more syllables | Pynte, 1974 |
| Longer when there is a single fixation on a word rather than two fixations | Kliegl, Olson, and Davidson, Chapter 19, this volume |
| Shorter on a letter than on dot or space in three-fixation sequence | Arnold & Tinker, 1939 |
| Shorter at the end of a return sweep | Huey, 1908 |
| Shorter when they are the final fixations on lines | Rayner, 1977 |

*(continued)*

of whether or not these local variations are examples of immediate control; that is, whether the fixation durations and the following saccade lengths are being influenced or controlled on the basis of information obtained during those very fixations. The problem of establishing the existence of immediate control is more difficult than simply demonstrating that local characteristics of texts influence eye movement patterns. It is always possible that the information having the effect was acquired from the periphery during a prior fixation, rather than during the present one. Thus, in order to establish the existence of immediate control it is necessary to know on what fixation certain information was in fact acquired by the reader.

The recent development of eye movement contingent display techniques has

TABLE 5.1 *(Continued)*

| | |
|---|---|
| Shorter when they are at the beginning and ends of words, rather than in the center | O'Regan, 1980 |
| Shorter on fixations prior to and following regressions | Stern, 1978 |
| Shorter prior to wide blank spaces in the text | Abrams and Zuber, 1972 |
| Shorter in the region between sentences | Rayner, 1975a |
| Influenced by the length and frequency of words not directly fixated | Kliegl, Olson, and Davidson, Chapter 19, this volume |
| *Saccadic movements are* | |
| Longer when a longer word lies to the right of the fixated word | O'Regan, 1979 |
| Longer following a fixation on a longer word | O'Regan, 1979 |
| Shorter when erroneous letters lie in the near periphery or when peripheral letters are replaced by a grating | McConkie and Rayner, 1975, 1976a; McConkie and Underwood, 1981; O'Regan, 1980; Rayner and Bertera, 1979; Rayner, Inhoff, Morrison, Slowiaczek, and Bertera, 1981; Rayner and Pollatsek, 1981 |
| Shorter, and with more regressions, in regions of text that are more important | Shebilske and Fisher, 1981 |
| More likely to be regressive if the text is shifted to the left during a saccade | O'Regan, 1981; McConkie, Zola, and Wolverton, 1980 |
| *Fixations are less likely to be centered on* | |
| The word *the* than on a three-letter verb | O'Regan, 1979, 1980; Rayner, 1977 |
| The region between sentences | Rayner, 1975a |
| Blank areas in the text | Abrams and Zuber, 1972 |
| *Fixations are more likely to be centered on* | |
| The centers of words rather than the ends | Rayner, 1979; O'Regan, 1981; Zola, 1981 |
| A short word if the word to the left is longer | Rayner, 1979 |
| A letter if it is in a word of medium length rather than longer or shorter | Rayner and McConkie, 1976 |
| A prior context sentence after encountering a pronoun | Carpenter and Just, 1977 |

made it possible to investigate this issue. It is now possible to make changes in the text display, contingent upon the reader's eye movements, thus ensuring that certain stimulus information was in fact not available to the reader until a particular fixation of interest, or a particular time during that fixation. If the information in question is then found to have an influence on the duration of that fixation, or on where the eyes go during the next saccade, this is evidence of immediate control. The danger in using this technique, of course, is that the stimulus change itself might in some way be producing the differential effects, a problem that requires great care in the selection of control conditions.

A few studies presently available meet this strict criterion for demonstrating immediate control of eye movements. The duration of a fixation can be increased if errors or gratings occur in the text on that fixation (Rayner & Pollatsek, 1981;

Underwood & McConkie, 1981), if the fixated word is different from what that word was on the prior fixation (Rayner, 1975a), or if the text was shifted during the prior saccade so that the eyes are not centered at the text location they normally would have been (O'Regan, 1981; McConkie, *et al.*, 1980). The latter manipulation also influences the immediately following saccade. In addition to demonstrations of immediate effects, there are also clear instances of delayed effects, where manipulations on one fixation influence the following fixation or the saccade following it (Rayner & Pollatsek, 1981; Underwood & McConkie, 1981). Thus, both immediate and delayed effects have been demonstrated, and a goal of future research must be to establish the conditions under which each occurs.

So far all studies that have provided unambiguous demonstrations of the presence or absence of immediate effects on eye movements during reading have employed stimulus manipulations involving gratings, errors, and shifting of the text, a point noted by Levy–Schoen & O'Regan (1979). There is not yet a conclusive demonstration of variables in normal text encountered during a given fixation influencing the duration of that fixation or the following saccade. Although it seems highly probable that some of the local effects noted in Table 5.1 are indeed immediate in nature, the final evidence is not yet in.

The issue of whether or not eye movements are primarily under immediate control is an active one in theories of reading. Some have argued there is not sufficient time during a fixation for such immediate control to occur (Bouma, 1978; Bouma & deVoogd, 1974; Kolers, 1976; Shebilske, 1975). Others have opted for a strong immediacy assumption (Hochberg, 1970; Hochberg, 1976; Just & Carpenter, 1980; McConkie, 1979) which often plays a critical role in their theories. Investigation on this issue should be lively during the next few years.

## 4.  INFORMATION ON WHICH THE SPATIAL DECISIONS ARE MADE

In considering the nature of eye movement control during reading in 1970, Hochberg noted that there are two sources of information that might be employed in determining where the eyes should move next. The first was visual information, primarily that from the periphery since the eyes typically (but not always) travel to a region not located foveally on the last fixation. Use of this source of information was labeled Peripheral Search Guidance, or PSG. The second was knowledge of language patterns that reduces uncertainty about the not yet fixated text, and which therefore might influence where the eyes are sent next. This source of influence was called Cognitive Search Guidance, or CSG. Hochberg proposed beginnings of a theory of reading based on the combined use of these two sources of information to gain processing efficiency, primarily through: (*a*) minimizing the amount of visual information required from words for their recognition, thus permitting more effective use of peripheral visual information: (*b*) optimizing the locations of the fixations using PSG and CSG; and (*c*) reducing the amount of visual processing required by suggesting that readers use their knowledge to form hypotheses that are tested against visual information. The CSG–PSG distinction is further clarified in a later publication (Hochberg, 1976). Whether or not later writers have accepted Hochberg's analysis-by-synthesis basis for perceptual processing, all have accepted as a fundamental distinction that between visual versus cognitive sources of information used in guiding the eyes, and the controversy has centered around whether neither of these is used (recognizing the possibility of only global control operating), whether one predominates, or whether both are involved (Bouma, 1978; Carpenter & Just, 1977; R. N. Haber, 1976; Kennedy, 1980; Kolers, 1976; Rayner & McConkie, 1976) and if both, how the combining occurs. Other possible sources of control include the establishment of a basic scanning routine that provides the general pattern required for reading (Levy–Schoen, 1981) and the possibility that the states of perceptual or cognitive processes can themselves be a basis for eye movement control (Rayner & McConkie, 1976).

a. **Visual Information in Spatial Control.** The primary contender at the present time for the use of purely visual information guiding the eyes is found in the "preferred viewing position" hypothesis (Rayner, 1979; O'Regan, 1981) which indicates a tendency for readers to fixate toward the centers of words (slightly before the centers of long words). Rayner suggests that the basis for eye guidance may be simply to send the eyes to the middle of the word beyond the last one identified. The fact that many fixations were not at the expected location, however, was of some concern, and three possible explanations were put forward: inaccuracy in the guidance system, lack of preciseness in the intended positioning of the eyes, or other semantic and/or syntactic factors (as yet unspecified) that may override this basic algorithm. This hypothesis is also closely allied with the observations that readers tend to send their eyes further when a long word lies to the right of their fixation location than when shorter words do (O'Regan, 1979) and that an initial fixation early in a long word is frequently followed by a short forward saccade whereas an initial fixation toward the end of a long word is frequently followed by a regression (O'Regan, 1980). Apparently whether one or two fixations are needed to recognize a long word depends on where the initial fixation lies, suggesting an efficiency in fixating near the center.

It should be pointed out that here, as with other eye fixation tendencies, the observation of a pattern in the data is not itself proof that guidance is based on an attempt to achieve that pattern. For instance, the fact that extreme letters in a word are more easily identified due to less lateral masking (Bouma, 1973) indicates that any theory suggesting that the eyes are sent to a region where identification did not previously succeed would predict that more fixations would be centered on the internal parts of words.

A second aspect of strictly visual control of eye positions is a tendency to avoid fixating on blank regions in the text (Abrams & Zuber, 1972) including the region between sentences (Rayner, 1975a).

**b. Cognitive Information in Spatial Control.**    One example of cognitive control is found in recordings of regressive movements. Readers sometimes move directly to a relevant previously read word when some processing difficulty is encountered (Carpenter & Just, 1977). Apparently the location of the word was retained and that information was used to guide the eyes.

It has often been suggested that language constraints are involved in spatial control; good readers presumably do not need to fixate highly constrained words, either because they can be identified in peripheral vision, or because they can be identified on the basis of cognitive information alone and visual analysis is not necessary (O'Regan, 1979; Hochberg, 1970; R. N. Haber, 1976). However, this notion has been challenged by one study that found no difference in the fixation patterns on a word under high and low constraint conditions (Zola, 1981).

**c. Combined Visual and Cognitive Information in Spatial Control.**    At present, the most frequently stated position on eye movement guidance in reading involves a combination of visual and cognitive information. For instance, optimal eye position may be selected on the basis of some combination of knowledge of language constraints and of patterns available in peripheral vision (Hochberg, 1970), or language constraints may increase the likelihood of recognizing certain words in the periphery, thus leading such words not to be fixated (R. N. Haber, 1978b; McClelland & O'Regan, 1981; McConkie, 1979; O'Regan, 1979; Rayner, 1979; Rumelhart, 1977). In this latter proposal, the combination of visual and cognitive information enhances peripheral recognition, thus allowing longer saccades, but is not specifically used in the spatial decisions themselves. This may be why the visual region within which erroneous letters disrupt reading is the same for poor fifth-grade readers as for college students (Underwood, 1981), yet the college students make longer saccades. If average saccade length reflects the region of perceptibility rather than visibility (O'Regan, 1979), this increased saccade length may reflect a more efficient use of peripheral visual information by the more skilled readers (Hochberg, 1970).

Finally, it may be that semantic preprocessing of peripheral visual information may aid in eye guidance (Neisser, 1967), but present evidence makes this possibility unlikely (Inhoff & Rayner, 1980; Kolers & Lewis, 1972).

### 5.   BASES FOR TEMPORAL DECISIONS

Gilbert (1959) suggested that fixations have three purposes: (1) to allow transmission of the visual stimulus while the eyes are at rest; (2) to provide a period free from interfering stimuli; and (3) to provide time to comprehend the ideas and relations involved. The first two purposes suggest that there may be some minimum time required for basic perceptual processes to occur in fixations; the third suggests that most will be longer than the minimum, the length of which should then be related to the time required for comprehension of the ideas and relations to occur. However, Gilbert did not deal with the question of what event triggers the initiation of the next saccade. Although Table 5.1 makes it clear that many local factors influence the durations of fixations (characteristics of the word fixated, characteristics of the next word, characteristics of the language context) it is still not clear just how much of the processing induced by a word or words perceived during a fixation has been accomplished by the point of no return on that fixation, nor just what it is that signals the fixation termination.

As an example, Zola (1981) found that the initial fixation on a word was 23 msec shorter when it was highly constrained by the prior context than when it was less highly constrained, an amount comparable to the facilitation in recognition time that Tulving and Gold (1963) obtained when appropriate contextual constraint was introduced. Thus, this indicates some efficiency in processing resulting from the language constraints. However, the nature of the mechanism underlying this savings is still not known. For example, it may be that in any of several ways, recognition of the critical word was sped up by the constraints, thus reaching sooner the processing state that triggers a saccade. Or it may be that once the word was recognized it was also noted that it fit easily with the developing structure, so less processing time was allotted. Or it may be that during the prior fixation the fact that this was a region of high constraint (low information value) was detected, and thus a shorter fixation was planned at the next location.

Although recent research has documented local effects on the durations of fixations, so far it has ignored the nature of the mechanism producing this variability. This fact has a bearing on attempts to use eye movement data as a basis for estimating the time required to process different segments of text, a topic that will be briefly discussed later.

### 6.   THE BASIS FOR SMALL SACCADES

One phenomenon that has been largely ignored in reading research, and that is something of an embarrassment to most present views of eye movement control, is the existence of small saccades. Why is it that readers at times move their eyes such a short distance that the new region fixated was within the fovea on the prior fixation? It seems unlikely that the level of visual detail available from that region on the prior fixation failed to permit adequate discrimination among letters, or that it would be anticipated that critical new information would be available there that was not accessible on the prior fixation. The typical way of dealing with short saccades is to ignore them. This is done in either of two ways. First, for most equipment there is a limit on the size of the saccade that can be reliably detected. The definition of a saccade is often set in the data reduction program in a way that eliminates small saccades; for instance, Just and Carpenter (1980) declare the eyes to be in a fixation until they move outside a three-character window around that fixation location. How small a saccade can be detected depends on such factors as the noise level of the equipment and the sampling rate (McConkie, Zola, Wolverton, & Burns, 1978). Second, the investigator may choose to ignore detected saccades if they are less than a certain length (O'Regan, 1979) or if they do not take the eyes out of some region of interest (Just & Carpenter, 1980).

The only available evidence on the frequency of microsaccades during reading (saccades of 11.6 min. of arc or less, which is about ½–¾ of a letter position in most displays used for eye movement research) indicates that for one subject they occurred on 1.7% of fixations and for a second, on 4.8% of fixations (Cunitz & Steinman, 1969). On fixations containing these microsaccades, median fixation durations were 535 and 520 msec, in contrast to 285–305 msec for fixations with no microsaccades. Furthermore, time from onset of the fixation to the onset of the microsaccade was 275 and 295 msec, very similar to the normal fixation time for these subjects. These authors claim that small saccades do not improve visibility, since low-velocity drifts are sufficient to accomplish that purpose and that, like larger saccades, they are scanning movements, made when a subject searches for very fine detail in a fixation target. Thus, they make no dichotomy between microsaccades and larger saccades.

This argument seems reasonable for a subject attempting to fixate a small target or to examine a display made of very fine detail. It loses its credibility in reading, however, where the level of detail needed to discriminate among letters and words is not very fine, certainly not fine enough to require half-letter or smaller saccades.

There seem to be two other possible explanations. One suggested by Cunitz and Steinman (1969) is that when examining a display for fine detail, small saccades are made that are "peripheral indicators of small changes in attention within a very circumscribed portion of the visual field [p. 691]." Thus, there may be a link between attention and the saccadic eye movement system close enough so that certain (perhaps discrete) movements of attention result in a small change in eye position, even when that change itself is not functional (McConkie, 1979). A second explanation is that the eye movement system operates with some base frequency of movement. That is, there may be some natural tendency for the eyes to move every 200–300 msec, and if the perceptual system has not called for such a movement by then a discharge occurs to move the eyes anyway. In this case, the eyes would only be moved a short distance so as not to interfere with ongoing perception. This explanation seems most compatible with Levy–Schoen's suggestion of a preestablished basic scanning routine for reading, described earlier. Another bit of compatible evidence is that when the text is masked with a grating during the early part of a fixation, readers sometimes initiate small eye movements even though there is really no useful stimulus pattern to attend to for reading (Rayner & Pollatsek, 1981). At the present time, there seems to be no basis for selecting among these or other possible explanations of small saccades. However, the existence of small saccades raises the issue of whether every saccade is purposeful, initiated for the purpose of sending the eyes to some location where added visual information is needed, or whether some are elicited on some other basis.

Whatever the basis for small saccades, their effect on certain aspects of our data should not be overlooked. Obviously, the durations of fixations reported from an experiment depend to some extent on what is taken to be a saccade. To ignore some saccades (as is usually technically necessary since the smallest saccades cannot be reliably detected with most equipment available for reading research) is to report longer fixations than actually occur. How much longer the average fixation duration is depends on the size of the saccades ignored, since the higher the threshold is set, the more are ignored, and hence the more "contaminated" fixation durations are included in the distribution. From Cunitz and Steinman's data, it appears that the primary effect of ignoring small saccades is to increase the number of fixations with long durations, thus increasing the positive skew in fixation duration distributions. It is also the case the such aspects of the data as the number of fixations made in reading a passage, the average length of saccades, and the number of regressive movements made are influenced by the saccade threshold of the study.

## 7.   THE BASIS FOR REGRESSIVE MOVEMENTS

Although most eye movements during reading are either rightward along the line or leftward and down to the next line, a considerable number cast the eyes against this normal progression, seeming to take the eyes back for a reexamination of earlier seen information. The question arises as to whether these regressive movements and the fixations that precede and follow them are perceptually any different than those bounded by forward saccades, or whether the basic perceptual processes are the same but these saccades are simply induced under different cognitive circumstances. There are differences in the eye movement patterns associated with regressions: The average duration of fixations prior to regressive saccades is shorter than those prior to forward saccades (Hawley, et al., 1974; Kliegl, et al., Chapter 19 of this volume); the average length of regressive saccades is shorter than that for forward movements (Taylor, 1971); and the fixation following a regression can also be shorter than normal (Hawley et al., 1974). Whether these differences reflect differences in the perceptual processes associated with these fixations is not presently known.

Most speculation has focused on the conditions under which regressive eye movements occur. For example, it may be that regressions are stimulated by inaccuracies in eye positioning, habits formed in early stages of learning to read (Taylor, 1971), comprehension failures (Shebilske, 1975), failure of recognition to be completed by the time the eyes are scheduled to move on (Bouma, 1978), the need for additional time for the reader to learn and remember high priority information (Shebilske & Fisher, 1981), anticipations (Russo, 1978) or the failure to confirm expectations (Wildman & Kling, 1978), or certain semantic factors (Carpenter & Just, 1977). It is obvious that very creative studies are going to be required to establish, and distinguish among, these and other similar alternatives.

As with forward saccades, the control of regressions can be immediate. Encountering errors left of the center of fixation can induce an immediate regression (Underwood & McConkie, 1981), as can shifting the text to the left during a saccade (O'Regan, 1981; McConkie, et al., 1980). The length of regressions that commonly follow return sweeps of the eyes depends on the position of the immediately prior fixation relative to the left edge of the text; this correlation was .97 for 36 instances produced by a subject whose data were available to me. At the same time, there are times when encountering errors has no effect on the immediately following saccade, but only on saccades following that (Underwood & McConkie, 1981).

Thus, both immediate and nonimmediate effects have been observed in the control of regressive saccades, but as yet there is no unambiguous evidence for immediate effects based on semantic and other higher level processing. This remains a challenge for the future.

## III.   Perception during a Fixation in Reading

Given that the eyes have been sent to some particular location, there next arises a set of issues about the nature of the perceptual processes occurring during the fixation (or perhaps, more properly, during the period of time that the mind is responding to the visual information provided by that fixation). First, it should be noted that although the visual system is sensitive during saccadic eye movements (Uttal & Smith, 1968) the type of visual detail needed to support reading is not acquired during those periods (Wolverton, 1979). Although there is some decrease in the sensitivity of the visual system immediately prior to and following each saccade (Volkman, 1976; Remington, 1980) this reduction is not sufficient to preclude perception of such high-contrast stimuli as are typically encountered in reading (Wolverton, 1979; Rayner et al., 1981). Thus, reading is based on perception of stimulus patterns available during fixations, and the visual system is sensitive throughout the period of the fixation.

The issues to be dealt with in this section have been divided into two groups, those involving the functional stimulus and those dealing with the dynamics of perception during a fixation.

### A.   The Functional Stimulus during a Fixation

An empirical issue, quite apart from questions of how perceptual processes proceed during a fixation, concerns just what aspects of the textual stimulus array that falls on the reader's retina during a fixation affect the reading process. This is the problem of identifying the functional stimulus. In considering this problem, it is first necessary to establish just what aspects of the stimulus pattern are actually available to the reader. Because of the small size of the fovea, the region providing the highest degree of visual resolution, together with the loss of acuity in more peripheral regions, different aspects of the visual pattern are available at different retinal locations. Furthermore, there are interactions within the visual system that result in letters located further into the periphery sometimes being more easily identified than letters closer to the fovea (Bouma, 1973). Although Bouma and his colleagues have contributed greatly to understanding on these issues, much work remains to be done so that the limits on what visual information is actually available to the reader might be fully known. This is needed to enable investigators to distinguish between failure to utilize stimulus information because it is not resolved by the visual system and because it was not attended.

In discussing the functional stimulus in reading, two basic issues will be considered. First, from what visual region is information of various sorts acquired during a fixation, and second, within this region what aspects of the visual pattern are used.

## 1. THE PERCEPTUAL SPAN DURING READING

The perceptual span will be defined as that region around the center of vision within which some aspect of visual detail of interest is used in reading (or affects the reading process). From this definition, it is clear that this region must be assessed for each aspect of visual information of interest. Furthermore, it is possible that this region changes as the nature of the task or of the text display changes. Thus, it is necessary to specify the nature of the information being studied and the nature of the task and stimulus characteristics for the concept of a span to be most useful.

To better understand what is being measured in studies that attempt to measure the perceptual span, it is necessary to make some further distinctions (Underwood & McConkie, 1981). It is possible that the region attended on different fixations varies, so the "span" is not the same from fixation to fixation. It is further possible that different regions are attended at different times during a single fixation. Thus, we must distinguish among three "spans." The *momentary span* is that region attended at some moment during a fixation, the *individual fixation span* is a region consisting of all those regions attended during a particular fixation, and the *perceptual span* encompasses all the individual fixation spans, though, of course, it may be coterminous with none of them. Thus, the perceptual span, as measured in present studies, may not necessarily indicate the region being perceived during particular fixations, or at any particular moment. Furthermore, this points up a weakness in our present techniques for measuring the perceptual span, which typically involve modifying some aspect of the text pattern at some peripheral visual location during certain or all fixations and observing whether this has any effect on reading, as indicated by eye movement patterns or reading rates. Whether or not a study reveals the use of some aspect of the stimulus at some retinal location depends on three factors: the frequency with which that aspect of the information is used at that location, the nature and size of the effects modifying this aspect of the text has on reading, and those characteristics of the design of the study that affect its sensitivity in detecting the types of changes in behavior being produced. Thus, if certain information is utilized from a particular region only occasionally and the method used to modify that information produces relatively small changes in behavior, or if the design of the sutdy is weak in its ability to reliably detect such changes, then the study will underestimate the size of the perceptual span for that information. In fact, it is quite possible that our studies will consistently underestimate the span for most types of information, especially if its use at the most extreme locations occurs but rarely.

Finally, it should be pointed out that demonstrating that visual information is being utilized from a certain peripheral region during fixations does not establish that words in that location are being identified on those fixations. Certain aspects of the text may be useful in eye guidance, in providing information about upcoming text that will facilitate its processing, or for purposes other than actual text identification. Also, the lack of use of certain visual information does not establish that words in that region were not identified, since it is logically possible that they may have been identified on the basis of contextual information. Thus, at the present time there is no well-established relationship between what information is utilized from given peripheral regions and whether words are identified in those regions.

**a. Perceptual Spans to the Right of the Fixation Location.**    Initial studies on the perceptual span question that utilized eye movement contingent display control techniques (McConkie & Rayner, 1975; Rayner, 1975a) suggested that different aspects of the visual pattern were being utilized at different distances into the periphery, with word length, word shape, and initial and final letters being acquired and used further out than internal letters. In more recent work, it has been established that replacing the text in the periphery with a square-wave grating, thus removing all information other than an indication of where the line lies and perhaps what its end point is, has no effect on reading if it is no closer than 14 character positions to the right of the fixation location (Rayner, Inhoff, *et al.*, 1981; Rayner & Bertera, 1979). This suggests that some more detailed aspects of the stimulus are typically acquired and used up to about 14 letter positions, though it is possible that the very noticeable, homogeneous pattern presented by the grating may have been having some effect of its own perhaps by influencing the subjects' reading strategies (O'Regan, 1980).

At the other extreme, distinctions among letters may not be made more than about six letters to the right (Underwood & McConkie, 1981; McConkie, 1978) with uppercase letters being perceived somewhat further than this (O'Regan, 1980). Fifth-grade children, both those reading at and above their grade level and those reading below, appear to acquire and use letter information from the same region as do college students (Underwood, 1981). Thus there is no evidence that the region within which letters are identified increases as reading skill develops (Stewart–Lester & Lefton, 1981).

Studies in which subjects are asked to read under conditions in which foveal information is masked (Rayner & Bertera, 1979) so that only peripheral visual information is available, indicate that little information beyond occasional letters (typically initial and final letters of words), word length, and the like can be acquired from words lying as much as six letter positions from the fixation location. Furthermore, studies designed to determine whether subjects can gain semantic, phonetic, or other such information from words in similar peripheral locations have failed to find such influences (Inhoff & Rayner, 1980; Rayner *et al.*, 1978; Rayner, McConkie, & Zola, 1980). These studies again indicate the narrowness of the region within which the type of visual detail normally considered to be the basis for reading can be obtained.

Although considerable progress has been made in this area, further work is needed to explore individual differences and the effects of text and task factors and to determine whether there is indeed variability in the individual fixation spans and momentary spans as people read.

**b. Perception to the Left of the Fixation Location.** The perceptual span for letter information lies asymmetric with respect to the fixation location, extending less far to the left than to the right (McConkie & Rayner, 1976a). This asymmetry is greater than can be accounted for strictly on the basis of visibility of letters and words (Bouma, 1978) and has been attributed to attentional processes (McConkie, 1979). The fact that the region perceived during fixations by Israeli readers extends further to the left as they read Hebrew than as they read English (Pollatsek, Bolozky, Well, & Rayner, 1981) adds further evidence for the attentional explanation. There is evidence that the region perceived during a fixation begins at the beginning of the presently fixated word, if it is within four letter positions to the left of the fixation location, or at about four letters to the left if the word extends beyond that point (Rayner, Well, & Pollatsek, 1980). It has been suggested that the reason the perceptual span seems to extend such a short distance to the left of the fixation location in readers of English is that when a saccade is made the eyes are sent to a location just beyond that where the text has been identified, and hence text to the left has already been perceived (McConkie, 1979).

**c. Variability in Individual Fixation Spans.** There is some evidence that individual fixation spans of a reader vary from fixation to fixation, but there is no basis yet for determining the degree to which this occurs. Present evidence indicates that the leftmost extent of the span may be determined by where the fixated word begins (Rayner, Well, & Pollatsek, 1980) and that whether one detects errors in the periphery may depend partially on the location of the fixation in the sentence (Rayner, 1975b). When the text is masked and removed during occasional saccades as subjects are reading and they are asked to report the last word read, they sometimes report the last word fixated and sometimes a word or two to the right of it (Hogaboam, 1979).

There are a number of reasons why variability in individual fixation spans might be expected. Retinal factors such as lateral masking influence whether a given letter or letter combination will be visible at the same retinal location on different fixations (Bouma, 1978). If perception is in word units then the individual spans will tend to be determined by the locations of word boundaries (Rayner, Well, & Pollatsek, 1980). Language constraints may influence how far into the periphery visual information is acquired and used (Haber, 1976; Hochberg, 1970; Wanat, 1971), though this has not been clearly demonstrated in reading.

Another likely possibility is that variability in individual fixation spans arises from different fixations serving different functions. It has been speculated that on the fixation at the end of a return sweep, followed by a regression, the only information attended has to do with the location of the left edge of the line of text, so a corrective movement can be made. However, Hogaboam has found in pilot studies that when the text is masked and removed following such fixations subjects can typically report the word fixated. The observation that on fixations in the region between sentences subjects are less likely to be influenced by errors in the periphery raises the possibility that such fixations may not have visual analysis as their primary purpose (Rayner, 1975b). When people read along with a slowly paced oral rendition of a passage, they make cycles of regressive and forward saccades (Levy–Schoen, 1981). Some of these fixations may be for the purpose of biding time rather than for visual analysis. Finally, some fixations preceding and following regressions may have a somewhat different function than those bounded by forward saccades (Just & Carpenter, 1980; McConkie, Hogaboam, Wolverton, Zola, & Lucas, 1979). We have observed many instances in which a reader regressed back to a word that, in the interim, had been changed, and even though fixating the word directly, shows no evidence of perceiving that a different word is in that location.

Finally, the individual fixation spans may vary for reasons related to temporal characteristics of the visual system described earlier. As indicated, the eyes are probably advanced prior to completing processing of the visual information available on any given fixation; in fact, the full visual array may be available in the visual centers for about 60 msec after a saccade is initiated, the time required for the saccade-associated stimulus changes to reach the brain. Thus, what is seen on one fixation may depend on how far processing has proceeded prior to the time the visual information arrives from the next fixation, which may in turn reflect processing difficulties encountered.

The possibility of variability in individual fixation spans raises the question of just how flexible readers are in their ability to read using information from different retinal regions. Bilingual Israeli–English readers show some flexibility as they change languages (Pollatsek et al., 1981). However, other information suggests that although it is true that the controls for eye movements and attention are not identical, there is a close relationship between where the next fixation will be and where one attends (Rayner, et al., 1978; Remington, 1980). When a normally used region of the visual field is masked, readers do not seem to be able to easily change and read from a different region (McConkie & Rayner, 1976a; Rayner et al., 1981).

It is sometimes assumed that the lengths of saccades, which are quite variable, are related to the size of the region being perceived (McConkie, 1979; Taylor, 1971). At present there is little evidence on this point (but see Hogaboam, 1979). In further work on this issue, it will probably be important to distinguish between the region where certain visual information is available and the region where words are identified. For instance, a word at a given retinal location may be identified on one encounter but not on another, not because of differences in the visual information available from it but because of language constraints. It may be that where the eyes are sent is related more closely to identification than to the individual fixation span.

## 2. ASPECTS OF THE STIMULUS USED IN READING

Various claims have been made about just what aspects of the stimulus serve as the basis for reading. Some have suggested that each letter is encountered and in some sense identified (Geyer, 1970; Gough, 1972); others have argued that due to the redundancy of the language, or to frequency of experience with certain patterns, identification can occur on the basis of partial information: word length, characteristics of the word shape, or information from only certain letters, and so forth (Rummelhart, 1977; Smith, 1971). This controversy raises questions about what aspects of the visual pattern within the perceptual span region are perceived and utilized in reading. There is good evidence that information such as word length or shape can facilitate guessing what word might be next in the text (L. R. Haber *et al.* 1981) and that errors that change the shapes of words can be detected more easily (Haber & Schindler, 1981), indicating that these types of information can be used when needed. The question, of course, is whether they are regularly used in reading and whether finer detail is sometimes ignored.

Actually, there are two issues to discuss. First is the question of whether full use is made of the available visual information in the regions attended; is it possible for the reader to extract only certain visual information needed for the decisions at hand and ignore the rest, as has so often been suggested. Second is the question of whether language constraints allow identification of words in the periphery to occur when only partial information is available.

**a. Selective Attending to Available Information.**     One of the most frequently made assumptions in theories of visual perception during reading is that, by some means, the reader is able to selectively attend to certain information that is of greatest value in the present context (Brown, 1970; L. R. Haber & R. N. Haber, 1981; Rumelhart, 1977). It is assumed that in so doing, efficiency is gained through maximizing the use of available language information and minimizing the perceptual processing that is required. If this is true, then which aspects of the text serve as the functional stimulus may be highly variable, depending on the context at the time and the degree and perhaps nature of the constraints in operation. Determining whether there is such variability in the functional stimulus is probably one of the most critical questions in the area of perception during reading, since it has played such a central role in recent theorizing. One study designed to detect whether skilled readers fail to process internal letters of highly constrained words found no evidence of this expected selectivity (Zola, 1981).

**b. Identification on the Basis of Partial Information.**     Even if readers do not selectively ignore available information they may identify words on the basis of less than full visual detail where that detail is not available, for instance, in the visual periphery. In fact, gaining this ability is thought by some to be a primary means by which reading fluency is achieved (L. R. Haber & R. N. Haber, 1981; Hochberg, 1976). From an information-theory perspective, the context, an initial letter, and a few global characteristics of a word are often sufficient to uniquely specify the word among the set of relatively common English words (R. N. Haber & L. R. Haber, 1981). The question, however, is whether this actually serves as a sufficient stimulus for reading. The research reviewed earlier, indicating that visual detail more coarse grained than that on which letter distinctions are made is available and used in the periphery, suggests that this might be the case. However, it is also possible that such information is not being used for identification directly, but rather that it is used for eye guidance, and in some way facilitates identification of information on the next fixation (Rayner, 1978b; Rayner et al., 1978; Rayner, McConkie, & Zola, 1980). Some evidence for identification on the basis of incomplete information is found in studies where the text is masked and removed during certain saccades, and subjects report the last word read (Hogaboam, 1979). Readers sometimes report words as much as two or more to the right of the last word fixated, words that had been some distance into the periphery. Whether this normally occurs during reading or only when required by the task of reporting words remains a question for further investigation.

## B.  The Dynamics of Perception

In addition to knowing what aspects of the visual stimulus serve as the functional stimulus for reading, it is necessary to know the dynamics within which this information is utilized. This will be discussed as two sets of issues: When during the fixation is information being acquired and used, and what is the nature of the perceptual processes involved.

### 1.  CHRONOLOGY OF PERCEPTUAL EVENTS

Another issue in the understanding of perception during reading is whether different types of perceptual activities occur at different times during a fixation, and whether different aspects of the stimulus pattern are processed at different times during a fixation. These issues are the topic of Chapter 3 in this volume, presented by members of our laboratory (Wolverton & Zola).

It has been suggested that the acquisition of visual information occurs early in a fixation, leaving the remainder of the fixation time for processing for comprehension and deciding where to send the eyes next (Gough, 1972). Just & Carpenter (1980) included this as a separate stage in their model, labeled "Get New Input." This view has been bolstered by evidence that people can read short sentences when they are available for only the first 50 msec of each fixation just as accurately as when they are continuously available (Rayner, et al., 1981). Wolverton and Zola (Chapter 3 of this volume) argue against this view.

To deal with this issue it is necessary to make a clear distinction between when it is that the information becomes available to the brain, which will be referred to as *registration,* and when the language processes are modified by the presence of that information, which will be referred to as *utilization.* Registration is simply a matter of transmission of retinal encodings to the brain, and this, of course, occurs early in the fixation. However, our observations have led us to believe that utilization may occur at any time throughout the period that visual information is available from a fixation. Although it may be possible for a reader to adopt a strategy by which reading can take place with the visual information available for only 50 msec of each fixation as efficiently (though not as easily, from my experience) as with a continuous view of the text, this may not be the normal case in reading. Rather, readers frequently report having read stimuli present only later in the fixaton, beyond even 100 msec. It seems possible that utilization occurs throughout the time the information is available, as needed to support the ongoing comprehension processing, though this possibility has not been established by firm evidence.

If there are stages during a fixation (i.e., times when characteristically different perceptual activities are carried out, such as visual input, testing hypotheses, generating hypotheses, calculating where to send the eyes, etc.) then the fixation must be regarded as psychologically fundamental in the reading process. The fixations become the basic time periods of mental activity, and regular cycles occur with respect to them. This may in fact be the case, but an alternative should also be considered (McConkie, 1979). Suppose that utilization occurs throughout the fixation, as needed by the comprehension processes. Reading is then a continuous process with visual information being utilized whenever appropriate for advancing an understanding of the text, and the fixation loses much of its psychological primacy. At this level, there are no fixation linked stages, since the nature of the mental activity is driven by the nature of the language processing occurring rather than by eye movement characteristics. At some lower level, the problems of ensuring that the eyes are in appropriate locations are handled without specific direction from the language processing taking place. In the saccade control there are obviously some events that must occur at specific times: Registration occurs early in the fixation, and at some point final information is provided to the saccadic system as to where to move next. These events, however, are peripheral, and may have very little effect on the more central cognitive processes taking place.

The purpose of this discussion has been to try to highlight one additional issue in our understanding of perception in reading: whether the eye movement activity that we monitor is a fundamental activity from which the higher mental processes are timed and sequenced, or whether they are incidental to the more fundamental processes and simply reflect patterns that are necessary to provide the mind with the information needed for reading.

**a. Utilization from Different Regions at Different Times.** There are several reasons, and some evidence, for expecting that visual information from different regions within the area perceived on a fixation are utilized at different times. Foveal stimulus patterns seem to have their effect earlier than more peripheral patterns, for instance (McConkie & Underwood, 1981; Rayner *et al.*, 1981; Underwood & McConkie, 1981). Whether this is due to differences in transmission times (Bouma, 1978), to the use of peripheral information only later when eye movement decisions are called for (Rayner *et al.*, 1981), or to a general tendency for readers to attentionally proceed along the line of text during a fixation (McConkie, 1979) requires investigation.

### 2.  THE PROCESSES OF PERCEPTION DURING READING

As has been evident from prior discussion, a wide range of proposals have been made concerning the nature of the perceptual processes during reading. Some view reading as involving letter by letter input followed by various stages of analysis of the information to gain its meaning (Geyer, 1970; Gough, 1972); others view it as primarily creating and testing hypotheses from previously encountered information and knowledge of language plus perhaps some peripheral visual information (Goodman, 1976; R. N. Haber & L. R. Haber, 1981; Hochberg, 1976; Russo, 1978); still others see it as involving the simultaneous operation of many processes, stimulated by information in a common memory space and entering the results back into that space (Rumelhart, 1977; Just & Carpenter, 1980). No attempt will be made here to review the various theories of perception during reading. The only point to be made is that these theories differ in the nature and timing of the processes assumed to be occurring during reading, and as a result make different predictions on the various issues that have been, and will yet be raised in this chapter, issues concerning what serves as the functional stimulus and when the information is utilized, what information is used in determining the location of the next fixation, and what information is carried over from one fixation to the next during reading. Thus, advancing knowledge on these issues will not only provide a basis for judging the strengths and weaknesses of present theories, it will also force reconsideration of the types of mechanisms that might underlie perception during reading, and will place constraints on future theories.

## IV.  Perception across Successive Fixations

In reading, as in most other visual tasks, a person makes several fixations per second, with each fixation providing a somewhat different view of the world. How the mind integrates information from successive fixations in a coherent, stable impression of the world is an issue of long standing in the field of psychology (Cumming, 1978; Huey, 1908), and underlies several questions about perception during reading, specifically. First, however, some differences between reading and many other visual tasks should be noted.

In most visual perception, the goal is to gain information about, or form a representation of, the figural characteristics of the stimulus array: shapes, spatial relations, and transformations of these over time. However, in reading the figural aspects of the stimulus pattern are simply a vehicle by which the person attempts to understand the message communicated by the text; the visual shapes are of little intrinsic interest except in the case of certain forms of poetry or graphic design. It is not the shapes of letters, words, sentences, or paragraphs that are important to retain, as is evident to anyone inspecting text written in a language he or she has not learned. At the same time, perception of the image of the page, which will be referred to here as the "scene" of the text, may be useful in reading in ways other than simply providing the visual features for the identification of individual words and of sentence punctuation, paragraphing, etc.

It has been suggested that the frequent regressions made by less skilled readers have the effect of presenting the text to the mind in an inappropriate order, leading to confusions in understanding (Taylor, 1971). Others have argued that this is not the case, but rather that the mind "smooths over" such erratic sequences, and although the eyes may fixate the words in some order other than that of the textual sequence, the fundamental perception is in the spatial sequence which maintains the normal language order (Kolers, 1976). This smoothing over process could be mediated by a mental image of the page which is to some degree independent of the fixation order (given that the necessary degree of visual detail is available in the text region where reading is directly occurring). This suggests the existence of a mental representation of an image of the text, to which each fixation contributes, and which is in turn the basis on which further reading processes depend (McConkie & Rayner, 1976b). It should be noted that neither the degree to which the mind can tolerate variations in exposure sequence to the text and still maintain comprehension and whether this ability is one developed as part of the development of reading skill, nor whether this depends on a spatial image of the text has been explored. Furthermore, although this is an appealing notion in that it provides a nice account for several aspects of perception during reading, recent studies have questioned it.

Traditionally, two explanations have been given for how images from successive fixations might be integrated into such a composite mental representation (Cumming, 1978). One possibility is that this integration depends on knowledge of the length and direction of the saccade: The image from the new fixation is mentally displaced a direction and distance to compensate for this new viewing position, and it then matches and is integrated with the image constructed from previous fixations. The other possibility is that saccade information is not needed: The new image is simply justified with the old on the basis of pattern similarity.

If images are justified on the basis of knowledge of saccades, then great disruption should be produced if during a saccade the text were to be shifted so that the following fixation was not centered at the place in the text where it was originally destined. However, shifting the text in this manner to right or left by two to three letter positions is not detected by readers (Bridgeman, Hendry, & Stark, 1975; O'Regan, 1981; McConkie et al., 1980) and although changes are induced in the eye movement pattern by this manipulation, they do not appear to indicate the type of disruption that would be expected (McConkie et al., 1980).

If integration occurs on the basis of pattern similarity, on the other hand, then similarity of the visual pattern from one fixation to the next would be critical. This was tested by having people read passages printed in AlTeRnAtInG cAsE, and changing the case of every letter during certain saccades, so successive visual images would not be similar (McConkie & Zola, 1979). These changes were not noticed by the readers, and had no effect on their eye movement patterns. Similar results were found in a word identification study (Rayner, McConkie, & Zola, 1980). Thus, if justification of images is based on visual similarity, this cannot be at the level of similarity of letter or word shapes. In pilot studies we have found that this result is not peculiar to text in alternating case. When subjects read text in which only 1/5 of the letters are capitalized they do not notice the fact that just which letters are capitalized is being changed from fixation to fixation. Furthermore, changing spacing between words is not detected. Thus, it is not clear at this time what aspects of visual similarity might be used as a basis for justifying an image from one fixation with some generalized prior image.

Turning to another related issue, it has often been suggested that information from the same word may be obtained on more than one fixation (i.e., that successive individual fixation spans may overlap) (R. N. Haber, 1976; L. R. Haber & R. N. Haber, 1981; Hochberg, 1976; Rayner *et al.*, 1981; Smith, 1971). This may allow information gained from the visual periphery on one fixation to facilitate perception of a word brought into foveal vision on the next fixation (Rayner, 1978b); it may provide a second opportunity to test a hypothesis but this time with greater detail (Hochberg, 1976); or it may reinforce perception of words in other ways (Bouma, 1978; Smith, 1971). A series of studies employing a multiple-fixation word identification task demonstrated that information acquired from a word in the periphery on one fixation can reduce the time required to name the word on the next (Rayner, 1978b; Rayner *et al.*, 1978; Rayner, McConkie, & Zola, 1980), though this may only occur when the set of words being used is known in advance by the subjects (McClelland & O'Regan, 1981; Paap & Newsome, 1981). Interference from having a word change from one fixation to the next during reading has also been reported (Rayner, 1975a; O'Regan, 1980). These results are all consonant with the notion that perceptual images are integrated across fixations.

On the other hand, recent studies in our laboratory have caused us to wonder whether such integration exists. If sentences are written in which either of two words differing in a single letter are appropriate at a given word location (e.g., *leaks–leans*), and the distinguishing letter is changed from fixation to fixation during reading, subjects are unaware of this and it produces no effect on the eye movement patterns (McConkie, 1978). Apparently the words are not being read on two successive fixations, or one would expect the change in meaning to be detected. If groups of four words differing in only two letter positions are identified (e.g., *mushy, musty, gushy,* and *gusty*), and sentences are written into which any of the words fit appropriately, the word can be switched from one fixation to the next without the reader's awareness, as well (McConkie, Zola, Blanchard, Wolverton, 1982).

The difference between studies in which changes in words causes detectable problems and these studies where it does not lies in the fact that in the latter studies any combination of letters the subject obtains from the screen at one time or another provides a readable rendition of the text. In the earlier studies, this was not the case. Thus, it seems likely that changing letters and words from one fixation to the next is not itself a detectable event during reading; the only question is whether the text (letter sequence) as perceived yields an appropriate meaning. This in turn suggests that information carried across fixations during reading may not be of the form of global perceptual images so much as of local letters or words (McConkie & Zola, 1979; Rayner, McConkie, & Zola, 1980).

At this point, then, there is reason to doubt that perceptual images are being integrated during reading in the manner described earlier. Both bases for such integration have been questioned, and it is not clear exactly what type of information is being carried across fixations at a perceptual level. This raises questions about the relation of perception in reading to that of viewing scenes and events, and thus about what one learns perceptually in learning to read. These questions would be easier to deal with if more were known about perception in viewing scenes. But assuming that a composite image is formed when perceiving pictures, in learning to read does one just develop a further way of using visual information from that image, or could it be that one learns a different way of responding to visual patterns, learning to attend to and use local detail for the purpose of reading, perceiving the meaning communicated, rather than forming composite images. The time is right for applying eye movement contingent research techniques to the study of perceptual learning in learning to read.

## V.  Obtaining Information about Mental Processes from Eye Movement Data

One motivation for studying eye movements and perception in reading has been the hope that, once this is understood better, it may be possible to use eye movement data to test hypotheses about higher mental processes. It may be that eye movement data can even yield a word-by-word indication of processing time (Just & Carpenter, 1980; McConkie et al., 1979). However, there are complexities in achieving this that must be recognized. For example:

1. When the eyes are centered on a word, it is not necessarily only that word that is being seen on that fixation.
2. The period of time spent fixating a word is not the actual time spent processing it, though there is a relationship between these times.
3. The length of the saccade following a fixation is probably not being directed on the basis of the full processing of the information utilized from that fixation, and just what aspects of the information are coming into play in that decision is not known.

4. Regressions are not necessarily stimulated by information gained on the fixations immediately prior to them, but can be the result of visual patterns on fixations previous to that.
5. Correlations in the language itself can easily mislead us in attempting to establish the cause of certain eye movement patterns.
6. As with any psychological research, averaged measures may not be an appropriate representation of the nature of the effect of a variable in individual instances.

Further clarification of the relationship between eye movements and cognitive processes involved in reading is an important goal for future research.

Despite these difficulties, eye movement data are proving useful in studying cognitive processes. Their use is fully justified in several situations. First, eye movement data can provide measures of reading time over larger regions of text (regions that require several fixations). Second, the existence of differences in eye movement patterns as a result of some text or display manipulation is evidence for the existence of processing effects of some sort, and the pattern of the differences can be a basis for speculating about the nature of those effects. Third, locating the time at which eye movement patterns are first affected by some variable places contraints on the time when the processes differentially affected by the different conditions took place. The existence of lagged effects on eye movement behavior makes it important that we recognize that the processes have occurred at least by the point at which differences are observed in the data; they may have occurred earlier. Thus, in several important ways, eye movement records can provide useful data in the study of cognitive processes in reading.

## VI. Concluding Comments

Considerable progress has been made in the study of perception during reading in recent years. New findings have been advanced, and issues have been clarified. Much of this progress has resulted from research involving the recording of eye movements, and particularly controlling aspects of the text display contingent upon those eye movements. With the base that has now been laid in both technology and theory, we can anticipate even greater progress in the future. We can expect to see answers coming forth on many of the issues raised in this chapter, and to see these research techniques extended to study children learning to read and people having reading difficulty. I hope this work will lead to the identification of specific types of perceptual difficulties where they exist, and may suggest standard diagnostic techniques. Finally, it seems likely that the general approach being taken in the study of perception during reading will be extended to the perception of complex scenes and events as electronic graphics technology develops.

# References

Abrams, S. G., & Zuber, B. L. (1972). Some temporal characteristics of information processing during reading. *Reading Research Quarterly, 8,* 42–51.

Andriessen, J. J., & deVoogd, A. H. (1973). Analysis of eye movement patterns in silent reading. *IPO Annual Progress Report, 8,* 30–35.

Arnold, D. C., & Tinker, M. A. (1939). The fixation pause of the eyes. *Journal of Experimental Psychology, 25,* 271–280.

Bouma, H. (1973). Visual interference in the parafoveal recognition of initial and final letters of words. *Vision Research, 13,* 767–782.

Bouma, H. (1978). Visual search and reading: Eye movements and functional visual field: A tutorial review. In J. Requin (Ed.), *Attention and performance VII.* New York: Erlbaum.

Bouma, H., & de Voogd, A. H. (1974). On the control of eye saccades in reading. *Vision Research, 14,* 273–284.

Bridgeman, B., Hendry, D., & Stark, L. (1975). Failure to detect displacement of the visual world during saccadic eye movements. *Vision Research, 15,* 719–722.

Brown, R. (1970). Psychology and reading. In H. Levin & J. P. Williams (Eds.), *Basic studies in reading.* New York: Basic Books, Pp. 164–187.

Carpenter, P. A., & Just, M. A. (1977). Reading comprehension as eyes see it. In M. Just & P. Carpenter (Eds.), *Cognitive processes in comprehension.* Hillsdale, New Jersey: Lawrence Erlbaum, Pp. 100–139.

Cumming, G. D. (1978). Eye movements and visual perception. In E. C. Carterette & M. P. Friedman (Eds.), *Handbook of perception* (Vol. 9). New York: Academic Press, Pp. 221–255.

Cunitz, R. J., & Steinman, R. M. (1969). Comparison of saccadic eye movements during fixation and reading. *Vision Research, 9,* 683–693.

Geyer, J. J. (1970). Models of perceptual processes in reading. In H. Singer & R. B. Ruddell (Eds.), *Theoretical models and processes of reading.* Newark, Delaware: International Reading Association.

Gilbert, L. C. (1959). Speed of processing visual stimuli and its relation to reading. *Journal of Educational Psychology, 55,* 8–19.

Goodman, K. S. (1976). Behind the eye: What happens in reading. In H. Singer & R. B. Ruddell (Eds.), *Theoretical models and processes of reading.* Newark, Delaware: International Reading Association.

Gough, P. B. (1972). One second of reading. In J. F. Kavanagh & I. G. Mattingly (Eds.), *Language by ear and by eye.* Cambridge, Massachusetts: MIT Press.

Haber, L. R., & Haber, R. N. (1981). Perceptual processes in reading: An analysis-by-synthesis model. In F. I. Pirozzolo & M. C. Wittrock (Eds.), *Neuropsychological and cognitive processes in reading.* New York: Academic Press.

Haber, L. R., Haber, R. N., & Furlin, K. R. (in press), Word length and word shape as sources of information in reading. *Reading Research Quarterly.*

Haber, R. N. (1976). Control of eye movements during reading. In R. A. Monty & J. W. Senders (Eds.), *Eye movements and psychological processes.* Hillsdale, New Jersey: Erlbaum, Pp. 443–451.

Haber, R. N. (1978). Visual perception. *Annual Review Psychology, 29,* 31–59.

Haber, R. N. (1983, in press). The impending demise of the icon: A critique of the concept of iconic storage in visual information processing. *Behavioral & Brain Sciences.*

Haber, R. N., & Haber, L. R. (1981). The shape of a word can specify its meaning. *Reading Research Quarterly, 13,* 334–345.

Haber, R. N., & Schindler, R. M. (1981). Error in proofreading: Evidence of syntactic control of letter processing? *Journal of Experimental Psychology: Human Perception and Performance, 7,* 573–579.

Hartje, W. (1972). Reading disturbances in the presence of oculomotor disorders. *European Neurology, 7,* 249–264.

Hawley, T. T., Stern, J. A., & Chen, S. C. (1974) Computer analysis of eye movements during reading. *Reading World, 13,* 307–317.

Hochberg, J. (1970). Components of literacy: Speculations and exploratory research. In H. Levin & J. P. Williams (Eds.), *Basic studies on reading*. New York: Basic Books.

Hochberg, J. (1976). Toward a speech-plan eye-movement model of reading. In R. A. Monty & J. W. Senders (Eds.), *Eye movements and psychological processes*. Hillsdale, New Jersey: Erlbaum, Pp. 397–416.

Hogaboam, T. W. (1979). *The relationship of word identification and eye movements during normal reading*. Paper presented at the twentieth annual meeting of the Psychonomic Society, Phoenix, Arizona, November.

Huey, E. H. (1908). *The psychology and pedagogy of reading*. New York: Macmillan.

Inhoff, A. W., & Rayner, K. (1980). Parafoveal word perception: A case against semantic preprocessing. *Perception and Psychophysics, 27*, 457–464.

Just, M. A., & Carpenter, P. A. (1978). Inference processes during reading: Reflections from eye fixations. In J. W. Senders, D. F. Fisher, & R. A. Monty (Eds.), *Eye movements and the higher psychological functions*. Hillsdale, New Jersey: Lawrence Erlbaum. Pp. 157–174.

Just, M. A., & Carpenter, P. A. (1980). A theory of reading: From eye fixations to comprehension. *Psychological Review, 87*, 329–354.

Kennedy, A. (1980). Reading sentences: Some observations on the control of eye movements. In G. Underwood (Ed.), *Strategies of information processing*. London: Academic Press, Pp. 217–233.

Kolers, P. A. (1976). Buswell's discoveries. In R. A. Monty & J. W. Senders (Eds.), *Eye movements and psychological processes*. Hillsdale, New Jersey: Erlbaum, Pp. 373–393.

Kolers, P. A., & Lewis, C. L. (1972). Bounding of letter sequences and the integration of visually presented words. *Acta Psychologica, 36*, 112–124.

Levy–Schoen, A. (1981). Flexible and/or rigid control of oculomotor scanning behavior. In D. F. Fisher, R. A. Monty, & J. W. Senders (Eds.), *Eye movements: Cognition and visual perception*. Hillsdale, New Jersey: Erlbaum Associates, Pp. 299–314.

Levy–Schoen, A., & O'Regan, K. (1979). The control of eye movements in reading. In P. A. Kolers, M. E. Wrolstad, & H. Bouma (Eds.), *Processing of visual language*. New York: Plenum Press, Pp. 7–36.

McClelland, J. L., & O'Regan, K. (1981). Expectations increase the benefit derived from parafoveal visual information in reading. *Journal of Experimental Psychology: Human Perception and Performance, 7*, 634–644.

McConkie, G. W. (1978). *Where do we read?* Paper presented at the annual meeting of the Psychonomic Society, San Antonio, Texas, November.

McConkie, G. W. (1979). On the role and control of eye movements in reading. In P. A. Kolers, M. E. Wrolstad, & H. Bouma (Eds.), *Processing of visual language*. New York: Plenum Press, Pp. 37–48.

McConkie, G. W., Hogaboam, T. W., Wolverton, G. S., Zola, D., & Lucas, P. A. (1979). Toward the use of eye movements in the study of language processing. *Discourse Processes, 2*, 157–177.

McConkie, G. W., & Rayner, K. (1975). The span of the effective stimulus during a fixation in reading. *Perception and Psychophysics, 17*, 578–586.

McConkie, G. W., & Rayner, K. (1976). Asymmetry of the perceptual span in reading. *Bulletin of the Psychonomic Society, 8*, 365–368. (a)

McConkie, G. W., & Rayner, K. (1976). Identifying the span of the effective stimulus in reading: Literature review and theories of reading. In H. Singer & R. B. Rudell (Eds.), *Theoretical Models and Processes of Reading* (2nd edition). Newark: Delaware: International Reading Association. (b)

McConkie, G. W., & Underwood, N. R. (1981). *Some temporal characteristics of perception during a fixation in reading*. An unpublished manuscript, (Available from George W. McConkie, Center for the Study of Reading, 51 Gentry Dr., Champaign, IL 61820).

McConkie, G. W., & Zola, D. (1979). Is visual information integrated across successive fixations in reading? *Perception and Psychophysics, 25*, 221–224.

McConkie, G. W., Zola, D., Blanchard, H. E., & Wolverton, G. S. (1982). Perceiving words during reading: Lack of facilitation from prior peripheral exposure. (Technical Report No. 243). Urbana: University of Illinois, Center for the Study of Reading.

McConkie, G. W., Zola, D., & Wolverton, G. S. (1980). *How precise is eye guidance?* Paper presented at the annual meeting of the American Educational Research Association, Boston, Massachusetts, April.

McConkie, G. W., Zola, D., Wolverton, G. S., & Burns, D. D. (1978). Eye movement contingent display control in studying reading. *Behavior Research Methods and Instrumentation, 10,* 154–166.

Neisser, U. (1967). *Cognitive psychology.* New York: Appleton.

O'Regan, K. (1979). Saccade size control in reading: Evidence for the linguistic control hypothesis. *Perception and Psychophysics, 25,* 501–509.

O'Regan, K. (1980). The control of saccade size and fixation duration in reading: The limits of linguistic control. *Perception and Psychophysics, 28,* 112–117.

O'Regan, K. (1981). The "Convenient Viewing Position" hypothesis. In D. F. Fisher, R. A. Monty, & J. W. Senders (Eds.), *Eye movements: Cognition and visual perception.* Hillsdale, New Jersey: Lawrence Erlbaum.

Paap, K. R., & Newsome, S. L. (1981). Parafoveal information is not sufficient to produce semantic or visual priming. *Perception and Psychophysics, 29,* 457–466.

Pollatsek, A., Bolozky, S., Well, A. D., & Rayner, K. (1981). Asymmetries in the perceptual span for Israeli readers. *Brain and Language, 14,* 174–180.

Pynte, J. (1974). Readiness for pronunciation during the reading process. *Perception and Psychophysics, 16,* 110–112.

Rayner, K. (1975). Parafoveal identification during a fixation in reading. *Acta Psychologica, 39,* 271–282. (b)

Rayner, K. (1975) The perceptual span and peripheral cues in reading. *Cognitive Psychology, 7,* 65–81.(a)

Rayner, K. (1977). Visual attention in reading: Eye movements reflect cognitive processing. *Memory & Cognition, 4,* 443–448.

Rayner, K. (1978). Eye movements in reading and information processing. *Psychological Bulletin, 85,* 616–660. (a)

Rayner, K. (1978). Foveal and parafoveal cues in reading. In J. Requin (Ed.), *Attention & performance VII.* New York: Erlbaum, Pp. 149–161. (b)

Rayner, K. (1979). Eye guidance in reading: Fixation locations within words. *Perception, 8,* 21–30.

Rayner, K., & Bertera, J. H. (1979). Reading without a fovea. *Science, 206,* 468–469.

Rayner, K., Inhoff, A. W., Morrison, R. E., Slowiaczek, M. L., & Bertera, J. H. (1981). Masking of foveal and parafoveal vision during eye fixations in reading. *Journal of Experimental Psychology: Human Perception and Performance, 7,* 167–179.

Rayner, K., & McConkie, G. W. (1976). What guides a reader's eye movements? *Vision Research, 16,* 829–837.

Rayner, K., McConkie, G. W., & Ehrlich, S. (1978). Eye movements and integrating information across fixations. *Journal of Experimental Psychology: Human Perception and Performance, 4,* 529–544.

Rayner, K., McConkie, G. W., & Zola, D. (1980). Integrating information across eye movements. *Cognitive Psychology, 12,* 206–226.

Rayner, K., & Pollatsek, A. (1981). Eye movement control during reading: Evidence for direct control. *Quarterly Journal of Experimental Psychology, 33A,* 351–373.

Rayner, K., Well, A. D., & Pollatsek, A. (1980). Asymmetry of the effective visual field in reading. *Perception and Psychophysics, 27,* 537–544.

Remington, R. W. (1980). Attention and saccadic eye movements. *Journal of Experimental Psychology: Human Perception and Performance, 6,* 726–744.

Rumelhart, D. E. (1977). Toward an interactive model of reading. In S. Dornic (Ed.), *Attention and performance VI.* Hillsdale, New Jersey: Erlbaum.

Russo, J. E. (1978). Adaptation of cognitive processes to the eye movement system. In J. W. Senders, D. F. Fisher, & R. A. Monty (Eds.), *Eye movements and the higher psychological functions.* Hillsdale, New Jersey: Erlbaum, Pp. 89–112.

Shebilske, W. (1975). Reading eye movements from an information-processing point of view. In D. Massaro (Ed.), *Understanding language*. New York: Academic Press.

Shebilske, W. L., & Fisher, D. F. (1981). Eye movements reveal components of flexible reading strategies. In M. L. Kamil (Ed.), *Directions in reading: Research & instruction*, 30th Yearbook of the National Reading Conference.

Smith, F. (1971). *Understanding reading*. New York: Holt, Rinehart and Winston.

Stern, J. A. (1978). Eye movements, reading, and cognition. In J. W. Senders, D. F. Fisher, & R. A. Monty (Eds.), *Eye movements and the higher psychological functions*. Hillsdale, New Jersey: Erlbaum. Pp. 145–155.

Stewart–Lester, K. J., & Lefton, L. A. (1981). Information extraction from the parafovea: A developmental study. *Journal of Experimental Psychology: Human Perception and Performance, 7,* 624–633.

Taylor, S. E. (1971). *The dynamic activity of reading: A model of the process* (Research Information Bulletin No. 9). New York: Educational Developmental Laboratories.

Tulving, E., & Gold, C. (1963). Stimulus information and contextual information as determinants of tachistoscopic recognition of words. *Journal of Experimental Psychology, 66,* 319–327.

Underwood, N. R. (1981). *The span of letter recognition of good and poor readers* (Technical Report No. 251). Urbana: University of Illinois, Center for the Study of Reading.

Underwood, N. R., & McConkie, G. W. (1981). *The effect of encountering errors at different retinal locations during reading.* Unpublished manuscript. (Available from George W. McConkie, Center for the Study of Reading, 51 Gentry Dr., Champaign, IL 61820.)

Uttal, W. R., & Smith, P. (1968). Recognition of alphabetic characters during voluntary eye movements. *Perception and Psychophysics, 3,* 257–264.

Volkmann, F. C. (1976). Saccadic suppression: A brief review. In R. A. Monty & J. W. Senders (Eds.), *Eye movements and psychological processes*. Hillsdale, New Jersey: Erlbaum, Pp. 73–83.

Wanat, S. (1971). *Linguistic structure and visual attention in reading*. Newark, Delaware: International Reading Association.

Wildman, D., & Kling, M. (1978). Semantic, syntactic and spatial anticipation in reading. *Reading Research Quarterly, 14,* 128–164.

Wolverton, G. S. (1979). *The acquisition of visual information during fixations and saccades in reading.* Paper presented at the annual meeting of the American Educational Research Association, San Francisco, California, April.

Woodworth, R. S. (1938). *Experimental Psychology*. New York: Henry Holt.

Zola, D. (1981). *The effect of redundancy on the perception of words in reading* (Technical Report No. 216). Urbana: University of Illinois, Center for the Study of Reading. September

Keith Rayner

# 6

# The Perceptual Span
# and Eye Movement Control
# during Reading[1]

## I.  Introduction

A great deal of recent research has utilized a technique developed by McConkie
and Rayner (1975) to investigate the characteristics of the perceptual span in
reading. In these experiments, the eye movements of subjects were recorded and
display changes were made on a cathode-ray tube (CRT) from which the subject
was reading that were contingent upon the subject's eye position. In general, the
results of a large number of experiments (Den Buurman, Boersema, & Gerrissen,
1981; McConkie & Rayner, 1975; Ikeda & Saida, 1978; O'Regan, 1980; Rayner,
1975; Rayner & Bertera, 1979; Rayner, Inhoff, Morrison, Slowiaczek, & Bertera,
1981; Rayner, Well, & Pollatsek, 1980) have indicated that for readers of English
the perceptual span extends from the beginning of the currently fixated word (but
not more than three or four characters to the left of fixation) to about 15 characters to the right of fixation. To the right of fixation, different types of information
are acquired. Information useful for identifying the meaning of a word is obtained
within the foveal region and the beginning of the parafoveal region. More gross
types of information, such as word shape or specific letter information, that do not
lead directly to word identification are acquired slightly further to the right of
fixation than is information leading to word identification. Word length information, which is useful in guiding eye movements to the next location, is acquired
out to about 15 character spaces to the right of fixation. For readers of Hebrew,

[1]Preparation of this chapter was supported by grant HD12727 from the National Institute of Child
Health and Human Development.

EYE MOVEMENTS IN READING:
PERCEPTUAL AND LANGUAGE PROCESSES

the perceptual span is asymmetric to the left of fixation (Pollatsek, Bolozky, Well, & Rayner, 1981).

Although there has been considerable research on the perceptual span and many of the effects just described have been replicated in several experiments, there remain a number of unanswered questions about the characteristics of the effective visual field during reading. In this chapter, I will focus on some recent research in our laboratory dealing with (*a*) further characteristics of the perceptual span; and (*b*) timing constraints related to programming eye movements during reading.

## II.  The Perceptual Span

Virtually all of the research previously conducted on the perceptual span using the "moving window" technique developed by McConkie and Rayner (1975) has defined the window area in terms of character spaces and the integrity of words has not been considered. However, if the perceptual span corresponds to whole-word boundaries, then previous studies may have either underestimated or over-estimated certain aspects of the perceptual span region. In particular, estimates of the region from which subjects obtain information useful for word identification could be particularly influenced by the fact that in prior research the window has been defined in terms of character spaces. Hence, we (Rayner, Well, Pollatsek, & Bertera, 1982) have compared reading performance when the experimentally de-fined window area to the right of fixation was defined in terms of number of characters visible (i.e., available in the display) with reading performance when the window area to the right of fixation was a fixed number of words. In each of the former conditions, the number of words visible to the right of fixation varied from fixation to fixation and parts of words were often visible, whereas in each of the latter conditions the number of words visible to the right of fixation was constant, but the number of letters varied from fixation to fixation. If on the average the same number of letters are presented in the letter and word window conditions and integrity of words is important, the latter conditions should pro-duce better reading performance. If the integrity of words is not important, then there should be little difference.

Table 6.1 shows examples of the different conditions and the reading rates for the whole word windows compared with the reading rates when the window was defined in terms of letters. The sizes of the windows defined in terms of letters were determined by estimating the average number of letters that would be visible to the right of fixation under the conditions in which the window was determined by word boundaries. As can be seen in Table 6.1, there were basically no dif-ferences between equivalent window sizes determined by number of letters and window sizes determined by word boundaries. More detailed analyses of the data revealed that performance in conditions in which word integrity was maintained could be predicted very accurately from simply knowing how many letters on the

TABLE 6.1
Different Conditions and Reading Rate Associated with Each[a]

| Window size | Sentence | Reading rate (wpm) |
|---|---|---|
| Control | An experiment was conducted in the lab | 348 |
| 0W (3.7) | An experiment xxx xxxxxxxxx xx xxx xxx | 212 |
| 1W (9.6) | An experiment was xxxxxxxxx xx xxx xxx | 309 |
| 2W (15.0) | An experiment was conducted xx xxx xxx | 339 |
| 3W (20.8) | An experiment was conducted in xxx xxx | 339 |
| 3L | An experimxxx xxx xxxxxxxxx xx xxx xxx | 207 |
| 9L | An experiment was xxxxxxxxx xx xxx xxx | 308 |
| 15L | An experiment was conducxxx xx xxx xxx | 340 |
| 21L | An experiment was conducted in txx xxx | 342 |

[a] The values in parentheses correspond to the average number of letters visible in the W condition. The dot represents the fixation point.

average were visible. On the other hand, performance in conditions in which the window was defined in terms of number of characters visible could not be understood in terms of the number of words completely visible.

## A. Partial Information Acquisition within the Visual Field

Our finding that the effective visual field to the right of fixation is determined by the number of letters visible and is not contingent on the preservation of word integrity suggests that in reading subjects acquire partial word information from the parafovea. Such a conclusion is consistent with previous research (Rayner, 1975; Rayner & Bertera, 1979) that has found that word shape and beginning letters of words are obtained from parafoveal vision. The conclusion is also consistent with the results of experiments (Rayner, 1978b; Rayner, McConkie, & Ehrlich, 1978; Rayner, McConkie, & Zola, 1980) in which a word or letter string was initially presented in parafoveal vision and when the subject made an eye movement to the stimulus it was replaced by a word which the subject named. The general conclusion reached from those studies was that visual information is not integrated across eye movements (see also McConkie & Zola, 1979 for a reading situation). Rather, subjects acquire information about the beginning letters of the parafoveal word that is useful in identifying the word to be named following the saccade. It is important to note that the results of the experiments indicated that the beginning letter information existed in the form of an abstract code rather than in a visual or phonological form.

Given the finding that partial information about the beginning letters of words facilitated naming of the word and given the implication from some of our prior research that partial information about words is useful in reading, we (Rayner, Well, Pollatsek, & Bertera, 1982) asked subjects to read text when (1) only the word fixated was visible and every other letter to the right of fixation was replaced by another letter; (2) the word fixated and the word to the right of fixation was visible and every other letter was replaced by another letter; or (3) the word fixated was visible and partial information about the word to the right of fixation was visible. In all of the conditions, all of the information to the left of fixation was visible. In the third condition, either one, two, or three letters of the word to the right of fixation were visible. Table 6.2 shows examples of the different conditions and the reading rates associated with each. As seen in Table 2, when the first three letters in the word to the right of fixation were visible and the

TABLE 6.2
Different Conditions and Reading Rate Associated with Each[a]

| Window condition | | Reading rate (wpm) | |
|---|---|---|---|
| | | Exp. 1 | Exp. 2 |
| Similar letters | | | |
| 0W | An experiment was ecmbnefob rm fko tsd. | 251 | 238 |
| 0W + 1 | An experiment was ccmbnefob rm fko tsd. | 281 | |
| 0W + 2 | An experiment was combnefob rm fko tsd. | 286 | |
| 0W + 3 | An experiment was conbnefob rm fko tsd. | 301 | 290 |
| 1W | An experiment was conducted rm fko tsd. | 329 | 295 |
| Dissimilar letters | | | |
| 0W | An experiment was tybalpelm la enp ots. | 234 | 208 |
| 0W + 1 | An experiment was cybalpelm la enp ots. | 232 | |
| 0W + 2 | An experiment was cobalpelm la enp ots. | 242 | |
| 0W + 3 | An experiment was conalpelm la enp ots. | 265 | 256 |
| 1W | An experiment was conducted la enp ots. | 312 | 270 |

[a]See Rayner, Well, Pollatsek, and Bertera (1982) for details of the differences between Experiment 1 and Experiment 2. The dot represents the fixation point.

remainder of the letters in the word were replaced by visually similar letters, reading rate was not different from when the entire word to the right of fixation was visible. We take this as strong evidence that partial word information is utilized during reading and that an individual word may be processed on more than one fixation. These conclusions suggest that any methodology that equates the time spent fixating on a word with the processing time for that particular word (Just & Carpenter, 1980) is in error. That is, restricting the rightmost extent of the window to the right boundary of the currently fixated word reduced reading speed to under half the normal rate, implying that significantly more information than the fixated word is extracted on many fixations. However, since the area that information is extracted from is relatively small, careful analyses of eye movement patterns can reveal interesting things about on-line processes in reading (e.g., Ehrlich & Rayner, 1981; Frazier & Rayner, 1982; Just & Carpenter, 1980).

Of primary interest is our finding that partially correct information facilitated reading. We found that visually similar letters that gave partially correct information about the letters they replaced facilitated reading (in comparison to having dissimilar letters outside the window area) as did the correct beginning of the word to the right of fixation. Furthermore, there appears to be an interaction between the types of partial information, since the facilitative effect of the visually similar letters was most pronounced in conditions where only the beginning of the word to the right of fixation was correct.

We believe that the results of our experiments are consistent with a model in which:

1. Some internal representation of a word is activated when there exists evidence for the word.
2. Feature information from parafoveal vision (or further away from fixation and hence of lower visual quality) contributes less activation than foveal information.
3. Identification of the word occurs when the activation achieves some threshold level (Ehrlich & Rayner, 1981; Morton, 1969).

According to such a model, partial word information obtained on fixation $n$ could facilitate reading in two ways. It could contribute activation sufficient to result in identification or it could merely increase activation (i.e., "prime" the word) so that the threshold is more readily reached when additional information is obtained on fixation $n + 1$. Since we have found that the availability of partial word information facilitates reading without resulting in many misidentifications, it seems reasonable to assume that the threshold for identification is set relatively high.

The finding that reading performance did not differ between the condition in which the word fixated and the word to the right of fixation were both visible and the condition in which the word fixated and the first three letters of the word to the right of fixation were visible (but the other letters of the word were replaced with visually similar letters) further suggests that partial information obtained from the word to the right of fixation is used in reading. It should be noted that on some fixations, subjects undoubtedly identified the entire word to the right of fixation. For example, when the word to the right of fixation was short it is highly likely that it was identified since the eye movement records indicate that such words were skipped a high proportion of the time. But when the word to the right of fixation was five letters or longer, there was no difference in the probability of fixating it between the two conditions.

Although it appears that subjects were obtaining partial information from para-foveal words, it is also clear that the processing of partial information was operating at an unconscious level. Although subjects in the Rayner, Well, Pollatsek and Bertera (1982) studies were often aware that parafoveal words were replaced by other letters (when only the fixated word was visible), they were not aware that letters had been replaced on every fixation. When the word to the right of fixation or the first three letters of the word to the right of fixation (with other letters replaced with visually similar letters) were visible, subjects were not aware of the letter replacements. As is clear in Table 6.1, their reading rate was slightly slower than when two or more words to the right of fixation were visible, yet it is an interesting fact that subjects showed no conscious awareness of the letter substitutions when letter information in the fovea was preserved.

## B.  Sequential versus Parallel Processing of Letters in an Eye Fixation

An issue that has been central to much theory and debate on word recognition and reading has focused on the extent to which letter processing occurs in a left-to-right serial manner. The results of many studies dealing with the presentation of isolated words seems to have led most researchers to the conclusion that serial models are not satisfactory, and they have opted for models in which letter information is processed in parallel. For reading of connected discourse, there have been numerous suggestions (Geyer, 1970; Gough, 1972) that during an eye fixation there is an internal sequential scan of the text at the rate of approximately 10 msec per character. In other words, during the fixation the mind's eye sequentially processes each letter in the text in a left to right fashion. When the eyes move, the sequential scan begins again for the currently fixated region.

The idea of a sequential scan of the text is intriguing (see McConkie, Chapter 5 of this volume and Wolverton & Zola, Chapter 3 of this volume), but there is little evidence to support such a claim. However, the idea is consistent with a couple of findings in some of our results. First, in a study in which we (Rayner et al., 1981) masked foveal vision a certain amount of time after the beginning of each fixation, we found that parafoveal information seemed to be utilized only after some initial foveal processing had been completed. Second, in an experiment reported by Rayner and Pollatsek (1981) subjects were asked to read text and at the beginning of each fixation a foveal mask was presented for a certain amount of time before the text appeared. Under some conditions in this experiment, foveal vision was completely masked but the information in parafoveal vision remained visible. In other conditions, both foveal and parafoveal vision were masked. In the former conditions, subjects could have processed the parafoveal information while the foveal mask was present and hence could have read faster than in the conditions in which both foveal and parafoveal vision was masked. However, we found no difference between the two conditions, again indicating that information in parafoveal vision is useful only after some initial foveal processing has occurred.

Both of the results discussed above are consistent with the notion that there is some type of sequential processing of text. However, in an attempt to test the Geyer hypothesis more explicitly, we (Slowiaczek & Rayner, 1982) have sequentially masked out letters at various rates during an eye fixation in an attempt to determine if we could find support for the idea that letters are scanned at the rate of approximately 10 msec each. In the first experiment, either the 7 or the 15 characters in the center of vision were masked all at once after 30, 50, or 90 msec or the characters were masked at the rate of 10 msec per letter from the inside character out or the outside character in. Table 6.3 shows an example of an inside–out mask as well as the results of the experiment. In both the inside–out and the outside–in conditions, the first characters masked were not affected until 30 msec had passed in the fixation. Thus, in the example shown in Table 6.3, the three characters in the center of vision were masked after 30 msec, then one character on each side was masked after 10 msec, and the two most extreme characters were masked 10 msec after that. As seen in Table 6.3, consistent with our prior work (Rayner et al., 1981), when the text was exposed for only 30 msec prior to the onset of the mask, reading performance deteriorated somewhat. However, we found no difference between the condition in which the entire center of

**TABLE 6.3**
**Example of Sequential Seven-Character Mask and the Results of the Experiment[a]**

thXXXXXXXine featured a story about films     50 msec

theXXXXXine featured a story about films     40 msec

the XXXazine featured a story about films     *Time*     30 msec

the magazine featured a story about films     $f_1$

| Delayed seven character mask | Reading rate (wpm) | Delayed fifteen character mask | Reading rate (wpm) |
|---|---|---|---|
| 30 | 223 | 50 | 289 |
| 30,40,50 | 281 | 50,70,90 | 280 |
| 50 | 279 | 90 | 306 |
| 50,40,30 | 238 | 90,70,50 | 293 |

[a]No mask reading rate is 346 wpm.

vision was masked after 50 msec and the condition in which the center of vision was masked sequentially from left to right (inside–out). If the mask moved from the outside in, reading performance was impaired. As can also be seen in Table 6.3, the control condition in which there was no mask resulted in faster reading rates than any of the experimental conditions. The difference between the 50-msec mask conditions and the control no-mask conditions in the Slowiaczek and Rayner (1982) study was greater than in the Rayner *et al.* (1981) study, but all other results are consistent.

One possible explanation for the results of the sequential masking study is that letters in the center of vision (in the fovea) are internally scanned one at a time at the rate of approximately 10 msec per character. However, an alternative explanation occurred to us. That is, perhaps even the central three characters are processed in the same amount of time as all the others, but because some initial processing is done on these characters when they are in the parafovea on fixation *n*, not as much time is needed when they fall in the fovea on fixation *n* + 1. This makes sense especially if the characters that are in the center of fixation or that are masked the most quickly are the ones that are just beyond the mask in the parafovea on the previous fixation. If so, the advantage of the central three characters under the sequential masking situation should go away if the parafovea were masked on each fixation so that preliminary processing of the letters beyond the mask region was impossible. We ran an experiment in which a seven-character window moved in synchrony with the eye and the seven characters in the center of vision were masked from inside out or outside in. Table 6.4 shows the results of the experiment. Under the conditions in which the parafoveal letters

### TABLE 6.4
### Example of Seven-Character Window with Delayed Sequential Mask and the Results of the Experiment

Seven-character sequential mask 30, 40, 50

          xxxxxxxxxxxxxxxxxxxxxxxxxxxxxxxxxxxxxxxxxxxxx                     50 msec

      xxexxxxxzxxxxxxxxxxxxxxxxxxxxxxxxxxxxxxxxxxx                           40 msec

    xxe xxxxazxxxxxxxxxxxxxxxxxxxxxxxxxxxxxxxxxxx                            30 msec

xxe magazxxxxxxxxxxxxxxxxxxxxxxxxxxxxxxxxxxx                                 f₁

| Mask delay (msec) | Reading rate (wpm) |
| --- | --- |
| 30 | 122 |
| 30,40,50 | 130 |
| 50 | 150 |
| 50,60,70 | 156 |
| No mask | 200 |

were masked, we found that reading performance in the sequential masking situation was the same as in the condition in which the entire window area was masked after 30 msec and both of these conditions resulted in poorer reading performance than when the entire window area was masked after 50 msec.

The results of the second Slowiaczek and Rayner (1982) experiment indicate that there is not a sequential scan of the material in the fovea; rather the letters are processed more rapidly because of some preliminary processing that occurred when they were in parafoveal vision on the prior fixation. This conclusion is in basic agreement with the results of the experiments described in the prior section which indicated that partial information is acquired from parafoveal vision and that some letters have already received some prior processing.

## C.  Summary of Perceptual Span Research

The work that we have recently completed on the perceptual span indicates that readers acquire useful information out to about 15 characters to the right of fixation. It appears that spatial information about word length is acquired furthest from fixation and that this information is useful in guiding eye movements to the next location. Specific letter information appears to be acquired no more than two words to the right of fixation. When the currently fixated word and two words to the right of fixation are visible to the reader, reading performance is no different from that in a condition in which the entire line is visible provided the spaces between words are left intact. Furthermore, we have found that the field of effective vision is better defined in terms of the number of letters visible on each fixation than in terms of the number of words visible. Reading performance when word integrity was maintained could be predicted from knowing how many letters were visible, but performance when the window was defined in terms of number of letters could not be predicted in terms of the number of words visible. The implication of this result is that partial information is acquired from words in parafoveal vision. In fact, when we compared performance in a condition in which the fixated word and the word to the right of fixation were visible with a condition in which the fixated word and the first three letters of the word to the right of fixation (with remaining letters replaced with visually similar words) were visible, we found that reading performance did not differ. This result implies that on many fixations the fixated word is processed along with the first few letters of the upcoming word. This preliminary letter processing of the beginning of the upcoming word presumably speeds up the reading process so that readers can read considerably faster when this partial information is available than when it is not. Of course, if the next word is a short word, having three letters visible beyond the fixated word would allow words of three or fewer characters to be processed on that fixation without the word ever being fixated. Such a conclusion is consistent with the fact that short words are fixated much less frequently than longer words in reading text (Rayner & McConkie, 1976).

Finally, although we have found some evidence that parafoveal information is utilized after the foveal information has been processed, we have not found evidence consistent with the notion that letters are scanned at the rate of approximately 10 msec per letter. In one experiment, we did find results that were consistent with the idea that the letters in the center of vision are scanned at the rate of 10 msec per letter. However, in a subsequent experiment we found that the effect disappeared when the letters in parafoveal vision were masked on each fixation such that the only letters available were those in the center of vision. We take the fact that there was no evidence for a scan when the parafoveal letters were masked as evidence for the fact that letters falling in the center of vision on fixation $n$ received some preliminary processing on fixation $n - 1$ when they were in parafoveal vision. Again, this conclusion is consistent with our other observations that partial information is acquired from the beginning of words falling in parafoveal vision.

## III.   Timing Constraints and Programming Eye Movements

Although the results of research concerning the characteristics of the perceptual span have been quite consistent across a number of laboratories, work on the characteristics of programming of eye movements has been quite controversial. Some researchers (e.g., Bouma & deVoogd, 1974) have assumed that the time necessary to encode words and then direct the eye movement is slow enough so that the text actually viewed on a fixation only makes its presence felt no sooner than one fixation later. According to this view, there simply is not sufficient time during a fixation to process the text and program the eye movement contingent upon that processing. Since the typical eye movement latency is 175–200 msec and the average fixation during reading is about 200–250 msec, it is assumed that it would be unfeasible to program eye movements based on only the first 50–75 msec on each fixation.

Others (e.g., Just & Carpenter, 1980; McConkie, 1979; Rayner, 1979b; Rayner & McConkie, 1976) have suggested that the decisions of how long the eye is to remain at a fixation and where to move next are directly controlled by information extracted from the text processed on the current fixation. Just and Carpenter (1980) have suggested that the estimate of 175–200 msec for eye movement programming time is too long and that something in the neighborhood of 50 msec is more reasonable. That is, the estimate of 175–200 msec is often obtained from tasks in which the subject is fixating on a target and the target suddenly jumps to another position. The time for the eye to move to the new location of the target is measured as the latency period. This situation, Just and Carpenter suggest, is vastly unlike the situation in reading in which the eye is making a series of movements (usually in a left to right direction).

In essence then, Just and Carpenter suggest that the oculomotor reaction time of the eye in an ongoing task like reading has been considerably overestimated. In another vein, it is worth noting that Rayner *et al.* (1981) presented a visual mask a certain amount of time after the onset of a fixation and found that if the mask was delayed 50 msec or longer, reading was not appreciably hampered. Thus, it is possible that much of the visual information necessary for reading can be acquired during the first 50 msec of a fixation, leaving the remainder of the fixation period to complete programming the next eye movement and for higher level linguistic processing. The point is that if one accepts either 50 msec for stimulus encoding time (Rayner *et al.*, 1981) or 50 msec for eye programming time, then direct control of eye movements based on the information extracted from the text processed on the current fixation is possible.

## A.  Direct Control of Eye Movements

In an attempt to determine if direct control of eye movements occurs during reading, Rayner and Pollatsek (1981) asked subjects to read text as a window moved in synchrony with their eye movements. One finding that has been very consistent in the prior research using the "window" technique is that as window size decreased, the average saccade length decreased. However, rather than the decrease being due to moment to moment changes in programming the saccade, one could easily argue that the results were due to some type of global strategy in which the reader realized that there was a small window on each fixation and accordingly adjusted the saccadic behavior to move a shorter distance on each saccade than when a larger window was available. Hence, Rayner and Pollatsek (1981) made the size of the window variable from fixation to fixation so that on any given fixation the size of the window was different from previous window sizes, yet the reader was not consciously aware of the size of the window on any fixation.

The interesting question in the experiment was whether or not subjects would be able to adjust the length of the saccade to correspond to the information available within the window on the current fixation. As seen in Table 6.5, there was no difference in the length of the saccade for any given window size between the fixed window condition in which the size of the window was constant from fixation to fixation and the variable window condition in which the size of the window varied from fixation to fixation. This result demonstrates that the length

TABLE 6.5
Mean Saccade Length in Fixed and Variable Window Condition[a]

|  | Window size (characters) | | |
| --- | --- | --- | --- |
|  | 9 | 17 | 33 |
| Fixed window | 4.6 | 5.9 | 6.9 |
| Variable window | 5.0 | 5.9 | 6.8 |

[a]From Rayner and Pollatsek (1981).

of the saccade is influenced by the characteristics of the information available on the current fixation. However, it was also found that the size of the window on the prior fixation also influenced the length of the saccade. That is, if the window on fixation $n$ was 17 characters, subjects tended to move their eyes a greater distance if the window on fixation $n - 1$ was 33 characters than if it was 9 characters. In fact, the effects due to the size of the window on fixation $n - 1$ were as strong as were those of fixation $n$ suggesting that the determination of where to look next is made on the basis of a combination of the information available from the current fixation and from the preceding fixation.

In a subsequent experiment, Rayner and Pollatsek (1981) delayed the onset of the text by presenting a visual mask at the end of each saccade. The duration of the mask varied between 25 and 300 msec but was constant on a given trial. We found that as text delay increased, fixation duration increased; although the overall linear fit of the fixation durations was quite good, it did appear that the eye overadjusts its delay for the short text delay conditions. Again, it could be argued that subjects were adjusting the duration via a global strategy; that is, on the first couple of fixations the subject realized that the text delay was long and so set up a global program so as to have longer fixation durations. Thus, in another study, Rayner and Pollatsek (1981) compared performance when the text delay was variable from fixation to fixation. Table 6.6 shows the results of the experiment. As in the prior experiment in which saccade length was compared for fixed and variable windows, there was no difference between the fixed and variable text delays, suggesting that fixation durations are directly controlled on a moment to moment basis. However, just as we had to qualify the conclusion with regard to saccade length, it was also necessary to qualify this conclusion because in the conditions in which the text delay was long (over 200 msec) subjects moved their eyes a high percentage of time (18% when the text delay was 200 msec and 43% when the text delay was 300 msec) prior to the onset of the text. The finding that fixation duration is increased less than the text delay for short delays together with the presence of fixations shorter than the text delay (in the long text delay conditions) suggests that certain decisions to move the eye are programmed either before the fixation begins or are programmed during the fixation but without regard to the visual display fixated on.

TABLE 6.6
Mean Fixation Duration for Variable and Fixed Delays[a]

|  | Delay (msec) | | | |
|---|---|---|---|---|
|  | 25 | 50 | 75 | 100 |
| Fixed delay | 247 | 253 | 264 | 283 |
| Variable delay | 252 | 259 | 266 | 274 |

[a]From Rayner and Pollatsek (1981).

The general thrust of the experiments reported by Rayner and Pollatsek (1981) is that there is direct control of eye movements on a moment to moment basis and that the characteristics of the text on the current fixation influences where the reader will look next and when the eye movement occurs. However, it is also clear that information from the previous fixation influences these decisions as well. Rayner and Pollatsek (1981) concluded that the results of their experiments provide support for a mixed control model of eye movements in reading in which decisions about when and where to move the eyes are based on information from the current fixation, the prior fixations, and possibly other sources.

## B.  Temporal Factors in Programming the Eye Movement

Much of the research on the characteristics of saccades during reading has demonstrated that word length characteristics are important in guiding the eye movements. The data (as reviewed by Rayner, 1978a, and Rayner & Inhoff, 1981) indicate that fixation locations are related to word length patterns in the text and that the reader is quite sensitive to space information. First, there is a differential probability that a letter within a word will be fixated as a function of the length of the word the letter is in: The probability is higher that a letter in a word 4–7 letters long will be fixated than if the letter is in a shorter or longer word (Rayner & McConkie, 1976). Second, the length of the word to the right of the currently fixated word has an influence on the length of the subsequent saccade (O'Regan, 1975; Rayner, 1979a): If the word to the right of fixation is longer, the eye tends to jump further than if a shorter word is there (unless the word is very short, in which case it will often be skipped altogether). Third, locations of fixations within words are not random but tend to follow a pattern such that the reader tends to fixate on a preferred viewing location. The preferred viewing location tends to be between the middle and beginning of the word; the preferred viewing location in a 5-letter word is the second letter and for a 10-letter word it is the fourth letter (Rayner, 1979a). Finally, experiments in which spacing between words in the parafovea and periphery is filled in (so that the reader has no information about the length of words to be fixated in parafoveal vision) have demonstrated that reading is severely impaired by the obliteration of the space information (Ikeda & Saida, 1978; McConkie & Rayner, 1975; O'Regan, 1975; Rayner & Bertera, 1979; Rayner et al., 1981; Spragins, Lefton, & Fisher, 1976). The closer to foveal fixation that word spacing is destroyed, the more severe is the reading impairment. All of these factors combine to make it very clear that where the eye fixates next in reading is related to word length and spacing between the words in the text.

The work described in the preceding sections also implies (as does the fact that the length of the word to the right of fixation influences saccade length) that the information about word length patterns to the right of fixation on the current fixation influences how far the eye will move. Furthermore, the work of Rayner *et al.* (1981) suggests that readers can take advantage of the visual information in the text very early in the fixation to program the next eye movement. As indicated previously, Rayner *et al.* presented a homogeneous masking pattern that appeared in foveal vision and moved in synchrony with the eye movements or was delayed in its onset for various amounts of time at the beginning of each fixation. It was found that if the onset of the mask was delayed for 50 msec on each fixation then the reading rate was only slightly slower in the control condition in which no mask was presented and the rate did not differ from conditions in which the onset of the mask was delayed for 100 or 150 msec. Thus, the results of this experiment suggest that readers can extract most of the useful information in reading, including the information needed to program the eye movement, during the first 50 msec of a fixation.

In an attempt to examine more explicitly the relationship between the use of word length and the timing factors involved in programming eye movements, Pollatsek and Rayner (1982) have conducted some studies in which the spaces between words to the right of fixation were filled in a certain amount of time into each fixation. The spaces between the words were filled in with random letters, digits, or one of two types of masking gratings. One type of grating was a small segment of the visual mask used previously in the Rayner *et al.* (1981) study and consisted of a square wave grating that filled the space between successive words. The other type of masking grating was separated so that the region above and below the spaces between words was filled in but the actual spaces were preserved. This condition was a control condition used to determine if the occurrence of a stimulus a certain amount of time into the fixation in and of itself resulted in disruption of the reading process. In one condition, all of the spaces between words to the right of fixation were filled in. In a second condition, the space between the word currently fixated and the word to the right of fixation was left intact, but all other spaces were filled in. The spaces were filled in 25, 50, 100, or 150 msec after the beginning of fixation. In the control conditions, the spaces were never filled in or they were filled in throughout the entire fixation. Table 6.7 shows the reading rates in two separate experiments in which the spaces between words were filled at a certain point in the fixation.

One result that is clear from the experiments is that if the space between the currently fixated word and the word to the right of fixation is left intact, filling in the rest of the spaces between words has very little effect after 50 msec. This result is consistent with results reported previously by Rayner *et al.* (1981). However, a somewhat different pattern emerges when the space next to fixation is filled in. Whereas reading performance reached asymptote at 50 msec in the conditions in which the space next to the fixated word was preserved, when that space was filled in reading performance never did reach asymptote and was always poorer than in the control condition. It is also clear from Table 6.7, that the characteristics of the space filler have an effect on the amount of disruption. Letters result in more disruption than digits, which in turn result in more disruption than the gratings. It is probably the case that whatever inconsistency there is between the Rayner *et al.* (1981) study and the data of Wolverton and Zola

TABLE 6.7
Reading Rate in the Pollatsek and Rayner (1982) Experiments[a]

**Experiment 1**

| | | | Delay | | |
|---|---|---|---|---|---|
| | 0 | 25 | 50 | 100 | 150 |
| Letters | | | | | |
| All filled | 130 | 174 | 212 | 237 | 270 |
| First preserved | 272 | 267 | 290 | 310 | 307 |
| Digits | | | | | |
| All filled | 179 | 216 | 247 | 279 | 297 |
| First preserved | 269 | 280 | 313 | 312 | 315 |

**Experiment 2**

| | | Delay | |
|---|---|---|---|
| | 25 | 50 | 100 |
| Letters | | | |
| All filled | 183 | 208 | 272 |
| First preserved | 274 | 306 | 332 |
| Gratings | | | |
| All filled | 238 | 271 | 287 |
| First preserved | 282 | 322 | 336 |
| Separated gratings | | | |
| All filled | 309 | 338 | 335 |
| First preserved | 344 | 333 | 340 |

[a] The reading rate in a control condition for Experiment 1 averaged 312 wpm and for Experiment 2 averaged 346 wpm.

(Chapter 3 of this volume) is at least partially due to the characteristics of the masking pattern used. Note that the results of the Pollatsek and Rayner (1982) study also make it clear that the disruption in reading when spaces are filled can be localized to actually filling the spaces. The separated grating condition (even when the space next to fixation was involved) had a slight disruption effect when the pattern appeared 25 msec into the fixation, but no other effect.

Pollatsek and Rayner (1982) concluded that filling in the space next to fixation not only interferes with programming the next eye movement, but it also interferes with word recognition processes both by obscuring the right-hand boundary of the word and by interfering with processing the final letters of the word. We also concluded that filling in all the spaces but the first space primarily interferred with programming the next eye movement. Thus, we proposed (see also Rayner & Pollatsek, 1981) a two-process model of eye movement control in reading. One process decides approximately where the eye should move to, largely utilizing word boundary information, and usually making the decision by 50 msec after the beginning of the fixation. The other process identifies foveal words and letters, and on a typical fixation, the eye movement is made with a latency of about

125–175 msec after the decision has been made where to send the eyes. However, if the mechanism monitoring foveal word identification has difficulty, it may postpone the forward eye movement or even program a regression. The first-space preserved conditions in the Pollatsek and Rayner (1982) study appear to be chiefly influencing the first process; whereas the all-filled conditions appear to be influencing both processes.

An alternative position to that proposed by the two-process model of Rayner and Pollatsek (1981) would be that the programming for a new eye movement begins about 50 msec after the beginning of the fixation and the exact details about where to move to are determined throughout the fixation. In its simplest form, such an alternative closely corresponds to the preprogramming model described by Vaughan (Chapter 23 of this volume). According to such a model, the duration of any fixation is determined prior to the beginning of the fixation. It would take more sophisticated explanations to work out a model in which the programming of the next eye movement begins roughly 50 msec into the fixation with more precise details about when and where to move filled in throughout the fixation. Hence, at the moment, I believe that the results of the experiments described in this section can most parsimoniously be explained by the two-process model of Rayner and Pollatsek (1981).

One final point should be made with respect to the Pollatsek and Rayner (1982) findings. As indicated above, we found that in the all spaces filled condition that filling in spaces interferes with reading at delays of greater than 50 msec. This seems inconsistent with the findings of Rayner *et al.* (1981) mentioned earlier. The Rayner *et al.* findings suggest either that all of the useful letter information is extracted from the fovea in 50 msec or that it is transferred to a "buffer" storage by then and the information in that store is unaffected by masking. For either interpretation of the Rayner *et al.* data, it is difficult to see why filling in the spaces (especially with gratings that are segments of the masking stimulus used by Rayner *et al.*) should have an effect at 100 msec or greater, since the visual information appears to be irrelevant at that time. One possible explanation is that readers usually spend the last 150 msec or so of each fixation primarily doing nonvisual processing (such as syntactic and higher level semantic processing), but that some visual events could disrupt this processing and cause the visual system to recompute the visual information processed. A uniform stimulus such as the square wave grating mask used by Rayner *et al.* might not have that power, since the visual system might be able to dismiss it as noise; whereas a stimulus that is still recognizably text, but with word boundaries altered, might not be as easy to ignore.

## C.   Eye Movement Latency in the Reading Situation

The final issue to be touched upon in this chapter concerns the actual oculomotor reaction time of the eye in a task like reading. As indicated earlier, Just and Carpenter (1980) have suggested that the typical estimate of 175–200 msec for saccadic latency is an overestimation of the oculomotor reaction time during reading. They argue that the estimate is typically based on a situation in which subjects are fixating (with their eyes in "cement") on a target stimulus (a cross or an asterisk) that is suddenly displaced in the visual field. The subject is instructed to move to the new target location as soon as possible. Just and Carpenter have suggested that this situation is unlike the normal reading situation in which the reader is constantly making eye movements and these movements are generally in a left to right manner. They further suggest that there is not much spatial uncertainty in the reading situation since the reader typically moves from the center of one word to the center of the next word. One problem with their argument is that the distance the eye moves is not simply from the middle of one word to the middle of the next. Many words are not fixated (as pointed out in this volume by Hogaboam, Chapter 18) and although there appear to be preferred viewing locations in words (O'Regan, 1980, Rayner, 1979), it is also the case that fixations are not all on the preferred location (as pointed out by McConkie, Chapter 5 in this volume).

Another problem with the Just and Carpenter suggestion is that in tasks that can be thought of as simulating the reading situation without the necessity of encoding stimuli, one still ends up with an estimate of approximately 175–200 msec for the oculomotor reaction time of the eye. For example, Arnold and Tinker (1939) asked subjects to sequentially fixate on each target of an array presented on a screen as quickly as they could. This task simulates the reading situation in that the subject is moving from left to right and there is no spatial or temporal uncertainty. Arnold and Tinker measured the time from the start of one fixation to the onset of the next eye movement as the oculomotor latency and again found average latencies in the range of 175–200 msec (see also Salthouse & Ellis, 1980).

In some experiments using somewhat more sophisticated techniques than those of Arnold and Tinker, we (Rayner, Slowiaczek, Clifton, & Bertera, 1982) asked people to quickly move their eyes from left to right under conditions of spatial uncertainty, temporal uncertainty, or spatial and temporal uncertainty. In a control condition, we asked subjects to move their eyes as quickly as they could fixating each of seven targets placed unequal distances apart but in the range approximating normal saccade lengths in reading. Average latencies in the task were approximately 210 msec. In the condition in which there was temporal and spatial uncertainty, subjects fixated on the initial target location (target $n$) and the next fixation target ($n + 1$) appeared. When they moved their eyes to target $n + 1$, target $n + 2$ appeared, and so on. The location of the next target could be anywhere from 1–4° to the right of the prior target, thus creating spatial uncertainty. Temporal uncertainty was created by delaying the onset of one of the seven targets by 50 or 150 msec on each trial. For targets not delayed, the average latency was again about 210 msec. For the targets that were delayed, the average latency was 260 msec in the 50 msec delay condition and 375 msec in the 150 msec delay condition.

In the condition in which there was only temporal uncertainty, the entire array was presented to the subject, but the subject was told to only make an eye movement to the next target when a square (serving as a temporal cue) surrounded the target. The onset of the cue was randomized and we found a latency of about 185 msec for the onset of the saccade following the onset of the cue. In the spatial uncertainty condition, subjects were presented with a new target for fixation every 400 msec, but the exact spatial location was not indicated. In this condition, the average latency was 181 msec. Thus, we found evidence that latencies were shorter when there was only temporal or spatial uncertainty than when there were both types. However, as in a number of previous experiments in which subjects were required to sequentially fixate on a number of target locations, we found that the average latencies were in the range of 175–225 msec. Thus, it appears that an acceptable account of eye movement factors during reading will have to contend with the fact that the oculomotor reaction time of the eye is relatively long considering the average length of fixations in reading.

## D. Summary of Timing Constraints and Programming Eye Movements Research

The work that we (Rayner, Slowiaczek, Clifton & Bertera, 1982) have completed dealing with the timing factors involved in programming eye movements during reading suggests that the simple oculomotor reaction time in reading averages roughly 175 msec. Consistent with work done on simple eye movement latencies, we find most of the latencies ranging between 100 and 300 msec. In the final section of this chapter I will attempt to relate this finding to some of the other findings concerning temporal factors in information acquisition during a fixation and programming the next eye movement.

We (Rayner et. al, 1981) have also found evidence to indicate that much of the information necessary for reading can be acquired during the first 50 msec of an eye fixation. This is not to say that information is not acquired at other points in time during the fixation. In fact, we have found that parafoveal information is processed only after the foveal information has been processed first. In experiments in which a visual mask moved in synchrony with the eye (Rayner et al., 1981) and in which the text in the center of vision was delayed in its onset by the presentation of a visual mask at the end of each saccade (Rayner & Pollatsek, 1981), we found that readers apparently were unable to take advantage of text in the parafovea until after the foveal information was available. Thus, our results at this point lead us to the conclusion that most of the information necessary for reading can be obtained from the foveal region during the first 50 msec of a fixation and that information in parafoveal vision is processed later in the fixation. However, it is also apparently the case that information presented to the foveal region throughout the fixation influences processing. Thus, if a change in the text presented in the fovea occurs at any point in the fixation, reading will be disrupted (Pollatsek & Rayner, 1982; Wolverton & Zola, Chapter 3 of this volume).

Finally, we (Rayner and Pollatsek, 1981) have found evidence that indicates that information available on the current fixation influences both the duration of the current fixation and the length of the subsequent saccade. On the other hand, we also found some evidence consistent with the notion that some fixations are preprogrammed and that information available on fixation $n - 1$ has as strong an influence on the subsequent saccade as does the information available on fixation $n$. In this regard it is also worth noting that in other experiments in our laboratory (Ehrlich & Rayner, 1981; Frazier & Rayner, 1982) it has been observed that the characteristics of text encountered on the current fixation influenced fixation duration not only for the current fixation but also for the next fixation. Thus, although it is clear that the information encountered on the current fixation influences the duration of the fixation and the following saccade, it is also clear that there are lag effects from the prior fixation (see also McConkie, Chapter 5 of this volume; O'Regan, 1980).

## IV.   Process Monitoring in Reading

The general characteristics of the experiments and the results described in this chapter lead toward a model of reading that has been referred to as a process monitoring model (cf., McConkie, 1979; Rayner, 1979b; Rayner & Inhoff, 1981; Rayner & McConkie, 1976). This model assumes that some mechanism is monitoring the various activities of the reading process and that eye movements are determined by this mechanism and influenced by the characteristics of the text. In short, fixation duration and saccade length are influenced by the cognitive processing state of the reader and by the characteristics of the visual patterns in the text.

During the fixation in reading, the reader is able to obtain information from a region extending from the beginning of the currently fixated word (but no more than 3 characters to the left of fixation) to about 15 characters to the right of fixation. It should be noted that this estimate is indeed an average and there could well be variability in the extent of the effective visual field just as there is variability in the length of the saccade (Rayner & McConkie, 1976) and as we have demonstrated in a number of experiments, the type of information that the reader is able to obtain varies directly with the distance from the fixation point. In the center of vision (the foveal region) and perhaps the beginning of the parafoveal region, readers are able to obtain the type of information that leads directly to word identification. However it is clear that information obtained from parafoveal vision is primarily partial information about words located there that cannot directly be used to access the meaning of that particular word. Rather, that partial information (about specific letters) is used on the subsequent fixation to identify the word. Slightly further into parafoveal vision (and extending out to 15 characters to the right of fixation), readers are able to acquire word length information that is useful in determining where to fixate next.

Elsewhere, we (Rayner, McConkie, & Zola, 1980; Rayner, Well, Pollatsek, &

Bertera, 1982) have proposed that readers engage in some type of preliminary letter identification on fixation $n$ for the beginning letters of words falling in parafoveal vision. That is, the reader tries to identify words as far to the right of fixation as possible and when acuity limitations and/or lateral masking factors make it impossible to correctly identify a word, the reader makes preliminary letter identifications of the letters beginning the next words. We further suggested that for words that cannot be completely identified, preliminary letter identification of the first three letters occurs. Thus, for example, the reader may be able to unambiguously identify (at an unconscious level) the first letter as a $p$, that the second letter is an $a$, $o$, $e$, or $c$, and that the third letter is an $l$, $t$, or $f$. Given that the text is presented in lower case, it is not at all surprising that a number of experiments (McConkie and Rayner, 1975; Rayner, 1975; Rayner & Bertera, 1979; Rayner, Well, Pollatsek, Bertera, 1982) have found what looks like evidence that word shape information is obtained from parafoveal vision. In reality, it might simply be that the preliminary letter identification process biases the results toward letters that are visually similar (Rayner, McConkie, & Zola, 1980). Hence, it seems that results indicating that word shape is a useful cue obtained from parafoveal vision are really due to the fact that word shape is a product of the letter features comprising the word.

Our experiments (Rayner et al., 1981) also suggest that much of the information necessary for reading can be acquired during the first 50 msec of a fixation. It is certainly the case, as suggested previously, that other information can be acquired throughout the fixation. In fact, presenting certain types of information foveally disrupts reading throughout the fixation (Pollatsek & Rayner, 1982) and the parafoveal information seems to be processed only after the foveal information has been processed. Although this latter statement implies some clear left to right processing, we (Slowiaczek & Rayner, 1982) found no evidence that letter information in the fovea is scanned at the rate of 10 msec per letter.

It appears that during the first 50 msec of the fixation, the reader determines a tentative region to fixate next. This determination is made on the basis of the word length characteristics of upcoming words and some estimate of how far to the right of fixation words can be identified. The mechanism monitoring the reading process makes this determination primarily on the basis of word length patterns close to fixation. Thus, if two short words fall in the center of vision, the eyes will be sent beyond the word to the right of fixation because both words can be identified on that fixation. On the other hand, if the next word is a long word, the eyes will be sent to the preferred viewing location (on average) to maximally process the content of that location. Occasionally, the eyes will be sent too far (or not far enough) which will cause adjustments in the fixation location (O'Regan, 1980).

When the determination of where to go next has been made (and we believe this is done fairly early in the fixation), the movement is programmed with an oculomotor latency of approximately 125–175 msec. During the time that the program for the saccade is being put into effect, higher level processing activities are under way. The meaning of the fixated word is accessed and various higher order syntactic and semantic processes are undertaken. There is clear evidence (see Rayner, 1978a; Ehrlich & Rayner, 1981) that the characteristics of the word being fixated influences the fixation duration. What is less clear is the extent to which all activities related to that word are completed prior to the eye moving from that word. In fact, other data collected in our laboratory and described elsewhere in this volume implies that certain syntactic and semantic processes related to that word are still occurring after the eyes have left that particular word and have moved to a new location. It is also the case that while readers are engaged in higher level activities with respect to the fixated material, lower level processes are occurring with respect to the nonfixated material. The reader tries to get as much useful information from as far to the right of fixation as possible. Given acuity limitations and lateral masking constraints, for words outside the center of vision the reader is able to extract via preliminary letter identification only partial information. However, this partial information obtained on fixation $n$ is useful in more quickly accessing the meaning of that word on fixation $n + 1$ when the word is directly fixated. As should be evident from this discussion, words are processed when they lie just to the right of fixation. Such an argument is quite consistent with the fact that words longer than seven characters are fixated about 95% of the time whereas the probability of fixating on a shorter word decreases as word length decreases.

Our proposal is that the process monitoring activities involved in accessing the lexicon are generally quite consistent with the oculomotor latency so that the meaning has usually been obtained for the fixated word by the time that the eye movement occurs. Syntactic parsing strategies (Frazier & Rayner, 1982) may also be well underway during the fixation, but it is probably the case that certain higher level semantic integration processes are not completed by the time the saccade occurs. It may also be the case that on some occasions, such as when the word fixated is extremely rare (or unusual) or when a nonword is presented in the text, fixation duration is lengthened and the subject moves the eye to a new location to try and use contextual information to determine the meaning of the word. This brings up the interesting question of what happens when fixations are lengthened. In essence, I have been arguing that information input to the process monitoring system occurs during the first 50 msec or so and that an eye movement will occur with a latency of approximately 125–175 msec thereafter. Thus, a certain amount of the variability in fixation duration is due to variability in programming the eye movement. However, it is well known (Rayner & McConkie, 1976) that many fixations fall into the range of 225–450 msec and that a fair percentage of fixations exceed 450 msec. One possibility is that once the program has been set up for the movement, the reader can put the move on "hold" when difficulty arises in accessing the meaning of the fixated word. Hence, the reader continues searching the lexicon until the meaning of the word is found, or the reader decides to move on and use contextual information to disambiguate the meaning. In either case, the process monitoring mechanism holds until sufficient information is available and then moves to the location already programmed. The alternative is that the reader "aborts" the initially planned saccade staying in the new location to get more information and then programs a new saccade (perhaps to the originally planned location if the lexical search is successful and, perhaps, a new saccade if unsuccessful).

According to these two alternatives, in one situation the reader holds on executing the saccade and in the other condition aborts the saccade and programs a new one contingent on some type of resolution or the decision that context might help. Note that in the latter condition, the abort command would not necessarily have to come at the end of the oculomotor latency. The decision to abort could come at any time during the fixation. In fact, there is good reason based upon double-step experiments with simple stimuli (Komoda, Festinger, Phillips, Duckman, & Young, 1973) to assume that if the abort decision came within 50–100 msec prior to the actual movement the reader would have to move to the planned location and then program a new movement. In such cases, it may be that although the reader cannot alter the movement to the previously determined location, he or she might be able to start programming the location for fixation $n + 2$ at the end of fixation $n$. In such a case, the duration of fixation $n + 1$ would be relatively brief. Such reasoning is certainly also consistent with the finding that fixations prior to regressions tend to be shorter than other fixations (cf., Rayner, 1978a). At the present time, I know of no evidence to distinguish between these two alternatives and it is quite possible that both types of activities are likely to occur during reading depending upon the particular context and timing factors involved.

In summary, I have tried to sketch some of the characteristics of the research carried on in our laboratory dealing with (a) the perceptual span; and (b) timing constraints related to programming eye movements. Although much progress has been made in understanding the perceptual processes during reading, many of the conclusions are only tentative. Additional focused research on various aspects of perceptual processes in reading will be necessary to completely unravel the fascinating mystery.

# References

Arnold, D., & Tinker, M. A. (1939). The fixational pause of the eyes. *Journal of Experimental Psychology, 25,* 271–280.

Bouma, H., & deVoogd, A. H. (1974). On the control of eye saccades in reading. *Vision Research, 14,* 273–284.

Den Buurman, R., Boersema, T., & Gerrissen, J. F. (1981). Eye movements and the perceptual span in reading. *Reading Research Quarterly, 16,* 227–235.

Ehrlich, S. F., & Rayner, K. (1981). Contextual effects on word perception and eye movements during reading. *Journal of Verbal Learning and Verbal Behavior, 20,* 641–655.

Frazier, L., & Rayner, K. (1982). Making and correcting errors during sentence comprehension: Eye movements in the analysis of structurally ambiguous sentences. *Cognitive Psychology, 14,* 178–210.

Geyer, J. J. (1970). Models of perceptual process in reading. In H. Singer & R. B. Ruddell (Eds.), *Theoretical models and processes of reading*. Newark, Delaware: International Reading Association.

Gough, P. B. (1972). One second of reading. In J. F. Kavanagh & I. G. Mattingly (Eds.), *Language by ear and by eye*. Cambridge, Massachusetts: MIT Press.

Ikeda, M., & Saida, S. (1978). Span of recognition in reading. *Vision Research, 18*, 83–88.

Just, M. A., & Carpenter, P. A. (1980). A theory of reading: From eye fixations to comprehension. *Psychological Review, 87*, 329–354.

Komoda, M. K., Festinger, L., Phillips, L. J., Duckman, R. H., & Young, R. A. (1973). Some observations concerning saccadic eye movements. *Vision Research, 13*, 1009–1020.

McConkie, G. W. (1979). On the role and control of eye movements in reading. In P. A. Kolers, M. E. Wrolstad, & H. Bouma (Eds.), *Processing of visible language 1*. New York: Plenum Press.

McConkie, G. W., & Rayner, K. (1975). The span of the effective stimulus during a fixation in reading. *Perception & Psychophysics, 17*, 578–586.

McConkie, G. W., & Zola, D. (1979). Is visual information integrated across successive fixations in reading? *Perception & Psychophysics, 25*, 221–224.

Morton, J. (1969). Interaction of information in word recognition. *Psychological Review, 76*, 165–178.

O'Regan, J. K. (1975). Structural and contextual constraints on eye movements in reading. Unpublished doctoral dissertation, University of Cambridge, 1975.

O'Regan, K. (1980). The control of saccade size and fixation duration in reading: The limits of linguistic control, *Perception & Psychophysics 28*, 112–117.

Pollatsek, A., Bolozky, S., Well, A. D., & Rayner, K. (1981). Asymmetries in the perceptual span for Israeli readers. *Brain and Language, 14*, 174–180.

Pollatsek, A. & Rayner, K. (1982). Eye movement control in reading: The role of word boundaries. *Journal of Experimental Psychology: Human Perception & Performance, 8*, 817–833.

Rayner, K. (1975). The perceptual span and peripheral cues in reading. *Cognitive Psychology, 7*, 65–81.

Rayner, K. (1978). Eye movements in reading and information processing. *Psychological Bulletin, 85*, 618–660. (a)

Rayner, K. (1978). Foveal and parafoveal cues in reading. In J. Requin (Ed.), *Attention and performance VII*. Hillsdale, New Jersey: Erlbaum. (b)

Rayner, K. (1979). Eye guidance in reading: Fixation locations in words. *Perception, 8*, 21–30. (a)

Rayner, K. (1979). Eye movements in reading: Eye guidance and integration. In P. A. Kolers, M. E. Wrolstad, & H. Bouma (Eds.), *Processing of visible language 1*. New York: Plenum Press. (b)

Rayner, K. (1981). Eye movements and the perceptual span in reading. In F. J. Pirozzolo & M. C. Wittrock (Eds.), *Neuropsychological and cognitive processes in reading*. New York: Academic Press.

Rayner, K., & Bertera, J. H. (1979). Reading without a fovea. *Science, 206*, 468–469.

Rayner, K., & Inhoff, A. W. (1981). Control of eye movements during reading. In B. L. Zuber (Ed.), *Models of oculomotor behavior and control*. Boca Raton, Florida: CRC Press.

Rayner, K., Inhoff, A. W., Morrison, R. E., Slowiaczek, M. L., & Bertera, J. H. (1981). Masking of foveal and parafoveal vision during eye fixations in reading. *Journal of Experimental Psychology: Human Perception and Performance, 7*, 167–179.

Rayner, K., & McConkie, G. W. (1976). What guides a reader's eye movements? *Vision Research, 16*, 829–837.

Rayner, K., McConkie, G. W., & Ehrlich, S. (1978). Eye movements and integrating information across fixations. *Journal of Experimental Psychology: Human Perception & Performance, 4*, 529–544.

Rayner, K., McConkie, G. W., & Zola, D. (1980). Integrating information across eye movements. *Cognitive Psychology, 12*, 206–226.

Rayner, K., & Pollatsek, A. (1981). Eye movement control during reading: Evidence for direct control. *Quarterly Journal of Experimental Psychology, 33A*, 351–373.

Rayner, K., Slowiaczek, M. L., Clifton, C. E., & Bertera, J. H. (1982). Latency of sequential eye movements. Unpublished manuscript, 1982.

Rayner, K., Well, A. D., & Pollatsek, A. (1980). Asymmetry of the effective visual field in reading. *Perception & Psychophysics, 27,* 537–544.

Rayner, K., Well, A. D., Pollatsek, A., & Bertera, J. H. (1982). The availability of useful information to the right of fixation in reading, *Perception & Psychophysics, 31,* 537–550.

Salthouse, T. A., & Ellis, C. L. (1980). Determinants of eye fixation duration. *American Journal of Psychology, 93,* 207–234.

Slowiaczek, M. L., & Rayner, K. (1982). Sequential masking during eye fixations. Unpublished manuscript, 1982.

Spragins, A. B., Lefton, L. A., & Fisher, D. F. (1976). Eye movements while reading spatially transformed text: A developmental study. *Memory & Cognition, 4,* 36–42.

J. Kevin O'Regan

# 7

# Elementary Perceptual and Eye Movement Control Processes in Reading

## I.   Introduction

The work I will report on here is motivated by a hypothesis that I formulated in some earlier papers (O'Regan, 1975, 1979, 1980). I called the hypothesis the "linguistic control" hypothesis of eye movements in reading, but it would be clearer to call it the "visual plus linguistic" hypothesis. The idea is that at each instant during reading, the size of the next saccade to be made by the eye is determined by the size of the region of "perceptibility" around the momentary fixation point. The size of this zone is determined by two sources of information, visual and linguistic. *Visual information* concerns the features of the letters present around the point of regard. This information allows the letters to be identified only in a fairly small zone, called the zone of "visibility." If *linguistic information*, notably information about the words that exist in the language, is added to the visual information, then the added constraints allow more letters to be identified than are in the zone of "visibility." I called this larger zone where letters can be identified the zone of "perceptibility." When linguistic constraints are very strong, the zone of perceptibility will be much bigger than the zone of visibility. When there are no linguistic constraints (as for example in random letter strings), the two zones will be of the same size. In all cases, the "visual plus linguistic" control hypothesis says that at each saccade, the eye jumps to the end of the region of perceptibility, since this is where no more information can be gathered.

My previous research has tested the "visual plus linguistic" control hypothesis in reading by manipulating variables such as the length and the identity of words in noncentral vision (O'Regan 1975, 1979, 1980), and the effect of context (Mc-

EYE MOVEMENTS IN READING:
PERCEPTUAL AND LANGUAGE PROCESSES

Clelland & O'Regan, 1981a, 1981b), and syntax (Holmes & O'Regan, 1981). However, controlling linguistic variables is difficult, and the variability of eye movement behavior in reading makes it hard to find effects. In this chapter I would like to present a different, more theoretical approach, in which I try first to find out how much purely "visual" information is available at each fixation, and then to see what happens when the "linguistic" information is added.

I start with a simple model of letter-in-string visibility. This leads to a prediction about how the visibility of letters changes when the reading distance is changed. I then try to generalize the prediction to saccade size and fixation duration in reading. When the linguistic information coming from the constraints in the lexicon are added to the visual information, a further prediction can be made about where the eye should fixate and how long it should fixate within a word. Finally I review some work being done by Ariane Lévy–Schoen and Zoi Kapoula which is more concerned with the way eye movements reflect the processing of visual information coming from noncentral parts of the retina.

## II.  The Visibility of Letters: Implications for Eye Movements

### A.  A Simple Model of Letter-in-String Perception

Psychologists have done much work on the perception of letters of the alphabet and on how the letters fall into confusion classes. Ergonomists have studied the influence of lighting conditions, type font, spacing, size, and color on letter visibility. However I know of no account in the psychological literature that tries to predict letter visibility from the known facts about visual psychophysics including acuity, contrast sensitivity, masking, and contour interaction, etc. Taking a first step in this direction, I propose a very naive model of letter-in-string perception based purely on what is known about retinal acuity, not taking into account effects due to contrast and contour interaction (though the latter will be mentioned later).

### B.  The Facts about the Fovea

In reading research people often think of the fovea as being the approximately 1–2° central part of the visual field where acuity is sufficiently high for clear vision of letters to be possible. Implicit in this view is the idea that within the fovea the eye's resolution is high and constant, and that acuity only starts to get worse when we move out of the fovea. Psychophysical acuity measurements show this to be false: Acuity drops off rapidly and continuously starting from an eccentricity of zero and going to an eccentricity of 10–15° from the center of regard (cf. Anstis, 1974; Jacobs, 1979). As can be seen from Jacobs's (1979) overview of the acuity literature, the smallest angular distance between two parts of a stimulus that can be resolved by the eye (i.e., the reciprocal of acuity) is not a steplike function of the eccentricity of the stimulus; it is a continuous linearly increasing function of the eccentricity of the stimulus. This fact will be used as the first postulate of the simple model to be described.

An idealization of the data reviewed by Jacobs (1979) is shown in Figure 7.1(a). Based on this idealization, I will posit that the minimum angle of resolution ($r$ radians) at an eccentricity $\phi$ radians is

$$r = k\phi + r_0$$

where $r_0$ is the resolution at the center of the eye.

The second postulate of the model involves the notion of what I call the "grain" size of a type font. Figure 7.1b shows the the eye fixating the letter X. In order for the off-center letter C to be distinguished from, say, an O, the part of the eye that it projects onto must have a power of resolution sufficient to distinguish the C's

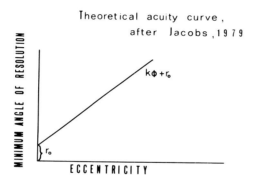

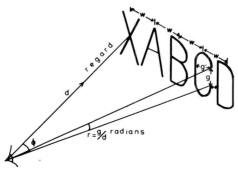

**FIGURE 7.1.** (a) *Theoretical acuity curve, after Jacobs, 1979.* $r_o$ *is the resolution of the eye at its center,* $\phi$ *is eccentricity from the eye's center.* (b) *Hypothetical situation with eye at distance* d *from the page, fixating the letter X. The letters are of width* w *(including spacing). The letter C is at eccentricity* $\phi$ *radians. The gap in the C is of size* g *cm, subtending g/d radians at the eye.*

distinguishing characteristics (e.g., that there is a space in the $C$'s contour, and that it is separate from the $D$. The size of these distinguishing characteristics will vary of course, but assume that for a given type font and spacing between the letters, *on average*, they have a size $g$, which I call the grain size for the given type font. Note that the average value for $g$ will depend to some extent on the spacing between the letters and on the whole set of letters used: It makes no sense to speak of the "distinguishing" characteristics of an individual letter. Also note that being an aspect of the type font itself, $g$ is a linear measure, not an angular measure (i.e. it is measured in centimeters not in degrees or radians).

How far away from the point of regard will a letter within a string be recognizable? Taking as an approximation that $d$ is large compared to $g$, the calculation in Figure 7.2 shows that the maximum excentricity at which a letter with grain $g$ can be recognized is

$$\phi_{max} = (g/dk) - r_0/k$$

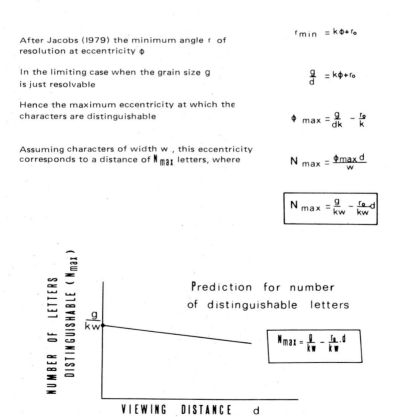

After Jacobs (1979) the minimum angle $r$ of resolution at eccentricity $\phi$

$$r_{min} = k\phi + r_0$$

In the limiting case when the grain size $g$ is just resolvable

$$\frac{g}{d} = k\phi + r_0$$

Hence the maximum eccentricity at which the characters are distinguishable

$$\phi_{max} = \frac{g}{dk} - \frac{r_0}{k}$$

Assuming characters of width $w$, this eccentricity corresponds to a distance of $N_{max}$ letters, where

$$N_{max} = \frac{\phi_{max} d}{w}$$

$$\boxed{N_{max} = \frac{g}{kw} - \frac{r_0 d}{kw}}$$

Prediction for number of distinguishable letters

$$\boxed{N_{max} = \frac{g}{kw} - \frac{r_0 \cdot d}{kw}}$$

NUMBER OF LETTERS DISTINGUISHABLE ($N_{max}$)

VIEWING DISTANCE $d$

**FIGURE 7.2.** *Calculation of the number of letters visible on each side of the fixation point in the situation of Figure 7.1b.*

This can be expressed in character spaces if the letters are assumed to have total width $w$ ($w$ includes spacing). In that case, the number of letters that can be seen on one side of the point of regard is

$$N_{max} = (g/kw) - (r_0/kw)d$$

This is a straight line with gradient $-(r_0/kw)$ cutting the $y$ axis at $(g/kw)$. Obviously if the constant $r_0/kw$ is small, then the slope of the line will be small, that is, the number of letters visible on either side of the fixation point will not depend strongly on the viewing distance.

## C.    Contour Interaction

It is well known that, particularly in noncentral vision, the visibility of a letter flanked by other letters is much less than the visibility of the letter on its own. This observation is often attributed to Woodworth and Schlossberg (1954). The phenomenon, and other phenomena concerning the mutual inhibition of contours in noncentral vision, has been studied by several authors (Andriessen & Bouma, 1976; Banks, Bachrach, & Larson, 1977; Banks, Larson, & Prinzmetal, 1979; Bouma, 1970, 1973; Chastain & Lawson, 1979; White, 1981). There is some debate about whether the phenomena can be explained purely in terms of the way acuity decreases in the parafovea, or whether an active inhibitory effect must be postulated. Bouma's (1970) finding that contour interaction acts over very large distances shows that a pure acuity explanation cannot be sufficient. For this reason the model of letter-in-string perception presented above can only be considered a first approximation. However, it should be noted that the contour interaction effects acting over short distances are nevertheless probably taken into account by the model. This is because Jacobs (1979) shows that the same linear relation between minimum angle of resolution and eccentricity holds even when the stimulus used for the acuity test is laterally flanked by bars. The only effect of the bars in Jacobs's data is to increase $k$ and $r_0$ by a factor of up to 2, depending on the closeness of the bars. From Jacobs's curves typical values for the case when a Landolt C is flanked by bars are $k = 0.01$ and $r_0 = 0.0001$ radians. If we insert these values into the equations of the model above, and assume, for instance, that the grain size $g$ is about one-tenth the character width $w$, with $w$ about 2.5 mm, then the $y$ intercept is at 10, and the gradient is $-.04$. This means that the model predicts that the number of letters visible on each side of the fixation point is nine when the eye is at distance 25 cm from the page, and this number decreases by one letter every time the eye moves back by $1/.04$, or about 25 cm.

## D.    An Experiment to Test the Model Directly

The direct measurements we have done of letter-in-string visibility show that subjects cannot see nine letters, but only at most four or five, on either side of the fixation point. Moreover this number falls off more slowly with viewing distance than one every 25 cm, reaching at most the rate of one every 75 cm. This would be compatible with a value of $k$ of .02 or .03 instead of Jacobs's .01. The fact that we may require a greater value of $k$ than Jacobs may be related to increased lateral masking in our experiments: In our experiments the test letter was embedded in a string of other letters, whereas in Jacobs's experiments there was only one masking bar on each side of the Landolt C. The experiment we have done is as follows.

The purpose was to try to measure directly the visibility of off-center letters in strings of letters. We would have liked to flash up a string of letters for a time too short for eye movements and ask the subject to report a letter at a given eccentricity. Unfortunately when we tried to use a nearby marker to indicate which letter was to be reported, the subjects were totally unable to tell which letter the marker was pointing to. Not only was there a problem of lateral masking, but more important, it seems that position information in noncentral vision is too poor to differentiate the letter spacing used. We therefore adopted another procedure. Instead of embedding the test letter in a string of other *letters*, the test letter was embedded in a string of *digits*. This provided contour interaction effects similar to those produced by letters, but nevertheless subjects were easily able to pick out the test letters among the digits. Any of the 26 letters of the alphabet could occur at each eccentricity. The upper graphs in Figure 7.3 show, for two subjects, the probability of correctly reporting such an embedded test letter as a function of its eccentricity, measured in character spaces from the fixation point. In each graph there are four curves, corresponding to four viewing distances between 30 and 90 cm that were used. It can be seen that the the four curves corresponding to the four viewing distances are very similar. Increasing the viewing distance gives very little loss in visibility.

To compare with the predictions of the model, it is necessary to find the maximum eccentricity at which letters were still visible at each viewing distance. This can be obtained from the upper graphs by finding the intersect of the four curves with the dotted line corresponding to the chosen 50% visibility criterion. These intersects have been plotted for the two subjects in the lower graph. Two further subjects' data are also shown (MR and BB), and the open circles are the means for all four subjects. The mean gradient is $-.013$ characters per cm. This means that a subject moving back by 75 cm will see one less letter on each side of the fixation point. This is a somewhat slower loss in visibility than predicted from the Jacobs data, and may be related to the fact that in the present conditions the density of lateral contours is greater than in Jacobs's experiment.

There are, of course, problems with the model and how to best validate it. In particular, the model assumed that a letter was or was not recognizable, whereas our results are based on the 50% threshold probabilities of correct response. Also, estimation of these 50% thresholds could be done in a more sophisticated way, and more data must be gathered (in the graphs shown, each point corresponds to each letter of the alphabet being presented only twice). Finally, no effort was made in the model to take into account the subjects' global familiarity with the letter font.

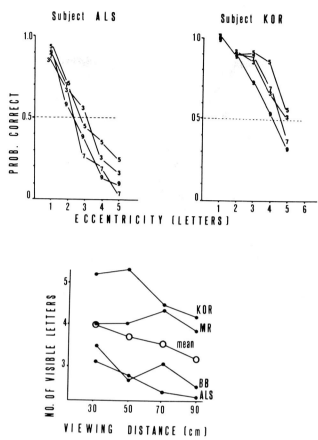

**FIGURE 7.3.** *Upper graphs: the probability of correctly reporting a letter appearing at a given eccentricity (measured in letterspaces) from the fixation point (results for subjects ALS and KOR). In each graph there are four curves labeled 3,5,7, and 9, corresponding to reading distances of 30, 50, 70, and 90 cm. The dotted line corresponds to the 50% visibility criterion. Lower graph: estimation of the number of letters visible with criterion of 50% on each side of the fixation point. The curves labeled ALS and KOR have been obtained from the intersects of the dotted lines in the upper graphs. Similar estimations for two other subjects are also shown. The open circles show the means for the four subjects.*

This undoubtedly accounts for the differences in the heights of the curves in the lower graph of Figure 7.3. Further work may enable a better fit to be found between the predictions and the data. We are currently trying to manipulate more closely factors that we suspect should influence the grain size, such as letter spacing. Still it is gratifying that such a simple model has given some insight into letter-in-string visibility. In particular it has served to point out the important fact that the number of letters clearly visible around the fixation point is to a large extent independent of the viewing distance.

## E.   Extension of These Results to
## Saccade Size in Reading

All models of eye movement control in reading assume that the size of saccades is linked to the size of the perceptual span: If overall fewer letters can be seen at each fixation, then saccade sizes should be smaller. Since we have found in the previous experiment that viewing distance has little effect on the number of letters that can be seen, it follows that saccade size (measured in letters) in reading should also be largely independent of reading distance.

We asked each of six subjects to read six paragraphs. Each paragraph was read at one of six different reading distances between 25 and 90 cm. We asked the subjects questions afterwards to ensure good comprehension. We used a latin square design to obviate effects due to presentation order and paragraph difficulty. Figure 7.4 shows the mean progression sizes made by the subjects: As predicted, there is very little difference in saccade size across different reading distances.

Interestingly the fact that reading distance does not affect the number of fixations per line made in reading had already been noted by Javal (1879) and Huey (1900), and a similar result for changes of letter size had been noted by Gilliland (1923). However no recent confirmation has existed until the present work and that described by Morrison (Chapter 2 of this volume). The finding is important because it implies that in reading research it is more reasonable to measure saccade size and eccentricities in character spaces than in degrees, since in that way reading distance is not a critical factor.

Another interesting question to ask is: What will be the effect of viewing

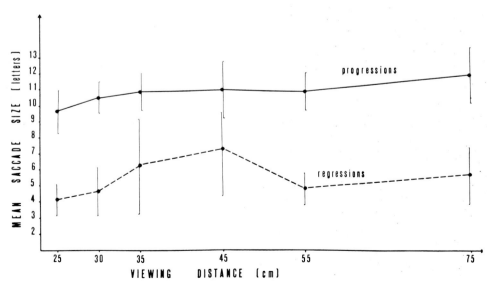

**FIGURE 7.4.** *Mean saccade sizes in letterspaces as a function of reading distance. Results for six subjects. Vertical bars are .05 confidence intervals.*

distance on fixation durations? I offer the following tentative hypothesis. The model of letter-in-string visibility defines the number of letters around the fixation point that can be identified, but this identification can be more or less difficult, depending on the nearness of the letters' distinctive features to the eye's threshold acuity. It seems reasonable to suggest that fixation duration should increase as we get nearer to threshold. To simplify, consider only the resolution at the point of regard, which is $r_0$. The letters have grain $g$, subtending an angle of $g/d$ radians, so we predict fixation duration to be inversely proportional to the difference between the two, that is, to

$$1/[(g/d) - r_0].$$

This is an increasing function of $d$ that becomes infinite at the critical distance $g/r_0$, where reading is no longer possible. The gradient of the function for each $d$ is inversely proportional to $g$. We therefore predict that fixation duration should increase as reading distance increases, and that this should happen faster the smaller the grain size of the typefont is. Figure 7.5 shows mean fixation durations measured in the present experiment. The prediction of increasing fixation duration is confirmed. We are doing similar experiments to see if the slope of the curve changes in the predicted way when different letter spacings are used.

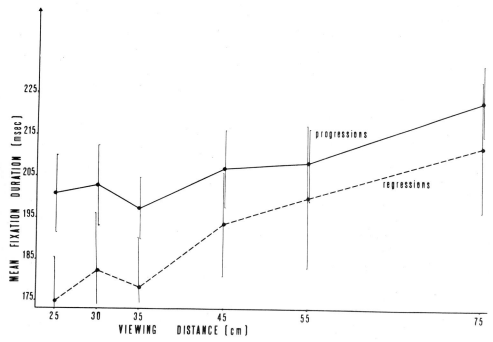

FIGURE 7.5. *Mean fixation durations in msec as a function of viewing distance. Results for six subjects. Vertical bars are .05 confidence intervals.*

## F.   The Addition of Lexical Constraints

The two studies discussed earlier were derived from the model of letter-in-string perception, where no linguistic constraints were used to disambiguate the letters. We are also doing some work to find out how adding linguistic (in particular lexical) constraints increases the perceptual span, and how this influences fixation duration on words.

The result of the visibility study described earlier shows that generally letters further than three or four character spaces from the fixation point cannot be identified from purely visual information. Yet in reading, the average saccade size is of the order of seven or more character spaces. This means that at the average fixation in reading, three or more letters are not seen clearly. It seems reasonable to suppose that this is possible because linguistic constraints make many letters redundant. The strongest constraints on letters act within words, and so we have chosen to look more closely at the way the linguistic constraints act within words.

Take the case of long words, and suppose that only three letters of the type font being used can be seen clearly on either side of the fixation point. Then to see all the letters in the word would require two fixations to be made on the word. In fact the eye will often make only one fixation, and this fixation tends to be just left of the middle of the word (cf. Dunn–Rankin, 1978; O'Regan, 1981; Rayner, 1979). This is easy to understand when we consider that the structure of the lexicon is such that if we know the first six or seven letters of a word, and if we know its length, then often this suffices to determine the word uniquely (this was noted already in O'Regan, 1979). If the eye lands near the third or fourth letter of the word, then the first seven letters of the word will fall into the zone of clear vision. The length of the word can be estimated fairly accurately from information in noncentral vision (Schiepers, 1979). Thus visual information, when added to lexical constraints, should enable the word to be identified when the eye fixates near the third or fourth letter of the word.

But there are exceptional cases where the lexical constraints of a word are such that knowing the beginning of the word gives little information about the end. Examples would be words starting with a fairly long prefix like *inter-* or *super-*, and long verbs where grammatical information must be obtained from the last letters. The hypothesis I put forward is therefore the following. If during reading, the eye falls on a position in a word where the seven or so letters that are visible permit the word to be uniquely determined (by the use of whatever linguistic constraints are available), then the eye need not make another fixation in the word. But if the eye falls on a region of the word where visual combined with linguistic information does not permit the word to be uniquely determined, then another fixation must be made in the word. This hypothesis was put forward in O'Regan (1980, 1981), where it was called the "convenient viewing position" hypothesis. The difference with Rayner's (1979) "preferred viewing position" idea is that here I add the notion that if the eye does not fall on the "correct" place in the word, there is a penalty. I will discuss the possible nature of the penalty later.

The experiments we are doing are as follows. The subject sits in front of a display screen fixating a point. A word appears which the subject has to say out loud as quickly as he or she can. The experimenter rejects trials in which the subject hesitates or says the wrong word. The computer measures naming time from appearance of the word to the first sound emitted by the subject. The words are of length 5, 7, 9, and 11 characters. They appear on the screen displaced with respect to the fixation point in such a way that the subject's eye is centered at a chosen position in the word, which can be the first, third, fifth, up to the eleventh letter of the word. We used a latin square design: Each of between three to six groups (depending on word length) of 20 words is seen by different subjects in different positions. In this way naming times for different positions can be compared for words of a given length without worrying about possible effects due to the pronounceability or frequency of the words.

Figure 7.6 shows mean naming times for 12 subjects as a function of the fixation position. The effect of position fixated is obvious: There is a definite advantage in fixating near the third letter of the word, whatever its length.

I was very surprised that the effects in this experiment were so strong, stronger

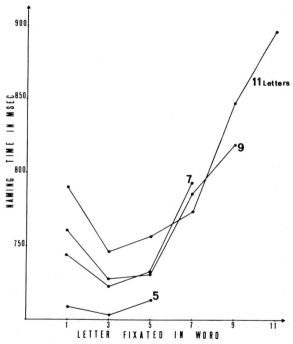

**FIGURE 7.6.** *Naming time for words as a function of the position in the word that the eye was fixating. The four curves marked 5, 7, 9, 11 correspond to results for words of lengths 5, 7, 9, and 11 letters. Each data point corresponds to a mean calculated over 20 words and over 4, 3, 2, and 2 subjects (for word lengths 5, 7, 9, and 11, respectively).*

in fact than the differences in pronounceability of the word groups (the effects exist for each subject individually despite the latin square design). The finding is important not only from a theoretical point of view; it also shows that fixation position in tachistoscopic word recognition experiments is an important factor to control. I have not seen this mentioned in the literature.

How can the data be interpreted? Is the convenient-viewing-position hypothesis supported? First, it is important to consider possible alternative explanations. To begin with, note that the data cannot be explained in terms of a simple left to right pronunciation strategy: It might be argued that the experiment merely measures the time it takes the subjects to recognize the first letter cluster and start pronouncing the words. In that case it is obvious that there should be a time saving when subjects' eyes are positioned at the beginning of the word. But note that if this were true: (1) words of all lengths would be pronounced equally quickly; (2) fixating the first letter of a word would be quicker than fixating the third. Neither of these results were obtained. Word length has a strong effect on naming time, and naming times when fixating the first letter are significantly **slower** than when fixating the third letter.

Another possible hypothesis might be that the experiment is really measuring the time it takes subjects to identify and start saying the first **syllable** of the word. The results then show that it is quicker to fixate near the third letter of the syllable than near the other earlier or later letters, so there is a "convenient viewing position" within syllables, at least. But again, why, even when fixated at the third letter, do the first syllables of long words take longer to name than those of short words. Surely there is no inherently greater difference in the average pronouncability of long words' first syllables compared to short words' first syllables. It must be concluded that more than just the first syllable of the words are being visually processed.

Finally, one can take the strongest version of the convenient viewing position hypothesis and say that since information in a word is generally contained in its first letters, this is where the subject should fixate to be able to name the word quickly. If his eye lands somewhere else, there is a penalty, and he takes longer to name the word. To be sure that the results are really caused by the interaction of linguistic constraints with visual information, we are currently doing another experiment, where the words being used have been specially chosen so that linguistic constraints are very poor at the beginning of the word. In this case the convenient viewing position should be near the end of the word instead of near the beginning. If this result is not found, then we must go back to the weaker version of the convenient-viewing-position hypothesis and say that naming of words is done syllable by syllable, but that within the first syllable a convenient viewing position also exists. In that case it would be interesting to manipulate constraints within the first syllable. We are also removing the naming task altogether so that effects are more likely to reflect purely perceptual processes. Instead of measuring naming time, we are measuring fixation duration in a word comparison task, thereby minimizing left–right scanning strategies and artifacts related to programming the naming response.

We now consider the penalty when the eye does not land at the convenient viewing position. The most obvious possibility is that when the subject's eye is in the "wrong" place, he or she has to make two fixations in the word instead of just one. An interesting question arises: What will be the durations of these two fixations? The data I have assembled from several sources (cf. O'Regan, 1981) shows that each of the two fixations will be 10–40 msec shorter than the fixation that would have been made at the convenient viewing position. It is as though when the eye is in the wrong place, it cuts short its fixation and makes another fixation elsewhere. Word identification can occur either in one long fixation or by a kind of distributed processing in which two shorter duration fixations are made.

But now suppose that the eye lands just a tiny bit away from the ideal convenient viewing position. Surely it would then not make a second fixation in the word. Rather I would expect it to make a slightly longer duration fixation while more effort is expended in visual processing and in probing lexical knowledge.

Summarizing the preceding points: There may be two opposing tendencies affecting fixation durations. If only one fixation is made in a word, then its duration will be longer the further the fixation is from the convenient viewing position. But if two fixations are made, their durations will be short (and perhaps we could say their durations will be shorter the further the fixation is from the convenient viewing position). The fact that there is a mixture of cases here— sometimes a fixation will be long, sometimes short, depending on where the eye lands—may explain why Rayner (1979) found no dependence of fixation duration on word length. My experiments have always been done in conditions where the preceding and following context in the short or long word being studied is kept the same, thereby decreasing the variability in landing positions. Several predictions made by this kind of argument were verified in O'Regan (1981). We are doing further experiments both to find out what the penalty is for not landing at the convenient viewing position, and to confirm that this position is really related to the way intraword lexical constraints interact with visual information.

## III.    Distributed Processing in Ocular Scanning

### A.    Using Peripheral Vision to Save Time

As witnessed by the last paragraphs, when trying to understand moment-to-moment variations in saccade size and fixation duration in reading, we quickly run into the problem of not knowing how processing of visual information is distributed from one fixation to the next. Does the eye compensate variations in its landing position by changing fixation duration? When is it profitable for the eye to make do with poor quality information from noncentral vision, and when is it profitable to cut short a fixation and make a saccade?

To study such questions in detail Ariane Lévy–Schoen has done work using very simple distributed processing situations involving nonlinguistic symbol identification or comparison tasks. Figure 7.7 shows an example of a typical experi-

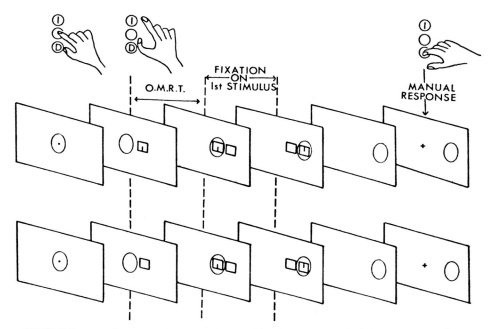

**FIGURE 7.7.** *Typical sequence of events in A. Lévy-Schoen's experiments. Each frame represents what is visible on the display screen at successive moments during an experimental trial. The circle indicates the position the subject is fixating on the screen (the circle is not visible to the subject). A trial is initiated by the subject lifting a finger from the central button, and terminated when he or she presses one of the two other buttons to indicate a response of "identical" or "different". O.M.R.T.: Oculomotor Reaction Time. In the upper sequence the distinguishing line segment in the first stimulus form is present while the subject is still fixating the center of the screen, whereas in the lower sequence the distinguishing line segment is absent.*

mental setup. The subject's task is to compare two forms which both appear either on the right or left, and make a same–different response by pressing a button. The display is made contingent on the subject's eye movements in such a way that the second form only appears after the subject has fixated the first. The reason for forcing such a definite eye scanning sequence is to try to remove effects due to scanning strategy that might influence fixation durations. Such effects will be mentioned in Zoi Kapoula's experiment later. Findlay (1982) has also shown that saccadic latencies are related to the precision of fixation required of the subject. The experiments presented above also show the strong dependence of fixation duration on even small changes in fixation position (it should not be forgotten that the acuity of the eye has dropped to half its central value at an eccentricity of only 30–103 min. of arc—cf. Jones & Higgins, 1947, and Ludvigh, 1941, both cited by Anstis, 1974).

Ariane Lévy–Schoen has been using her highly constrained situations to study the interaction of central and noncentral visual information as well as the time course of this interaction. A summary of the conclusions that can be drawn from a number of studies is as follows:

1. Noncentral vision can be used to gain time on the next fixation. This effect is classic, and has been known since Dodge (1907). Keith Rayner, George McConkie, Ariane Lévy–Schoen, and I have all been studying it since before 1975.

2. Better use is made of this peripheral information when it is always available: When experiments manipulating noncentral information are done in blocked designs rather than mixed designs, the time gain achieved through the presence of the noncentral information is greater.

3. The time spent during a fixation analyzing noncentral information does not seem to prolong the fixation. It is as though parallel processing of noncentral information takes no extra effort.

4. There is some suggestion that false information gathered in noncentral vision does not provoke a loss in time, even though true information provokes a gain.

5. Information can be gathered at a fixation from its very onset: There is no oculomotor "clearing-up" period.

6. Delaying the appearance of centrally presented information does not provoke an equal delay in fixation duration. The eye tends to move on to the next fixation even if processing is not quite finished. There seems to be a drive to keep moving the eyes.

## B. How Eye Positioning Is Affected by Peripheral Visibility

This experiment, part of Zoi Kapoula's PhD thesis (cf. Kapoula, 1982), extends the results of the preceding work to a situation that is more like reading in the sense that fixation locations are now variable. However the experiment still avoids the problems of interpretation that arise when the material to be read has linguistic structure. The subject had to scan a line containing a series of simple symbols, counting the number of occurrences of a target symbol. The symbols were spaced out in an unpredictable fashion on each line, at spacings of 4,8,12, or 24 letter spaces. The main thing we were looking for was a correlation between the length of each saccade and the duration of the following fixation. We expected this because when a large saccade is made, the peripheral information available about the element being saccaded toward is poorer than when a small saccade is made. Several workers have sought but not found such correlations in reading (Andriessen & de Voogd, 1973; Rayner & McConkie, 1976), and it seemed to us that the reason might be that in reading, linguistic processing might be the dominant contributor to fixation durations and would mask any such subtle perceptual effects. This is why we used the simple, nonlinguistic counting task.

The first kind of symbol we used were O's and 8's, one of which was designated as the the target. We chose these symbols on the basis of pretests so that their visibility declined gradually as their eccentricity from the fixation point increased, attaining chance level around an eccentricity of 24 character spaces from the fixation point. Curve A in Figure 7.8 shows the fixation durations made on the

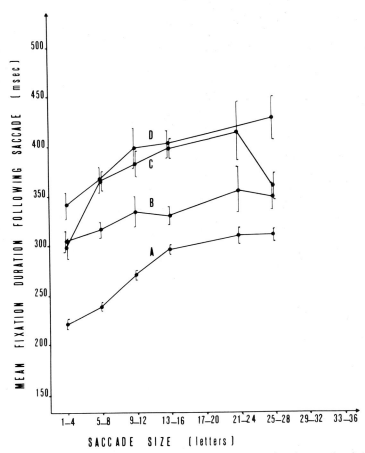

**FIGURE 7.8.** *The mean fixation duration for fixations that follow saccades of a given length (measured in letterspaces). Vertical bars are .05 confidence intervals. A: The subjects were scanning sequences of spaced out O's and 8's (distinguishable at a peripheral eccentricity of up to 12 letterspaces) and counting the number of occurrences of a target symbol. B and C: scanning stimulus pairs that were distinguishable only up to an eccentricity of 4 letterspaces. D: Subjects counting a series of similarly spaced crosses.*

symbols as a function of the length of the preceding saccade. We were very happy to find the long sought correlation of fixation duration with preceding saccade size, and we interpreted it as being caused by the fact that less use is made of noncentral vision when the eye makes a large saccade. To strengthen the finding we designed two other types of symbols whose visibility declined much faster in noncentral vision: Beyond about four character spaces from the point of fixation they could not be distinguished. We expected that except when preceded by four-character saccades, fixation durations should be uniformly long for all preceding saccade sizes. The curves are plotted as B and C in Figure 7.8. Contrary to prediction the correlation looked substantially the same as for the easily visible 0 and 8 symbols. An explanation for the effect having nothing to do with peripheral preprocessing must therefore be sought. Perhaps some sort of oculomotor recovery period is involved: The eye takes longer to recover from a large saccade than from a small one. If this were true, the same effects should be found when no identification of the symbols being scanned is necessary. We therefore did another experiment in which subjects only had to fixate each symbol once, moving from left to right. So that very little visual processing would be done on each symbol, we only used one kind, namely, crosses. Curve D in the figure shows the results: The correlation is found again. At first view it seems therefore that the correlation has nothing to do with the intake of noncentral information. However, further work by Zoi Kapoula, in which accurate and inaccurate fixation sequences are considered separately, shows that two mechanisms give rise to the correlations found here. One is preprocessing of information in peripheral vision, and the other is the requirement of making accurate fixation sequences. When symbols are easily visible in noncentral vision, the eye tends to single out the target symbols for counting, jumping over the nontarget symbols, or at least analyzing them by groups. Under these circumstances peripheral preprocessing is done and saccade size–fixation duration correlations are found because of this preprocessing. But when the symbols are hard to see in noncentral vision, the eye fixates each symbol with great precision, a large number of correction saccades are made, and correlations are found related to oculomotor control.

## IV.   Conclusion

The purpose of the work related to reading that I have been doing with others is to try to define the elementary perceptual and motor processes involved in reading. The idea of the experiments is to test the limits of the oculomotor control system: How quickly can information from noncentral vision be used in controlling eye behavior? While ultimately directed at reading research, the experiments use much simpler tasks than reading itself. In this way we try to isolate those effects related purely to limitations in how eye movements can be controlled, without having to worry about effects related to linguistic processing. While the work reported takes as a working hypothesis that eye movements can be controlled from moment to moment during reading, we are also looking at the degree to which such moment to moment control is subject to an overall eye movement program (Lévy–Schoen, 1981). We hope that ultimately our approach of moving up from the elementary processes will be of use to researchers studying other aspects of reading.

### ACKNOWLEDGMENTS

The work reported here was done in collaboration with A. Lévy–Schoen, Z. Kapoula, I. Czaczkes, D. Gabersek, and B. Brugaillère in the Groupe Regard in Paris.

# References

Andriessen, J. J., & Bouma, H. (1976). Eccentric vision: Adverse interactions between line segments. *Vision Research, 16*, 71–78.

Andriessen, J. J., & de Voogd, A. H. (1973). Analysis of eye movement patterns in silent reading. *IPO Annual Progress Report, 8*, 30–35.

Anstis, S. M. (1974). A chart demonstrating variations in acuity with retinal position. *Vision Research, 14*, 589–592.

Banks, W. P., Bachrach, K. M., & Larson, D. W. (1977). The asymmetry of lateral interference in visual letter identification. *Perception & Psychophysics, 22*, 234–240.

Banks, W. P., Larson, D. W., & Prinzmetal, W. (1979). Asymmetry of visual interference. *Perception & Psychophysics, 25*, 447–456.

Bouma, H. (1970). Interaction effects in parafoveal letter recognition. *Nature, 226*, 177–178.

Bouma, H. (1973). Visual interference in the parafoveal recognition of initial and final letters of words. *Vision Research, 13*, 767–782.

Chastain, G., & Lawson, L. (1979). Identification asymmetry of parafoveal stimulus pairs. *Perception & Psychophysics, 26*, 363–368.

Dodge, R. (1907). An experimental study of visual fixation. *Psychological Review Monograph Supplement, 35* (8).

Dunn–Rankin, P. (1978). The visual characteristics of words. *Scientific American, 238* 122–130.

Findlay, J. M. (1982). Global visual processing for saccadic eye movements. *Vision Research, 22*, 1033–1046.

Gilliland, A. R. (1923). The effect on reading of changes in the size of type. *Elementary School Journal, 24*, 138–146.

Holmes, V., & O'Regan, J. K. (1981). Effects of syntactic structure on eye fixations during reading. *Journal of Verbal Learning and Verbal Behavior, 20*, 417–430.

Huey, E. B. (1900). On the psychology and physiology of reading. I. *American Journal of Psychology, 11*, 283–302.

Jacobs, R. J. (1979). Visual resolution and contour interaction in the fovea and periphery. *Vision Research, 19*, 1187–1196.

Javal, K. E. (1879). Essai sur la physiologie de la lecture. *Annales d'Oculistique, 82*, 243–253.

Kapoula, Z. Le contrôle des mouvements des yeux: information périphérique et régulation d'un programme d'exploration oculaire semblable à celui de la lecture. Doctoral dissertation, Université de Paris 5, 1982.

Lévy–Schoen, A. (1981). Flexible and/or rigid control of oculomotor scanning behavior. In D. F. Fisher, R. A. Monty, & J. W. Senders (Eds.), *Eye movements: Cognition and visual perception*. Hillsdale, New Jersey: Erlbaum, pp. 299–314.

McClelland, J. M., & O'Regan, J. K. (1981). Expectations increase the benefit derived from parafoveal visual information in reading words aloud. *Journal of Experimental Psychology: Human Perception & Performance, 7*, 634–644. (a)

McClelland, J. M., & O'Regan, J. K. (1981). On visual and contextual factors in reading: A reply to Rayner and Slowiaczek. *Journal of Experimental Psychology: Human Perception & Performance, 7*, 652–657. (b)

O'Regan, J. K. (1975). *Constraints on eye movements in reading.* Unpublished doctoral dissertation, University of Cambridge.

O'Regan, J. K. (1979). Eye guidance in reading: Evidence for the linguistic control hypothesis. *Perception & Psychophysics, 25* (6), 501–509.

O'Regan, J. K. (1980). The control of saccade size and fixation duration in reading: The limits of linguistic control. *Perception & Psychophysics, 28*, 112–117.

O'Regan, J. K. (1981). The convenient viewing position hypothesis. In D. F. Fisher, R. A. Monty, & J. W. Senders (Eds.), *Eye movements: Cognition and visual perception*. Hillsdale, New Jersey: Erlbaum.

Rayner, K. (1979). Eye guidance in reading: Fixation locations within words. *Perception*, 8, 21–30.

Rayner, K., & McConkie, G. (1976). What guides a reader's eye movements? *Vision Research*, 16, 829–837.

Schiepers, C. W. (1979). Global attributes in visual word recognition, Part 1. Length perception of letter strings. *Vision Research*, 19, 1343–1349.

White, M. J. (1981). Feature-specific border effects in the discrimination of letter-like forms. *Perception & Psychophysics*, 29, 156–162.

Woodworth, R. S. & Schlossberg, H. (1954). *Experimental psychology*. Holt, New York.

.

Arnold D. Well

# 8

# Perceptual Factors in Reading

## I.  Introduction

The chapters by McConkie, Rayner, and O'Regan (Chapters 5, 6, and 7, respectively) all reflect the considerable progress that has recently been made in understanding perceptual factors in reading. However, the chapters differ considerably in scope and emphasis.

Both McConkie and Rayner deal primarily with the study of individuals engaged in some approximation to normal reading for comprehension. This should not be surprising since many of the recent advances in understanding perceptual processing in normal reading are due to developments in eye movement research that they pioneered. Techniques in which characteristics of the visual display can be altered contingent on the position of the eye have been used creatively and have proved to be extremely valuable.

The McConkie chapter is a comprehensive review of issues related to the control of eye movements, perception during a fixation, and perception across fixations in reading. A number of issues are examined in detail and our current level of understanding is evaluated in terms of a large body of research including some of the most recent work coming out of the Center for the Study of Reading at the University of Illinois. Rayner's chapter is more focussed on recent developments at the University of Massachusetts and deals primarily with studies that have added to our knowledge of the perceptual span and the programming of eye movements during reading.

Unlike McConkie and Rayner, who have concentrated on normal or almost normal reading, O'Regan primarily deals with "elementary" perceptual and eye

EYE MOVEMENTS IN READING:
PERCEPTUAL AND LANGUAGE PROCESSES

movement processes. That is, with the exception of two studies in which saccade lengths and fixation durations during reading for comprehension are recorded in order to determine whether these measures are sensitive to viewing distance, the work reported deals with situations that are much simpler than actual reading. Examples of this work include studying the identifiability of individual letters as a function of eccentricity, the speed with which words can be named as a function of fixation location, and the extent to which noncentral visual information can facilitate comparison of nonlinguistic stimuli when that information is subsequently fixated.

The merits of studying reading by first studying tasks simpler than reading are open to some debate and the issue is discussed briefly by McConkie. The assumption underlying this perspective must be that the more elementary perceptual aspects of reading operate with a minimal amount of adjustment and direction from higher order processes, and so function in normal reading in much the same way as they do when studied in isolation. Pollatsek and I have argued elsewhere (Well & Pollatsek, 1981) that lower level aspects of reading can be studied in a meaningful fashion without necessarily addressing higher level linguistic variables in detail. However, if one is interested in the study of normal reading, it would seem highly desirable to be as creative as possible in studying individuals actually engaged in normal reading. I think the most important recent findings in the field of reading have followed from developments in eyetracking methodology and computer-generated displays that have allowed the study of perceptual processing during the actual reading of text for comprehension.

## II.  The Perceptual Spans in Reading

I find the work on the perceptual span in reading to be particularly interesting because this area is one in which recent developments in eye movement research have resulted in so much progress that one is tempted to say that most of the interesting questions have already been answered. There is no question that we have amassed a very impressive body of knowledge about the effective visual field during reading. Yet, upon detailed examination, it seems that there is room for further refinement in our thinking about the perceptual span and that important and difficult questions remain.

McConkie defines the perceptual span as the region around the center of vision within which some aspect of visual detail of interest is used in reading or affects the reading process. It is clear from this definition that different perceptual spans must exist for different kinds of visual information used in reading. Numerous techniques have been used to estimate the effective visual field during reading and the estimates obtained have been dependent on the techniques used (Rayner, 1981). Some of the most important recent work has used the "moving window" technique developed by McConkie and Rayner (1975) in which the experimenter has control of the amount of visual information available to the reader at any given moment, even though the reader is able to make normal eye movements.

Initially, altered or mutilated text is displayed on a cathode-ray tube (CRT), but as soon as the reader fixates a portion of the text, a region around fixation (the "window") is changed to normal text. That is, within the window text is preserved while outside the window the text is mutilated. When the eye moves to a new point of fixation, the window within which text is unmutilated follows along. With this technique the perceptual span is operationally defined in terms of how close to fixation the boundaries of the window can be brought before reading performance differs from a control condition in which only normal text is presented. For example, consider the case in which the window extends $n$ character spaces to the right of fixation and the mutilation outside of the window consists of replacing letters by other letters such that the shapes of words are preserved. If reading in this condition is as good as in the normal-text control, we would conclude that the perceptual span for specific letter information extends no further than $n$ characters to the right of fixation. Using variations on this and related procedures (e.g., varying the nature of the text mutilation outside of the window, having a mask follow the eye rather than a window) a number of interesting results have been obtained.

Experiments employing the moving window technique (e.g., McConkie & Rayner, 1975; Rayner & Bertera, 1979; Rayner, Inhoff, Morrison, Slowiaczek, & Bertera, 1981) have suggested that readers acquire useful visual information no further than 15 character spaces to the right of fixation. Information acquired furthest out is word length or word boundary information which can be used to parse the visual display into words and is useful in programming eye movements. Information about specific letters can be acquired no further than 10 character spaces to the right of fixation and Underwood and McConkie (1981) and McConkie (1978) report that distinctions among lowercase letters cannot be made more than about six letters to the right.

Although previous work has usually confounded number of characters and visual angle, work reported in this volume by Morrison (Chapter 2) and by O'Regan (Chapter 7) suggests strongly that the appropriate metric is indeed number of characters. Further, comparisons of reading performance when the window consists of either a fixed number of letters or a fixed number of words indicate that the perceptual span is better defined in terms of character spaces than words (Rayner, Well, Pollatsek, & Bertera, 1982). When varying amounts of visual information were made available to the right of fixation, it was found that preserving all the letters of a word was of no special benefit beyond making more letters available.

It has also been found that the perceptual span is asymmetric (McConkie & Rayner, 1976) and for normal reading of English extends no further to the left of fixation than four character spaces or to the beginning of the currently fixated word if that is less (Rayner, Well, & Pollatsek, 1980). When, however, information to the right of fixation is restricted, subjects will acquire information further to the left than the beginning of the currently fixated word (Rayner et al. 1982). We are as yet unable to say whether this change in the perceptual span is attentional in nature or is merely a concomitant of the lower reading rates and longer fixation durations that occur when information to the right of fixation is restricted.

We have, however, demonstrated that the asymmetry of the perceptual span in normal reading is largely an attentional phenomenon. For readers of Hebrew, the perceptual span is asymmetric to the left (i.e., extends further to the left of fixation than to the right) and for Hebrew–English bilinguals the direction of the asymmetry depends on which language is being read (Pollatsek, Bolozky, Well, & Rayner, 1981).

I think that this comprises an impressive package of knowledge about where during reading visual information is acquired. It should be noted, however, that the effective visual field during reading may well vary from moment to moment and we do not yet know very much about this kind of variability.

McConkie argues for distinguishing among three spans: (1) the *momentary span*, defined as the region of text attended at some moment during a fixation; (2) the *individual fixation span*, consisting of the region included in at least one momentary span during a fixation; and (3) the *perceptual span*, a region encompassing all the individual fixation spans. It is this latter span that should, in principle, be revealed by the moving-window technique, although as McConkie points out, depending on the importance of a particular kind of visual information at a given eccentricity and the frequency with which it is used in reading, the overall perceptual span for that kind of visual information will tend to be underestimated.

Although I agree that the overall perceptual span will be underestimated, the measures that are psychologically most important, and are in fact the measures that most people understand as the perceptual span in reading, are the momentary and individual fixation spans, and these will be overestimated by the moving-window procedure. How much these spans will be overestimated depends on how much variability there is from moment to moment and from fixation to fixation in the effective visual field.

There is some evidence that visual information is acquired from different portions of the text at different times during a fixation. Slowiaczek and Rayner (1982) did not find evidence for a sequential scan within windows of 7 or 15 characters centered about fixation. However, Rayner *et al.* (1981) found that most information within a symmetric 17-character window is acquired during the first 50 msec of fixation whereas information further from fixation is obtained over a much longer period. It is unlikely, however, that one would want to say that the momentary span after 50 msec did not include the central 17 character positions, since we know that changing information in this region well after 50 msec has an effect on reading (e.g., Pollatsek & Rayner, 1982). There is also evidence suggesting that the individual fixation span varies as a function of the redundancy of the text. Ehrlich and Rayner (1981) have shown that high levels of contextual constraint cause readers to skip fixations of words and to be less sensitive to visual features encountered in central vision. Subjects were less likely to be aware of a misspelling introduced into a target word that was directly fixated in high contextual constraint than in low-constraint conditions.

If one assumes that there is a considerable amount of variability in individual fixation spans, it follows that the interpretation of work in which the overall perceptual span is the dependent variable will be complicated. It seems reasonable, for example, to expect that we will soon see more work in which the new eye tracking methodology is applied to the study of individual differences in reading. McConkie reports work done by Underwood (1981) in which good and poor fifth graders as well as college students served as subjects. Although this work is not described in detail, it was found that the visual region within which erroneous letters disrupted reading was the same for poor fifth-grade readers as for college students, although the latter group had, on the average, longer saccade lengths.

It is not clear what to make of this finding. More proficient readers might be expected to have larger individual fixation spans and therefore larger overall perceptual spans. On the other hand, although the individual fixation spans of poorer readers may on the average be shorter, they also may be more variable in size and to some extent in location. This variability would also lead to a large overall perceptual span. Fairly large perceptual spans for poor readers would also be consistent with their longer fixation durations. Given these problems, the perceptual span may not be a very satisfactory variable to consider in the study of individual differences in reading, at least until more is learned about fixation-to-fixation variability. In this regard, studies such as that of Ehrlich and Rayner (1981) in which the region from which information is acquired has been shown to vary as a function of the strength of contextual constraint seem to me to be particularly useful.

Finally, there seems little reason to expect that measures of the perceptual span and mean saccade length should be closely coupled. As indicated earlier, the former represents the *union* of the individual fixation spans whereas the latter represents the *average* of individual saccade lengths. Moreover, saccade length is not only influenced by the information available on the current fixation (i.e., the size of the window) but also as strongly by the information available on the preceding fixation (Rayner & Pollatsek, 1981). Also, it has been suggested that saccade length may reflect the region within which sufficient visual information is acquired for words to be identified, given the support of the linguistic context. Our recent experiments do not identify the perceptual span with a region of "perceptibility" defined in this way. We have found that the perceptual span extends to a region from which partial word information is acquired (Rayner *et al.*, 1982). That is, the visual information acquired on the current fixation may not be sufficient to result in identification of a word in the parafovea but will "prime" or increase activation of the internal representation of the word so that identification can be more readily achieved when additional information is acquired on the next fixation.

In summary, we have acquired an impressive amount of knowledge about the overall perceptual span during the past few years. However, the momentary and individual fixation spans are most important psychologically, and we have yet a good deal to learn about them.

## III.   Integration of Information across Fixations

Although one might almost be tempted to say that most of the interesting questions about the overall perceptual span have been answered, no similar temptation exists with regard to the issue of integration of visual information across fixations. How the mind integrates information from successive fixations during reading and forms a stable and coherent representation of the text remains one of the most difficult and important problems to be addressed in future research.

The position held by McConkie and Rayner in 1976 was that integration took place by means of an "integrative visual buffer." On each fixation, visual information from the parafovea and periphery would be stored in the buffer and would later be integrated with the information added to the buffer when those regions of text were later fixated. Integration of the old and new information could be based on knowledge about how far the eye had moved and on the similarity of the visual information acquired on different fixations. However, as discussed by McConkie, Chapter 5 in this volume, a number of studies have subsequently produced evidence that is inconsistent with the notion of an integrative visual buffer.

McConkie, Zola, and Wolverton (1980) and O'Regan (1981) have shown that displacements of the text to the right or left by several character positions during a saccade are not noticed by readers, although McConkie et al. did observe some changes in eye movement behavior. These findings seem quite inconsistent with the idea that integration of visual information across fixations depends heavily on detailed information about how far the eyes have been programmed to move.

Another series of experiments suggests that integration of old and new information does not occur simply on the basis of justification of similar or identical visual information. McConkie and Zola (1979) presented lines of text in alternating case and instructed subjects to read the text for understanding of the basic content so as to be able to answer comprehension questions. During some saccades, the case assignments were reversed (e.g., MaNgRoVe became mAnGrOve). During other saccades, no case changes were made. Switches of case assignment were not noticed by readers and had no effect on eye movements. In addition, Rayner, McConkie, and Zola (1980) used words displayed in letters of alternating case and found that a word displayed in the parafovea facilitated the naming of the same word following an eye movement to that position, regardless of whether case assignments were switched or not. McConkie briefly reports several interesting pilot studies that further strengthen the case against an integrative visual buffer. In one study, a display in which only occasional letters were capitalized was used. Changes from fixation to fixation in which letters were capitalized were not detected. In a second study, changes in the spacing between words from fixation to fixation in a display in which interword spacing was irregular were not detected by readers.

Although the idea of an integrative visual buffer seems untenable, there are clear demonstrations that information obtained from the parafovea on one fixation

can facilitate word naming and identification on the next fixation (e.g., McClelland & O'Regan, 1981; Rayner, McConkie, & Ehrlich, 1978; Rayner, McConkie,
& Zola, 1980; Rayner *et al.*, 1982). One possibility is that little integration of
*visual* information takes place across fixations in reading (at least for text which is
unusual in some fashion, such as that incorporating alternating case or irregular
interword spacing) and that the information that *is* integrated across fixations is at
a more abstract level. In this respect, reading may be quite different from other
types of visual tasks. The goal in reading, at least for competent readers engaged in
reading for comprehension, is to abstract the meaning of the text, not to attend to
visual details. Integration of information across fixations in reading may be
achieved not so much by means of a *visual* buffer but rather through an "integrative letter information buffer."

Consider as a first approximation model of the visual processing of a word in
reading one that has a series of levels of detectors. First the word must be isolated
from the rest of the display, or at a minimum the left-hand boundary of the word
must be located. Certain features are then extracted from positions in the text
relative to the left boundary and information from features in the same character
positions is combined to activate letter detectors. As evidence about letters begins
accumulating, it can be used in the identification of the word. Knowledge about
orthography can be represented in the model by inserting a level of letter–cluster
detectors between the letter detectors and the word detectors. A word presented
in isolation would be identified when some weighted sum of the inputs from letter
and letter–cluster detectors exceeded a threshold. Contextual information could
be accommodated in the model by lowering the identification threshold or increasing the activation of the word detector so that less visual information would be
required for identification. In terms of such a model, a word in the parafovea
would generate activity in a series of letter detectors whose activity was justified
with respect to the beginning of the word. This activation, in combination with
contextual information might be sufficient to identify the word on the current
fixation, and if not, would facilitate identification of the word when it was fixated
on the next fixation.

Integrating of old and new information would take place by "lining up" the
patterns of letter detector activation localized with respect to the left boundary of
the word. The alternating-case data could easily be accommodated in this formula-
tion if either (1) lowercase letter information generated at least some activation in
uppercase letter detectors and vice versa (this would seem to be a distinct possibility since for many letters there is considerable overlap of features for upper-
and lowercase versions of letters, and in any event one would expect these detectors to be hooked up in some fashion); or (2) there was a layer of "abstract letter
detectors" represented in the system that received input from case-specific letter
detectors. The outputs of these abstract letter detectors would contain information about the identities but not about the visual details of letters. I do not mean to
imply that case-specific information is completely lost or unimportant in reading

normal text. Readers obviously can discriminate between upper- and lowercase letters, and strings like *Ruth* and *FBI* have meanings that *ruth* and *fbi* do not. I am suggesting, however, that evidence about the identifies of letters is available, and at least for alternating case and other unusual forms of text, it is this information that is primarily used in integrating information from fixation to fixation.

Coltheart (1981) has argued strongly that there is a component in the reading system that is capable of assigning abstract letter identities (ALIs) to letters and gives it a prominent role in his model of reading aloud and comprehending single words. As support for the existence of ALIs, Coltheart cites studies demonstrating that responses to a word or nonword can be facilitated by prior presentation of a stimulus sharing at least some of the letters in the same position, even if the letters were presented in the opposite case (e.g., Evett & Humphreys, 1981; Rayner, McConkie, & Zola, 1980; Scarborough, Cortese, & Scarborough, 1979). Other evidence adduced comes from work with brain-damaged individuals. For example, a conduction aphasic who had a very severe impairment of the ability to derive phonology from print was shown to be able to perform without error in a same–different matching task with nonwords in which the two items in the pair differed in case (e.g., ANER–aner or ANER–aneg). Since neither direct visual matching (because of case differences) nor semantic information (because the strings were not words) could be used to perform the task, and since the patient was unable to generate phonological code from print, the conclusion is that some additional abstract code must be involved. Other evidence is provided with work from deep dyslexics (Saffran, 1980). Moreover, the ALI cannot simply be regarded as the name of the letter. The phonological dyslexic A.M. could match uppercase letters to their lowercase equivalents, but his naming of single letters was much impaired.

Taken together, these lines of evidence suggest strongly that there are components in the reading system capable of extracting and of using a code based on abstract letter identities. It seems reasonable to speculate that this code is used in reading, since what is important in reading is the identification of words, and according to the model sketched out earlier, words are identified on the basis of the activity of letter detectors (it should be noted that the activation of a letter detector can contribute to the identification of a word without the letter itself having to be identified). With the exception of information about the capitalization of the first letters of certain words, information about the detailed visual characteristics of letters would generally seem to serve little purpose in reading and therefore may not play much of a role in the integration of information across fixations.

More research along the lines of McConkie's pilot studies would be useful. It should be determined if visual information plays a more important role in the integration of information across fixations in text that is more nearly normal than alternating-case text. Experiments involving the reading of alternating-case text have proved interesting, but it is not obvious that the processes involved in reading alternating-case text are exactly the same as those involved in reading normal text.

# IV.  Concluding Comments

One cannot fail to be impressed both by the recent progress that has occurred in the understanding of perceptual processing in reading and by the difficulty of some of the problems that remain. In my discussion, I have addressed two major areas: the perceptual span, an area in which the progress is perhaps more obvious than the remining problems, and integration of information across fixations, an area in which I believe the reverse to be true.

Although many difficult problems remain, I am extremely encouraged by the current state of activity in the field. There is a general feeling that a great deal of progress is being made and, significantly, much of this progress is based on experiments with individuals actually engaged in reading for comprehension. Although the wedding of sophisticated eye tracking equipment and computer generated displays has already been used effectively, I believe the potential of this technology is just beginning to be realized. The chapters in this section have given some indication of the work remaining to be done. I would expect in the next few years not only to see progress with respect to the basic perceptual issues in reading, but also in linguistic issues, work with individual differences, the development of reading, and related perceptual issues in scene perception. In particular, contrasting the findings from work in reading and in complex scene perception should lead to deeper insights in both domains.

# References

Coltheart, M. (1981). Disorders of reading and their implications for models of normal reading. *Visible Language 15*, 245–286.

Ehrlich, S. F., & Rayner, K. (1981). Contextual effects on word perception and eye movements during reading. *Journal of Verbal Learning and Verbal Behavior 20*, 641–655.

Evett, L. J., & Humphreys, G. W. (1981). The use of abstract graphemic information in lexical access. *Quarterly Journal of Experimental Psychology, 33A*, 325–350.

McClelland, J. L., & O'Regan, K. (1981). Expectations increase the benefit derived from parafoveal visual information in reading words aloud. *Journal of Experimental Psychology: Human Perception & Performance 7*, 634–644.

MConkie, G. W. (1978). Where do we read? Paper presented at the annual meeting of the Psychonomic Society, San Antonio, Texas, November.

McConkie, G. W., & Rayner, K. (1975). The span of the effective stimulus during a fixation in reading. *Perception & Psychophysics 25*, 221–224.

McConkie, G. W., & Rayner, K. (1976). Asymmetry of the perceptual span in reading. *Bulletin of the Psychonomic Society 8*, 365–368.

McConkie, G. W., & Zola, D. (1979). Is visual information integrated across successive fixations in reading? *Perception & Psychophysics 25*, 221–224.

McConkie, G. W., Zola, D., & Wolverton, G. S. (1980). How precise is eye guidance? Paper presented at the annual meeting of the American Educational Research Association, Boston, Massachusetts, April.

O'Regan, K. (1981). The "Convenient Viewing Condition" hypothesis. In D. F. Fisher, R. A. Monty, & J. W. Senders (Eds.), *Eye movements: Cognition and visual perception*. Hillsdale, New Jersey: Lawrence Erlbaum.

150                                                                                      Arnold D. Well

Pollatsek, A., Bolozky, S., Well, A. D., & Rayner, K. (1981). *Brain and Language 14*, 174–180.
Pollatsek, A., & Rayner, K. (1982). Eye movement control in reading: The role of word boundaries. *Journal of Experimental Psychology: Human Perception & Performance, 8*, 817–833.
Rayner, K. (1981). Eye movements and the perceptual span in reading. In F. J. Pirozzolo & M. C. Wittrock (Eds.), *Neuropsychological and cognitive processes in reading.* New York: Academic Press. Pp. 145–165.
Rayner, K., & Bertera, J. H. (1979). Reading without a fovea. *Science 206*, 468–469.
Rayner, K., Inhoff, A. W., Morrison, R. E., Slowiaczek, M. L., & Bertera, J. H. (1981). Masking of foveal and parafoveal vision during eye fixations in reading. *Journal of Experimental Psychology: Human Perception & Performance 7*, 167–179.
Rayner, K., McConkie, G. W., & Ehrlich, S. (1978). Eye movements and integrating information across fixations. *Journal of Experimental Psychology: Human Perception & Performance 4*, 529–544.
Rayner, K., McConkie, G. W., & Zola, D. (1980). Integrating information across eye movements. *Cognitive Psychology 12*, 206–226.
Rayner, K., & Pollatsek, A. (1981). Eye movement control during reading. Evidence for direct control. *Quarterly Journal of Experimental Psychology, 33A*, 351–373.
Rayner, K., Well, A. D., & Pollatsek, A. (1980). Asymmetry of the effective visual field in reading. *Perception & Psychophysics 27*, 537–544.
Rayner, K., Well, A. D., Pollatsek, A., & Bertera, J. H. (1982). The availability of information to the right of fixation. *Perception & Psychophysics, 31*, 537–550.
Saffran, E. M. (1980). Reading in deep dyslexia is not ideographic. *Neuropsychologia 18*, 219–233.
Scarborough, D. L., Cortese, C., & Scarborough, H. S. (1979). Frequency and repetition effects in lexical memory. *Journal of Experimental Psychology: Human Perception & Performance 3*, 1–17.
Slowiaczek, M. L., & Rayner, K. (1982). Sequential masking during eye fixations. Unpublished manuscript. (Available from Department of Psychology, University of Massachusetts, Amherst.)
Underwood, N. R. (1981). *The span of letter recognition of good and poor readers.* (Tech. Rep.). Urbana: University of Illinois, Center for the Study of Reading.
Underwood, N. R., & McConkie, G. W. (1981). The effect of encountering errors at different retinal positions during reading. Unpublished manuscript. (Available from Center for the Study of Reading, University of Illinois.)
Well, A. D., & Pollatsek, A. (1981). Word processing in reading. *Visible Language 15*, 287–308.

# III
# Eye Movements
# and Context Effects

Wayne L. Shebilske and Dennis F. Fisher

# 9

# Eye Movements and Context Effects during Reading of Extended Discourse

## I. Introduction

This chapter concentrates on two theoretical topics: (1) effects of context on comprehension, a central issue in contemporary psycholinguistics; and (2) effects of comprehension on eye movements, a main consideration of this volume. We will briefly sketch relevant issues and then present a framework for bringing them together in studies of eye movements during reading of extended discourse.

Psycholinguists distinguish three contexts that come into play during textbook reading:

1. *Situational context* is the sum total of nonlinguistic external stimuli that act upon a reader, including: (*a*) task demands (e.g., reading as quickly as you can); (*b*) purpose (e.g., reading for pleasure, general knowledge, exam preparation, or term paper research); and (*c*) presentation mode (e.g., reading from a book or TV screen). Ignoring situational context can lead to a lack of external validity. For example, Spache and Spache (1977) argued that Davis (1968) isolated skills that have little or no relevance outside of the taking of reading tests.

2. *Conceptual context*, which is a reader's background knowledge at the moment of reading, includes: (*a*) concepts given in earlier parts of a text; (*b*) a reader's prior knowledge within a specific domain; and (*c*) a reader's general world knowledge. A college text and a tenth-grade text that we reviewed differed, for example, in assumptions about prior knowledge on Darwin's Theory of Evolution. A reader who does not understand Darwin's theory could easily understand the tenth-grade discussion of speciation but, in contrast, would have had to struggle through the college discussion of speciation. Texts also differ in the extent to

EYE MOVEMENTS IN READING:
PERCEPTUAL AND LANGUAGE PROCESSES

which they require readers to draw pragmatic inferences, are inferences based upon world knowledge (cf. Flood, 1981).

A famous example of pragmatic inference is Bransford, Barclay, and Franks's (1972) "Three turtles rested on a floating log and a fish swam beneath it" from which readers infer that the fish swam beneath the turtles. Good writers avoid tedious and clumsy exposition by purposely leaving gaps for readers to fill, but sometimes authors leave gaps that are too wide. For instance, a tenth-grade biology text relied on students' knowledge of brown bears and polar bears to communicate the idea that geographical isolation can maintain distinctness between species. Readers remembered the example, but they either never made the inference about geographical isolation or they forgot it. The bear example was one of many ineffective examples. In fact, Twohig (1982) improved the text's recallability by leaving out examples that made poor use of conceptual context.

3. *Linguistic context* is the particular letters, words, and sentences that, because of the particular way that they are arranged, provide three kinds of information: (*a*) *orthographic information* based upon rules for combining letters within words; (*b*) *syntactic information,* based upon rules for combining words within sentences; and (*c*) *semantic information,* based upon a word's minimal or dictionarylike definition (Miller, 1972). These redundant sources of information supplement visual information used to recognize words (cf. Massaro, 1975). Textbook publishers control linguistic context to some extent with readability formulas (Fry, 1968). Readability levels depend upon sentence length, which indirectly influences syntactic context, and upon word familiarity, which indirectly influences semantic and orthographic contexts. Many researchers have investigated linguistic contexts in an effort to link eye movements to recognition processes. We will not review that research in this chapter because it is taken up in detail elsewhere (McConkie, Chapter 5 of this volume).

The important issue for psycholinguists is not whether, but how, context affects comprehension. Most psycholinguistic theories break language processing into subprocesses that perform specific operations such as extracting physical features, encoding words, encoding sentences, and so on. Psycholinguistic theorists agree that context influences the final outcome, which is assumed to be an integrated conceptual representation, but they disagree about how. Some argue, for instance, that nonlinguistic contexts influence higher order conceptual processing stages, but not lower order processing stages. Theories making this assumption are called "bottom-up" theories (e.g., Forster, 1979; Swinney, 1979; Tanenbaum, Leiman, & Seidenberg, 1979). Others argue that nonlinguistic contexts influence conceptual processes which in turn influence linguistic processes. On this account, output from higher order conceptual processes can serve as inputs to lower order linguistic processes. Such theories are called "top-down" theories (e.g., Morton, 1969; Newell, 1980; Riesbeck & Schank, 1978; Schank & Abelson, 1977; Schvaneveldt, Meyer, & Becker, 1976).

## II.  Comprehension and Eye Movements

Despite a long history of research that seems disappointing with respect to the goal of using eye movements to analyze language processes, we believe that eye movement data can be brought to bear on the nature of context effect in comprehension. Why has it been so difficult to learn about language processes from eye movement records? McConkie (1979) suggested that progress has been blocked because it is not known: (1) what part of the text is actually being "seen" during a fixation; and (2) what relationship exists between eye movements and the cognitive processes. We submit that another hinderance has been that, until recently, researchers have inadequately quantified aspects of text that might be relevant to the ways readers control their eye movements. In this section, we discuss how we are attempting to break through these barriers.

### A.  Eye Movements and Visible Language

McConkie (Chapter 5 of this volume) and Rayner (Chapter 6 of this volume) developed a paradigm that enables them to measure information processed in a single fixation during reading. Since their research is reviewed at length in this book, we will not go into it here except to note that it has greatly clarified the relationship between eye movements and perceptual processes occurring during reading.

We attempt to shed light on higher order language processes by observing interrelationships between eye movement patterns, subject and situational factors, formal and perceived text structures, and the understanding of conceptual content in typical classroom reading assignments. We then draw inferences about language processes from the observed interrelationships without assuming specific models of language processing or of eye movement control. A theoretical foundation guides our observations, of course, so we will briefly outline that framework.

We make a heuristic distinction between recognition processes and comprehension processes (cf. Shebilske & Reid, 1979). Recognition processes are operations that map output from the eyes onto *linguistic units*, that correspond to letters, syllables, clauses, and sentences. Comprehension processes link linguistic units with *conceptual units*, and they map lower order concepts, which correspond to words, clauses, and sentences, onto higher order concepts, which correspond roughly to the headings one would put down in outlining a text. We are in no way committed to a specific model of how these processes interact. We realize that all levels of processing may operate in parallel and in noncanonical orders (Levelt, 1978; Newell, 1980; Winograd, 1972). At this point our distinction is intended only as a guideline for placing emphasis in our research. As mentioned earlier, theorists tend to agree that the end product in reading is an internal conceptual representation. We are using eye movements to explore the comprehension processes that go into structuring that conceptual representation. Our focus is drawn to higher level comprehension processes because we believe that they account for important differences between skilled and unskilled readers (cf. Gibson & Levin, 1975).

Our use of the phrase *structuring conceptual representations* shows another of our theoretical orientations. We conceive of comprehension as a dynamic process in which people draw inferences that go well beyond the literal or direct meaning of a text (Bransford & Johnson, 1973; Clark, 1978). We therefore believe that what a reader sees in a text is as important as what an author writes in it (Estes & Shebilske, 1980; Shebilske, 1980). As a result, we quantify potentially relevant aspects of text by means of our readers' perceptions. We ask our readers to analyze texts in various ways that allow us to assess: (*a*) their perceptions of text structure; (*b*) their impressions of how a text relates to specific task demands; and (*c*) their awareness of how a text relates to what they already know. We balance this "top–down" viewpoint with a "bottom–up" viewpoint, which is reflected in our concern for the way in which stimulus information affects visible language processing. We have, for instance, studied the effects of special typographies on comprehension (Fisher, 1979b; Shebilske & Rotondo, 1981).

Our concern with "bottom–up" processing is also reflected in our critique of Just and Carpenter (Shebilske & Fisher, 1982) and in our own analysis of eye movements dynamics. Just and Carpenter make an eye–mind assumption, which implies that language processes influence eye movements directly; we leave open the possibility that language processes sometimes influence eye movements indirectly. Shebilske (1975) distinguished between Directly Regulated Scanning (DRS) and Indirectly Regulated Scanning (IRS). In DRS, eye movements come under direct control of language processes as when a reader decides to skip a very long word that appears frequently or when a reader decides to reread an important list of names. In IRS, the brain processes one word while the eyes look at another. High level brain processes operate upon the contents of a buffer that holds categorical information, whereas the eye and brain load new information into the buffer (cf. Bouma & deVoogd, 1974). The contents of the buffer influence eye movements as follows: When the buffer is full, or nearly full, the eyes slow down; when the buffer is empty, or nearly empty, the eyes speed up. Characteristics of stimulus information influence the rate at which information can be read into the buffer; comprehension processes influence the rate at which information is read out of the buffer; consequently, both indirectly affect eye movements. Rayner (1978) reviews ample evidence that language processes influence eye movements, but the data collected to date leaves open the possibility that readers operate in an IRS mode, which is periodically interrupted by DRS control. The possibility of IRS control makes inferring language processes from eye movements difficult but not impossible. We designed a system of eye movement analysis that allows us to get at language processes without assuming a direct link between the two. In the next section, we will describe how we use our paradigm to analyze situational and conceptual context effects.

## B.  Eye Movements and
## Contextual Effects on Comprehension

A flexible reader can be thought of as one who adapts reading rate and approach to fit situational, conceptual, and linguistic contexts. Educators know that a high degree of adaptability is associated with superior reading, but they do not know how flexible readers adapt (Harris & Sipay, 1975; Rankin, 1974). Similarly, psycholinguists know that context affects comprehension, but they do not know how. Direct inquiries into how people adapt reading to fit different contexts suggest that many important contextual influences are beyond introspection (Gibson & Levin, 1975). Researchers have therefore developed a variety of experimental tasks and dependent measures that enable them to observe how context affects reading behavior (Levelt, 1978; Olson & Clark, 1976). They infer from these observations the nature of adaptable reading of extended discourse. The most naturalistic task, of course, is silent reading of extended discourse. With an unobtrusive eye monitor, one can record a wealth of observable behavior during this task. In the next section, we review old and new experiments that provide direct records of rate adjustments during silent reading in various contexts. As a step toward understanding cognitive operations underlying flexible reading, we attempt to characterize adjustments readers make in each context.

## III.   Situational Contexts

Reading experiments have scrutinized three kinds of situational contexts having to do with: (1) format; (2) goals; and (3) repeated exposures. We will review each of these in turn.

## A.  Format

Tinker's (1951) work especially concerns flexibility in eye movement dynamics as a function of typography. He observed dramatic changes in fixations as shown in Table 9.1. We begin our review with his intriguing results as a warning that researchers must not lose sight of the physical form in which information is presented. A text's physical format may limit the range of adjustments that readers can make to other contextual variables. Conversely, individual language skills may constrain the kinds of adjustments that can be made to changes in typography. Fisher and his associates (Fisher, 1975; Fisher & Lefton, 1976; Lefton & Fisher, 1976) have found developmental trends, for example, in the kinds of adjustments readers make to altered typographies. Fisher (1979a) interprets these trends in terms of different language processing skills available to readers who are at different developmental levels. The possibility of interactions between typographical variables and other contextual variables (cf. Fisher & Montanary,

TABLE 9.1
Typographical Variations and Fixation Duration[a]

| |
|---|
| *Line width* |
| (6 point): 13 picas, 233.3 msec, vs. 5 picas, 266.6 msec; +33.3 msec; +14.3% |
| (6 point): 13 picas, 230.8 msec, vs. 36 picas, 239.8 msec; +9.0 msec; +3.9% |
| (10 point): 19 picas, 222.6 msec, vs. 9 picas, 240.4 msec; +17.8 msec; +8.0% |
| (10 point): 19 picas, 218.2 msec, vs. 43 picas, 226.6 msec; +8.4 msec; +3.8% |
| *Size of type* |
| (19 picas): 10 point, 226.2 msec, vs. 6 point, 242.4 msec; +16.2 msec; +7.2% |
| (19 picas): 10 point, 226.3 msec, vs. 14 point, 212.6 msec; −13.7 msec; −6.1% |
| (22 vs. 16 picas): 11 point, 224.9 msec, vs. 8 point, 234.4 msec; +9.5 msec; +4.2% |
| (22 vs. 14 picas): 11 point, 240.0 msec, vs. 6 point, 260.0 msec; +20.0 msec; +8.3% |
| *Type face* |
| Scotch Roman, 239.6 msec, vs. Old English, 242.6 msec; +3.0 msec; +1.3% |
| *Type form* |
| Lowercase, 233.3 msec, vs. all capitals, 212.8 msec; −20.5 msec; −8.8% |
| *Color print* |
| Black on white, 228.0 msec, vs. red on green, 261.0 msec; +33.0 msec; +14.5% |
| *Black versus white print* |
| Black print, 244.0 msec, vs. white print, 238.0 msec; −6.0 msec; −2.5% |
| *Optimal versus nonoptimal* |
| 10 point, 19 pica line width, 2 point leading, black on white, 225.4 msec, vs. 6 point, 34 pica line width, set solid, white print on black background, 239.5 msec; +14.1 msec; +6.3% |

[a]Adapted from Tinker (1951), p. 475.

1977) is especially important today when many eye movement researchers present texts in special formats on CRT monitors or on projection screens. One precaution that we might consider taking is to compare reading from these special displays to reading from printed pages of text. Researchers are in a better position to generalize when a detailed analysis of recall and reading times shows that the same level of comprehension is achieved in the same amount of time for texts presented in different formats.

## B.   Goals

Anderson (1937) compared eye movements of college students who read short paragraphs (10–12 lines) for three different purposes: (1) "read as you normally read such material" (neutral instruction); (2) "read to obtain a knowledge as complete and detailed as possible from one reading" (detail instruction); (3) "read to secure only the general idea of the contents" (gist instruction). Anderson's subjects included 50 good readers (highest decile on the *Iowa Silent Reading Test*) and 50 poor readers (lowest quartile on the *Iowa Silent Reading Test*). Reading according to neutral instruction revealed expected differences between groups. The good readers read faster, made fewer regressions, had longer interfixation distances, and shorter fixation durations. Both groups responded appropriately to detail instruction; they read slower, made more regressions, and had shorter interfixation distances and longer fixations durations. Good readers made better adjustments than poor readers but the differences were slight. The most dramatic result came in response to gist instruction. Whereas both groups might be expected to speed up and to use more efficient eye movement patterns, in fact, only good readers responded in this way. They read faster, made fewer regressions, and had shorter fixation durations than they did for neutral instruction. Poor readers responded in the opposite direction! They read slower, made more regressions, and had longer fixation durations. Anderson (1937) offered the following explanation:

> Effective reading for the general idea is a highly refined skill which presupposes a mastery of certain reading fundamentals, i.e., accurate perception, word recognition, vocabulary, and sentence meaning. Unless these elementary skills function with a minimum of effort, the reader will fail to make the psychological transition which reading for the general idea requires. Good readers, in whom the specific skills are well developed, succeed. . . . Poor readers, because they are so engrossed in problems of an elemental nature, tend to read all material in about the same way. . . . If they try to comply with the instructions, their efforts lead to ineffectual attempts and finally to mental confusion [p. 17].

Anderson's hypothesis had two components:

1. Good readers learn to automate lower order recognition skills (cf. La Berge & Samuels, 1974; Fisher, 1979a, 1979b)
2. Good readers learn a higher order comprehension skill, which involves rapid abstracting of gist (cf. Shebilske, 1980).

Anderson's experiment raises many important questions. For example, does every individual adjust every eye movement parameter that was changed in group averages? Do readers learn to adjust all parameters at once, or do they first adjust one, say duration, and later learn to adjust others? Where in a text do readers slow down or speed up? That is, with respect to what textual characteristics do readers modulate their scanning? What is the relationship between one's ability to adjust to different purposes for reading and one's ability to adjust to other task demands? These questions remain today.

Shebilske and Reid (1979) addressed the question about flexibility with respect to different task demands. They measured eye movements of 12 college students who read 400-word stories for two different purposes: (1) "read as you would normally read such a story for recreation—you will not be tested" (recreational reading); (2) "read these stories in preparation for a detailed short-answer test" (rigorous reading). The students adjusted their reading in a way that was comparable to Anderson's neutral instructions and detail instructions. Shebilske and Reid took the experiment a step further by comparing the magnitude of the same individual's adjustments in two other tasks.

One of the other tasks was reading a 1900-word narrative for recreation (no test). Readers adjusted their reading by slowing down for sentences that had to be integrated with three or more other sentences to form a macroproposition. The magnitude of a student's adjustment on this task was correlated with the magnitude of the student's flexibility with respect to purpose for reading on the first task.

The same students performed a third task, reading Raygor's (1970) standardized test of flexibility. Raygor's test measures flexibility in terms of a reader's ability to modulate reading rate with different levels of passage difficulty while reading in preparation for a test. Students' abilities to adapt in this third task were not correlated with abilities to adapt in the first two tasks. These results are consistant with a view that flexibility is composed of fundamental component processes, some (but not all) of which are interrelated. One individual might be more flexible with respect to difficulty than with purpose; other individuals might show flexibility in terms of purpose. It remains for future experiments to specify cognitive processes that underlie these individual differences.

Rothkopf (1978) also raised questions about individual differences in adaptability to purpose for reading. He analyzed the effect of task demand on eye movements during goal-guided reading. He used electronystagmography to record eye movements of 18 high-school students who read a 1500-word passage on oceanography with or without advanced learning goals. An example of a learning goal was: *What do the Mediterranean, Baltic, and Adriatic seas have in common?* Answers were always contained in single sentences, which Rothkopf called goal relevant; all other sentences were called background. The text was divided into 12 slides with one goal-relevant sentence per slide. Six students memorized goals for half the slides; six other students memorized goals for the other slides; and the remaining six students tried to learn as much as possible about the passage without receiving any specific goals. Group averages indicated that students recalled material better when it was goal relevent than when it was background. Eye movements were analyzed in the hope of revealing how students accomplished this improvement.

The eye movement records were not precise enough to indicate when subjects were reading goal-relevant sentences and when they were reading background. Rothkopf was therefore forced to develop a special "subtraction technique" to estimate eye movement patterns generated by goal processing. He first averaged certain fixation parameters over entire pages noting differences between pages with goal-relevant sentences and pages without goal-relevant sentences. He then estimated eye movement characteristics generated by goal processing on slides containing goals by subtracting out eye movement characteristics generated by background processing. He estimated the latter from slides containing all background sentences. Statistical tests of group averages suggested that goal processing involves more rereading of lines, more fixations per line, and more time per fixation resulting in more time spent on goal-relevant sentences. Each component of these scanning patterns is consistent with the possibility that readers devoted more processing resources to goal processing in an effort to increase goal-relevant competance.

Rothkopf also applied the "subtraction technique" to individual data and made a case for the position that readers respond in highly individual ways. Some did more rereading; some made more fixations; some made more regressions; some did all three during goal processing; and some showed no differences between goal processing and background processing. The individual scanning patterns were not associated with goal-relevant competence. In fact, readers who slowed down the most for goal-relevant sentences did not improve their goal-relevant competence any more than readers who did not slow down. Rothkopf concluded that time consuming goal-processing activities do not improve goal-relevant competence and therefore are essentially superstitious behaviors. He concluded further that eye movements may not reveal fundamental psychological processes during reading because scanning patterns include many ineffective components.

Rothkopf's group data, must be interpreted cautiously because it is rarely wise to generalize from group to individual performance especially when the optimal metric may not yet be available. Yet, the group data are important because they indicate a normative tendency to adapt scanning patterns in response to goal-relevant material. The observed pattern of adaptability is consistent with adjustments readers make whenever they perceive information to be important (Shebilske & Fisher, 1981).

Rothkopf's analyses of individual data are questionable on methodological grounds. His "subtraction technique" is based upon an oversimplified assumption that differences between goal slides and background slides are due to adjustments made during goal processing. The technique is accurate only if a reader's background processing is uniform. If, on the other hand, a reader adjusts background processing on goal slides, those adjustments are erroneously attributed to changes in goal processing. The experimental design made the uniformity assumption plausible for average group comparisons but not for individual comparisons.

Group comparisons were controlled for differences between background material by means of a cleverly counterbalanced design (goal slides for half the subjects were background slides for the other half and vice versa). Individual comparisons lacked this control because they were based on the assumption of uniform background processing between slides even though the background material differed from slide to slide. We therefore have no way of knowing the extent to which individual differences were caused by differences between materials. Many variables that might have differed between materials have been shown to affect recall. For example, ideas conducive to imagery are more memorable (Montague & Carter 1973; Yuille & Paivio, 1969) as are ideas holding prominent positions in a text's structure (e.g., Beaugrande & Dressler, 1979; Deese, 1980; Frederiksen, 1975; Kintsch, 1974; Meyer, 1975; Norman, Rumelhart, & the LNR Research Group, 1975; Van Dijk, 1977). Possibly these variables have a smaller effect when they are in background material. Another study addressing this issue, however, (cf. Fairbrother 1981) found that perceived text structure greatly influences recall of background material. Thus, Rothkopf might have judged there to be individual differences in goal processing when there were in fact differences in background processing.

In summary, a number of experiments have shown that eye movements are influenced by purpose for reading. All of the experiments leave open important questions concerning individual differences and the effects of textual variables. These questions will possibly guide future experiments toward an understanding of cognitive processes underlying situational context effects and flexible reading.

## C.  Repeated Exposures

Judd and Buswell (1922) measured eye movements of students who reread a passage. The passage, which was taken from Thorndike's *Alpha Reading Test*, was a short expository on hay fever. The exact instructions were: "Read this paragraph through once silently. Read it very rapidly as you would read a newspaper article, just to find out what it is about." Immediately after the first reading the subjects were instructed: "Now read it again more carefully. When you finish, you will be asked questions about it." Fourteen sixth-grade pupils, five high-school pupils, and one college student were tested. Unfortunately, the design confounds repetition with purpose for reading so adjustments are difficult to interpret. Most students adjusted in a way that was consistent with adjustments found in response to Anderson's (1937) gist instructions. The most interesting results are from two subjects who did not adjust. Judd and Buswell (1922) describe them as follows:

> This pupil [Subject 94], like many another in the schools, does not exhibit any ability to comply with the direction to read a passage rapidly. All reading for such a pupil is a form of study [slow, careful reading]. . . . [Subject 102] is a good reader, but evidently little affected by the exhoration to study the passage carefully. Practical teachers will have no difficulty in recalling students of this type [p. 29].

These failures to adapt show not only an inability to comply with the instructions, but also an inability on the second reading to take advantage of what was learned on the first reading. We like to think of these failures as evidence of inappropriate skill acquisition not intellectual limitations.

These failures are of special concern when one considers that the complete cycle of studying school assignments usually involves more than one reading. At the University of Virginia, for example, we administered a study habits inventory and learned, among other things, that 57% of college students in our sample *frequently or always* study an assignment once when it is first given as homework and then, at a later date, review it one or more times in preparation for a test or class discussion. Another 36% use more than one session for some of their assignments, and only 6% *rarely or never* study an assignment in more than one session. Could it be that the latter group is similar to the two students in Judd and Buswell's study who seemed unable to take advantage of repeated exposures? Could students be taught to overcome this handicap? A first step in developing effective teaching methods is to learn more about how successful students take advantage of multiple exposures.

Surprisingly little is known about the effect of repeated exposure on subjective perception of text structure or on quality of comprehension and recall (cf. Frederiksen, 1975), because research designs calling for a single exposure to a text dominate the literature on comprehension even in experiments explicitly designed to investigate study habits (cf. Anderson & Armbruster, 1980). This lack of fundamental knowledge motivated us to explore effects of repeated exposure on reading strategies and recall, which we will discuss in the next section (see also Karmiohl & Shebilske, 1982).

## IV.  Conceptual Context

In this section we move from experiments that study relationships between eye movements and external variables to experiments that study eye movements and internal variables like the state of a reader's conceptual knowledge. Although it is impossible to get pure cases of each variable type, we are concerned with experiments that have internal conceptual variables as their primary focus. Experimenters cannot observe internal states directly, of course, so they measure some observable indicator. These indicators fall into two categories: (1) *formal*, which are based upon rules that link structural aspects of a text to structural aspects of a reader's internal conceptual representations; and (2) *behavioral*, which are based upon performance of subjects on tasks that are designed to reflect aspects of internal conceptual structures. Researchers have related eye movements to both kinds of measures.

### A.  Formal Measures

Texts have what Halliday (1970, 1973) called *thematic structure*, which reflects the author's judgment about what readers do and do not know at each point. Scinto (1978) attempted to relate eye movements to thematic structure by recording eye movements of five college students who read a 225-word narrative fable for the purpose of writing a précis. Modifying a notation developed by Danes (1974), Scinto (1978), divided passages into segments representing old and new information. For example, brackets mark old information and parentheses mark new information in his first two sentences, as follows:

(*There once was a man*) [*who*] (*loved money very much.*) [*He loved money*] (*so much*) (*that*) [*he*] (*would not spend a penny*) if [*he*] (*could help*) [*it*].

Subjects saw the text in a standard format without the brackets and parentheses. Scinto found that the mean duration of fixations on old information was significantly shorter than the mean duration of fixations on new information. This difference occurred in all five subjects and it held when word length was controlled. Scinto argued that readers terminate processing earlier for old information because it is more predictable.

Carpenter and Just (1977) also related eye movements to aspects of thematic structure. In three experiments, college students read paragraphs consisting of five sentences each. The students judged whether each successive sentence was consistent or contradictory with the previous sentences. Eye movements were monitored and gaze durations were computed on whole sentences instead of on words.

In one experiment, Carpenter and Just studied the effect of giving contradictory signals about old and new information. For example, one pair of sentences was:

*The ballerina captivated a musician in the orchestra during her performance. The one who captivated the trombonist was the ballerina.*

The second sentence is the critical one. It is a pseudocleft construction, which usually puts old information in the slot held by the word *trombonist* and new information in the slot held by the word *ballerina*. The sentence is mismatched with the first sentence in this example, because the trombonist is "new" and the ballerina is "old" with respect to the first sentence. A matched sentence would read *the one who the ballerina captivated was the trombonist.* Carpenter and Just found that students spent considerably more time on mismatched sentences and they spent more time looking back at the original sentence when it was mismatched. Although there are surface differences between matched and mismatched pairs of sentences, Just and Carpenter argue that the most relevant mismatch is not in the surface of the text, but in the *conceptual* representation of the reader. Under this assumption, the results suggest that conceptual context influences eye movements.

In a second experiment, Carpenter and Just studied the effect of *foregrounding* on the assignment of pronominal reference. For example, one pair of sentences was:

*The one who the guard mocked was the arsonist. He had been at the prison for only one week.*

The first sentence is a pseudocleft construction that foregrounds the *arsonist.* The second sentence contains an ambiguous pronoun, *he,* that could have two referents, *arsonist or guard.* Half of the paragraphs foregrounded with pseudoclefts as in the example; the other half used cleft constructions (e.g., *It was the arsonist who the guard mocked.*) to control for serial position, that is, the foregrounded word was first half of the time and second half of the time. Carpenter and Just found that readers made regressive eye fixations back to the preceeding line over 50% of the time when they encountered an ambiguous pronoun. Furthermore, when students did regress, they tended to look at the foregrounded word significantly more frequently. Carpenter and Just argued, as they did in the first experiment, that their manipulation affected attempts to structure a conceptual representation. Accordingly, their results add more support to the claim that conceptual context influences eye movements.

A third experiment attempted to understand comprehension processes in another way. The experimental manipulation is again described best in terms of an example. One sentence pair was:

*It was dark and stormy the night the millionaire was murdered. The killer left no clues for the police to trace.*

Another sentence pair was identical except that the verb *died* was used in place of *was murdered*. The verb *was murdered* entails the existence of an agent, a killer, whereas the verb *died* does not. Half of the opening sentences entailed an agent that was mentioned in the second sentence; half of them did not. Carpenter and Just found that students spent more time looking at the second sentence and more time looking back at the first sentence when the first sentence did not entail the agent in the second sentence. Carpenter and Just argue that case entailments speed up the construction of an internal conceptual representation. On this account, the results show another way in which conceptual context influences eye movements.

Carpenter and Just tested an additional group of five students in a control condition designed to show that the case entailment effects that were observed in the third experiment are not specific to the consistency–judgment task that was used in that experiment. The control condition used the same five sentence paragraphs as the third experiment. It required students to push a button as soon as they understood each sentence. The results were similar to those of the third experiment, suggesting that case entailmaent effects on eye movements can be generalized beyond the consistency–judgment task.

Stone (1979) argues that while Carpenter and Just's control task is better than their consistency–judgment task, it still does not reflect general reading processes. The control task forced students to understand each sentence before going on to the next, which is not necessarily the strategy that readers employ in more natural conditions. Ordinary discourse is far richer than the texts employed by Carpenter and Just. As a result, ambiguities that exist at one point in an everyday discourse are usually resolved latter in the text. Readers have the option therefore of resolving the ambiguity immediately or later. Stone's criticism is important because it stands at odds with Just and Carpenter's (1980) immediacy assumption.

Stone tested the immediacy assumption by measuring eye movements of 12 college students while they read two passages from *The Reader's Digest* condensed readers. One passage, "Remember the Alamo" had 1971 words; the other passage, "Appomattox: Epic Surrender" had 1516 words. Stone modified the passages slightly to contain 20 critical sentence pairs between them. In half the pairs, the first sentence entailed the agent in the second sentence; in the other half of the pairs it did not. Two material sets were created in a way that the same sentences were read with and without case entailment. The results were comparable to Carpenter and Just's. Students spent less time on a sentence containing an agent when the preceeding sentence entailed the agent. Stone concluded that the immediacy assumption is safe for the moment but future experiments should include putting ambiguities in unimportant parts of a discourse. The rationale is that readers may not resolve ambiguities immediately if the content is unimportant.

In summary, researchers in three different laboratories have used various formal measures of thematic structure to reflect aspects of conceptual context. All the data indicate that conceptual context affects fixation duration and regressions. It remains for future research to determine whether or not thematic structure affects interfixation distance as well.

Kintsch and Keenan (1973) asserted that a text's meaning can be represented as a hierarchically ordered list of micropropositions, and they used a formal grammar (Kintsch, 1974) to derive the hierarchy. They went on to show that their propositional structure captures interesting aspects of reading rate and recall.

In one experiment, students silently read short paragraphs, pressed a button when they had finished, and immediately recalled the paragraph in their own words. Kintsch and Keenan found that paragraphs of the same word length were read slower when they contained more micropropositions. Reading time increased about 1.5 sec per additional proposition for short paragraphs and about 4.5 sec per additional propositions for long paragraphs. Assuming that the propositional hierarchy reflects an internal conceptual representation, the results again suggest that conceptual context affects reading rate and hence eye movements. Apparently, the eyes slow down as comprehension processes accumulate propositions to a conceptual representation. The results also suggest that it takes longer to add propositions to a larger, more complex representation and that students were more likely to recall propositions that were high in the hierarchy that had required more processing time.

Kintsch and van Dijk (1978) elaborate further upon the nature of conceptual representations. They hypothesize that micropropositions are combined to form macropropositions. Van Dijk (1977) proposed a formal grammar for representing macropropositions in a hierarchical structure and outlined 25 macropropositions that summarize a 1900-word story from Boccaccio's *Decameron*. Some of the macropropositions summarized one or two sentences whereas others summarized as many as seven. Shebilske and Reid (1979) hypothesized that more processing resources are spent on forming macropropositions that summarize many micropropositions. They therefore predicted that the time required to read sentences containing the same number of micropropositions would increase as the number of sentences combined in one macroproposition increased, and this was confirmed by eye movement records taken on 12 college students who read Boccaccio's story for recreation. Apparently, the ratio of micropropositions to macropropositions is an important aspect of conceptual context.

The results of Kintsch and Keenan and those of Reid and Shebilske suggest that comprehension processes influence eye movements when they map surface units onto micropropositions and when they map micropropositions onto macropropositions. This conclusion is also supported by experiments that measure reading rates of sentences that are presented one at a time (e.g., Cirilo & Foss,

1980; Graesser, Hoffman, & Clark, 1980; Haberlandt, Berian, & Sandson, 1980; Meyer, 1977), and by eye movement experiments using behavioral measures to reflect conceptual context.

## B.    Behavioral Measures

Zola (1982) and Ehrlich and Rayner (1981) used a modified cloze procedure to measure the extent to which context constrained words. They then measured the influence of contextual constraint upon fixation duration and probability of fixation. Zola manipulated conceptual constraint on a word by changing an immediately preceeding adjective. The first part of one sentence, for instance, was: "Since movie theaters must have buttered popcorn to serve their patrons. . . ." The word *popcorn* is highly constrained in this sentence, as indicated by the fact that students predicted it 83% of the time when they were given the passage up through the word buttered. A second sentence was identical except that "buttered" was replaced with "adequate" making the target word, *popcorn,* less constrained, as indicated by students predicting it 8% of the time when they were given the passage up through the word *adequate.* Zola found in the main part of his experiment that highly constrained context did not reduce the probability that students fixated the target word, which was fixated 97% of the time, and it only slightly reduced fixation duration on the target word.

Ehrlich and Rayner hypothesized that effects of context may not be immediate, but may build up over time. They therefore manipulated context well in advance of a target word instead of manipulating only the immediately proceeding word. They developed high and low constraining contexts for each target word. In a modified cloze task similar to Zola's, students predicted the target word 93% of the time in the high constraint context and less than 15% of the time in the low constraint context (cf. Ehrlich, Chapter 11 of this volume).

In the eye movement part of the experiment, students read the passages in order to answer comprehension questions. These readers fixated the target word less frequently in the high constraint context (66%) then they did in the low constraint context (81%). They showed this difference even though the last fixation before the target word was about 5.5 character spaces to the left in both the high and low conditions. Furthermore, when readers did fixate the target word, the fixation durations were shorter in the high constraint condition (254 msec) than in the low constraint condition (221 msec). These results are evidence of conceptual context effects if it can be assumed that they are caused by differences in underlying conceptual representations. The results are important because they localize context effects with respect to a specific word. None of the other experiments discussed so far, with the possible exception of Just and Carpenter (1980), have narrowed conceptual context effects to the word level.

A warning is in order, however. Although pinning down context effects to scanning patterns generated around a specific word is valuable, it does not guarantee that the scanning changes are related to the processing of that word. We can illustrate this warning by taking Ehrlich and Rayner's explanation of their results. They suggest that "the quality of information picked up from parafoveal vision is constant independent of the level of constraint. However, information from para-foveal vision can be utilized more effectively in the high constraint condition because the threshold for identifying a parafoveal word is lower than in the low-constraint condition. Only in this sense, it may be assumed that the perceptual span region or the effective visual field in reading (Rayner, 1975) is somewhat variable depending on context [p. 654]." This account assumes that scanning changes were generated in a DRS mode of control.

Alternatively, the changes could have been generated in an IRS mode. A highly constraining context might have increased the general rate at which information is read out of a categorical storage buffer. As a result, readers could have increased their rate by increasing interfixation distance and by decreasing fixation durations on the target word or on other words in the target sentence.

One could test the DRS and IRS alternatives by masking the entire display while the eyes were in saccadic motion after the last fixation before a target word. According to Ehrlich and Rayner's DRS account, the terminus of that saccade should be directly related to what a reader could report on a probe recognition test following the mask. According to the present IRS account, it should not. Testing Ehrlich and Rayner's hypothesis could be critical with respect to a fundamental psycholinguistic issue introduced earlier, since the hypothesis is contrary to the idea that linguistic processes are sensitive only to inputs from preceeding stages of processing.

On either account, the procedure of combining cloze tasks with eye movement investigations could be a valuable paradigm. It could provide a way of comparing and constrasting the various conceptual context effects that we have discussed. Researchers might use cloze tasks, for instance, to investigate the effect of old—new thematic structures, foregrounding, case entailment, etc., on the pre-dictability of specific words. They could then determine whether or not equally predictable words generate the same eye movement dynamics even when the predictions are generated by means of different kinds of conceptual constraints. If equally predictable words generate different scanning patterns depending upon how the predictions are derived, then the differences would shed light on how comprehension processes affect eye movements. If, on the other hand, equally predictable words generate the same scanning patterns, then many conceptual context effects would boil down to one variable. One might then argue that a fundamental component of flexible reading is to reduce scanning of predictable words.

We have also developed an eye movement paradigm to analyze comprehension processes and context effects. We give students a battery of behavioral tests that reflect various aspects of conceptual structure of relatively long texts and take measures based upon the form of the text itself. The *HEL Oculometer* (cf. Lam-bert, Monty, & Hall, 1974) is used to measure eye movements of other students who read the texts silently with task demands as naturalistic as we can make them. We hypothesize the existence of a conceptual context effect when we observe a relationship between eye movements and one of our behavioral or formal measures. We then test that hypothesis by manipulating the context in which students read excerpts from our text.

We have measured eye movements of college graduates and community college students who read a 2866-word excerpt from a tenth-grade biology textbook (Biological Sciences Curriculum Study). Our behavioral and formal measures, which are described elsewhere (Deese, 1980; Rotondo, 1980; Shebilske & Rotondo, 1981), identified 74 "Meaning Units," and they quantified 18 characteristics of those units. The characteristics are listed in Table 9.2 and they are described in detail by Estes (1980).

In one experiment (Shebilske & Fisher, 1981), we asked two college graduates to read the biology passage as they would ordinarily read material for a homework assignment. We told them that they would be tested with detailed essay and multiple choice questions and that they would have an opportunity to reread the text before the test. Students read at their own pace pushing a button to advance slides to new pages. They read once, took a 10-min break, and then read again. A test of paraphrastic recall and a multiple choice test followed the second reading.

Recall on both tests and average reading rates proved to be comparable to those observed in previous experiments in which college students read from printed pages without their eyes monitored (cf. Shebilske & Rotondo, 1981). These results set the stage for our eye movement analyses, which we approached hierarchically, first analyzing macrolevel aggregates of eye movements and then measuring microlevel parameters of individual fixations.

The macrolevel analysis revealed modulations in reading rate per Meaning Unit

### TABLE 9.2
#### Meaning Unit (MU) Characteristics

1. MU recall equals proportion of subjects recalling MU
2. MU importance rating
3. Average importance of propositions in MU
4. Number of propositions in MU
5. Number of words in MU
6. Number of propositions essential to gist
7. Number of important propositions
8. Proportion of propositions essential to gist
9. Proportion of important propositions
10. Serial position in text
11. Serial position from beginning of section
12. Serial position from end of section
13. Serial position from beginning of paragraph
14. Serial position from end of paragraph
15. Number of zero-diameter clusters contained in MU
16. Proportion of subjects placing segment boundary at beginning of MU
17. Proportion of subjects placing segment boundary at end of MU
18. Old–new rating

as a function of Meaning Unit Characteristics. Students tended to slow down for important ideas and for ideas that contained new or unfamiliar material on the first reading. Difference scores between first and second readings were correlated with: (1) Meaning Unit Importance ratings; (2) average importance of propositions in Meaning Units; (3) number of propositions essential to the gist of a Meaning Unit; and (4) serial position of a Meaning Unit. The correlation with serial position indicates that subjects slowed down toward the end of the passage, which may have been because the end of the passage contained a high density of important Meaning Units. The overall pattern of correlations suggests that readers modulate their rate with familiarity on the first reading, spending more time on unfamiliar material, and with importance on the second reading, spending more time on important Meaning Units.

Our microlevel analysis probed the effect of importance on the first and second reading. On the first reading, the students read important and unimportant ideas at rates of 280 words per min (wpm) and 288 wpm, respectively. On the second reading, they read important ideas at a rate of 229 wpm (51 wpm slower) and unimportant ideas at the rate of 372 spm (84 wpm faster). On the second reading, important Meaning Units generated longer fixation durations and more regressions, but not larger interfixation distances. Specifically: (1) mean fixation durations were 276 msec for important Meaning Units and 240 msec for unimportant ones; (2) students made four regressions per Important Meaning Unit and one regression per Unimportant Meaning Unit; and (3) average interfixation distances were 8.6 characters for important Meaning Units and 9 characters for unimportant ones.

We are currently in the process of analyzing results of a follow-up experiment. We had 11 community college students read the same passage with the same instructions except that they were not told that they would be given an opportunity to reread the passage, and in fact we tested them after their first reading. For this chapter, we analyzed the results of six students who had reading rates and recall scores that were comparable to college students observed by Shebilske and Rotondo (1981).

Table 9.3 summarizes correlations between reading rate and Meaning Unit characteristics (see Table 9.2) for all six subjects and for the average rates of those subjects. The main finding is that Meaning Unit Importance (Characteristic 2) accounts for a fair amount of variance. The correlation was $r = .48$, $p < .001$ for average rates, and the correlations were substantial for nearly every student. Importance also accounts for other moderate correlations (Characteristics 3, 7, and 9). It may also account for serial position effects (Characteristics 10, 12, and 13), as mentioned earlier. The relationship between eye movements and importance is stronger in this experiment than it was in the first experiment on the first reading. We do not yet know whether this was owing to individual differences or to the fact that students in the first experiment knew that they would have a chance to review while students in the present experiment knew that they would be tested after the first reading. Perhaps students bear down on important material to a greater extent right before tests.

# TABLE 9.3
## Correlations and $p$ Values: Rate and Meaning Unit Characteristics

Meaning Unit Characteristic

| Subject number | | 1 | 2 | 3 | 4 | 5 | 6 | 7 | 8 | 9 | 10 | 11 | 12 | 13 | 14 | 15 | 16 | 17 | 18 |
|---|---|---|---|---|---|---|---|---|---|---|---|---|---|---|---|---|---|---|---|
| 1 | r | .16 | .17 | .07 | .27 | .26 | .06 | .26 | .34 | .003 | .001 | .20 | .08 | .44 | .14 | .30 | .29 | .05 | .12 |
|   | p | (.09) | (.08) | (.26) | (.01) | (.01) | (.31) | (.01) | (.001) | (.49) | (.49) | (.04) | (.24) | (.001) | (.11) | (.005) | (.006) | (.33) | (.16) |
| 2 | r | .22 | .41 | .24 | .06 | .03 | .20 | .19 | .09 | .26 | .31 | .03 | .19 | .001 | .04 | .11 | .03 | .22 | .10 |
|   | p | (.03) | (.001) | (.02) | (.30) | (.40) | (.04) | (.05) | (.22) | (.01) | (.003) | (.40) | (.06) | (.50) | (.35) | (.18) | (.41) | (.03) | (.19) |
| 3 | r | .11 | .30 | .18 | .05 | .04 | .08 | .13 | .02 | .18 | .25 | .09 | .13 | .05 | .21 | .09 | .14 | .02 | .21 |
|   | p | (.19) | (.004) | (.06) | (.33) | (.39) | (.25) | (.14) | (.42) | (.06) | (.02) | (.22) | (.14) | (.34) | (.03) | (.22) | (.12) | (.42) | (.03) |
| 4 | r | .23 | .22 | .02 | .04 | .04 | .07 | .12 | .07 | .02 | .03 | .39 | .26 | .15 | .03 | .16 | .17 | .11 | .29 |
|   | p | (.03) | (.03) | (.44) | (.35) | (.35) | (.29) | (.16) | (.28) | (.43) | (.41) | (.001) | (.01) | (.10) | (.40) | (.08) | (.07) | (.17) | (.01) |
| 5 | r | .16 | .26 | .22 | .06 | .07 | .05 | .15 | .14 | .20 | .07 | .06 | .10 | .16 | .21 | .11 | .09 | .15 | .003 |
|   | p | (.08) | (.01) | (.03) | (.30) | (.27) | (.34) | (.10) | (.12) | (.04) | (.28) | (.32) | (.20) | (.08) | (.03) | (.17) | (.22) | (.10) | (.49) |
| 6 | r | .28 | .34 | .16 | .04 | .04 | .16 | .13 | .08 | .09 | .12 | .15 | .11 | .10 | .005 | .02 | .20 | .19 | .14 |
|   | p | (.008) | (.001) | (.08) | (.37) | (.36) | (.08) | (.14) | (.24) | (.21) | (.16) | (.10) | (.17) | (.19) | (.48) | (.43) | (.04) | (.06) | (.12) |
| Average | r | .27 | .48 | .21 | .14 | .12 | .14 | .28 | .12 | .21 | .21 | .11 | .23 | .28 | .17 | .23 | .27 | .08 | .26 |
|   | p | (.01) | (.001) | (.04) | (.12) | (.14) | (.11) | (.007) | (.15) | (.04) | (.04) | (.18) | (.02) | (.008) | (.07) | (.02) | (.01) | (.24) | (.03) |

A number of other characteristics merit special attention in our future investigations. For example, the first experiment indicated a marginal tendency to spend more time on unfamiliar material and that tendency appeared again the present study (Characteristic 18). Reading rate was also related to Meaning Unit recallability (slower for more recallable, Characteristic 1) and to sharpness with which the beginning of a Meaning Unit was defined (slower reading for sharper boundaries, Characteristic 17). Finally, we will keep an eye on the correlation with Characteristic 15. It suggests that students read a Meaning Unit slower when it contains many zero-diameter cluster units, which are groups of words that were never divided when we asked readers to divide a passage into Meaning Units. Rotondo (1980) and Shebilske & Rotondo (1981) speculate that zero diameter clusters may reflect subunits that are used to construct Meaning Units. Accordingly, the present result tentatively suggests the hypothesis that students slow down when they have to integrate many subunits to form a Meaning Unit.

The hypothesis most strongly suggested by our results is that readers adapt their scanning rate according to how important they perceive a Meaning Unit to be with respect to the passage as a whole. They scan faster when they judge a Meaning Unit to be unimportant with respect to the author's main message and slow when they judge it to be important. We hypothesized therefore that Meaning Unit Importance reflects an aspect of conceptual context that influences scanning patterns. Our hypothesis predicts that differences between Important and Unimportant Meaning Units would disappear if the units were read separately out of the larger context.

Alternatively, one could argue that reading rates differed as a function of importance because of surface differences in vocabulary and syntax. This alternative hypothesis predicts that reading rates would differ between Important and Unimportant Meaning Units even if the units were read isolated from the larger context.

We tested our hypothesis against the alternative with a control condition in which six community college students read 9 Important Meaning Units and 9 Unimportant Meaning Units, and 42 filler units on various topics. The Important and Unimportant Meaning Units were selected to match serial position in the text, word length, and number of propositions. We told students to read units one at a time and then to read a line of alphanumeric symbols that was printed between each unit. We told students that we would test only some of the ideas, but that they had to read each one carefully, because they would not know if a unit would be tested until they finished it. We tested 12 units immediately after students finished reading them. We told students that they could forget the other units.

On the average, students recalled 9 out of the 12 tested units correctly. Their reading rate on the 9 Important Units was 118.1 wpm; their rate on Unimportant Units was 118.5 wpm. In contrast, the 9 Important Units were read in context at the rate of 213 wpm, and the 9 Unimportant Units were read in context at the rate of 254 wpm. These results support our hypothesis that perceived importance of Meaning Units is an aspect of conceptual context that influences reading rate.

Our next step was to analyze the eye movement dynamics that generated the observed differences in reading rates between Important and Unimportant Meaning Units. Table 9.4 summarizes the results for all six students in our main experiment. The results are fairly consistent across subjects showing that Important Meaning Units were read with longer fixation durations, more regressions, and about the same interfixation distances. These eye movement patterns are apparent in the fixation patterns shown in Table 9.5.

The interesting contrasts in Table 9.5 are between the first two Meaning Units, which are unimportant, and the last one, which is important. Subject 2 read the first two at rates of 406 and 361 wpm respectively, and the last one at 242 wpm. Table 9.3 indicates that Subject 2, like our other subjects, typically slowed down for important information. The subject's fixation pattern reflects eye movement dynamics that underlie this tendency.

To analyze those dynamics we use parameters that are based on well-established facts about reading eye movements and vision. The eyes make saccadic movements from one fixation point to another. The duration of each fixation is no less than 85 msec because of limitations in the oculomotor system's reaction time. The eyes reach velocities as high as 175° per sec during movements and meaningful visual input is virtually wiped out during these rapid movements (cf. Shebilske, 1975). The language processor consequently receives a sequence of discrete inputs during fixations. Fixation patterns are therefore related to when and where readers have an opportunity to process information. Table 9.5 illustrates three parameters that are often used to analyze fixation patterns: fixation duration, interfixation distance, and regressions.

We interpret these parameters as follows:

1. *Fixation duration* is often taken as an index of processing time (cf. Shebilske, 1975). The average fixation durations in Table 9.5 were 230 msec and 213 msec

TABLE 9.4
Eye Movement Dynamics of Students Reading Important and Unimportant Meaning Units[a]

| Subject number | Reading rate (wpm) | | Number of regressions | | Duration of forward fixations (msec) | | Interfixation distance (characters) | |
|---|---|---|---|---|---|---|---|---|
| | Important | Unimportant | Important | Unimportant | Important | Unimportant | Important | Unimportant |
| 1 | 228 | 266 | 5.44 | 1.44 | 241 | 219 | 8.76 | 9.24 |
| 2 | 247 | 290 | .56 | 1.56 | 283 | 261 | 7.82 | 10.32 |
| 3 | 253 | 285 | 2.70 | 1.60 | 280 | 243 | 6.50 | 8.96 |
| 4 | 286 | 337 | 3.67 | 1.89 | 271 | 259 | 10.22 | 10.34 |
| 5 | 140 | 181 | 12.22 | 6.00 | 238 | 235 | 10.74 | 9.44 |
| 6 | 194 | 237 | 3.44 | 4.78 | 281 | 248 | 9.42 | 9.96 |
| Average | 225 | 266 | 4.67 | 2.88 | 266 | 244 | 8.91 | 9.71 |

[a]Values are averaged across Meaning Units. Passage was from a biology textbook, 2866 words.

## TABLE 9.5

Fixation patterns of Subject 2 reading Meaning Units 29, 30, and 52. Meaning Units are divided by slashes in the text. Meaning Units 29 and 30 are unimportant; and Meaning Unit 52 is important. The numbers that are directly above the lines of print indicate the location and serial order of each fixation. The numbers above each fixation number indicates fixation duration. The actual stimulus slides contained about 10 double-spaced lines. The distance between lines and some words is increased here to accommodate the numbers.

```
  556    150   183    283    316        250 350 100   133    216    183            150
   1      2     3      4      5          6   8   7     9      11     10             12
```
*Or we might pick out likenesses in the number of legs and lump together all organisms with four legs: frogs,*
```
  167                         333    216 366 117    133    167    283 300
   13                         14     16  15  17     18     19     20  21
```
*alligators, mice, lions./ Or we might classify organisms according to where they live, lumping together those*
```
 233    183    300    366   167 200   233
  22     23     25     24    26  27    28
```
*that are found in human households: dogs, geraniums, canaries, rats, fleas.*
```
       233   133 233    266         383    216 133    300        200 133 117 266 183 333
        58    57  59      60          61     62 64      63         65  66  67  68  69  70
```
*In summary, then, we can say that a species is a population of individuals that are more or less alike and*
```
          500 600350 316 283 200 283    283 183 183
           79  71 78  80  72  77  74     737 5  7 6
```
*that interbreed and produce fertile offspring under natural conditions./*

for the first two units and 241 msec for the last one. The longer durations for important information is consistent with the overall averages given in Table 9.4. We conclude therefore that readers increase fixation durations when they slow down for important information. Presumably, the extra time allows them to perform additional processing on important information. An important next step will be linking increased durations to specific processing activities. If we could do that, we could analyze the extra processing activities done on important Meaning Units. We see no satisfactory way, however, to make this connection at the present time.

A major problem is that readers only fixate between ½ and ⅔ of the words in many reading situations. In Table 9.5, 51% of the words are fixated in the first two units and 57% are fixated in the last unit. These percentages are representative of percentages obtained in our experiment. They are also consistent with percentages found by other researchers (cf. Shebilske & Fisher, 1982). Another typical characteristic of the records in Table 9.5 is the fact that many content words are skipped (Shebilske, 1975). Notice, for example, that the reader skipped the words *four legs* in the second line. Did the reader process these words while looking at some other word? If so, how does one divide fixation durations into processing times for the fixated word and the other words? Perhaps the division of processing time can be estimated by averaging across subjects. Different readers skip different words so that almost every word is fixated by some subjects. Collapsing across subjects would therefore give an average duration for each word. One could assume that these group averages somehow indicate how individuals divide durations between fixated words and other words. This assumption is implicit when researchers compute "gaze durations" per word averaged across subjects and then conclude that they have analyzed moment-to-moment real time characteristics of reading (cf. Just & Carpenter, 1980). We are unwilling to make this assumption in our work. McConkie (this volume) is making progress that we hope will lead to a less speculative way to link increased durations to the specific supplementary processes that are allocated to important Meaning Units.

2. *Interfixation distance* is the metric that is often used to measure how readers space their fixations. Average interfixation distances are usually computed by averaging the distances between successive fixations. This metric did not function well for us. One can see at a glance in Table 9.5 that fixations are spaced quite differently in the important and unimportant units. It is especially interesting to notice that the reader skipped over trivia (e.g., *mice, lions, canaries, rats,* and *fleas*) in the unimportant units. Yet, average interfixation distances did not capture the apparent differences. In fact, the average interfixation distances are 9 characters for the first two units and 11 characters for the last unit, which is the opposite of what one would expect. The occurrence of regressions seems to contaminate interfixation distance scores. Therefore, until a better metric is developed, we will hold in abeyance conclusions about how readers modulate the spacing of their fixations when they slow down for important Meaning Units.

3. *Regressions* are movements from right to left within a line of print or movements to preceding lines. Shebilske (1975) argued that some regressions are caused by dysmetria in the oculomotor system whereas others are determined by the language processor. He suggested further that saccadic dysmetria is especially likely to cause regressions at the beginning of lines. The saccadic system undershoots the beginning of the line and then makes a regression to bring the eyes back to the intended location. A control condition in our experiment supported this hypothesis. We had each subject read a page of alphanumeric symbols that were printed in lines like text. The frequency of regressions at the beginning of lines was very similar for alphanumeric displays and for texts even though the language information was very different. We therefore distinguish between regressions at the beginning of lines and "other" regressions. The regressions listed in Table 9.4, for example, exclude regressions occurring at the beginning of lines. Table 9.5 is consistent with the general trend that we observed in "other" regressions. One and none were made, respectively, in the first two unimportant units and four were made in the important unit. The results are consistent with our contention that comprehension processes influence regressions. The regressions are concentrated on the words *produce fertile,* which are not difficult words for our subjects to recognize. They are, however, essential to the reader's underlying conceptual representation.

Taken as a whole our results tentatively suggest that a fundamental component of flexible reading is modulating rate and pattern of scanning with respect to perceived importance of Meaning Units. This component captures not only effects of conceptual context, but also effects of situational context since perceived importance is judged with respect to specific task demands.

## V.  Implications

Throughout this chapter we have pointed to theoretical implications for issues in psycholinguistics and to practical implications for teaching flexible reading in content area classrooms (Estes & Vaughan, 1981). One of the theoretical questions that we addressed was: Are linguistic processes autonomous in the sense of being sensitive only to inputs from preceeding stages of processing? We did not completely answer this question, but we did outline an approach for moving toward a more complete answer by combining aspects of several eye movement paradigms in order to test the autonomy hypothesis during reading of extended discourse.

One of the practical questions that we addressed was: What are the components of flexible reading? We hinted that eye movement studies support two possible components: (1) reducing scanning of predictable words; and (2) modulating scanning rate and pattern with respect to perceived importance of Meaning Units. If these components are verified, we think it will be possible to teach these to students as processing strategies as opposed to eye movement strategies. Our project is based upon the critical assumption that the mechanics of reading are largely controlled by the level of understanding and not the other way around. Therefore, the path of previous attempts to improve reading by improving the mechanics of eye movements (cf. Tinker, 1958) goes counter to our purpose. We believe, however, that if we can identify fundamental components of flexible reading that teachers will then be able to develop lesson plans for teaching these fundamental advanced reading skills.

## References

Anderson, I. H. (1937). Studies in the eye-movements of good and poor readers. *Psychological Monographs, 48*, 1–35.
Anderson, T. H., & Armbruster, B. B. (1980). *Studying.* (Tech. Rep. 155). Urbana: University of Illinois, Center for the Study of Reading.
Beaugrande, R., & Dressler, W. (1979). *Introduction to text linguistics.* London: Longman.
Biological Sciences Curriculum Study. (1963). *High school biology (green version)* (2nd ed.). Chicago: Rand McNally.
Bouma, H., & de Voogd, A. H. (1974). On the control of eye saccades in reading. *Vision Research, 14*, 273–284.
Bransford, J. D., Barclay, J. R., & Franks, J. J. (1972). Sentence memory: A constructive versus interpretive approach. *Cognitive Psychology, 3*, 193–209.
Bransford, J. D., & Johnson, M. K. (1973). Consideration of some problems of comprehension. In W. G. Chase (Ed.), *Visual information processing.* New York: Academic Press, pp. 383–438.
Carpenter, P. A., & Just, M. A. (1977). Reading comprehension as eyes see it. In M. A. Just & P. A. Carpenter (Eds.), *Cognitive processes in comprehension.* New York: Wiley.

Cirilo, R. K., & Foss, D. J. (1980). Text structure and reading time for sentences. *Journal of Verbal Learning and Verbal Behavior, 19,* 96–109.

Clark, H. H. (1978). Inferring what is meant. In W. J. M. Levelt & G. B. Flores d' Arcais (Eds.), *Studies in the perception of language.* New York: Wiley.

Danes, F. (1974). *Papers on functional sentence perspective.* Prague: Publishing House of the Czech Academy of Sciences.

Davis, F. R. (1968). Research in comprehension in reading. *Reading Research Quarterly, 3,* 499–544.

Deese, J. (1980). Text structure, strategies, and comprehension in learning from textbooks. In Robinson, J. (Ed.), *Research in science education: New questions, new directions.* Boulder: BSCS.

Ehrlich, S. F., & Rayner, K. (1981). Contextual effects on word perception and eye movements. *Journal of Verbal Learning and Verbal Behavior, 20,* 641–655.

Estes, T. H. (1980). *Properties of text producing comprehension.* Paper presented at the 30th annual meeting of the National Reading Conference, San Diego, December. (Available from Thomas Estes, McGuffey Reading Center, Rufner Hall, University of Virginia, Charlottesville, Va. 22901.)

Estes, T. H., & Shebilske, W. L. (1980). Comprehension: Of what the reader sees of what the author says. In Kamil, M. L. & Moe, S. J. (Eds.), *Twenty-ninth yearbook of the National Reading Conference,* pp. 99–104.

Estes, T. H., & Vaughan, J. L., Jr. (1981). *Reading and learning in the content classroom: Diagnostic and instructional strategies* (2nd ed.). Boston: Allyn and Bacon.

Fairbrother, H. (1981). *Comprehension of textbooks: Advanced organizers and perceived text structure.* Unpublished masters thesis, University of Virginia.

Fisher, D. F. (1975). Reading and visual search. *Memory & Cognition, 3,* 188–196.

Fisher, D. F. (1979). Dysfunctions in reading disability: There's more than meets the eye. In L. Resnick & P. Weaver (Eds.), *Theory and practice in beginning reading.* Hillsdale, New Jersey: Lawrence Erlbaum Associates. (a)

Fisher, D. F. (1979). Understanding the reading process through the use of transformed typography: PSG, CSG and Automaticity. In P. Kolers, M. E. Wrolstad & H. Bouma (Eds.), *Processing of visible language.* New York: Plenum Press. (b)

Fisher, D. F., & Lefton, L. A. (1976). Peripheral information extractions: A developmental examination of the reading process. *Journal of Experimental Child Psychology, 24,* 77–93.

Fisher, D. F., & Montanary, W. E. (1977). Spatial and contextual factors in beginning reading: Evidence for PSG–CSG complements to developing automaticity. *Memory and Cognition, 5,* 247–251.

Flood, J. (1981). Prose comprehension: A selected review of literature on inference–generation as a requisite for understanding text. In D. F. Fisher & C. W. Peters (Eds.), *Comprehension and the competent readers: Inter-specialty perspectives.* New York: Praeger.

Forster, K. I. (1979). Levels of processing and the structure of the language processor. In W. E. Cooper & E. C. T. Walker (Eds.), *Sentence processing.* New York: Wiley.

Frederiksen, C. H. (1975). Representing logical and semantic structures of knowledge acquired from discourse. *Cognitive Psychology, 1,* 371–458.

Fry, E. (1968). A readability formula that saves time. *Journal of Reading, 11,* 513–516.

Gibson, E. J., & Levin, H. (1975). *The psychology of reading.* Cambridge, Massachusetts: MIT Press.

Graesser, A. C., Hoffman, N. L., & Clark, L. F. (1980). Structural components of reading time. *Journal of Verbal Learning and Verbal Behavior, 19,* 135–151.

Haberlandt, K., Berian, C., & Sandson, J. (1980). The episode in story processing. *Journal of Verbal Learning and Verbal Behavior, 19,* 635–650.

Halliday, M. A. K. (1970). Language structure and language function. In J. Lyons (Ed.), *New horizons in linguistics.* Baltimore: Penguin Books.

Halliday, M. A. K. (1973). Explorations in the functions of language. London: Edward Arnold.

Harris, A. J., & Sipay, E. R. (1975). *How to increase reading ability: A guide to developmental and remedial methods* (6th ed.). New York: David McKay Company Inc.

Judd, C. H., & Buswell, G. T. (1922). Silent reading: A study of the various types. *Supplementary educational monographs*, (Vol. 23). Chicago: University of Chicago Press.

Just, M. A., & Carpenter, P. A. (1980). A Theory of Reading: From eye fixations to comprehension. *Psychological Review*, 87, 329–354.

Karmiohl, C. M. & Shebilske, W. L. (1982). *Behavioral vs. formal procedures of text analysis: Discourse style, task demands, and reading strategies.* Manuscript submitted for publication.

Kintsch, W. (1974). *The representation of meaning in memory.* New York: Wiley.

Kintsch, W., & Keenan, J. (1973). Reading rate and retention as a function of the number of prepositions in the base structure of sentences. *Cognitive Psychology*, 5, 257–274.

Kintsch, W., & van Dijk, T. A. (1978). Toward a model of text comprehension and production. *Psychological Review*, 85, 363–394.

La Berge, D., & Samuels, S. J. (1974). Toward a theory of automatic information processing in reading. *Cognitive Psychology*, 6, 293–323.

Lambert, R. H., Monty, R. A., & Hall, R. J. (1974). High-speed data processing and unobtrusive monitoring or eye movements. *Behavior Research Methods & Instrumentation*, 6, 525–530.

Lefton, L. A., & Fisher, D. F. (1976). Information extraction during visual search: A developmental progression. *Journal of Experimental Child Psychology*, 22, 346–361.

Levelt, W. J. M. (1978). A survey of studies in sentence perception: 1970–1976. In W. J. M. Levelt & G. B. Flores d' Arcais (Eds.), *Studies in the perception of language.* New York: Wiley.

Massaro, D. W. (1975). Primary and secondary recognition in reading. In D. W. Massaro (Ed.), *Understanding language: An information-processing analysis of speech perception, reading and psycholinguistics.* New York, Academic Press.

McConkie, G. W. (1979). On the role and control of eye movements in reading. In P. A. Kolers, M. E. Wrolstad, and H. Bouma (Eds.), *Processing of visible language* (Vol. 1). New York: Plenum Press.

Meyer, B. J. F. (1975). *The organization of prose and its effect on recall.* Amsterdam: North Holland.

Meyer, B. J. F. (1977). The structure of prose: Effects of learning and memory and implications for educational practice. In R. C. Anderson, R. Spiro, & W. E. Montague (Eds.), *Schooling and the acquisition of knowledge.* Hillsdale, New Jersey: Lawrence Erlbaum Associates.

Miller, G. A. (1972). English verbs of motion: A case study in semantics and lexical memory. In A. W. Melton & E. Martin (Eds.), *Coding processes in human memory.* Washington, D.C.: Winston.

Montague, W. E., & Carter, J. F. (1973). Vividness of imagery in recalling connected discourse. *Journal of Educational Psychology*, 64, 72–75.

Morton, J. (1969). The interaction of information in word recognition. *Psychological Review*, 60, 329–346.

Newell, A. (1980). Harpy, production systems and human cognition. In R. Cole (Ed.), *Perception and production of fluent speech.* Hillsdale, New Jersey: Erlbaum.

Norman, D. A., Rumelhart, D. E., & the LNR Research Group. *Exploration in cognition.* San Francisco: W. H. Freeman.

Olson, G. M., & Clark, H. H. (1976). Research methods in psycholinguistics. In E. C. Carterette & M. P. Friedman (Eds.), *Handbook of perception* (Vol. 7: *Language and speech*). New York: Academic Press.

Rankin, E. F. (1974). The measurement of reading flexibility: Problems and perspective. *Reading information series: Where do we go?* International Reading Association.

Raygor, A. L. (1970). *McGraw–Hill basic skills system: reading test* (manual). New York: McGraw–Hill.

Rayner, K. (1975). The perceptual span and peripheral cues in reading. *Cognitive Psychology*, 7, 65–81.

Rayner, K. (1978). Eye movements in reading and information processing. *Psychological Bulletin*, 85, 618–660.

Riesbeck, C. K., & Schank, R. C. (1978). Comprehension by computer: Expectation-based analysis of sentences in context. In W. J. M. Levelt & G. G. Flores d' Arcais (Eds.), *Studies in the perception of language.* New York: Wiley.

Rothkopf, E. Z. (1978). Analyzing eye movements to infer processing styles during learning from text.

In Senders, J. W., Fisher, D. F., & Monty, R. A. (Eds.), *Eye movements and the higher psychological functions.* Hillsdale, New Jersey: Lawrence Erlbaum and Associates.

Rotondo, J. A. (1980). *Clustering analysis of subjective partitions of text.* Paper presented at the National Reading Conference, San Diego, California, December.

Schank, R. C., & Abelson, R. P. (1977). *Scripts, plans, goals, and understanding: An inquiry into human knowledge structures.* Hillsdale, New Jersey: Erlbaum.

Schvaneveldt, R. W., Meyer, D. E., & Becker, C. A. (1976). Lexical ambiguity, semantic context, and visual word recognition. *Journal of Experimental Psychology: Human Perception & Performance,* 2, 243–256.

Scinto, L. F. (1978). Relations of eye fixations to old–new information of texts. In Senders, J. W., Fisher, D. F., & Monty, R. A. (Eds.), *Eye movements and the higher psychological functions.* Hillsdale, New Jersey: Erlbaum.

Shebilske, W. L. (1975). Reading eye movements from an information-processing point of view. In D. W. Massaro (Ed.), *Understanding language: An information-processing analysis of speech perception, reading, and psycholinguistics.* New York: Academic Press.

Shebilske, W. L. (1980). Structuring an internal representation of text: A basis for literacy. In P. A. Kolers, M. E. Wrolstad, & H. Bouma (Eds.), *Processing of visible language* (Vol. 2). New York: Plenum.

Shebilske, W. L., & Fisher D. F. (1981). Eye movements reveal components of flexible reading strategies. Kamil, M. L. (Ed.), 31st Yearbook of the National Reading Conference, Clemson, South Carolina.

Shebilske, W. L., & Fisher D. F. (1982). Understanding extended discourse through the eyes: How and why. In R. Gröner, D. F. Fisher, R. A. Monty, & C. Menz (Eds.), *Eye movements: An international perspective.* Hillsdale, New Jersey: Erlbaum.

Shebilske, W. L., & Reid, L. S. (1979). Reading eye movements, macro-structure and comprehension processes. In P. A. Kolers, M. E. Wrolstad, and H. Bouma (Eds.), *Processing of visible language* (Vol. 1). New York: Plenum Press.

Shebilske, W. L., & Rotondo, J. H. (1981). Typographical and spatial cues that facilitate learning from textbooks. *Visible Language,* 15, 41–54.

Spache, G., & Spache, E. (1977). *Reading in the elementary school.* Boston: Allyn & Bacon.

Stone, F. V. (1979). *The effect of textual cohesion of connected discourse.* Unpublished doctoral dissertation, University of Virginia.

Swinney, D. A. (1979). Lexical access during sentence comprehension: (Re) Consideration of context effects. *Journal of Verbal Learning and Verbal Behavior,* 18, 645–660.

Tanenbaum, M. K., Leiman, J. M., & Seidenberg, M. S. (1979). Evidence for multiple stages in the processing of ambiguous words in syntactic contexts. *Journal of Verbal Learning and Verbal Behavior,* 18, 427–440.

Tinker, M. A. (1951). Fixation pause duration in reading. *Journal of Educational Research,* 44, 471–479.

Tinker, M. A. (1958). Recent studies of eye movements in reading. *Psychological Bulletin,* 55, 215–231.

Twohig, P. (1982). *Effectiveness of examples in promoting comprehension of expository discourse.* Unpublished doctoral dissertation, University of Virginia.

van Dijk, T. A. (1977). *Text and context: Explorations in the semantics and pragmatics of discourse.* London: Longmans.

Winograd, T. (1972). Understanding natural language. *Cognitive Psychology,* 3, 1–191.

Yuille, J. C., & Paivio, A. (1969). Abstractness and the recall of connected discourse. *Journal of Experimental Psychology,* 82, 467–471.

Zola, D. (1982). The effects of context on the visual perception of words in reading. *Perception & Psychophysics,* in press.

Albrecht Werner Inhoff

# 10

# Attentional Strategies during the Reading of Short Stories[1]

## I.   Introduction

During reading we adjust our eye movements in response to textual charac-teristics. Hence eye movements seem to constitute a sensitive interface between the information processing structure of the reader and the text to be com-prehended. In this chapter both components will receive some consideration.

As a prerequisite for comprehension, Kant and other philosophers have argued for the necessity of abstract mental categories that serve to coordinate sensations into ideas. Without these categories, we would be unable to gain knowledge beyond mere "superficial" stimulus attributes. According to Kant, understanding occurs when we are successful in relating stimulus triggered sensations to idea categories. Similarly, the comprehension of text in reading may be contingent upon the reader's successful relation of incoming information to an appropriate "idea" or internal model. This will supply the reader with additional information which is not made explicit in the text itself, but which is necessary to arrive at a complete text interpretation. Recently, two major types of such internal models that guide the comprehension of text have been developed, notably models that relate the *content* of the text to the reader's available "knowledge base" (Minsky, 1977; Schank & Abelson, 1977) and theoretical conceptions that rest on the assumption that people also share tacit knowledge about the *structural organization* of text that serves to envelope incoming material (Bower, 1976; Johnson & Mand-ler, 1979; Mandler & Johnson, 1977; Thorndyke, 1977). *Content* and *structure* seem to substitute different types of story attributes (e.g., Minsky, 1977).

[1]Preparation of this chapter was supported by Grant BNS79-17600 from the National Science Foundation.

*EYE MOVEMENTS IN READING:*
*PERCEPTUAL AND LANGUAGE PROCESSES*

According to the former, *content* oriented position, readers use their familiarity with recurring situations and (causal) dependencies among the constituents of such situations to interpret text material. It is assumed that the reader's knowledge base is organized around a series of familiar situations (called scripts or frames) which are contacted once corresponding text is to be parsed. The latter, *structural* approach, holds that the position of the description of an event within a text partially determines its interpretation. For example, *John cried, because Mary said she loved Bill* carries the literal meaning that John cried because of Mary's speaking. However, our familiarity with the content of a situation like this suggests an interpretation that goes beyond the literal expression. We know that someone must be seriously hurt in order to start crying. If we arrive at such a conclusion, we may do so because we have successfully contacted an internal content frame. In addition we tend to weigh the sentence differentially, depending on its structural role. John's crying may end a story, may supply its setting, or may describe a (potentially unsuccessful) problem-solving technique. Which sets of conclusions the reader may draw depends on the sentence's structural roles. Hence, contact with internal frames that supply *content* and *structural* interpretations is essential to comprehension of the text material. However, it is also conceivable that accessing a "lovesick man" frame may cause an inappropriate and misleading sentence interpretation. John may have known all along about Mary's "secret" but it was only when she started to talk about it, that he began crying. It seems that prior contextual information is required, including information about the relationship between the three people, to successfully select the appropriate frame.

There is also text material that is not easily understood, even when the reader has accessed the appropriate frame. Words or phrases may be unknown to the reader, implausible, or contradictory, so that the reader finds no correspondence in the internal model. For example, upon reading about a school curriculum, the reader is well prepared to encounter the subjects of French and music, but would not expect the teaching of washing, especially if he or she has been informed about other subjects that were fairly predictable. How will the reader respond to such unexpected pieces of information? Are such text–frame discrepancies noticed immediately or only after subsequent statements have been evaluated? Once the discrepancy is discovered, how will the reader respond to it? Will a routine reprocessing suffice or will frame-distant text information require a qualitatively different process of meaning generation? The available literature, briefly presented below, cannot answer these questions. Hence, they constitute the major focus of my own investigation.

## II.  The Role of Content and Structure

A convincing case in favor of the effectiveness of *content* frames for text comprehension was provided by Bransford and Johnson (1972) in a series of sentences with or without a guiding frame (a picture or a story headline). The individual sentences were constructed so that they had no obvious connections with each other. However, when a frame was supplied that provided information not stated in the sentences, the text could be tied to a coherent theme. The observed frame effect was striking: Recall of the frame group far exceeded that of the controls. Similarly, Pichert and Anderson (1977) and Anderson and Pichert (1978) demonstrated that information that was not part of the text determined the reader's text evaluation (recall of text constitutents and a ranking of idea units) effects presumably due to the access of *content* frames.

Rumelhart (1975) and Mandler and Johnson (1977) compiled a general *structural analysis* for simple stories. They suggested a set of rewrite rules that were assumed to be available to the reader. For example, it was hypothesized that a story consists of the setting and the event structure. The setting introduces the protagonist and specifies time and location. The events (episodes) consist of a beginning, a story development, and an ending; each of these sections unfolds according to additional rewrite rules so that each statement of the story will hold a particular position within the overall *structure*. Mandler and Johnson (1977) showed that the recall performance of children and adults was indeed affected by the position assigned to statements by the story structure. Settings and beginnings were better recalled than story developments and endings. Converging results were reported by Glenn (1978), Gentner (1976), Graesser, Robertson, Lovelace, and Swinehart (1980), Meyers and Boldrick (1975), McKoon (1977), and others.

In each of the earlier investigations the effect of story *content* and *structure* was measured after the completed reading of the entire text. Other data are available that allow a closer look at the reading performance (Cirilio & Foss, 1980; Graesser, Hoffman, & Clark, 1980; Haberland, Berian, & Sandson, 1980). For example, Graesser, Hoffman and Clark showed that stories with familiar topics are read at a faster rate than stories with unfamiliar topics, and Cirilio and Foss demonstrated that an identical sentence consumed different amounts of reading time, depending on its structural assignment. Sentences in central structural position required longer reading times than more peripheral controls.

This brief review indicates that earlier studies have tended to rely on the reader's recall performance, implying that the product or result of story comprehension was investigated rather than the process of comprehension itself. The more recent data concerning the reader's use of frames during encoding used relatively coarse dependent variables like reading time per sentence and therefore supply only global indices. Hence, the available data do not reveal whether readers stay in immediate contact with their internal frame or whether this consulting takes place in a delayed manner, for example, only after a whole sentence has been read. Only an online recording of the reader's encoding behavior could reveal such strategies.

The following section discusses the reader's response to different degrees of text–frame correspondence, in particular, how the reader allocates mental resources to safeguard text comprehension.

## III. The Allocation of Mental Effort Depending on the Availability of Story Frames

Friedman (1979) hypothesized that the encoder engages in different encoding strategies depending on the availability of frame knowledge, and that when the encoder can contact the content frames successfully, information evaluation occurs in a relatively automatic manner. However, Friedman suggests, when the knowledge base cannot be consulted, procedures that require the allocation of mental resources are invoked. A trade-off between the success of frame exploitation and the degree to which automatic encoding is possible. The more frame deviant the stimulus attributes, the more effortful processes Friedman expected to be. She obtained longer initial fixation durations for unpredictable picture elements than for highly predictable controls and further observed that subjects in a recognition test generally noticed only changes that had been made to unpredictable elements. From this she concluded that effortful processes resulted in longer encoding operations and stronger memory traces (or an episodic tagging) and that the availability of frame knowledge was effectively guiding the investment of cognitive resources. However, pictures may be encoded differently than text material: "Pictures are often held to be a class of objects that stands in clear contradistinction to the class of objects which are words [Friedman, 1979, p. 318]," so that an extrapolation to the reading situation cannot be readily made.

Indeed, Britton, Westbrook, and Holdredge (1978) seemed to show that the reading of easy passages consumed more mental effort than the comprehension of difficult material. Britton, Holdredge, Curry, and Westbrook (1979) replicated the finding using identical stories for the easy and difficult passages. In each of the two studies a click detection technique was applied to measure mental effort; one to three clicks were presented at randomly determined text positions and click detection was found to be delayed for easier text conditions. Britton *et al.* (1978) argued that in reading easy passages the cognitive processor is filled optimally whereas breakdowns occur for difficult material which results in a temporary unloading of the processor. This was suggested to leave increased mental capacity available for the secondary task, and fast reaction times were the result. Britton, Holdredge, Curry, and Westbrook (1979) further specified that once an internal frame is successfully contacted ("the apperceptive mass called up by familiar topics") cognitive capacity will be filled leaving little extra resources for the execution of the secondary task.

Since alternative theoretical formulations relating *content* (semantic) text characteristics to the immediate mental operations of the reader are lacking at the present time, the research deserves a more detailed evaluation. This need is enhanced by the fact that a different theoretical position has been advocated for picture perception (Friedman, 1979) and because the interpretations provided by Britton *et al.* (1978) and Britton, Holdredge, Curry, and Westbrook (1979) are somewhat counterintuitive. For example, it is not obvious why a collapse of the central processor should result in an effective unbinding of mental resources;

furthermore, why should the processor break down less frequently in the frame condition if contacting an internal frame increases the allocation of mental effort?

A closer look at the experiments reveals that some of the results may be open to alternative interpretations. For example, Britton, Holdredge, Curry, and Westbrook (1979) had subjects read passages that were meaningless without a title or guiding idea (the stories were taken from Bransford & Johnson, 1972). Both conditions resulted in about equal reading rates, which suggests, provided an equal number of saccades were executed, that an equal amount of information was to be parsed during each fixation. As indicated, title stories, which allowed a successful frame contact, were responded to more slowly in the secondary task than the no-title, incomprehensible controls. However, the subjects may have been engaged in quite different types of reading. In the title condition, readers were trying to read for meaning, whereas they may have resigned from meaning generation in the no-title trials and may have solely concentrated on the secondary task; in this case the experiment would have only demonstrated that *content* frames mediate story understanding and that comprehension processes may consume mental resources.

Britton, Meyer, Simpson, Holdridge and Curry (1979) investigated the effect of *structural* story attributes upon the reader's allocation of mental resources. An identical paragraph was embedded in different passages so that it occupied either a more central or more peripheral position according to a structural analysis. As before, click detection was used to measure the allocation of mental resources. Although recall rate confirmed the structural assignment of the paragraphs, that is, a more central position resulted in a higher recall rate, there was no indication that the more central paragraph required longer reading times, and, furthermore, there was no evidence that different amounts of cognitive resources were allocated. (Note that this is in contrast with results obtained by Cirilio & Foss, 1980; both data sets were collected in a reading situation.)

Based on this present state of research, the issue of how the reader responds to different degrees of text frame correspondence clearly remains unresolved. The data available are, in part, contradictory, and a closer inspection reveals that critical questions could not be addressed due to the insensitivity of the methods employed.

The present investigation was performed to gain insight into the role of internal frames and context information for story comprehension as it occurs in reading, that is, during the encoding of individual text components. Further, the reactions of the reader to different degrees of text–frame correspondence were investigated. Two experiments were designed to separately assess the role of *content* frames and tacit *structural* knowledge.

The reader's fixation durations provided an on-line measure of the encoding behavior. Fixations have repeatedly been shown to be valid indicators of text related mental activities (e.g., Rayner, 1978). However, the measure employed to estimate the investment of mental resources deserves a more extensive justification.

# IV. The Measurement of
# Resource Allocation (Attention)

Friedman (1979) claimed that fixation durations per se were a valid indicator of the mental effort invested during the encoding of visual stimuli. If this is true, short fixations for words with high frequency counts and for highly predictable text elements would indicate automatic encoding and long fixations, which might be recorded for words with low frequency counts and unpredictable words, would suggest effortful processes. However, long fixations could be due to different factors: For example, a rare word may require the reader to engage in a more extensive sampling of visual information, whereas an unexpected word may require the reader to rearrange the interpretation of a particular phrase or sentence. The processes may differ in the amount of mental resources required, although they may both result in longer fixations. Hence, resource allocation has to be estimated separately from the reader's encoding behavior if fixation durations serve as the dependent variable. The click (probe) detection technique (e.g., Britton, Westbrook & Holdredge, 1978; Britton, Holdredge, Curry, & Westbrook, 1979; Britton, Meyer, Simpson, Holdredge, & Curry, 1979) seems to be relatively problematical in achieving this. Presenting clicks randomly and deciding in a post hoc fashion whether they were presented at long (or short) fixations does not seem to be appropriate. This is because probe presentation may occur at different processing stages during an individual fixation.

Alternatively, Logan (1978, 1979) suggested a concurrent task to measure attention. He argued that loading a STM buffer (secondary task) would reduce the mental capacity available for the primary task. This capacity reduction will only interfere with a primary task if effort is to be invested for its execution. This implies that a concurrent task will interfere with encoding operations (fixations) only if they are indicative of effortful processes; complementarily, no such interference due to a secondary task is expected to occur for fixations if they reflect automatic encoding.

This poses the question of which concurrent task will be the most appropriate. Logan required his subjects to store digits as a secondary task; the primary tasks were relatively simple and required the subjects to make discriminations at a subsemantic level. Storing digits or words in STM while being engaged in a relatively complex reading task may yield some problems; for example, if the reader were to store digits, and the text was about calculations, an observed interference between story comprehension and secondary task might be due to semantic interference rather than because of a competition for processing resources.

In the present study a concurrent task has been devised that increases processing load during each fixation duration. At the same time semantic interference is excluded. This is accomplished by moving a small visual mask in synchrony with the reader's eyes. Rayner, Inhoff, Morrison, Slowiaczek, and Bertera (1981) observed that a mask applied to only one focal letter reduced reading rate drastically while leaving the remainder of the text completely legible.[2]

To investigate the role of *content* frames, four stories were selected from Lewis Carroll's *Alice in Wonderland* (Experiment 1) and four other stories were taken from Mandler and Johnson (1977) to observe effects of story *structure* (Experiment 2).

In the experiments, subjects' eye movements were monitored by a computer based, highly sensitive eye movement recording system as they looked at a cathode-ray tube (CRT). The individual short stories were presented line by line and subjects were instructed to read each line of text and press a button upon its successful comprehension. The button press resulted in an erasure of the text and its replacement with a fixation marker at the beginning of the line. Upon the reader's return to the fixation marker a new line of text was provided and the reading cycle was repeated until the whole story was read. The computer recorded individual fixation durations at the respective fixation positions. In the trials involving the application of the secondary task, a one-letter mask was moved in synchrony with the reader's eyes.

In Experiment 1, different degrees of story content–frame correspondence were assumed to occur. The text excerpts (see Table 10.1) have the characteristic that part of the text content conforms to the reader's expectations. For example, upon asking what subjects were taught at school, Alice may answer "French and music." Here French and music are in agreement with the reader's knowledge about school curricula. On the other hand, highly predictable elements alternate with unexpected statements. For example, after having asked Alice about her subjects, the interrogator may continue: "How about washing?" Here we may be prepared to encounter a question; however, the content of the question is highly unexpected. There is no world knowledge that ties the subjects of French, music, and washing to a grammar school curriculum. At the same time, both expected and unexpected information has to be integrated throughout the story, since it is the interplay of these expectation conform and nonconform elements that gives the stories their particular (and sometimes peculiar) meaning.

To obtain an objective measure of text–frame correspondence, individual words were rated for their predictability within the story context. Based on this, a group of high-, medium-, and low-predictable items were selected. Figure 10.1a shows the pattern of results obtained. The data reveal that total viewing time per word was a function of predictability. As expected, low frame conform elements required longer encoding operations than more predictable controls. Furthermore, Figure 10.1a demonstrates that predictability interacted with the secondary task

---

[2]This manipulation is intended to tap the amount of reader's resource allocation (or processing "intensity"). Friedman (1979) advanced such a view. Automatic processes were suggested to operate in a top–down fashion. Here the internal frame is the predominant means by which the meaning of a word is generated. In this case a one-letter mask will carry little interference with respect to word identification. In contrast to this, effortful processing is regarded as bottom–up. Memorial structures are less effective and a more detailed stimulus evaluation has to take place. Under these circumstances a one letter mask should strongly interfere with (bottom–up) word identification, that is, it results in a highly increased reading time for frame discrepant words.

**TABLE 10.1**
Modified Text Excerpt from "Alice in Wonderland"

"we learned french and music"
"and washing?" asked the biber.
"certainly not" answered alice.
"then yours wasn't a really good school"
said the biber,
in a tone of great relief.
"now at ours, they had,
at the end of the bill,
french, music, and washing extra".
"and what were the regular courses?"
asked alice curiously.
"reeling and writhing, of course,
and then the different branches
of arihmetic; for example,
ambition, distraction, uglification",
exclaimed the biber.
"but I suppose you know
what to beautify is?"

employed: low-predictable words were more interferred with than high-predict-able components.

To test whether the effect reflected the reader's text–frame contact or merely

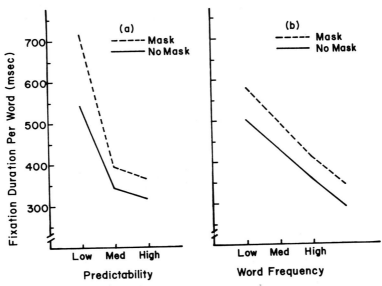

**FIGURE 10.1.** *Total fixation duration per critical word. Three different levels of predictability and word frequency were investigated under a no-mask and a one-letter mask condition.*

the stage of word identification, high, medium, and low frequency words were selected from the word pool that had been rated for predictability. There was a strong effect of word frequency; low frequency words consumed longer reading times than high frequency controls. However, as Figure 10.1b shows, there was virtually no indication that frequency interacted with the secondary task. A separate scoring, in which reading time per letter was the basic unit of analysis, revealed virtually identical results. Hence, the predictability effect suggests that readers contact frames on line, that is, during the encoding of individual words, and that arriving at a semantic interpretation, presumably by contacting the internal frame, constitutes a more complex process than simple word identification. Words have to be integrated and interpreted and the reader may encounter passages that cannot be readily understood; under such circumstances a relatively effort consuming process has to be initiated to arrive at a text interpretation.

Unfortunately, predictability and word frequency were correlated in the present study; in addition, the question may be raised whether total viewing time per word may conceal a more intricate strategy of information evaluation. For example, predictability effects may be restricted to a more frequent reprocessing of low predictable items. To explore this possibility, high and low predictable words were scored separately for low and high frequency words. One evaluation scored only the forward fixations on the word only, whereas the second scoring included all fixations and interword regressions. The data are shown in Table 10.2. Again, predictability and word frequency affected the reader's encoding behavior. Low predictable and low frequency items consumed more encoding time. This suggests that text frames are indeed controlling the encoding of individual words. The data also reveal that the interaction of the secondary task and predictability was significant only when regressive fixation time was included.

The results indicate that identification and interpretation of individual text components, such as words, are supported by an efficient and successful frame contact. This process occurs in a fairly automatic manner. On the other hand, highly unpredictable text elements consume relatively long reading times and result in excess of regressions. This may indicate that the reader is engaged in establishing a meaning generation that goes beyond the frame representation. In

### TABLE 10.2
#### Fixation Times of Critical Words

| | High frequent | | | | Low frequent | | | |
|---|---|---|---|---|---|---|---|---|
| | High predictability | | Low predictability | | High predictability | | Low predictability | |
| No mask | 274 | (254) | 402 | (351) | 320 | (281) | 576 | (464) |
| Mask | 301 | (253) | 553 | (430) | 402 | (322) | 787 | (513) |

[a]Values indicate fixation durations per critical word. The first value represents total fixation duration; values in parentheses indicate the initial fixation duration, i.e. excluding regressive fixations.

this case, the reader is not able to automatically assign meaning. Rather, the frame deviant item may engage the reader in the task of generating a new unprecedented interpretation or modifying a prior assessment. These processes are relatively unique and the reader may have to invest attentional resources to safeguard their execution.

Experiment 2 was performed to qualify the effect of *structure* upon the reader's encoding behavior. Only three of the four stories could be analyzed due to loss of data for the fourth story. Four sections (levels) were differentiated for each story: setting, beginning, goal path, and ending. Total reading time per level was calculated. Since the sections varied in length, reading times per individual letter of each section were obtained. Figure 10.2 shows the data. The results indicate that *structure* modified the reader's encoding behavior. Analogous to the Mandler and Johnson findings (1977), settings and beginnings required longer encoding operations than goal path and ending sections. The secondary task interacted with *structure* for subjects as a random variable but not for stimuli, suggesting that the comprehension of settings and beginnings may have required more resource allocation than the reading of goal paths and endings. There were virtually no regressions during the reading of the Mandler and Johnson stories.

## V.   Conclusion

On the basis of the experiments carried out to this point, I would like to propose a tentative view of the reader's parsing strategy in reading short prose

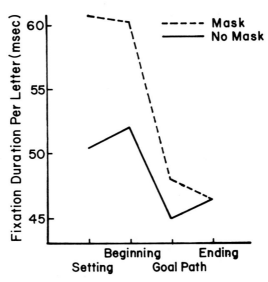

FIGURE 10.2. *The effect of story structure upon the reader's fixation duration with and without a one letter mask.*

passages. It seems that the reader is engaged in a text interpretation performance while reading individual text components. The interpretation is assumed to be guided by prior context and an immediate text–frame contact. Word identification and word interpretation influence the reader's encoding behavior. Both occur fairly automatically, as long as the text remains predictable or frame (content) conform. If the reader fails to hold on to a frame conform interpretation, refixations tend to occur. Then effortful processing occurs, presumably because a new text interpretation has to be generated. In addition, *structural* characteristics of the story may control the reader's encoding strategy. Particular text sections, like settings and beginnings, required more encoding time than more constrained text sections. These findings are in essential agreement with Friedman's (1979) hypotheses, although the assumption that long fixation durations indicate effortful processes per se was not supported. On the other hand, the present data argue against some theoretical perspectives taken by Britton *et al.* (1978) and Britton, Holdredge, Curry, and Westbrook, (1979) although the effect of structure was replicated (Britton, Meyer, Simpson, Holdredge, & Curry, 1979).

# References

Anderson, R. C., & Pichert, J. (1978). Recall of previously unrecallable information following a shift in perspective. *Journal of Verbal Learning and Verbal Behavior 17*, 1–12.

Bower, G. H. (1976). Experiments on story understanding and recall. *Quarterly Journal of Experimental Psychology 28*, 511–534.

Bransford, J. D., & Johnson, M. K. (1972). Contextual prerequisites for understanding: Some investigations for comprehension and recall. *Journal of Verbal Learning and Verbal Behavior 11*, 717–726.

Britton, B. K., Holdredge, T. S., Curry, C., & Westbrook, R. D. (1979). Use of cognitive capacity in reading identical texts with different amounts of discourse level meaning. *Journal of Experimental Psychology: Human Learning & Memory 5*, 262–270.

Britton, B. K., Meyer, B. J. F., Simpson, T. S., Holdredge, T. S., & Curry, C. (1979). Effects of the organization of text on memory: Tests of two implications of a selective attention hypothesis. *Journal of Experimental Psychology: Human Learning & Memory, 5*, 496–506.

Britton, B. K., Westbrook, R. D., & Holdredge, T. S. (1978). Reading and cognitive capacity usage: Effects of text difficulty. *Journal of Experimental Psychology: Human Learning & Memory 4*, 582–591.

Carroll, L. *Alice's Adventures in Wonderland*. London: The New English Library Limited.

Cirilio, R. K., & Foss, D. J. (1980). Text structure and reading time for sentences. *Journal of Verbal Learning and Verbal Behavior, 20*, 96–109.

Friedman, A. (1979). Framing pictures: The role of knowledge in automatized encoding and memory for gist. *Journal of Experimental Psychology: General 108*, 316–355.

Gentner, D. (1976). The structure and recall of narrative prose. *Journal of Verbal Learning and Verbal Behavior 15*, 411–418.

Glenn, C. G. (1978). The role of episodic structure and of story length in childrens' recall of simple stories. *Journal of Verbal Learning and Verbal Behavior 17*, 229–247.

Graesser, A. C., Hoffman, N. L., & Clark, L. F. (1980). Structural components of reading time. *Journal of Verbal Learning and Verbal Behavior 19*, 135–151.

Graesser, A. C., Robertson, S. P., Lovelace, E. R., & Swinehart, D. M. (1980). Answers to why-questions expose the organization of story plot and predict recall of actions. *Journal of Verbal Learning and Verbal Behavior 19*, 110–119.

Haberland, K., Berian, C., & Sandson, J. (1980). The episode schema in story processing. *Journal of Verbal Learning and Verbal Behavior 19*, 635–650.

Johnson, N. S., & Mandler, J. M. (1979). A tale of two structures: Underlying and surface forms in stories. *Poetics, 9*, 51–86.

Logan, G. D. (1978). Attention in character-classification tasks: Evidence for automaticity of component stages. *Journal of Experimental Psychology: General 107*, 32–63.

Logan, G. D. (1979). On the use of a concurrent memory load to measure attention and automaticity. *Journal of Experimental Psychology: Human Perception & Performance, 5*, 189–207.

Mandler, J. M., & Johnson, N. S. (1977). Remembrance of things parsed: Story structure and recall. *Cognitive Psychology 9*, 111–151.

Meyers, L. S. and Boldrick, D. (1975). Memory for meaningful connected discourse. *Journal of Experimental Psychology: Human Learning & Memory 1*, 584–591.

McKoon, G. (1977). Organization of information in text memory. *Journal of Verbal Learning and Verbal Behavior 16*, 247–260.

Minsky, M. (1977). Frame-system theory: In P. N. Johnson-Laird & P. C. Watson (Eds.), *Thinking;* Cambridge University Press.

Pickert, J. W. & Anderson, R. C. (1977). Taking different perspectives on a story. *Journal of Educational Psychology, 69*, 309–315.

Rayner, K. (1978). Eye movements in reading and information processing. *Psychological Bulletin 85*, 618–660.

Rayner, K., Inhoff, A. W., Morrison, R. E., Slowiaczek, M. L., & Bertera, J. H. (1981). Masking of foveal and parafoveal vision during fixations in reading. *Journal of Experimental Psychology: Human Perception & Performance 7*, 167–179.

Rumelhart, D. E. (1975). Notes on a schema for stories. In D. G. Bobrow & A. Collins (Eds.), *Representation and understanding: Studies in cognitive science.* New York: Academic Press, pp. 211–236.

Schank, R., & Abelson. (1977). *Scripts, plans, goals and understanding.* Hillsdale, New Jersey: LEA.

Thorndyke, P. W. (1977). Cognitive structures in comprehension and memory of narrative discourse. *Cognitive Psychology 9*, 77–110.

Susan F. Ehrlich

# 11

# Contextual Influences on Eye Movements in Reading

## I.  Introduction

Data from a number of sources have shown that the linguistic constraints of context can influence word perception. For example, the semantic and syntactic characteristics of text have been shown to influence reading errors (e.g., Otto, 1977; Stevens & Rumelhart, 1975). Generally, these errors reveal that readers use both visual features from the page and expectations based on information from earlier in the text to identify words. A number of eye movement studies are discussed here which provide insight into the mechanisms for this integration. Studies of the influence of the constraint of context on the location of upcoming fixations and on fixation duration are reviewed. The fixation duration measure has provided information about word processing time and sensitivity to visual features under varying conditions of constraint.

## II.  Word Identification versus Word Interpretation

To set the theoretical stage for this discussion, two different types of word recognition will be distinguished. The first will be termed word *identification* and the second will be termed word *interpretation* (Ehrlich, 1981). Identification refers to the singling out of an element within the lexicon. Mechanisms for this singling out process have been suggested by a number of researchers (e.g., Meyer, Schvaneveldt, & Ruddy, 1975; Morton, 1969). In Morton's (1969) model, for

EYE MOVEMENTS IN READING:
PERCEPTUAL AND LANGUAGE PROCESSES

example, the elements within the lexicon, called logogens, have threshold values associated with them. Information from a number of different sources can influence the level of activation of a logogen. When certain types of information come in from the perceptual systems and from other contextually influenced systems, the activation of a particular logogen will reach threshold and it will fire, thus proclaiming itself the word that is currently being read. Each logogen in the lexicon has a number of different feature lists associated with it, including a phonological feature list, a graphic feature list, a semantic feature list, and perhaps a syntactic feature list. The logogen will fire when it receives evidence of a sufficient number of the relevant features.

The second kind of word recognition, word *interpretation,* refers to the establishment of the relationship between the word on the page and the other concepts that have appeared earlier in the text. In other words the interpretation of a word is established when its discourse function is established. It seems self-evident that this kind of recognition is the ultimate goal of word recognition in prose. The nature of this integration process has been discussed by researchers in the area of mental representation (Anderson, 1976; Anderson & Bower, 1973; Kintsch, 1974; Kintsch & Vipond, 1978). It is generally assumed that words are incorporated into a "conceptual" or "propositional" network which represents the functional relations of concepts and propositions (truth-bearing "statements" of relationships between concepts).

It is important to note that word identification and word interpretation are potentially independent. On occasion, a new representation for a concept may be created within the reader's conceptual network on the basis of information already residing in memory, whether or not a particular item has been singled out within an independent lexicon. Schank (1972) has argued that such creation of memory representations for inferred concepts is a pervasive aspect of language comprehension. On the other hand, the singling out of an element within the lexicon may occur without establishing the function of that word within the discourse.

Notice that the processes used to construct a conceptual network might actually take precedence over processes used to single out words in the lexicon. If a reader is having difficulty establishing the discourse function of a word that appeared before the word that is currently being fixated, some of the reader's limited attentional capacity may be required to create inferential links between that earlier word and the concepts that have already been incorporated into the network (Kintsch & Vipond, 1978). This effort may "distract" the comprehension component so that it fails to monitor the element in the lexicon that is activated by the currently fixated word. The hypothesis that problems in interpretation may interfere with correct recognition of subsequent words has received some support from studies of reading errors (Isaksen & Miller, 1976; Otto, 1977).

On the other hand, conceptual processing of context could potentially influence activation levels of the elements in the lexicon, according to the word detector theories. It seems likely that priming would be dependent on input provided by the comprehension processes that build the conceptual network. If the comprehension component monitors the lexicon for items that are to be inserted into the network, such monitoring may be focused on the subset of lexical elements that are consistent with the current requirements of the network. For example, the comprehension component may be "on the look out" for words that are particular parts of speech or words that have particular semantic characteristics. Those words that are being monitored may thus have lowered thresholds for identification.

We can see that context might influence eye movements in a number of ways. If context dictates insertion of a concept into the conceptual network, it is possible that visual analysis of a word that references that already established concept may be foregone. Readers may simply skip fixation of highly constrained words. High levels of constraint may also function to reduce fixation durations either because less complete visual analysis is required or because less work is required to establish the correct discourse function for the constrained word.

## III.  Contextual Influences on Visual Feature Analysis

Although it is possible that high levels of constraint may decrease sensitivity to visual features, there are a number of sources of data that run counter to this argument. For example, the influence of context on speed of recognition of tachistoscopically presented words decreases with age and reading ability (Perfetti & Roth, 1980; West & Stanovich, 1978). It has also been shown that for adults, the influence of contextual constraint is weak when the words in question are presented clearly and for unconstrained durations (eg., Becker & Killion, 1977; Stanovich & Pachella, 1977). These studies suggest that readers *can* depend on contextual constraint to compensate for deficiences in visual input but that for adults, visual analysis takes precedence over contextual analysis for undegraded words, presumably because of the automaticity and speed of perceptual analysis. Notice, however, that in the studies where the dependent measures are speed or accuracy of recognition, the goal presented to the subject is accurate word *identification*. Because the subject is not necessarily attempting to construct a conceptual representation of the content of the text, priming that may be dependent on such comprehension processes may not be evidenced. The inferential processes that may play a role in appropriate *interpretation* of words may not be engaged.

## IV.  Evidence from Studies of Eye Movements

The eye movement studies described here address the degree to which context influences visual sensitivity. It has been noted that context could allow readers to skip fixation of words that are highly constrained. This kind of effect cannot be examined with the word recognition paradigms which use speed or accuracy of recognition as dependent measures. It is also important that in the eye movement studies, accurate word identification is not required of the subject. Subjects are often asked to read the passages for meaning. This more natural goal may trigger the use of word recognition strategies that are different from those used in the word recognition procedures. Accurate *identification* may be deemphasized whereas accurate understanding of conceptual relationships may take precedence.

A study reported by O'Regan (1979) provides evidence for the hypothesis that linguistic factors influence whether or not particular words will be directly fixated. In that study, O'Regan presented subjects with sets of sentences to read and monitored their eye movements. One of the important findings that he reported was that the length of saccades was dependent on both the length of the word that was currently being fixated and on the length of the upcoming word. As the length of these words increased, the saccade length increased, suggesting that subjects were programming their eye movements so they would fixate on the most informative spot within the upcoming word. More important for our purposes was the fact that readers were less likely to make fixations on particular types of words. O'Regan held the part of the sentence preceding the critical word constant and found that readers were more likely to skip fixation of the article *the* than they were to skip fixation of a three letter verb like *met*. The data from this experiment suggested that information from peripheral vision (in combination with the information from the preceding part of the sentence) was sometimes sufficient to cause the subject to skip fixation of the critical word. Presumably this was because the identities of the more frequent words were established to a sufficient level of confidence to allow less complete visual analysis.

Zola (1982; see also McConkie & Zola, 1981) carried out a study that was a direct attempt to examine whether high levels of contextual constraint would influence subjects' eye movement patterns. He presented subjects with paragraphs that differed in the extent to which particular words were constrained to occur in particular positions. The pairs of passages that were used were identical except for an adjective that determined the degree of contextual constraint for the upcoming word. In a pair of paragraphs about the movie industry, for example, the adjective *adequate* preceded the word *popcorn* in the low-constraint condition, whereas the word *buttered* preceded *popcorn* in the high-constraint condition. It was independently established that subjects could guess the identity of the target words 83% of the time in the high-constraint paragraphs but only 8% in the low-constraint paragraphs. Zola recorded eye movements as subjects read the passages with either the constraining or the neutral adjectives. In some conditions, Zola made letter substitutions in the target words that followed the adjectives. He was interested in determining if subjects would be less sensitive to the letter substitutions under the conditions of high constraint. Zola looked at the probability of fixating on the target words and fixation durations on the targets. In general, the results showed that the influence of contextual constraint was very weak. The level of constraint had no influence on the probability of fixating the target word (97% across all conditions). Also, the fixation durations on the target words were longer for words with letter substitutions, independent of the level of constraint. The only significant effect of context was that fixation duration was significantly longer on the target words in low constraint (237 msec) compared to the targets in high constraint (221 msec).

These results provided little support for the idea that context influences the degree of visual feature analysis and the data seem to conflict with the results of word recognition studies in which visual features were degraded (Morton, 1969; Tulving & Gold, 1963). In Zola's study, the visual features of the words were clearly presented for periods of time that were controlled by the subject's own fixations. The results of Zola's study also seem to be inconsistent with reading error data that has been collected for children (Biemiller, 1970; Goodman, 1965; Weber, 1970) for adults with reading problems (Otto, 1977), or under conditions where text is artificially manipulated (Kolers, 1970). In all of these studies, context has been found to influence the nature of reading errors. However, in all of these cases, direct visual analysis may have been more difficult than depending on context to isolate word identity. It has already been noted that the influence of constraint on word recognition decreases with age and reading ability and with the completeness of the visual stimulus (see Ehrlich, 1981, for a review). Nevertheless, our common experience suggests that there *are* certain circumstances where proficient readers may misidentify words on the basis of contextual constraint.

An experiment by Ehrlich and Rayner (1981) has provided some information about such cases. This study was similar to the study reported by Zola in many respects. High and low constraint paragraphs were developed for particular target words and letter substitutions were introduced in the target words for some conditions.

However, the experiment differed from Zola's along a number of important dimensions. First, the constraint for the target word was manipulated more globally. In the high-constraint paragraphs, semantic and conceptual information throughout the preceding text provided constraint for the target word. More important, the concept that was referenced by the target word was established for the reader earlier in the paragraph either by a direct reference or indirectly through a natural inference that was essential for understanding the paragraph. A high-constraint paragraph for the word *shark* is presented in Table 11.1. The context established the general function of the target word within the discourse prior to any visual analysis. This being the case, local syntactic and semantic clues just prior to a target word would have been sufficient to lead the reader to "know"

**TABLE 11.1**
**High Constraint**

He saw the black fin slice through the water and the image of sharks teeth came quickly to his mind. He turned quickly toward the shore and swam for his life. The coast guard had warned that someone had seen a shark off the north shore of the island. As usual, not everyone listened to the warning.

that this already established concept was about to come up. The predictability of the target words as determined by a modified cloze procedure was 93% across the high constraint paragraphs.

Another way in which the two studies differed was in terms of the lengths of the target words. Zola used seven- and eight-letter words whereas we used five-letter words. Rayner and McConkie (1976) have established that words that are seven to eight letters long will be fixated 95% of the time whereas words that are five letters long will be fixated 64% of the time. In part, this may be because more of a shorter word can fit within the region of high acuity when the center of fixation is not directly on that shorter word.

The third important difference between the two experiments concerns the influence of the letter substitutions on the target word. In our experiment, the letter substitutions, which occurred with equal probability in either the first, middle, or last letter position of the word, created alternative words (night–right, horse–house, steak–steal). The word *sharp* replaced the word *shark* in the paragraph presented in Table 11.1. Subjects' sensitivity to the letter substitutions resulted in the identification of a word that was anomalous for both the high and low constraint paragraphs. This was an advantage because it assured increased fixation durations on the words when the letter substitutions were taken into account during perceptual analysis. Also, subjects were likely to remember seeing the anomalous words later on because they were inconsistent with the text.

The three major measures of interest were probability of fixating on the target word, fixation duration on the target word, and probability of remembering the existence of the anomalous word in a postsession debriefing. Contrasting with the experiment reported by Zola, strong effects of contextual constraint were found for all three measures. Table 11.2 shows the probability of fixating the target word as a function of the level of constraint and as a function of whether or not there was a letter substitution. Subjects were more likely to make forward fixations on target words under low constraint conditions and an even stronger effect was found when regressive fixations were taken into account. Subjects were also more likely to fixate words with letter substitutions, suggesting that this information was available to the subjects in parafoveal vision and that it influenced the locations of the subsequent fixations.

The fixation duration data for control words and for words with letter substitutions are presented in Table 11.3. For those control words that did receive direct

**TABLE 11.2**
**Probability of Fixating on the Target Word**[a]

|  | High constraint | Low constraint |
| --- | --- | --- |
| Control | .51 (.54) | .62 (.71) |
| Misspelling | .56 (.73) | .79 (.87) |

[a]Values in parentheses include regressions.

TABLE 11.3
Average Fixation Duration on the Target Word[a]

|  | High constraint (msec) | Low constraint (msec) |
|---|---|---|
| Control | 221 (248) | 254 (305) |
| Misspelling | 313 (476) | 324 (541) |

[a]Values in parentheses indicate total reading time for the target word.

fixations, average fixation duration was significantly longer for the low constraint conditions. The effect size was substantially larger (33 msec) than that found by Zola (16 msec). It was also found that for the conditions with letter substitutions, the probability that the subjects remembered seeing the anomalous words at the end of the session was higher for the low-constraint condition (.86) than for the high-constraint condition (.64), confirming that the subjects were indeed less sensitive to the letter substitutions under conditions of high constraint.

It is of interest that for 43% of the cases where the subjects did *not* fixate the target words, they still reported awareness of the letter substitutions in the postsession debriefing. These must have been cases where the subjects gained information concerning the letter substitution from parafoveal vision. Also of interest is the fact that for 13% of the total number of cases, subjects were *unaware* of the letter substitutions even though the target word in question was directly fixated (88% of these cases were in the high constraint condition). These cases seem to reflect a block of the influence of visual features in central vision on word recognition. Fixations on anomalous words that the subjects did not remember were substantially shorter than on such words that the subjects did remember (251 msec vs. 316 msecs, respectively). When regressive fixations were added to the forward fixations, the differences were even larger (278 msec vs. 497 msec). These data thus provide strong evidence that subjects were sometimes insensitive to letter substitutions that were directly fixated.

In a second experiment (Ehrlich & Rayner, 1981), two alternative words were included in high-constraint context. The target in the first condition was highly predictable as in Experiment 1. The target for the second condition was not predictable but it *was* consistent with the ideas in the paragraph. (The counterpart to this condition in Experiment 1 was a word that was anomalous in the high-constraint context). The number of forward fixations on the target was the same for both conditions. However, more regressions were made to the unpredictable target, which also received longer fixation durations.

Both experiments showed that under the special conditions of highly redundant, in fact repetitive context, visual analysis of five-letter words is reduced either because such words are not directly fixated or because visual sensitivity is reduced when such words are directly fixated. It remains to be seen if these effects would also be found for words that are longer than five letters. Possible mechanisms supporting such effects have been outlined in the introduction to this chapter. It was suggested that a restricted set of items in the lexicon may be monitored, having the effect of lowering the identification threshold for those items. If this were the case, fewer visual features would be required in order to single out a particular element that is to be incorporated into the conceptual network. Although logogens that are outside the set of monitored elements may receive appropriate perceptual inputs, the sensitivity to those logogens would be lower. When the syntactic and semantic constraints of context are weak (there is no information that could be used to limit the set of monitored elements) each element would have equal status and selection would have to be made on the basis of visual feature analysis.

It should be kept in mind that in the Ehrlich and Rayner study, the referent of the target word had been established for the subject earlier in the text. It is possible that this repetitive structure is required to produce the fixation location and strong fixation duration effects that were found.

It is also important that subjects were consistently sensitive to visual features in parafoveal vision. When letter substitutions influenced the overall shapes of words, subjects were less likely to skip fixation of those words, suggesting that visual feature analysis plays at least some role in directing saccades under such conditions of high constraint.

One possibility is that visual feature analysis is inhibited under conditions of high constraint. This alternative seems unlikely if we assume that feature analysis is so practiced as to be automatic. It is unclear why effort should be put into inhibiting an essentially effortless activity. However, automatic visual analysis of inconsistent words might be blocked from affecting ultimate identification because the anomalous words that are activated are not being monitored.

The eye movement studies reviewed here lend support to two hypotheses concerning the influence of context on visual feature analysis. First, such features may not be fixated directly because the word's identity has been previously established on the basis of inputs from the comprehension system in combination with visual features obtained from parafoveal vision. Second, analysis of visual features may be outweighed in the process of selection within the lexicon because such features influence word detectors which are not within the set of detectors that are being monitored by the comprehension system. Both types of reduction of visual sensitivity are hypothesized to be dependent on the comprehension processes that are used to build a conceptual representation of the text and may only be evidenced under conditions where this comprehension goal is presented to the subject.

ACKNOWLEDGMENTS

The author thanks Miriam Schustack and Keith Rayner for comments on an earlier version of this chapter.

# References

Anderson, J. R. (1976). *Language, memory, and thought*. Hillsdale, New Jersey: Erlbaum.

Anderson, J. R., & Bower, G. H. (1973). *Human associative memory*. Washington, D.C.: Winston.

Becker, C. A., & Killion, T. H. (1977). Interaction of visual and cognitive effects on word recognition. *Journal of Experimental Psychology: Human Perception & Performance, 3*, 389–401.

Biemiller, H. (1970). The development of the use of graphic and contextual information as children learn to read. *Reading Research Quarterly, 6*, 75–96.

Ehrlich, S. F. (1981). Children's word recognition in prose context. *Visible Language, 15*, 219–244.

Ehrlich, S. F., & Rayner, K. (1981). Contextual effects on word perception and eye movements during reading. *Journal of Verbal Learning and Verbal Behavior, 20*, 641–655.

Goodman, K. (1965). A linguistic study of cues and miscues in reading. *Elementary English, 42*, 639–643.

Isakson, R. L., & Miller, J. W. (1976). Sensitivity to syntactic and semantic cues in good and poor readers. *Journal of Educational Psychology, 68*, 787–792.

Kintsch, W. (1974). *The representation of meaning in memory*. Hillsdale New Jersey: Erlbaum.

Kintsch, W., & Vipond, D. (1978). Reading comprehension and readability in educational practice and psychological theory. In L. G. Nilsson (Ed.), *Memory: Processes and problems*. Hillsdale New Jersey: Erlbaum.

Kolers, P. A. (1970). Three stages of reading. In H. Levin & J. Williams (Eds.), *Basic studies in reading*. New York: Basic Books.

McConkie, G. W., & Zola, D. (1981). Language constraints and the functional stimulus in reading. In A. M. Lesgold & C. A. Perfetti (Eds.), *Interactive processes in reading*. Hillsdale, New Jersey: Erlbaum.

Meyer, D. E., Schvaneveldt, R. W., & Ruddy, M. G. (1975). Loci of contextual effects on visual word recognition. In P. M. A. Rabbitt & S. Dornic (Eds.), *Attention and performance* (Vol. 5) London: Academic Press.

Morton, J. (1969). Interaction of information in word recognition. *Psychological Review, 76*, 165–178.

O'Regan, K. (1979). Saccade size control in reading: Evidence for the linguistic control hypothesis. *Perception & Psychophysics, 25*, 501–509.

Otto, J. (1977). Reading cue utilization by low-achieving freshmen. *Journal of Reading Behavior, 9*, 71–83.

Perfetti, C. A., & Roth, S. (1981). Some of the interactive processes in reading and their role in reading skill. In A. M. Lesgold & C. A. Perfetti (Eds.), *Interactive processes in reading*. Hillsdale, New Jersey: Erlbaum.

Rayner, K., & McConkie, G. W. (1976). What guides a reader's eye movements? *Vision Research, 16*, 829–837.

Schank, R. C. (1972). Conceptual dependency: A theory of natural language understanding. *Cognitive Psychology, 3*, 552–631.

Stanovich, K. E., & Pachella, R. G. (1977). Encoding, stimulus–response compatibility, and stages of processing. *Journal of Experimental Psychology: Human Perception & Performance, 3*, 411–421.

Stevens, A. L., & Rumelhart, D. E. (1975). Errors in reading: Analysis using an augmented network model of grammar. In D. A. Norman, D. E. Rumelhart, & the LNR Research Group (Eds.), *Explorations in cognition*. San Francisco: Freeman.

Tulving, E., & Gold, C. (1963). Stimulus information and contextual information as determinants of tachistoscopic recognition of words. *Journal of Experimental Psychology, 66*, 319–327.

Weber, R. M. (1970). First graders' use of grammatical context in reading. In H. Levin & J. Williams (Eds.), *Basic studies in reading*. New York: Basic Books, 1970.

West, R. F., & Stanovich, K. E. (1978). Automatic contextual facilitation in readers of three ages. *Child Development, 49*, 717–727.

Zola, D. (1982). The effect of redundancy on the perception of words in reading. *Perception & Psychophysics*.

Philip B. Gough

# 12

# Context, Form, and Interaction

## I.   Introduction

We knew that context had significant effects on the recognition of isolated words in contrived tasks like tachistoscopic recognition (e.g., Tulving & Gold, 1963), word naming (e.g., Stanovich & West, 1979), and lexical decision (e.g., Fischler & Bloom, 1979). Now we know that context has comparable effects on eye movements in silent reading. Context influences the probability of fixating a word, at least if the word is short (e.g., Ehrlich, Chapter 11 of this volume). It then influences the duration of that initial fixation (Ehrlich, Chapter 11 of this volume; Inhoff, Chapter 10 of this volume). Finally, it affects the probability of regressing to the word (e.g., Ehrlich, this volume; Inhoff, this volume). Combining these effects, context considerably influences the total viewing time afforded a given word. Moreover, each of these effects is exaggerated if the word is degraded by altering (Ehrlich) or blanking (Inhoff) one of its letters. Perhaps the only specific question remaining is whether context influences "its own" eye movements: Are the fixations preceding (or following) a predictable word different from those surrounding a less predictable one?

But there remain unanswered three larger questions concerning context's influence on reading in general and eye movements in particular, two of them empirical, the third theoretical.

## II.   The Extent of Context Effects

The first question concerns the true extent of contextual influence on ordinary reading.

203

EYE MOVEMENTS IN READING:
PERCEPTUAL AND LANGUAGE PROCESSES

By this I do not mean the magnitude of obtainable context effects; there is no doubt that these can be considerable. For example, Kleiman (1980) found that a sentential context like *The cup was placed on the* . . . reduced lexical decision latency for the target *table* by 95 msec, or nearly 20%. And Inhoff (Chapter 10 of this volume) reports a difference of over 200 msec between the fixation durations of high versus low predictable low-frequency words when masked.

Nor do I question the potential variety of contextual influences on word recognition. As Shebilske and Fisher (Chapter 9 of this volume) point out, various kinds of contexts surrounding a word can be identified, ranging from the reader's background knowledge to the immediately prior word. It seems reasonable that any and all of these different contexts might facilitate word recognition, in the same or even different ways.

We have argued elsewhere (Gough, Alford, & Holley–Wilcox, 1981) that one difference in context must lead to different effects. This is the distinction between syntactic and semantic context, for their effects must have different time courses. Any effect of syntactic context must be labile, fast and transient, for syntactic context changes with each successive word. But the effect of semantic context must be stable, enduring across words, sentences, and paragraphs to facilitate the recognition and integration of appropriate word families.

But at the same time, it seems likely that the various kinds of context (e.g., the reader's background knowledge and the preceding words) must have a "final common path," for if they made independent contributions, then by the logic of additive factors word recognition could be speeded (or slowed) by hundreds of milliseconds. I take it to be a fact, and (as I will argue in what follows) a fact of fundamental importance for our understanding of reading, that, so long as the stimulus is not degraded, a skilled reader can recognize a totally isolated word (or pseudoword) so fast that improvement due to context can be counted in only a few milliseconds.

It seems reasonable to assume that this final common path to a target word can be indexed by the *predictability* of that word. Certainly the reader's background knowledge, earlier text, and local syntactic and semantic constraints should all affect predictability. So let us assume that predictability represents the sum total of contextual influences on a target word, and let us ask how facilitation varies with predictability.

There is no question that high levels of predictability are associated with strong facilitation effects. The context–target pairs used in every study of word recognition in context, from Tulving and Gold's (1963) "The skier was buried alive by the sudden *avalanche*" to Zola's (1982) "Since movie theaters must have buttered *popcorn* . . . ," used highly predictable target words, and these have produced the contextual effects with which we are all familiar. But at the same time, there are also indications that when predictability is not so high, the effects of context are diminished, if not altogether absent. For example, Fischler and Bloom (1979) report that when predictability falls below .90, they find no evidence of contextual facilitation of lexical decision.

The question then arises, how predictable are words in ordinary reading matter? To compare ordinary reading matter with materials like those of Tulving and Gold (1963), Pamela Holley–Wilcox and I drew the first sentence of at least nine words from each of 100 successive articles in the *Reader's Digest*, beginning with the issue of January 1978. We then gave the first eight words of each sentence to 100 introductory psychology students, and asked them to predict the ninth word. (Actually, 49 of the original 100 target words turned out to be function words, 51 content, so for symmetry's sake we drew one more of the former to replace one of the latter.) We then tallied the proportion of Ss predicting each of the 50 content and 50 function target words, with the results presented in Table 12.1.

Overall, the mean predictability of the ninth word in *Reader's Digest* sentences was almost exactly .25. But this is the average of predictability of function words (including pronouns) and content words (i.e., adjectives, nouns, verbs, and adverbs). The predictability of function words is approximately .40, but the predictability of content words, the targets of virtually every study of context, is only .10. Inspection of the distribution shows that not 1 content word in 50, drawn from ordinary reading matter, has a predictability as high as those typically used in context experiments. Fully 70% have a predictability less than the .15 characterized as "low constraint" by Ehrlich. And a predictability of zero—not one of 100 Ss correctly guessing the target—is virtually the mode.

The objection can be raised that these sentences were themselves lifted out of context, and that the predictability of words in running text might be higher. This is certainly a possibility, but there is little evidence to support it. When we (Gough *et al.*, 1981) asked a colleague to guess the first 100 words of each of 10 books, providing him with the complete prior context before each guess, he was

TABLE 12.1
Predictability of Words from Eight Words of Sentence-Initial Prior Context,
Drawn from the *Reader's Digest*

| Predictability | Number of target words | |
|---|---|---|
| | Content | Function |
| .00 | 17 | 4 |
| .01–.10 | 18 | 17 |
| .11–.20 | 4 | 8 |
| .21–.30 | 5 | 3 |
| .31–.40 | 4 | 4 |
| .41–.50 | 1 | 3 |
| .51–.60 | 1 | 1 |
| .61–.70 | 0 | 2 |
| .71–.80 | 0 | 3 |
| .81–.90 | 0 | 3 |
| .91–1.00 | 0 | 2 |
| Mean predictability = | .10 | .39 |

correct in almost exactly the same proportions of both content (.10) and function (.40) words.

I would submit these percentages: 40% for function words, 10% for content words, combining to yield 25% for the average word, for the record books as valid estimates of word predictability in ordinary reading matter. But whether or not they are accepted, it seems clear that our knowledge of the effects of context on word processing derives almost exclusively from studies of materials atypical of ordinary reading matter. The target words in these studies have always been *nouns*, virtually always in sentence-final position, and virtually always more predictable than any but the rarest word in normal text. It is worth remembering that nouns are only a proper subset of the content words, and taken as a whole, content words account for only a half of the words in running text. It is also worth remembering that the average sentence in a newspaper is over 20 words in length (Kucera & Francis 1967), so that if we study only sentence-final targets, we are ignoring 95% of printed words. In short, we have studied atypical targets.

It is almost certainly the case that as a result, we have overestimated the effects of context, and it is at least a possibility that the modal context has no effect at all. It is undeniable that context *can* have powerful effects on word recognition, but it remains an open question whther it usually does.

## III.   Context and Individual Differences

My second question concerns the importance of contextual effects in explaining differences in reading ability.

It has always seemed to me that at least there are essentially two views of reading. One view, which might be called the Simple View, is that reading amounts to little or nothing but (1) the translation of print into linguistic forms (i.e., decoding); and (2) the translation of those forms into meaning (i.e., comprehension). This view (which I believe I share with Flesch [1955, 1981], Liberman & Shankweiler [1979], and Rozin & Gleitman [1977]) begins with the observation that the child normally comes to reading with the ability to comprehend the language, so that the primary task of reading instruction is to teach decoding (cf. Gough & Hillinger, 1980). On this view, there are two basic components in reading. One is the ability to decode, the other is the ability to understand the (spoken) language. It follows that differences in reading ability must arise from one (or both) of these component abilities, so that a disabled reader is either a poor decoder, a poor comprehender, or both.

It is much harder to characterize the opposing view, for it is defined by opposition to the simple view ("There's more to reading than just decoding"). But I think its adherents include most "top–down" or "interactive" theorists of reading. Shebilske and Fisher appear to be advocating such a view when they argue that differences in reading "flexibility" are an important component of differences in reading ability. In support of this idea, they cite several studies to show that skilled readers make "better adjustments" to changes in reading purpose. This they interpret as evidence for differences in "processing strategies" which might profitably be taught to improve reading ability. But in each of the studies they cite, the supposed difference in "flexibility" was revealed when the poorer readers were unable to speed up under gist instructions, or when rereading the material. I would submit that this difference might be attributed not to a difference in strategy, but rather to a difference in one of the two simple components: either decoding or comprehension. That is, to read flexibly, you must be able to read fast, and it seems to me entirely possible that the good reader is not good because of being flexible; the good reader is flexible because of being good.

I would further submit that the available evidence argues against the idea of looking for context effects to explain the variance in reading ability. Stanovich (1980) has reviewed nearly a dozen studies comparing context effects in good and poor readers. In *no instance* has context been found to help good readers more than poor; if anything, poor readers make better use of context than good readers. Put differently, the most conspicuous difference between good and poor readers in confronting the printed word is in the speed and accuracy with which they read isolated words (cf. Gough, 1981). I think that the simple view, that deficient reading ability results from either a deficit in decoding or listening ability, remains to be disproven.

## IV. The Substance of Interaction

My final question concerns our theoretical understanding of context effects in reading.

The obvious significance of context effects on word recognition is that they refute a strictly "bottom–up" model of reading like that I offered a decade ago (Gough, 1972). I think it is important to examine exactly what this means.

The bottom–up model is a simple and straightforward application of the idea of serial processing to reading. To my mind, the idea of serial processing is one of the few theoretical ideas in cognitive psychology with any real explanatory power, and I would like to show why.

A completely developed serial model would involve five distinct assumptions. First, we make the basic serial assumption that there are two stages of processing, A and B, with the output of A ($0_a$) serving as input to B. Second, we assume that some set of one or more variables $V_a$ influences only stage A. Third, we assume that some other set of one or more variables $V_b$ influences only stage B. Fourth, we assume that we have one (or more) responses $R_b$ whose occurrence indicates the completion of the second stage of processing ($0_b$).

Thanks to Sternberg (1969), we are all familiar with the fact that these four assumptions entail the additivity of the effects of variables $V_a$ and $V_b$ on the latency of $R_b$, so that an interaction of these variables argues against the proposed serial model.

But I would maintain that there is a fifth assumption which we often add to the serial model, if only implicitly, and that it plays at least as important a role in our theoretical thinking as the others. This is the assumption that we have a response $R_a$, whose occurrence serves as index of the completion of the *first* stage.

The addition of this assumption yields two more entailments from the serial model. First, the first set of variables, $V_a$, should have identical effects on the latencies of $R_a$ and $R_b$. Second, the variable(s) $V_b$ should affect the latency of $R_b$ *but not $R_a$*.

Consider how this paradigm would be applied to reading. It seems natural (at least for a devotee of decoding) to assume that the first stage of reading is word recognition, and that its completion can be indexed by tasks like word naming or lexical decision. We acknowledge that context has important effects on reading, on things like the resolution of lexical (or structural) ambiguity, and on the comprehension and integration of sentences. But we suppose that these effects are located in a stage subsequent to immediate word recognition, and indexed by responses ($R_b$) like paraphrase, question answering, or even memory. So it should follow that context ($V_b$) should influence the latency of $R_b$, *but not $R_a$*. Context—at least some context—*does* influence the latency of responses like naming and lexical decision, and so the serial model is refuted.

Now I would argue that the case against the serial, bottom–up, model is far from complete. For one thing, as I have already argued, the evidence for context effects on word recognition arises almost entirely from the use of artificially predictive contexts. There is no doubt that the bottom–up model is wrong in these cases, but it is still possible that it correctly describes the situation in the usual case, where the target word is not predictable. For another thing, the evidence clearly indicates that the effects of context on word recognition increase with stimulus degradation, whether by random noise, contrast, letter deletion, or mis-spelling. But the other side of this coin is that the effects of context decrease with stimulus clarity. Eye movement researchers (and others) should remember that CRT displays, in comparison with virtually any magazine viewed under a 100-watt bulb, offer quite degraded stimuli, so that the context effects observed in the eye movement laboratory are almost certainly larger than those that might be obtained in the library. Finally, the effect of context has consistently been shown to *decrease* with reading ability. If we combine these functions, I find it possible to maintain the conviction that the skilled reader, reading ordinary text in good light, is virtually free from contextual influences and may be—most of the time—essentially bottom–up.

In fact, it seems to me that much of the eye movement literature tends toward the same conclusion. I well remember, a decade ago, hearing that eye movements in reading were all but random across a page. Now we have come to the point where Just and Carpenter (1980) can claim that the skilled reader fixates virtually every word on a page. Their critics will argue that the proportion may be as low as .5 or .67, but no current student of eye movements seems to challenge the view that reading proceeds essentially word by word, as a bottom–up model would have it. (At this point, I would tentatively suggest the possibility that the word *unfixated* in, for example, Ehrlich's study, might well have been "included" in an adjacent fixation. This possibility underscores the importance of examining not only fixations on the target itself, but also fixations on the material to the immediate left and right.

But suppose this argument is wrong. Suppose that the effects of context turn out to be not just occasionally potent, but instead to be ubiquitous. Then one could scarcely disagree with those who argue that reading is interactive.

But I am dissatisfied with the interactive models that we have been offered so far. I hope it is obvious that the explanatory power of an information processing model is not enriched by increasing the vividness of the adjectives used to describe it. Its explanatory power lies only in its structure, that is, the structural relationships it posits. So although an interactive theorist may describe the interaction of context and form as "dynamic" or "active" or even "graceful," the only real content of the claim is that the variables $V_a$ and $V_b$ do not influence distinct serial stages. But note what a cheap claim this is: If $V_a$ and $V_b$ influence the latency of $R_b$ anything but additively, then an interactive model must be right.

I wish it were as obvious to others as it is to me that an "interactive" model is nothing but the negation of the serial model. The serial model made a strong and interesting claim. If that claim is false, then the serial model is false and the interactive model is true. But the serial model did all the work: It yielded the falsified prediction. Until interactive models can be shown to yield new and falsifiable predictions, I see them as having no explanatory value at all.

Interactive theorists have shown little inclination (beyond describing the interaction in fulsome terms) to specify the nature of the interaction. Indeed, at least since Tulving, Mandler, and Baumal (1964), most discussions of the interaction of context with visual form seem to conflate, if not confuse, two distinct ideas about the confluence of these two potential information sources. One is that context and form provide separate and independent sources of information which are then simply combined—added—to determine the target word. The other is that the sources are *not* independent, that context not only provides information about the target but also influences the extraction of information from its visual form.

It should be clear that these two notions of "interaction" are quite distinct. The first, which I would call weak interaction, implies statistical independence—a lack of statistical interaction—between context and form, whereas the second (call it strong interaction) implies the opposite. Tulving, Mandler, and Baumal (1964) offered evidence for the latter; Gough, Alford, and Holley–Wilcox (1981), faulting their methods, presented evidence for the former. Whatever the truth, an interactive model should at least be clear on whether it claims strong or weak interaction, for then at least in this it would go beyond the serial model it supplants.

I would submit that the weakness of the interactive idea is that it concentrates on the interaction, to the neglect of the interacting factors. Let me illustrate my point with an analogy. Suppose I were to maintain that what we see is often influenced by what we hear; I take it that this is undeniable. So now I propose an interactive model of vision and hearing in which information from each source is combined (either "weakly" or "strongly") to yield perception. Now I would submit that such a model might well be true, in some vague (or even precise) sense, but it would tell us virtually nothing about either vision or hearing. It would surely be no substitute for a theory of vision, a theory of hearing, and a specification of how they interact.

In the same vein, I would maintain that an interactive theory of reading can never substitute for a theory of how we recognize the isolated word (i.e., how we read bottom–up), how we integrate those words (i.e., how we comprehend discourse), and how the two come together in skilled reading.

# References

Fischler, I., & Bloom, P. A. (1979). Automatic and attentional processes in the effects of sentence contexts on word recognition. *Journal of Verbal Hearing and Verbal Behavior, 18,* 1–20.

Flesch, R. (1955). *Why Johnny can't read—and what you can do about it.* New York: Harper and Row.

Flesch, R. (1981). *Why Johnny still can't read.* New York: Harper and Row.

Gough, P. B. (1972). One second of reading. In T. F. Kavanagh & I. G. Mattingly (Eds.), *Language by ear and by eye: The relationship between speech and reading.* Cambridge, Massachusetts: MIT. Pp. 331–358.

Gough, P. B. (1981). A comment on Kenneth Goodman. In M. L. Kamil (Ed.), *Directions in reading: Research and instruction.* Washington, D.C.: National Reading Conference. Pp. 92–95.

Gough, P. B., Alford, J. A., Jr., & Holley–Wilcox, P. (1981). Words and Contexts. In O. L. Tzeng & H. Singer (Eds.), *Perception of print: Reading research in experimental psychology.* Hillsdale, New Jersey: Erlbaum. Pp. 85–102.

Gough, P. B., & Hillinger, M. L. (1980). Learning to read: An unnatural act. *Bulletin of the Orton Society, 30,* 179–196.

Just, M. A., & Carpenter, P. A. (1980). A theory of reading: From eye fixations to comprehension. *Psychological Review, 4,* 329–354.

Kleiman, G. M. (1980). Sentence frame contexts and lexical decisions: Sentence-acceptability and word-relatedness effects. *Memory & Cognition, 8,* 336–344.

Kucera, H., & Francis, N. (1967). *A computational analysis of everyday English.* Providence: Brown University Press.

Liberman, I., & Shankweiler, D. (1979). Speech, the alphabet, and teaching to read. In L. B. Resnick & P. A. Weaver (Eds.), *Theory and practice of early reading* (Vol. 2). Hillsdale, New Jersey: Erlbaum. Pp. 109–134.

Rozin, P., & Gleitman, L. R. (1977). The structure and acquisition II: The reading process and the acquisition of the alphabetic principle. In A. S. Reber & D. L. Scarborough (Eds.), *Toward a psychology of reading: Proceedings of the CUNY Conference.* Hillsdale, New Jersey: Erlbaum. Pp. 55–142.

Stanovich, K. E. (1980). Toward an interactive-compensatory model of individual differences in the development of reading fluency. *Reading Research Quarterly, 16,* 32–71.

Stanovich, K. E., & West, R. F. (1979). Mechanisms of sentence context effects in reading: Automatic activation and conscious attention. *Memory & Cognition, 7,* 77–85.

Sternberg, S. (1969). The discovery of processing stages: Extensions of Donder's method. *Acta Psychologica, 30,* 276–315.

Tulving, E., & Gold, C. (1963). Stimulus information and contextual information as determinants of tachistoscopic recognition of words. *Journal of Experimental Psychology, 66,* 319–327.

Tulving, E., Mandler, G., & Baumal, R. (1964). Interaction of two sources of information in tachistoscopic word recognition. *Canadian Journal of Psychology, 18,* 62–71.

Zola, D. (1982). The effect of redundancy on the perception of words in reading. *Perception & Psychophysics.*

# IV
## Eye Movements and Language Processes I

Lyn Frazier

# 13

# Processing Sentence Structure[1]

## I.   Introduction

I will assume that providing an adequate theory of how people read is going to involve constructing a number of subtheories of the component processes of reading and an account of how these subtheories fit together, specifying how the component processes may interact. In recent years, considerable attention has been devoted to certain component processes of reading, including the perceptual aspects of reading, the representation of word meaning, lexical retrieval procedures, the effects of text structure and organization, and the ultimate memory representation for texts. Apart from an intense spurt of activity lasting roughly from the early 1960s to the mid-1970s, relatively less attention has been directed to the processing of sentence structure. What is worrisome to me is not so much the relative lack of investigation into this area in recent years, but the unstated implication in much of the psychological literature that no theory of this domain is even needed, at least with respect to the processing of ordinary everyday-variety sentences. At times, this view is explicitly expressed as follows: Normals assign relations to the words of the sentence on the basis of lexical constraints when these constraints lead to a unique analysis of the sentence. The implication of this view is that syntactic comprehension is possible in normal humans, but is only exploited as a last resort, when all other routes to successful comprehension have failed.

It may be true that purely syntactic comprehension—comprehension based

[1]Preparation of this paper was supported by grant BNS79-17600 from the National Science Foundation.

exclusively on knowledge of the permissable syntactic relations of the words of a sentence—is exceptional in the processing of the texts we encounter every day. But even if this is true, it is an uninteresting fact about the relative frequency of occurrence of different sentence types. What is at issue is not whether people typically must rely exclusively on syntactic information to figure out the relational aspects of the structure and meaning of a sentence, but whether the processing of syntactic structure is a component part of normal sentence processing and hence a proper domain for one of the subtheories of a theory of reading. Put somewhat differently, the question is whether we can construct a theory of reading on the assumption that having constructed an adequate theory of perceptual and lexical processes, on the one hand, and a theory of referential semantics, textual organization and the use of world knowledge, on the other, the two theories will meet.

The alternative is to assume that there is a crucial stage of grammatical processing which intervenes, that is, which takes place during normal reading for comprehension, though it is not necessarily temporally subsequent to lexical processing or temporally prior to the processing of referential relationships, world knowledge, and textual structure.

The first section of this chapter presents arguments for this latter position. The second section examines the value (and limitations) of the eye movement recording technique for helping us to construct the subtheory concerned with the processing of sentence structure. The third section argues for a particular theory of structural processing, based on some work Keith Rayner and I have been doing with the eye movement recording technique.

## II.   The Case for Structural Processing

It is often assumed that it is unnecessary to compute a structural representation of a sentence like *The man kicked the table.* The basic idea is that people can and do determine the underlying relations of the words in a sentence using lexical information and relevant world knowledge, for example, knowledge that people can kick tables, but tables do not kick people.

The lexical constraints hypothesis seems to have been entertained in various forms in the psychological literature, varying according to which lexical items were thought to contribute to the determination of semantic relations, what type of information was considered to be lexical information, and what type of semantic or pragmatic constraints were thought to be operative. In its strongest form, the hypothesis claims that the basic semantic relations of a sentence are determined exclusively on the basis of information carried by open class items, that is, nouns, verbs, adjectives, and adverbs. But clearly closed class items such as prepositions also influence the relations assigned to the words and phrases of a sentence, including prepositions which carry specific lexical semantic content (e.g., *to* and *on* in the sentences in (1) determine how many arguments are assigned to the verb *help*) and those that are more purely syntactic (e.g., *of* in *the destruction of the city*, specifies that *the city* corresponds to the theme of *destroy*).

(1) a. *The umpire helped the child to third base.*
   b. *The umpire helped the child on third base.*

Hence, it looks as though all words of a major lexical category are important to determining the semantic relations in a sentence, as are words drawn from the minor lexical categories, for example consider the role of *the* in disambiguating the sentences in (2).

(2)    *He showed her baby pictures.*
    a. *He showed her baby the pictures.*
    b. *He showed her the baby pictures.*

Grammatical formatives such as the possessive marker *'s* play a similar function in that they also delimit the semantic relations between the words of a sentence; in (3) only the presence or absence of the possessive marker on *men* can be used to distinguish between the semantic relations in (3a) and (3b).

(3) a. *Beware of rich men's friends and shysters.*
   b. *Beware of rich men friends and shysters.*

The above examples illustrate two points. First, they indicate that if the lexical constraints hypothesis is to alleviate the need for a detailed structural representation to be computed, it must claim that all lexical items and grammatical formatives are used in determining the relations in the sentence. There does not seem to be any principled class of items that can be ignored.

Second, it should be emphasized that it is not simply the presence of some grammatical formative that is important in determining the relations in a sentence; the *absence* of a grammatical formative is equally important. In sentence (2), the absence of a determiner permits the sentence to have two meanings, corresponding to those of (2a) and (2b). Similarly, in (3b) the absence of the possessive marker permits the noun phrase *rich men* to be interpreted as one of the arguments of *beware* (i.e., as one conjunct of a conjoined noun phrase). Thus the legitimate semantic relations in a sentence are affected by both the presence and the absence of grammatical formatives and therefore cannot be determined if any of the items in the sentence are ignored or overlooked since by definition an overlooked item and the absence of some item in the input string cannot be distinguished. Of course, one might try to detect only the absence of particularly crucial items, but identifying the position in a sentence where the absence of some item is crucial to the semantic relations of the sentence will itself involve computing a detailed syntactic analysis of the sentence.

In some sentences, it might appear that the possible semantic relations of the sentence could be determined without computing a syntactic analysis of the sentence. Consider a sentence like *Read newspapers editorials and essays.* At first it might appear that it is simply the fact that *read* selects for a human subject and an inanimate object which would permit the language processor to safely conclude that lexical constraints lead to a unique analysis of the relations in this sentence. But if we omitted the plural marker on *newspaper*, or changed the plural marker to the possessive marker, *newspaper* would no longer function as one of the arguments of the verb. This illustrates that there are many semantic roles that words and phrases can assume beyond those determined by the argument structure of verbs; thus, determining the set of possible semantic roles in a particular sentence (and whether lexical constraints will lead to a unique analysis of these roles) depends on detailed inferences about the structure of a sentence involving much more than the mere retrieval of the semantic restrictions on the argument of verbs.

We turn now to a more detailed examination of the specific information available in lexical entries; the purpose of the discussion is to determine whether fully exploiting this information in any way mitigates the need to construct a full structural representation of a sentence. We will assume that a lexical entry contains information about the phonological and orthographic form of a word, the morphological structure of the word, its lexical category, subcategorization information (what syntactic frame the word can be inserted into), selection restrictions, information about argument structure (e.g., how many arguments the word can take, and what their thematic roles are), and some type of semantic representation.

In any version of the Lexical Constraints hypothesis in which subcategorization information is exploited, it will be necessary to determine the lexical category of the words in the sentence. What lexical categories of an item in any particular sentence are permissable depends not only on lexical information about the possible categories of the item but also on the categories assigned to the other items in the sentence. Consider the string *The desert trains . . .* If *desert* is categorized as an adjective then *trains* must be categorized as a noun, as in (4a). But this constraint cannot be derived from lexical information; rather, it is a syntactic fact which follows from the constraint that a noun phrase must obligatorily contain a noun. If *desert* is categorized as a noun, then *trains* may be analyzed as a verb, as in (4b).

(4)  a. *The desert trains are always crowded.*
     b. *The desert trains people to be rugged.*

However, *trains* may not be analyzed as a verb if *desert* has been categorized as an adjective. One might try to capture such constraints lexically. For example, the lexical entry for an item that is ambiguous between an adjective and a noun categorization might specify that it should be labelled as an adjective if it occurs before a noun, but as a noun if it occurs before a verb. But of course this is false. This item might be a noun when it occurs before a noun, as in the conjoined noun phrase in *the desert trains people and dogs all bother me.* The point, of course, is that determining the proper lexical category of an item depends on an inferential chain involving the possible lexical categories of the items in the sentence, the category assigned to other items, and the possible syntactic configurations of the language. This is precisely the sort of inferential chain that the syntactic representation of a sentence encodes. Thus, this example illustrates the rather obvious fact that in many cases lexical information is only useful if a structural representation of the sentence is computed, thereby permitting useful syntactic constraints to be exploited. Lexical information about the category of an item is helpful largely by virtue of the constraints it places on the analysis of the other items in the sentence; yet these constraints would be unavailable if the language processor did not keep a record of its structural decisions, but rather directly assigned underlying semantic relations.

The same general point applies to the use of subcategorization information. Consider the sentences in (5).

(5)  a.  *After John died his girlfriend her mother and her father arrived.*
     b.  *After John left his girlfriend her mother and her father arrived.*

The fact that *die* cannot take a direct object could be determined simply on the basis of its subcategorization, and this in turn entails that the phrase *his girlfriend* cannot be analyzed as a constituent of the subordinate clause in (5a). In (5b), subcategorization information can be used to determine that *his girlfriend* can be analyzed as the direct object of *leave*. However if *his grilfriend* is analyzed as the direct object of *leave*, then that noun phrase cannot be interpreted as one of the conjuncts of the subject noun phrase of the main clause. Now the question is whether this constraint could be determined on the basis of lexical information. Perhaps we might say that a phrase may only be assigned to a slot in a single subcategorization frame. Thus, having assigned the phrase *his girlfriend* to the direct object slot of the subcategorization frame for *leave* the phrase would be unavailable to be assigned to some other role in the sentence. This "unique assignment" constraint would prevent the processor from making a dual assignment of the phrase *his girlfriend* in (5b). It would also prevent the phrase *the story* from being assigned as both the direct object of the verb *kill* and the direct object of the verb *tell* in a sentence like (6).

(6)  *The man told the girl that Sam killed the story.*

Thus, although lexical information about the subcategorization of words is not very informative by itself, together with some principles like the unique assignment constraint, it might potentially be used to specify many of the constraints on the possible relations in a sentence. Unfortunately, the unique assignment constraint is simply untenable. In a relative clause, such as that in (7), the head of the relative, *the book*, must be assigned to the direct object slot of the subcategorization frame for *buy* and to the direct object slot of the subcategorization slot for *lose*.

(7)   *Mark lost the book Sam bought.*

And of course there are lots of more complicated examples where a phrase must be assigned to a slot in more than one subcategorization frame, for example, sentences with parasitic gaps (*Who did John's talking to bother most?*), across-the-board extractions (*Who did John like and Mark hate?*), etc. Thus again we see that lexical information (this time, subcategorization information) is useful in large part because of the constraints it places on the analysis of the constituents of the sentence, but that these constraints are not available unless a structural representation of the sentence is computed.

Perhaps the most powerful lexical restrictions on the relations of a sentence stem from the selection restrictions and semantic representation of the words in the sentence. Thus we might ask whether these restrictions could often lead to a unique analysis of the semantic relations in a sentence. If one has already computed the set of grammatically licensed meanings of a sentence, then it is perfectly coherent to resort to a principle like semantic coherence or pragmatic plausibility to guide the selection of one particular meaning for the sentence. But without an already identified candidate set of grammatically licensed meanings to choose from, claiming that semantic coherence or pragmatic plausibility are used to assign semantic relations predicts that people compute sensible sentence meanings but do not determine whether the meaning they arrive at is a grammatically possible meaning for the particular sentence they have heard or read. In fact, this seems to roughly characterize what people do when they encounter multiply center-embedded sentences that are too difficult to correctly comprehend; however, multiply center-embedded sentences are the exception, not the rule.

Typically, people only report grammatically licensed meanings for sentences. For example, in a sentence like (8), the adverb *yesterday* and the locative phrase *at the races* may each by analyzed as a constituent of the embedded sentence where they modify *died*, or as constituents of the matrix sentence where they modify *claimed*; or *yesterday* may attach in the embedded sentences and *at the races* in the higher sentence.

(8)   *John claimed the gangster died yesterday at the races.*

It is not possible (unless the prepositional phrase is spoken with parenthetical intonation) for the adverb to attach in the higher sentence and the locative phrase in the lower sentence, since this would lead to crossed branches in the phrase marker of the sentence. One can change the semantic properties of the sentence as much as one likes to try to tempt people into the illicit crossing-branches analysis of the sentence, as in (9), but people will not report the more plausible meaning (where the gangster will die at the shootout), presumably because it is not grammatically licensed.

(9)   *John claimed the gangster will die yesterday at the shootout.*

People do not report the pragmatically tempting set of semantic relations if they correspond to an illegitimate structural representation that is not grammatically licensed.

I have argued that a theory of structural processing is a proper subdomain of a theory of reading, or any theory of language comprehension. People must compute a structural representation of a sentence in order to arrive at a grammatically licensed meaning of a sentence and they must utilize syntactic information to do so. Though the Lexical Constraints hypothesis superficially appears to offer an alternative to the claim that people compute a structural representation of a sentence, when we take the hypothesis seriously and examine its predictions in detail, we see that it does not permit the assignment of relations to be determined on the basis of purely lexical information. Further, the apparent computational savings stemming from not computing a structural representation of the sentence is illusory. It is bought at the expense of either (*a*) performing a series of ad hoc syntactic tests to determine the viability of an analysis of semantic relations based exclusively on available lexical and pragmatic constraints; or (b) incorrectly predicting that people assign grammatically illicit meanings to sentences containing pragmatically tempting relations that do not correspond to a well-formed analysis of the sentence.

## III.   The Eye Movement Recording Technique

Given that we need to include a theory of structural processing in an adequate theory of reading, how do we go about constructing that theory? Clearly we do not have a window into the language processing mechanism that would permit us to directly examine the internal workings of the language processor. Instead we must rely on data concerning the preferred interpretation of linguistic material, systematic processing errors, and data about the relative processing complexity of sentences to obtain evidence about the processing routines used in language comprehension.

The problem, of course, is that this type of data only takes us so far; it gives us direct information only about the output of the language comprehension (and inferential) system. A considerable body of psycholinguistic evidence suggests that detailed structural properties of sentences are no longer important (or even available in memory) shortly after a sentence has been processed. Hence, data concerning the ultimate output of the language comprehension system are of limited value in constructing a theory of structural processing. What we really need is data concerning the operations that take place during the processing of a sentence. This data will allow us to check our interpretation of findings based on end-of-sentence measures, for example, they will permit us to determine whether increases in processing load occur in the predicted region of the sentence. Further, they will allow us to test hypotheses about the precise timing of various processing operations and the effects of the availability of various types of information on the output of these operations. Presumably such data would also allow us to detect more subtle differences in processing complexity which may no longer be detectable by the time the end of a sentence has been processed. As theories of sentence processing become more refined, we must increasingly rely on these more subtle effects to check the predictions of a theory and to evaluate competing theories of sentence processing.

The major distinctive advantage of the eye movement recording technique is that it permits us to obtain evidence about what is happening during the comprehension of a sentence without significantly altering the normal characteristics of either the task or the presentation of materials. Subjects may simply read some linguistic material for comprehension. They need not perform some secondary task that might disrupt or alter the normal comprehension process, nor must the theorist worry about the relation between the secondary task and the primary task of comprehending linguistic material. I am not aware of any other available experimental psycholinguistic technique that fully shares these important advantages.

Despite the important advantages of the eye movement recording technique, it does have several drawbacks and limitations. One minor drawback of the technique (as well as being a major advantage) stems from the sheer amount of data that one collects. This can be a problem because one gets more information that can be interpreted if the investigator does not have a clear idea of what effects are expected and where in the eye movement record they are likely to show up (i.e., if one has some reason for performing a "fishing" expedition, I would suggest using a different technique.)

A more serious current limitation of the eye movement recording technique stems from the fact that one cannot be certain what material is being processed when. However, this problem is insurmountable only if the lag between the time when some portion of a sentence is fixated and the time when it is processed varies randomly. In this case, the eye movement recording technique would be no more useful as a measure of processing complexity than any other indication of global reading time. However, I am not aware of any evidence that this is the case. In this chapter I will present some evidence that indicates that the increase in processing complexity associated with the structural analysis of an item can be detected in the eye movement record as soon as that item has been fixated, though the effects of the increase in complexity may also extend beyond the fixations associated with that one item. This evidence provides one indication that the language comprehension device is structurally processing each word as it is read, though it may still also be concerned with deeper levels of analysis of preceding material.

Another limitation of the eye movement recording technique is the absence of explicit detailed theories of eye movement control (e.g., see discussion in Carpenter & Just, 1977; Rayner, 1978). There are still many open questions with respect to the factors that govern where people fixate, on the one hand, and for how long they fixate, on the other. Until these questions have been completely resolved, various precautions are in order when scoring the data. One precaution is simply to perform a number of different analyses of the data, to make sure that the outcome of the different analyses converge on a single coherent interpretation of the data and to exclude the possibility of trade-offs between different indicators of processing complexity. Similarly, it makes sense to perform rather fine-grained analyses of the data, to try to isolate potentially independent effects, for example, separating out initial fixations on an item from second pass fixations, analyzing within-word regressions separately from those that extend beyond a word, etc.

There are actually two reasons for performing this type of fine-grained analysis of the data. One is simply to verify the conclusions drawn from a particular study. The other reason is to determine whether different aspects of the eye movement data may not be providing us with a selective measure of different component processes of reading. At least in principle, it is possible that, say, the position of first pass fixations is determined primarily by perceptual characteristics of words (e.g., word length) under control of a mechanism that is largely independent of the language processing mechanism proper (cf. O'Regan, 1979; Rayner & Mc-

Conkie, 1976), at least in circumstances where processing complexity remains under some base-line level determined by the overall complexity of the text. By contrast, the factors governing the initiation of regressive eye movements (or perhaps some identifiable subset of them) and governing the position of second pass fixations might be due to nonperceptual aspects of processing, such as an incompatibility between currently fixated material and the chosen analysis of preceding material, or the need to find an antecedent for currently fixated material (cf. Carpenter & Just, 1977; Carpenter & Daneman, 1981; Holmes & O'Regan, 1981).

Much of the eye movement recording literature is at least compatible with the claim that linguistic factors govern the duration of fixations but not the position of first pass fixations. However one notable exception to the predictions of this selective measure hypothesis derives from a study by Mehler, Bever, and Carey (1967). They examined the effects of syntactic structure on readers' fixation patterns and concluded that readers fixate the beginnings of surface structure constituents. For example, in the ambiguous sentences in (10) and (11), subjects tended to fixate more often on the word *dog* when it was interpreted as the beginning of the noun phrase *dog candies*, as indicated in (11), than when it was interpreted as the head of the noun phrase *her dog*, as indicated in (10).

(10)     *They   gave   (her      dog)     can       dies.*
          14.3 3.5   3.7   2.6   8.7   2.1   10.3     9.8

(11)     *They   gave   her    (dog     can       dies).*
          13.5  3.6   7.9  3.6   14.3  2.8   10.4     10.7

However, first pass fixations were not measured separately from regressive fixations in this study, raising the possibility that the observed correlation between the position of fixations and the surface structure assigned to a sentence was due entirely to second pass fixations (as would be expected if readers who initially computed the contextually inappropriate meaning of a phrase regressed to the beginning of the ambiguous string to revise their initial analysis of it). Further, O'Regan (1975) was unable to replicate the findings of Mehler, *et al.* Finally, the hypothesized correlation is conceptually problematic since it is not clear how readers could determine either the position or the number of left brackets (beginnings of constituents) before they had performed an analysis of the structural consequences of the words they had not yet fixated. At best, it seems that the expected correlation should have been between the possible syntactic continuations of the string already analyzed and the pattern of fixations. But of course this predicts no difference in the first pass fixation pattern for the sentences tested in the Mehler, *et al.* study. Thus, although the hypothesis that there is a correlation between surface syntactic structure and readers' fixation patterns is interesting, there is not really evidence for the existence of such a correlation, especially with respect to first pass fixations.

Mehler, *et al.* also consider the effects of word syntax and observe that there is some suggestive evidence in their data for the existence of a correlation between the position of fixations and the morphological structure of words. The possibility that word level syntax is correlated with readers' fixation patterns clearly warrants further investigation. It is quite possible that readers have available to them a list of the bound morphemes in the language which would permit them to identify a considerable amount of morphological structure without performing anything but a perceptual analysis of the word string. The fact that the word level domain is much more local than the sentence domain implies that readers might have performed some preliminary structural analysis of the items in that domain before determining the location of an immediately following fixation. Though the existence of left recursion remains a problem in the case of word syntax, the problem is not as severe here as it is in the case of phrase and sentence level syntax, due to the relative size of the domains involved. These considerations suggest that further investigation of the selective measure hypothesis should examine the effects of word level syntax and phrase level syntax separately, as well as analyze first pass and second pass fixations separately.

As noted, the possible effect of syntactic structure on the position of first pass fixations and in turn on reading time and fixation duration measures can be controlled for by computing more global measures of reading time that should reflect any trade-off between reading times in the region of interest and in surrounding regions of the sentence. Thus unresolved questions about the eye movement recording technique in no way undermine its usefulness as an online measure of structural processing complexity; rather, they suggest that a variety of scoring methods should be employed in order to obtain an accurate profile of the processing complexity of sentences and to pin down more precisely the relation between different aspects of the eye movement record and readers' internal processing operations.

## IV.  A Garden-Path Theory of Sentence Comprehension

In this section I briefly describe some eye movement experiments we have conducted to further elaborate a particular theory of the structural processing that occurs during sentence comprehension. The theory claims that readers systematically construct a representation of the constituent structure of a sentence as the words of the sentence are encountered. Two strategies, late closure and minimal attachment, characterize the processor's preferred options at choice points where the well-formedness rules of the language would permit more than one structural analysis of the input lexical string. The late closure strategy states that items are preferably analyzed as a constituent of the phrase currently being processed. Hence, in a string like (12), the temporarily ambiguous noun phrase *a mile* will initially be analyzed as the object of the verb *jog*. In (12a) this decision will be compatible with subsequent context; in (12b) this decision will prove to be incompatible with subsequent items and hence the processor will have to revise its initial decision.

(12)    *Since Jay always jogs* **a mile** . . .
   a.  *Since Jay always jogs a mile* **this seems** *like a short distance to him.*
   b.  *Since Jay always jogs a mile* **seems like** *a very short distance to him.*
(13)    *Tom heard* **the latest gossip about the new neighbors** . . .
   a.  *I wonder if Tom heard the latest gossip about the new neighbors.*
   b.  *Tom heard the latest gossip about the new neighbors* **wasn't true.**

The minimal attachment strategy states that incoming words are incorporated into the phrase marker being constructed using the fewest nodes consistent with the well-formedness rules of the language. In (13) this predicts that the temporarily ambiguous phrase *the gossip about the new neighbors* will initially be interpreted as the direct object of the verb *hear*; interpreting it as the subject of a complement sentence would require postulating an additional S— node. In (13b), but not (13a), this decision will have to be revised when subsequent items are processed. Assuming that revising an incorrect analysis of the sentence is not cost free, these strategies predict greater processing complexity for the (b) than for the (a) versions of sentences (12) and (13).

I will refer to this theory as a garden-path theory of sentence comprehension since it claims that the processor is often led down the garden path, that is, that the processor frequently constructs an incorrect analysis of some portion of the sentence on the way to arriving at a correct analysis that is tenable for the entire sentence. Initial support for the garden-path theory and for the generality of the late closure and minimal attachment strategies derives from studies confirming their complexity predictions using a grammaticality-judgment task (cf. Frazier, 1978). The grammaticality-judgment task only provides an end of sentence measure of processing complexity. Using data from that technique, one can only infer that the increase in complexity associated with the garden-path versions of the sentences, for example, (13b) and (14b), is in fact due to the region of the sentence that was predicted to be incompatible with the chosen analysis of the temporarily ambiguous phrase. Localizing the increase in complexity to the predicted region of the sentence would provide more direct support for the theory.

The garden-path theory is underdetermined in many important respects. Though it makes rather explicit claims about the initial structural analysis of sentences, it does not specify the nature of the processing routines that are used to revise an initial incorrect analysis of some portion of the sentence. Further, the theory does not specify how the structural analysis of a sentence is influenced by nonsyntactic factors. For example, what happens when the syntactically preferred analysis of a string is less plausible on pragmatic grounds than some competing analysis of the string? Will pragmatic considerations dictate which analysis of the sentence is initially computed, or will they only influence the ease of arriving at the final correct analysis of the sentence? In general, how are syntactic preferences integrated with lexical preferences and semantic information, as they surely must be if we are to account for the ultimately preferred analyses of ambiguous sentences?

Keith Rayner, Marcia Carlson, and I conducted three eye movement experiments to investigate these questions. The first study was designed to localize the increase in processing complexity associated with the garden-path version of the sentences in (12) and (13) and to explore the reanalysis procedures used to recover from an incorrect analysis of the sentence. Recall that late closure and minimal attachment predict that the increase in complexity in the (b) version of the sentences should be associated with the processing of the disambiguating region of the sentences, which was defined as the two words immediately following the ambiguous region. If the predicted increase in complexity is observed in the disambiguating region of the sentence, indicating that the processor has detected an error in the initial analysis of the sentence, then the question is how the processor goes about correcting its erroneous analysis. One possibility is that it returns to the very beginning of the sentence and reprocesses the entire sentence over again, opting for alternative decisions at choice points. This "forward reanalysis hypothesis" predicts that regressive eye movements initiated from after the ambiguous region of the sentence should return to the very beginning of the sentence. Alternatively, the processor might automatically back up through the sentence once an error is discovered in the initial analysis of the sentence. This "backward reanalysis hypothesis" predicts that regressive eye movements should proceed systematically through the sentence from right to left until the ambiguous region of the sentence is encountered. One final possibility is that upon encountering an error in its chosen analysis of the sentence, the processor exploits whatever information it has about the ill-formedness of its initial analysis (e.g., the sentence is missing an obligatory noun phrase subject for this verb) in an attempt to diagnose the source of its error. This "intelligent reanalysis hypothesis" predicts that regressive eye movements initiated from after the ambiguous phrase should return directly to the ambiguous region of the sentence providing that the structure of the sentence is such that it provides an informative error signal that would permit the processor to infer the source of its error. (Our experimental sentences all contained potentially helpful information of this type.)

To test these predictions we instructed 16 subjects to read sentences like those in (12) and (13). Each subject read 16 closure sentences, 16 attachment sentences, and 64 distractor sentences. There were four versions of each experimental sentence: Two were consistent with the predictions of the above parsing strategies (one containing a short, one- or two-word, ambiguous phrase, one containing a longer ambiguous phrase); two were inconsistent (one contained a short ambiguous phrase and one contained a longer ambiguous phrase). The position and duration of each fixation was recorded as each subject read the sentences. (For a more detailed discussion of the methodology and results, see Frazier & Rayner, 1982.)

Various analyses of the data were performed. The most important findings are summarized in Table 13.1. As predicted, the reading time per character for the early closure and non-minimal-attachment versions of the sentences were longer than for the late closure and minimal attachment versions, respectively. As expected, the increase in processing complexity was observed in the disambiguating region of the garden-path versions of the sentence: The reading time per character in the disambiguating region was significantly longer than in either the ambiguous region of the sentence or the region of the sentence preceding the ambiguous phrase in the early closure sentences with long ambiguous phrases, but not in the late closure sentences. (The same pattern emerged in the sentences with short ambiguous phrases but did not quite reach significance.) In the non-minimal-attachment sentences, the reading time per character was also significantly longer in the disambiguating region than in either of the prior regions. In the minimal attachment sentences, the end of the ambiguous region coincided with the end of the sentence so this analysis could not be performed. An analysis of average fixation durations surrounding the point of disambiguation was also performed. We labeled the first fixation in the disambiguating region of the sentence as fixation $d$, we then computed the average fixation duration of fixation $d$, and of the two subsequent fixations. We compared the average duration of each of these fixations with the average duration of each of the three fixations immediately preceding fixation $d$. These data are presented in Panel C of Table 13.1. As expected, the fixations (even the very first) following the disambiguation point were significantly longer than the three preceding fixations in the garden-path sentences (i.e., early closure and non-minimal-attachment sentences) but not in the late closure sentences (again the minimal attachment sentences did not provide this comparison). This finding strongly suggests that readers immediately perform a structural analysis of fixated words, detecting any problem these words pose for the structural analysis assigned to preceding words of the sentence.

The pattern of regressive eye movements that extend beyond word boundaries is presented in Panel D of Table 13.1. The dominant type of regression was one initiated from the disambiguating region of the sentence landing in the ambiguous region of the sentence. Readers were likely to regress to the beginning of the sentence only when the eye movement was initiated from the very end of the sentence. Roughly half the regressions were initiated from the disambiguating region of the sentence; these ended in an earlier portion of the disambiguating region of the sentence or in the ambiguous phrase. The other major type of regression was one initiated from the very end of the sentence; these regressions typically ended in the ambiguous region or at the beginning of the sentence.

In our experimental sentences, the predictions of the intelligent reanalysis and backward reanalysis hypotheses can only be distinguished in the case of regressive eye movements initiated from some portion of the sentence following the disambiguating region: In such cases, there was no evidence of subjects systematically backtracking through the sentence, as would have been indicated by a series of right to left movements. Though the results of the regression-type analysis are difficult to quantify, the predominance of regressions directly to the ambiguous

## TABLE 13.1
### Eye Movement Data from Experiment 1

*Panel A* Mean reading time per character (msec)

|  | Early closure | Late closure | X̄ |  | Nonminimal attachment | Minimal attachment | X̄ |
|---|---|---|---|---|---|---|---|
| Long ambiguous phrase | 68 | 50 | 59 |  | 61 | 45 | 53 |
| Short ambiguous phrase | 57 | 55 | 56 |  | 51 | 49 | 50 |
| X̄ | 62.5 | 52.5 |  |  | 56 | 47 |  |

*Panel B* Mean reading time per character in different regions of the sentence

|  |  | Before ambiguity | Ambiguity | Disambiguity |
|---|---|---|---|---|
| Early closure long | First pass | 44 | 40 | 54 |
|  | Second pass | 21 | 32 | 48 |
|  | Total | 65 | 72 | 102 |
| Early closure short | First pass | 43 | 37 | 41 |
|  | Second pass | 18 | 37 | 41 |
|  | Total | 61 | 74 | 82 |
| Late closure long | First pass | 43 | 35 | 40 |
|  | Second pass | 12 | 15 | 23 |
|  | Total | 55 | 50 | 63 |
| Late closure short | First pass | 40 | 42 | 47 |
|  | Second pass | 16 | 27 | 22 |
|  | Total | 56 | 69 | 69 |

|  |  | Before ambiguity | Ambiguity | Disambiguity |
|---|---|---|---|---|
| Nonminimal long | First pass | 43 | 37 | 51 |
|  | Second pass | 17 | 22 | 30 |
|  | Total | 60 | 59 | 81 |
| Nonminimal short | First pass | 43 | 36 | 47 |
|  | Second pass | 10 | 15 | 23 |
|  | Total | 53 | 51 | 70 |
| Minimal long | First pass | 41 | 36 | — |
|  | Second pass | 7 | 7 | — |
|  | Total | 48 | 43 | — |
| Minimal short | First pass | 42 | 36 | — |
|  | Second pass | 8 | 12 | — |
|  | Total | 50 | 48 | — |

Panel C Average fixation duration on the three fixations before and the three fixations after disambiguation

| | (d−3) | (d−2) | (d−1) | (d) | (d+1) | (d+2) |
|---|---|---|---|---|---|---|
| Early closure long | 252 | 259 | 236 | 301 | 285 | 313 |
| Early closure short | 245 | 227 | 245 | 283 | 267 | 277 |
| Late closure long | 248 | 239 | 243 | 260 | 247 | 242 |
| Late closure short | 228 | 239 | 243 | 268 | 248 | 242 |
| Nonminimal long | 248 | 259 | 258 | 291 | 284 | 301 |
| Nonminimal short | 247 | 235 | 226 | 292 | 280 | 267 |

Panel D Regression proportions based on 222 regressions[a]

| Regression initiated from | | Eye movements ended | | | |
|---|---|---|---|---|---|
| | Beginning of sentence | Before ambiguity | In ambiguity | In disambiguity | Total |
| Disambiguating region | .03 (.01) | .04 (.03) | .33 (.36) | .12 (.11) | .52 (.51) |
| After disambiguating region | .01 (.02) | .04 (.03) | .06 (.05) | .04 (.05) | .15 (.15) |
| End of sentence | .18 (.17) | .03 (.03) | .10 (.12) | .02 (.02) | .33 (.34) |
| Total | .22 (.20) | .11 (.09) | .49 (.53) | .18 (.18) | |

[a]Values in parentheses are for early closure and nonminimal and nonminimal attachment sentences; 70% of the regressions in closure sentences were in the early closure version of the sentence; 72% of the regressions in attachment sentences were in the nonminimal attachment version of the sentence.

phrase, together with the absence of evidence indicating systematic backtracking, suggests that subjects were often able to diagnose the source of their error, as predicted by the intelligent reanalysis hypothesis.

These results provide further evidence for the garden-path theory of comprehension, together with the late closure and minimal attachment strategies. Readers have difficulty processing the disambiguating region of the garden-path version of the sentences, as indicated by longer reading times per character in this region of the sentence, longer average fixation durations and a higher probability of initiating a regressive eye movement. The results also provide some initial support for intelligent or selective reanalysis, clearly disconfirming the hypothesis that subjects always return to the very beginning of a sentence and reprocess the entire sentence whenever they encounter a problem with their initial structural analysis of it. We turn now to questions concerning the influence of pragmatic constraints on the initial structural analysis of sentences.

Let us return for a moment to the hypothesis that the language processor only constructs a structural analysis of a sentence when all other routes to successful comprehension fail. This predicts that the reading times associated with some sentence or portion of a sentence should be shorter when the relations of the words or phrases are plausible than when they are implausible since the processor either (1) does not have to compute a structural representation at all; or (2) only needs to check the structural relations to confirm the relations assigned on the basis of pragmatic plausibility constraints. Consider the sentences in (14) for example.

(14)  a.  ***The florist sent the flowers* was very** pleased.      (implausible)
      b.  *The performer sent the flowers was very pleased.*      (plausible)
      c.  *The performer who was sent the flowers was very pleased.*      (plausible)
      d.  *The performer sent the flowers and was very pleased with herself.*
          (implausible)
(15)  a.  *The florist sent the flowers*
      b.  *The performer sent the flowers*

In (14a), readers might exploit their knowledge that florists are likely to be senders of flowers to assign semantic or thematic relations to the ambiguous portion of the sentence, and in (14b) they might exploit the knowledge that performers are likely to be recipients of flowers to assign a different set of relations. If so, then subjects should assign the correct semantic relations to the sentences in (14b) and (14c) and should be garden pathed in sentences (14a) and (14d), where pragmatic considerations would lead to an incorrect set of semantic relations. In fact, Crain and Coker (1979) found that subjects' responses in a paraphrase verification task testing the interpretation of the sentence fragments in (15) revealed that subjects reported the reduced relative reading of (15a) only 16% of the time, but reported the reduced relative clause reading of (15b) 43% of the time. Thus, in their study, the pragmatic constraints in (15b) almost tripled the proportion of reduced relative clause readings assigned to the word string. Although this study provides initial support for the view that pragmatic constraints influence the processing of sentences, it is not relevant to the question of whether pragmatic considerations influence the processor's selection of an initial structural analysis of sentences. If the initial structural analysis of sentences is computed on the basis of syntactic preferences without regard for the likelihood of possible real world events, then we would expect readers to opt for the minimal attachment analysis of the ambiguous portions of (14a) and (14b) as well as of (14d); only in (14d) will the chosen (simple sentence) analysis turn out to be correct. Hence, this hypothesis predicts that readers should be garden pathed in both (14a) and (14b) but not in (14d). This would be reflected by longer reading times and longer fixation durations associated with the words immediately following the ambiguous phrase in (14a) and (14b) relative to (14c), which contains an unambiguous string with the same syntactic structure as (14a) and (14b), and relative to (14d) where the minimal attachment analysis turns out to be correct.

To test these predictions, 20 subjects were instructed to read sentences like those in (14). Each subject read 12 experimental sentences and 84 distractor sentences with varied syntactic structures. There were four versions of each experimental sentence, as illustrated in (14): One version contained a reduced relative clause with implausible semantic relations, as in (14a); one version contained a reduced relative clause with plausible semantic relations, as in (14b); one version contained an unreduced relative clause with plausible semantic relations, as in (14c); and the final version included a word string identical to the initial portion of the plausible reduced relative but in this sentence the string had to be assigned a structure corresponding to a simple active sentence, and thus the correct relations in the sentence corresponded to relatively implausible relations, as in (14d). The sentences were completely counterbalanced so that no subject saw more than one version of a sentence, and each subject saw an equal number of each sentence type. (For details of the experimental procedure and results, see Rayner, Carlson, & Frazier, in press.)

The most important results of the study are presented in Table 13.2. The results clearly support the predictions of the hypothesis that readers initially construct a structural analysis of the sentence based on syntactic preferences. Contrary to the predictions of the pragmatic constraints hypothesis, there is evidence that subjects are garden pathed in sentences like (14b), where pragmatic considerations would have led to a correct first analysis of the sentence. Further, there is no evidence that subjects are garden pathed in sentences like (14d), where pragmatic considerations would have led to an incorrect initial analysis of the ambiguous portion of the sentence. The total reading time per character for the different sentence types is presented in Panel A of Table 13.2. The first pass reading time per character measure shows no difference between sentence types, as predicted by the hypothesis that the processor follows its structural preference in all sentences regardless of pragmatic considerations. The crucial prediction concerns the reading time per character for the disambiguating region of the reduced relative clauses versus reading time in this region for the control sentences with the unreduced relative and the simple active versions of the sentence.

**TABLE 13.2**
**Eye Movement Data from Experiment 2**

*Panel A* Mean reading time per character (msec) (mean reading time per character for first fixations only are presented in parentheses)

| | | |
|---|---|---|
| Plausible reduced relatives | 47 | (33) |
| Implausible reduced relatives | 52 | (32) |
| Unreduced relative | 41 | (30) |
| Active | 34 | (29) |

*Panel B* Mean reading time per character in different regions of the sentence (mean reading time per character for first pass fixations only are presented in parentheses)

| | Before relative | | Relative | | Disambiguating region | |
|---|---|---|---|---|---|---|
| Plausible reduced relatives | 39 | (29) | 46 | (29) | 57 | (40) |
| Implausible reduced relatives | 41 | (32) | 55 | (29) | 60 | (36) |
| Unreduced relatives | 35 | (31) | 48 | (31) | 40 | (28) |
| Active | 34 | (29) | 34 | (28) | 35 | (29) |

*Panel C* Average fixation duration of the three fixations before and the three fixations after disambiguation

| | Before | After |
|---|---|---|
| Plausible reduced relatives | 213 | 250 |
| Implausible reduced relatives | 210 | 257 |
| Unreduced relatives | 218 | 224 |
| Active | 198 | 213 |

*Panel D* Number of regressions for each sentence type (based on 188 regressions)

| | Plausible reduced relative | Implausible reduced relative | Unreduced relative | Active |
|---|---|---|---|---|
| Regressions from in or after disambiguating region or to an earlier region in or before disambiguating region | 26 | 33 | 13 | 8 |
| Regressions from end of sentence to the region in or before disambiguating region | 21 | 22 | 16 | 23 |
| *Total regressions* | | | | |
| Initiated after ambiguous region ending in or before disambiguating region | 47 | 55 | 29 | 31 |
| Regressions within relative clause | 3 | 5 | 15 | 3 |
| Total | 50 | 60 | 44 | 34 |

Reading times for the initial portion of the sentence (up to and including the head of the relative clause), the relative clause itself (excluding the head of the relative clause), and the disambiguating region (the two words immediately following the relative) are presented in Panel B. It is clear that the reading times associated with the disambiguating region of the reduced relative clause sentences (14a) and (14b) are much longer than for the non-garden-path sentences. The average duration of the three fixations following the disambiguation point was significantly longer than the average of the preceding three fixations in the reduced relative sentences, but not in the other sentence types.

Regressive eye movements extending beyond a word boundary that were initiated from some region of the sentence following the ambiguous phrase are presented in Panel D of Table 13.2. As expected, there were more regressions in the reduced relatives than in any other version of the sentences.

The results of this study suggest that pragmatic constraints concerning the relative likelihood of various possible real world situations or events do not influence the processor's initial choice of a structural analysis of the lexical string. Thus the study further supports the conclusion arrived at in Section I that it is necessary to compute a structural analysis of sentences. Nevertheless it is clear from intuitive evidence that the real world likelihood of some situation or event does influence which of two or more grammatically licensed interpretations of a sentence people eventually tend to report. The next experiment represents an initial attempt to pin down the mechanism responsible for the influence of lexical preferences and pragmatic considerations on the ultimately preferred analysis of sentences.

Ford, Bresnan, & Kaplan (1981) argue that the momentarily preferred lexical form of a verb is responsible for determining the structural analysis assigned to ambiguous sentences like those in (16).

(16)  a.  *The woman wanted **the dress on that rack.***
      b.  *The woman positioned **the dress** on that rack.*

The basic idea is that the verb *position* prefers to take two arguments in its complement, an object and a locative phrase; whereas, the verb *want* prefers to take just a single argument. In Ford, *et al.*'s system these lexical preferences will determine the *initial* analysis assigned to sentences like those in (16) and thus will account for the difference in the preferred interpretation of the ambiguous portion of the sentences (see Ford, *et al.* for details of the actual parsing principles proposed to accomplish this).

I have argued elsewhere (Frazier, 1981) that a somewhat different mechanism is needed to account for the influence of lexical preferences and pragmatic plausibility. I appeal to a specialized processor, or "focused processor," that operates over the alternative forms stored in a lexical entry (presumably thematic structures) and selects the most plausible form based on world knowledge, knowledge about discourse function, and the like. The focused processor is distinct from the syntactic processor responsible for constructing a structural representation of the sentence, however the output of the focused processor can influence the operation of the syntactic processor. If the lexical structure selected by the focused processor is incompatible with the syntactic analysis assigned to the relevant portion of the lexical string, the focused processor's output will function as a signal to the syntactic processor that there is a potentially better analysis of that string. This signal will cause the syntactic processor to revise its analysis of that string (assuming that there is a syntactically well-formed analysis corresponding to the focused processor's proposal.)

Though the details of the focused processor's operation have not been worked out the basic hypothesis makes rather clear predictions about the processing of sentences like (17). Even though a verb like *see* probably does not prefer to take two arguments in its complement, the minimal attachment strategy predicts that the syntactic processor will initially opt for the minimal attachment analysis of the ambiguous prepositional phrase, where it will be interpreted as an argument of the verb, that is, as an instrumental phrase. (I am assuming that the "nonminimal attachment analysis" requires an extra noun phrase to be postulated, as implied by the phrase structure rule: NP → NP − PP.)

(17)   a. *The spy saw the cop **with binoculars** but the cop didn't see him.*
       b. *The spy saw the copy **with a revolver** but the cop didn't see him.*

In (17a) the minimal attachment analysis will correspond to the more plausible analysis of the prepositional phrase; however, in (17b) it does not and thus, by hypothesis, the focused processor will propose an alternative analysis to the syntactic processor, namely, an analysis where *the man with a revolver* forms a complex noun phrase. This predicts that readers should arrive at the more plausible, nonminimal attachment, interpretation of (17b), but that (17b) should be difficult to process relative to (17a).

To test these predictions, we asked 16 subjects to read sentences like those in (17). Each subject saw 12 experimental sentences and 84 distractor sentences. There were four versions of each experimental sentence: two where the semantic information in the prepositional phrase rendered the minimal attachment analysis the most plausible analysis (of these, one had a short prepositional phrase and one had a long prepositional phrase), and two where the non-minimal-attachment analysis was most plausible (again the length of the prepositional phrase was varied).

TABLE 13.3
Eye Movement Data from Experiment 3

| | Mean reading time per character (msec)[a] | | | |
|---|---|---|---|---|
| | Short | | Long | |
| Minimal attachment | 32 | (25) | 33 | (26) |
| Nonminimal attachment | 37 | (29) | 39 | (29) |

[a]Mean reading time for first pass fixations only are presented in parentheses.

As predicted, reading time per character is longer in the non-minimal-attachment sentences than in the minimal-attachment sentences. These data are presented in Table 13.3. These results provide initial support for the focused processor hypothesis, and argue against any theory that claims either that pragmatic considerations determine the first analysis assigned to an ambiguous sentence or that all structural analyses of a sentence are computed and then pragmatic considerations are used to simply select the most plausible analysis from this set.

## V.   Conclusions

I have argued that any adequate theory of reading must contain a subtheory concerned with the mechanisms and principles governing the processing of sentence structure. I argued that the lexical constraint hypothesis, the only reasonable alternative to computing a structural analysis of sentences, does not provide a coherent alternative to structural processing once the hypothesis is cast in a form explicit enough to be evaluated. I have tried to show that the hypothesis either (1) does not permit any aspects of the structure of the sentence to be ignored; or (2) it incorrectly predicts that people assign illicit meanings to sentences that in fact people correctly comprehend. Although this conclusion is unlikely to be surprising to most linguists, it seems to have often been overlooked in the psychological literature, where people seem to have used a post hoc analysis of sentences to argue that it was unnecessary to compute a structural analysis of particular sentences.

I argued that eye movement recording provides a valuable tool for gathering data about the online structural processing of sentences. Initial evidence suggests that reading times and the average durations of fixations in some region of a sentence provide a rather immediate reflection of an increase in processing complexity associated with that region of the sentence. However, whether the position of first pass fixations provides any evidence about the structural processing of sentences is still an open question.

I reported eye movement experiments that provided evidence for the garden-path theory of sentence comprehension. The outcome of the experiments further supported the conclusion that readers perform a systematic structural analysis of sentences. They also suggest that readers quickly compute the structural consequences of the word currently being fixated, typically immediately noting any incompatibility of the fixated word and the analysis assigned to preceding items. The experiments also suggest that the initial structural analysis of a sentence is not constructed on the basis of pragmatic considerations concerning the most likely relations of the words or phrases in a sentence. However the effects of semantic and pragmatic constraints are detectable using eye movement data: In the third experiment, the structural consequences of pragmatic factors were detectable in the eye movement record.

# References

Carpenter, P. A., & Daneman, M. (1981). Lexical retrieval and error recovery in reading: A model based on eye fixations. *Journal of Verbal Learning and Verbal Behavior, 20,* 137–160.

Carpenter, P. A., & Just, M. A. (1977). Reading comprehension as the eye sees it. In M. Just & P. Carpenter (Eds.), *Cognitive processes in comprehension.* Hillsdale, New Jersey: Erlbaum.

Crain, S., & Coker, P. (1979). A semantic constraint on syntactic parsing. Paper presented at the annual meeting of the Linguistic Society of America, Boston December.

Ford, M., Bresnan, J., & Kaplan, R. (1980). *A competence based theory of syntactic closure.* MIT Center for Cognitive Science Occasional Paper No. 14. To appear in J. Bresnan (Ed.), *The Mental Representation of Grammatical Relations.* Cambridge: MIT Press.

Frazier, L. (1978). On comprehending sentences: Syntactic parsing strategies. Unpublished doctoral dissertation, University of Connecticut. (Available from Indiana University Linguistics Club, 310 Lindley Hall, Bloomington, Indiana, 47401.)

Frazier, L. (1981). *Constraints, control and strategies in sentence comprehension.* Paper presented at the Sloan workshop on Modelling Human Parsing Strategies, University of Texas, Austin, March.

Frazier, L., & Rayner, K. (1982). Making and correcting errors during sentence comprehension: Eye movements in the analysis of structurally ambiguous sentences. *Cognitive Psychology, 14*(1), 178–210.

Holmes, V. M., & O'Regan, J. K. (1981). Eye fixation patterns during the reading of relative clause sentences. *Journal of Verbal Learning and Verbal Behavior, 20,* 417–439.

Mehler, J., Bever, T. G., & Carey, P. (1967). What we look at when we read. *Perception & Psychophysics, 2,* 213–218.

O'Regan, J. K. (1975). Structural and contextual constraints on eye movements in reading. Unpublished doctoral dissertation, University of Cambridge.

O'Regan, J. K. (1979). Saccade size control in reading: Evidence for the linguistic control hypothesis. *Perception & Psychophysics, 25,* 501–509.

Rayner, K. (1978). Eye movements in reading and information processing. *Psychological Bulletin, 85,* 618–660.

Rayner, K., Carlson, M., & Frazier, L. (1982). The interaction of syntax and semantics during sentence processing: Eye movements in the analysis of semantically biased sentences. *Journal of Verbal Learning and Verbal Behavior* (in press).

Rayner, K., & McConkie, G. W. (1976). What guides a reader's eye movements? *Vision Research, 16,* 829–837.

Alan Kennedy

# 14

# On Looking into Space

## I. Scanning Pictures

In a widely quoted study, Yarbus (1967) examined the way in which people looked at a painting (*The Unexpected Visitor* by Repin). Their eye movements were shown to be influenced by prior instructions. For example, asked to work out what had been going on, subjects scrutinized the heads and upper torsos of all the characters depicted. When asked to estimate how long the visitor had been away, subjects produced a series of saccades from the head of the visitor to those characters poised to greet him. The conclusion from this study, and from many others of a similar kind, is fairly obvious. In looking at pictures, the eye is directed systematically to those areas that will yield appropriate information. Although it is *possible* to shift attention without moving the eyes (Posner, 1980), in normal circumstances this is not done. The question is, what, if anything, drives these patterns of inspection? What, if anything, is their functional significance?

It has been argued that the sequence of eye movements might form in part the basis of memory for pictures (Noton & Stark, 1971). Thus, in a recognition task, detection of a match between a particular current sequence of eye movements and a sequence made during an earlier learning phase would serve to trigger a positive identification. The data on this point are, in general, equivocal or negative: The consistency in individual scanpaths is not strikingly high, and in any case it is hard to see how difficult discriminations could be handled by reference to such a stored sequence of inspections. What appears likely is that any obtained degree of consistency is, in part at least, a by-product of the scanpath induced by particular physical properties of a figure or by a particular configuration of objects. Two

EYE MOVEMENTS IN READING:
PERCEPTUAL AND LANGUAGE PROCESSES

classes of determining influence on the direction and location of eye movements may be isolated: (1) the presence of visual information in central and peripheral vision; (2) knowledge of possible shapes and orientations of objects, and of their possible combinations. The evidence on (1) is well documented (Nodine, Carmody, & Kundel, 1978; Parker, 1978; Walker-Smith, Gale, & Findlay, 1977). On (2) it may be noted that subjects often scan across large visual angles to locate points that would, prior to the saccade, have been available only in a very degraded form, since acuity falls off sharply from the narrow central region of foveal vision. For example, Nodine *et al.* report mean interfixation distances during the search for a hidden figure in a picture of from 4.4–4.9° of visual angle. In such circumstances it is likely that, in addition to physical properties of a display, subjects also make use of a kind of general spatial knowledge, such that once an object is identified its relative spatial coordinates will also be known. This is not to imply that the underlying memorial representation *is* a stored sequence of eye movements; rather, that the representation will allow for the integration of information in peripheral vision and help in directing successive saccades. Thus, having identified an object in a picture as a standing man, and, having "scaled" the representation within the picture as a whole, it may be possible to scan from head to toe accurately using general knowledge about the relative location of head and feet in standing figures. Under certain circumstances knowledge of this general kind has been shown to drive eye movements. For example, Cooper (1974) showed that the direction of gaze over an array of pictures could be influenced by a concurrent auditory stimulus. Similarly, if subjects are looking at an array of pictures and asked to name all the cars they know, their eyes are drawn to a picture of a car if one is present (Kahneman & Lass, 1973). The information gained by doing this is of little assistance in this specific task, but it appears that in gaining access to representations in memory, some features of the perceived world become more significant than others. Thinking about cars may involve imaginal processing, which in turn has its roots in perceptual activity, including patterns of inspection. Thus, if a congruent stimulus is actually present while a subject is engaged in thought, inspection is automatically triggered. The origins of this interdependence of thought and perception probably lie in the early experience of infants. There is a stage in the development of object concepts during which knowing *where* features lie in space appears necessary for learning *what* an object is. Significantly, in the study by Kahneman and Lass, cited earlier, subjects scanned to the positions previously occupied by relevant pictures, even if the stimulus array had been removed. Since, in the real world, static objects do not commonly disappear, it is normally helpful to retain knowledge of their relative spatial location over a period of time. (Although it is interesting to speculate where subjects in the Kahneman & Lass study might have looked if the relevant stimuli had been, at the point of removal, moving in the visual field). Not only the location of salient features of objects themselves but the spatial representation of many common configurations of objects must be represented in memory, and a highly evolved mechanism must exist for encoding this information. There is abundant anecdotal evidence of coding of this form. For example, in conversation someone may gesture to a chair previously occupied by the person who is the present focus of discussion; lecturers, in a similar fashion, sometimes point to blank blackboards, as if to conjure up the text that had recently been written there. This chapter is directed toward assessing the role such generalized spatial knowledge may play during skilled reading.

## II.   Eye Movements in Reading

Certain important distinctions must be drawn between looking at pictures and reading as means of acquiring knowledge. A written text (at least in an alphabetic script) that gives rise to a representation of some meaning, does not, *of itself*, convey spatial information. (Apart, that is, from curiosities like poems about butterflies which are themselves formed into a butterfly shape). To comprehend an object is to give rise to a particular memory representation, part of which may be, as Yarbus (1967) showed, spatial. However, in reading, as distinct from listening, the person is also confronted with a spatially extended stimulus: an array of letters and spaces. It is possible, therefore, to ask what relationships might obtain between properties of text and particular patterns of eye movement. Indeed, this question has been asked since the time of Javal (1879), and Huey (1908). The question is, in part, pitched at two levels since any relationship could be between eye movements and physical properties of the text, or between eye movements and whatever the text represents. However, it would be bizarre to expect eye movements characteristic of looking at say a boat or a donkey to be elicited by the **words** *boat* or *donkey*. The links between features of text and patterns of inspection are often discussed in terms of contrasts between the "physical" and the "semantic" or "linguistic," but these last two terms are at best metaphors. What is missing in looking at text as distinct from pictures are the conventions of graphical representation which preserve between elements of the object depicted relationships found in the object itself in the real world. Such conventions themselves, of course, differ widely, but all are distinct in this respect from writing. It is, therefore, very much an open question whether a reader's eye movement control mechanism makes use of the fact that the referents of what is read are accessed and understood while the eyes are directed to particular spatial locations.

Eye movement control during reading is probably influenced by (1) physical features, such as word length and the occurrence of interword spaces (O'Regan, 1980; Rayner, 1978); (2) a loose mapping of certain physical features of text to certain syntactic structures, for example the knowledge that some noun phrases have a characteristic shape (Ranklin & Barber, 1978; Wanat, 1976); and (3) alterations in the stimulus evidence needed for lexical access. Primed words may be identified in peripheral vision on less evidence than unprimed. If such processing occurs during a fixation it may influence either saccade extent or subsequent fixation duration (Kennedy, 1978b; Kennedy & Pidcock, 1981; Rayner, 1975).

It is useful to distinguish two phases of reading, which, following Yarbus, could be termed cycles. When a sentence is read for the first time (the first cycle), eye movements are under the control of a combination of the features just identified. These sources of influence are relatively small if normal reading is contrasted with a reading strategy that simply involves examining each line of text every six to eight characters. It is partly because the effects of text features on eye movements are small that the question whether *any* influence is exerted by them has persisted so long in the literature. The end product of the first cycle of reading is the construction of a memory representation of the text. In addition, spatial information is available about the position of some or all of the words within the array presented. This is effectively coded in terms of relative location on the page. Direct evidence on this issue will be presented later, but it should be evident that such information is bound to be extracted, given what is known about the role of eye movements in scanning objects and pictures, and the fact that reading as a skill is relatively late to develop. It would be surprising indeed if a unique and specialized eye movement control system developed solely for reading. A priori it is much more likely that scanning during reading takes advantage of earlier-developed eye movement control systems.

The second cycle of inspection takes place over an already encoded array. The subject has looked at virtually every word (Just & Carpenter, 1980). It will be claimed here that the subject also knows where each word is. It is in this second cycle that regressive eye movements occur. In contrast to the first cycle, regressive saccades are often large, perhaps spanning several degrees of visual angle. Regressions occur between lines (Just & Carpenter, 1978) and across large parts of a single line (Kennedy, 1978a; Kennedy, 1981), (see Figure 14.1). Eye movements of this type bear more resemblance to those found in picture scanning under certain kinds of instruction than to the patterns of eye movement typical of the first cycle. For example, Figure 14.2 shows one of my subjects attempting to

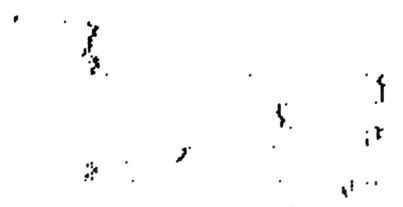

FIGURE 14.1. *A regressive saccade from the word* district *to the word* crime. *Note that time is in the vertical axis.* [*Data from Kennedy, 1978a.*]

FILL MEN FIRE MORTFIL .  SOCRATES IS A MAN .

**FIGURE 14.2.** *Pattern of inspection during reading of two terms of a syllogism. [Data from Kennedy, 1981.]*

understand the two premises of a syllogism, prior to making a judgment on a conclusion. Given such material, which can sometimes be rather difficult to grasp, these patterns of multiple inspection are not rare. To interpret regressive eye movements as a "holding operation," saving the processor from an "overload" of information, or as simply indexing poor reading ability, obviously misses an important point. Such refixations are not random, they are precisely located, and fall on some words rather than on others (Just & Carpenter, 1978, make a similar point). Further, regressive fixations appear to have a functional significance, and it is worthwhile speculating on what this might be.

## III.   Why Look at the Same Word Twice?

In one sense, the behavior of the subjects illustrated in Figures 14.1 and 14.2 is odd. The sentences are short and could easily be learned in one reading. It is not enough to say that cross references are called for, though this is certainly the case. What is in need of explanation is *why* subjects choose to look again at particular words which they have already inspected. Assume that a subject is asked to read:

*The drunken captain crossed the deck to the mate. He grasped the wheel . . .*

The object of the first cycle of reading is to establish a memory representation of the text such as that illustrated in Figure 14.3. The pronoun *he* presents a problem. It is not clear who grasped the wheel—the captain or the mate. Let us suppose that disambiguation is carried out by searching for potential referents and integrating them into the memory representation. (In the case presented here, of course, the pronoun cannot be disambiguated, although prior context, or some

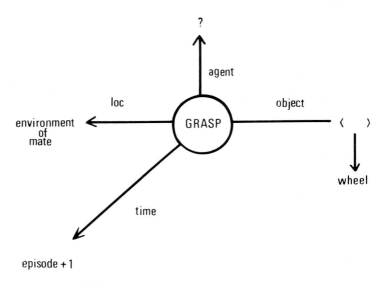

**FIGURE 14.3.** *Propositional representation of sentence.*

later information, may solve the problem. If an inappropriate connection is made, this will, when invalidated, trigger a further search). The search for referents could take place within the memory structure itself. If a text is very explicit this is possibly the normal mode. If the text is very allusive, however, large demands might be placed on memory since a number of potential referents and their possible relationships will need to be saved in a temporary store. One way of reducing this memory load is to use the spatial coordinates of selected items to direct eye movements. This has the effect of readdressing the system, since selected words will be presented visually for access to the mental lexicon. By cycling through a series of spatial coordinates in this way computational load would be reduced. Such a process argues for a division between thinking and looking. There is no requirement that information recycled in this way is processed to any depth, or necessarily integrated into the eventual final memory representation (Rosen, 1975): The pattern of refixations itself simply serves as an *aide-mémoire*. It is possible to go one step further. If comprehension is very difficult, and the reading task calls for a particular response (e.g., was the word *skipper* used in the ambiguous sentence quoted?), then the memory representation may be a very *inefficient* way of providing a correct answer. The goal of comprehension is to arrive at a coherent representation of the relationships between propositions, not a verbatim record. For responses of this kind the spatially addressable code will provide much more exact information. Thus, knowing *where* can be as useful as knowing *what* under some circumstances. The printed page functions like a stable map (in the sense used by Mackay, 1973), or as a memory addressed directly through spatial coordinates.

If this account of the function of the second cycle of reading is to be accepted, it gives a particular status to regressive fixations. It also gives rise to a number of relatively strong empirical predictions.

## IV.   A Spatially Addressable Memory Code

As Kolers (1976) recently pointed out, the peculiar nature of the visual input during reading, and the fact that it poses problems for theories of memory, was appreciated not long after the systematic study of eye movements first began (Judd & Buswell, 1922). "The visual system must keep track of the spatial frame of reference within which it is sampling contents, and keep track of the location within that frame that each sample is derived from." (Kolers, 1976, p. 390). What is involved is a three-way mapping: a temporal sequence of fixations; their spatial location; and a sequence of ideas. It appears striking that more or less the same train of thought can arise from quite different patterns of brief inspection of sequences of around six letters across a line of print. Perhaps less striking, though, when it is appreciated that the stability of the perceived world in general arises in a directly analogous fashion.

One obvious and strong prediction flows from this point of view. If the reader is *not* able to maintain a record of spatial coordinates, then reading will be significantly impaired. Further, the predicted impairment will be in comprehension, not necessarily in more peripheral components of the reading skill. I have recently examined this proposition in a series of experiments (Kennedy, 1982). Subjects read sentences in a self-paced presentation task, pressing a key in order to see one word at a time presented on the screen of a computer terminal. Three conditions of presentation were compared:

1. *central* presentation—each word appeared in the same location, centered on the screen
2. *sequential* presentation—each word appeared in its appropriate location across the screen. Thus, although only one word at a time was displayed, each was presented at the location it would have occupied had the sentence as a whole been displayed
3. *random* presentation—the words of sentences appeared in their correct order, but in random locations across a single horizontal line. This was achieved by scrambling the words into a random sequence and then presenting them one at a time in their new locations.

In both the central and random presentation conditions, information relating to relative location is disturbed. It is disturbed most, of course, in the central condition, where differential spatial coordinates cannot be used at all to "address" parts of the sentence.

The material employed consisted of quite difficult three-term syllogisms. For example:

(1)   *No musicians are tone deaf. Most musicians can sing.*
(2)   *Some people that can sing are not tone deaf.*

Twenty-four syllogisms were constructed, 12 sound, and 12 unsound. They were assigned using a latin square to different presentation conditions for different subjects. Order of presentation was balanced so that each condition followed every other an equal number of times. The two premises were presented, one word at a time, under one of the three conditions described above. The conclusion was then presented as a single line of text on the screen. Subjects were told to pace through the premises as quickly as they could, consistent with comprehension, and then to respond using one or the other of two buttons to indicate whether the conclusion was sound. Subjects were told to make this response as quickly as they could, consistent with accuracy. There was extensive practice on the task.

The prediction is that comprehension, as indexed by solution time, should be affected by the loss of spatial information in the central and random conditions. Some spatial information is, of course, available in the random condition; however, to keep track of random locations imposes a very heavy memory load, and it appears unlikely that subjects would be able simultaneously to memorize locations and comprehend the premises. Any spatial information stored would be less com-

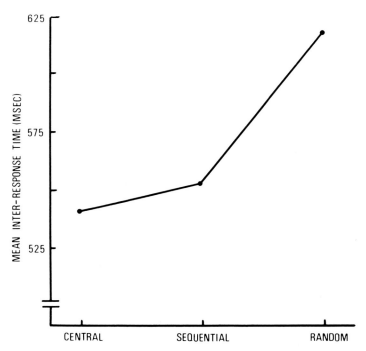

**FIGURE 14.4.** *Mean interresponse times under central, sequential, and random conditions of presentation of premises.*

plete than in the sequential condition. Thus, the predicted order of difficulty (indexed by solution time) is: central > random < sequential.

The mean interresponse times as subjects paced through the two premises are shown in Figure 14.4. The data are based on 12 subjects. These apparent differences were highly significant. The random presentation method produced slower responses than the other two, which did not differ.

Mean solution times are shown in Figure 14.5. It will be clear that the predicted order of difficulty is demonstrated. The differences in solution time between the sequential and random and the sequential and central conditions were statistically significant. The difference between the random and central conditions, although in the predicted direction, was not significant.

These findings are in conflict with those of Bouma and DeVoogd (1974). They employed a form of "line-step" presentation, in which text was moved in units of varying size over a steady fixation point. Both oral and silent reading was possible in this situation. However, it was less clear that the subjects understood what they read, ". . . . a difficulty is that attention is very much focused on keeping the eyes steady. Although this does not interfere with speed of reading, it is likely to interfere with memorizing." (Bouma & DeVoogd, 1974, p. 278). Assessing the soundness of the conclusion of a syllogism is a complex task calling for a high level of understanding.

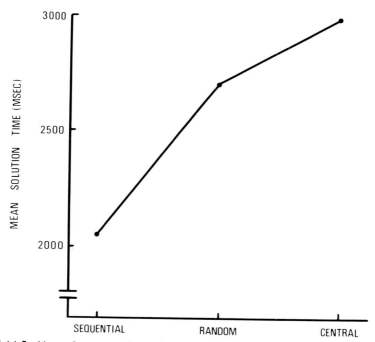

FIGURE 14.5. *Mean solution times for conclusions of syllogisms as a function of sequential, random, and central conditions of presentation of premises.*

If subjects in the sequential condition can take advantage of a spatially coded representation in arriving at a decision on the conclusion, it should be possible to demonstrate this directly by means of measured eye movement activity. The following experiment was carried out to study patterns of eye movements while subjects assessed the soundness of a set of syllogisms (see Kennedy, 1982). The material consisted of eight syllogisms, four sound and four unsound. They were constructed so that the two premises could be displayed in a single line on the point plotting display used in the eye movement apparatus (for details see Kennedy, 1980). Eye movements were recorded using a conventional infrared tracking system coupled to a computer. Horizontal movements of the left eye were recorded at a 100 Hz sampling rate.

The two premises were presented as a pair of sentences on a single line separated by a full stop. Subjects were allowed to read them freely until they understood them, at which point, by pressing a key, the display was terminated. After a delay of 500 msec an inspection point appeared at the left margin of the screen for 200 msec. The screen was then blank and subjects heard, through headphones, the conclusion, which they assessed by pressing buttons. Eye movements were recorded both while the premises were read, and also from the time the inspection point disappeared to the point when the button was pressed. When questioned later, subjects said they were unaware that eye movements might have been recorded while they were assessing the soundness of the auditorily presented conclusions. The experiment was described to subjects as being concerned with looking and listening.

**TABLE 14.1**
**Total Number of Fixations on Locations Occupied by Words in Visually Presented Premises During Assessment of Auditorily Present Conclusions[a]**

| No pigs can fly. Most pigs can grunt. | (Some things that grunt can't fly). |
|---|---|
| 8  10  6  11   4   3   1   0 | |
| Some trees are green. All trees are plants. | (Some plants are green). |
| 11  11  6   4   3   2   0   0 | |
| All eggs have shells. Some nuts have shells. | (Some nuts are eggs). |
| 8  14  8   5   2   0   1   2 | |
| All students can think. Rupert can think. | (Rupert is a student). |
| 8   12   7   7   1   0   2 | |
| Some cars are unsafe. All taxis are cars. | (Some taxis are unsafe). |
| 7  ,9   1   9   4   5   0   0 | |
| All fruit has seeds. The lime is a fruit. | (The lime has seeds). |
| 7   7   0   3   1   8   0   0   1 | |
| No snails can run. My pet cannot run. | (My pet is a snail). |
| 15   8   6   3   1   6   3   1 | |
| No men can fly. John is a man. | (John can't fly). |
| 7   12   4   1  , 3   3   1   4 | |

[a]Conclusions, derived from 7 subjects, are given in brackets, half are sound and half unsound.

The question of interest, of course, is whether during the solution of the syllogisms, subjects showed systematic patterns of eye movements, albeit that in this situation they would be scanning a blank screen. Table 14.1 shows the "words" fixated by seven subjects for the eight syllogisms. The "words" of course refer only to the locations occupied by those items when the two sentences were originally displayed: The data are derived from measurements made while subjects looked at a blank screen. As can be seen, in many cases subjects engaged in what appears to be a systematic inspection of particular locations. Some typical records are shown in Figure 14.6.

Although it might be felt that these data offer strong support for the notion of a spatially addressable memory, alternative accounts are possible. Ehrlichman, Weiner, and Baker (1974) and Weiner and Ehrlichman (1976) report increases in "ocular motility" while subjects responded to questions presented auditorily. (Although the claim is frequently made, their data suggested that it is not the case that subjects consistently scan in a particular direction when presented with verbal, as opposed to spatial, problems). A general increase in scanning eye movements takes place in this situation. Thus, the results shown in Table 14.1 and Figure 14.6 could arise as an artifact: Subjects may make fixations at random, and certain of these will fall across the positions previously occupied by words in the display. Although inspection of some of the patterns of eye movements makes this interpretation seem rather implausible (see Figure 14.6), it is necessary to consider at least two controls.

First, subjects' eye movements were monitored while all the material was presented auditorily. A different group of naive subjects was used. It is difficult to give this procedure face validity, since after extensive calibration of eye movement equipment, subjects expect to have some stimuli to look at. The difficulty was overcome in part by a dummy experiment in which visual material was presented initially and subjects were then left connected to the eye movement equipment while they completed "a short auditory test." The data were in general not scorable. Subjects either fixated a single point, or rotated their eyes outside the calibrated range of the equipment, or made scanning movements distributed in part outside the calibrated range and in part within it. In no case were data produced resembling those found in the main experiment.

A second control is provided by a statistical analysis of the data in Table 14.1. If these arise as a result of purely random eye movements, then the proportion of fixations on "characters" and on "spaces" in the display (again these terms refer to the items which occupied particular locations in the original display) should be equal. If, on the other hand, subjects are scanning to particular locations, then the time spent fixating "characters" should be significantly greater than that spent on "spaces." Measurements were made of the total number of eye movement samples falling between "word" and "space" boundaries. The obtained times were means of 18 msec per "space" and 32 msec per "character." This difference is statistically highly significant. In fact all subjects showed a difference in the same direction for all syllogisms.

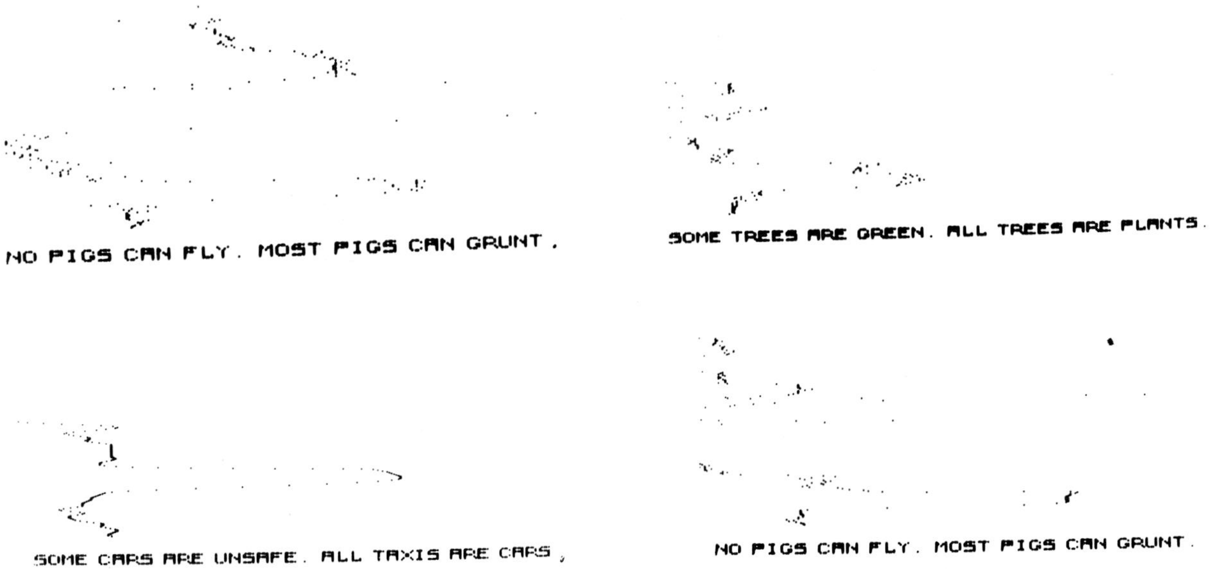

NO PIGS CAN FLY . MOST PIGS CAN GRUNT .

SOME TREES ARE GREEN . ALL TREES ARE PLANTS .

SOME CARS ARE UNSAFE . ALL TAXIS ARE CARS ,

NO PIGS CAN FLY . MOST PIGS CAN GRUNT .

**FIGURE 14.6.** *Examples of patterns of eye movements across a blank display. (Locations of words in the original display are indicated). Recordings taken during the solution of auditorily presented conclusions.*

# V.   Conclusion

Although the data presented comment in a novel fashion on the way sentences are processed during reading, there are a number of parallels in the literature. For example, Hall (1974) showed that subjects in a Sperling partial-report paradigm direct eye movements to the cued row after the display is terminated. Carpenter and Just (1978) speak of eye fixations as a "retrieval operation" in which information might be transferred from an internal memory system to Short Term Memory. They claim that eye fixations are correlated with memory retrieval because it "may be that the spatial position of an element plays an organizational role in visual tasks. The position of an element in space may be coded along with other attributes of the element, so that positional information may subsequently be used to index the element [p. 131]." Similarly, Kennedy (1978a) argued that increases in reading time when low frequency exemplars of a category had to be integrated resulted from the time spent in making large regressive eye movements, very exactly located, to reinspect the category name (see Figure 14.1).

On the other hand, several studies do not show adult readers producing frequent regressive eye movements. In particular, it has proved quite difficult to construct materials that will reliably trigger regressions. One obvious candidate here is the manipulation of anaphoric reference in text, yet the data so far are equivocal. Sometimes an ambiguous pronoun, for example, will serve to trigger a regressive eye movement to possible antecedents, at other times there may be no effect, or the reader may simply alter the duration of the current fixation.

A possible resolution of this conflicting evidence is to consider the interaction between the difficulty of the materials used and the reader's skill. The former relates to the density of allusion in the text. The latter relates to the ability of a reader to maintain a rich and internally coherent memory representation within which mental operations can be carried out.

The materials used in the present study come close to representing a limiting case in terms of complexity. The kind of eye movements they elicit (as in Figure 14.2, for example) are not typical of those produced by normal adults reading text. The argument presented in Section III suggests a threshold of complexity, below which readers need make no use of reinspections. The determining factor is not the linguistic function of particular words (e.g., that a pronoun relates to a certain antecedent), but the overall demand placed on working memory by, for example, unresolved ambiguities or numerous logical operators whose scope may be difficult to determine. It is thus not necessarily inconsistent with the notion of a spatially addressable memory that certain materials may fail to produce refixations.

Another variable influencing the occurrence of regressive eye movements is the reader's level of skill. Regressions are far more frequent in inexperienced readers; indeed, for the beginner they often occur *within* words. This is quite consistent with the argument presented here if it is appreciated that letter identification cannot alone determine word meaning, but must be taken along with a record of spatial location. One of the difficulties facing the learner is that not only must the identity of stimuli be determined, but also their relative position. Mason (1980) has recently argued that differences in reading skill may lie in precisely this domain: the ability to encode *where* information is located.

## References

Bouma, H., & de Voogd, A. H. (1974). On the control of eye saccades in reading. *Vision Research 14*, 273–284.

Carpenter, P. A., & Just, M. A. (1978). Eye fixations during mental rotation. In J. W. Senders, D. F. Fisher, & R. A. Monty (Eds.), *Eye movements and the higher psychological functions*, Hillsdale, New Jersey: Erlbaum.

Cooper, R. M. (1974). The control of eye fixation by the meaning of spoken language. *Cognitive Psychology 6*, 84–107.

Ehrlichman, H., Weiner, S. L., & Baker, A. H. (1974). Effects of verbal and spatial questions on initial gaze shifts. *Neuropsychologia, 12*, 265–277.

Hall, D. C., (1974), Eye movements in scanning iconic imagery. *Journal of Experimental Psychology 103*, 825–830.

Huey, E. B. (1908). *The psychology and pedagogy of reading*. New York: Macmillan.

Javal, K. E. (1879). Essai sur la physiologie de la lecture. *Annales d'Oculistique 82*, 243–253.

Judd, C. H., & Buswell, G. T. (1922). Silent reading: A study of the various types. *Supplementary Educational Monographs, 23*.

Just, M. A., & Carpenter, P. A. Inference processes during reading: Reflections from eye fixations. In J. W. Senders, D. F. Fisher, & R. A. Monty (Eds.), *Eye movements and the higher psychological functions*. Hillsdale, New Jersey: Erlbaum.

Just, M. A., & Carpenter, P. A. (1980). A theory of reading: From eye fixations to comprehension. *Psychological Review, 87*, 329–354.

Kahneman, D., & Lass, N. (1973). *Eye position in tasks of association and memory*. Unpublished manuscript, Hebrew University, Jerusalem. (Cited in D. Kahneman, *Attention and effort*. Englewood Cliffs: Prentice–Hall).

Kennedy, A. (1978a) Eye movements and the integration of semantic information during reading. In M. M. Gruneberg, R. N. Sykes, & P.E. Morris (Eds.), *Practical aspects of memory*. New York: Academic Press.

Kennedy, A. (1978b) Reading sentences: Some observations on the control of eye movements. In G. Underwood (Ed.), *Strategies of information processing*. New York: Academic Press.

Kennedy, A. (1980). Eye movements and reading (final report on SSRC Project HR6309). Lodged in British Lending Library.

Kennedy, A. (1982). Eye movements and spatial coding in reading. *Psychological Research*. In press.

Kennedy, A., & Pidcock, B. (1981). Eye movements and variations in reading time. *Psychological Research, 43*, 69–79.

Kolers, P. A. (1976). Buswell's discoveries. In R. A. Monty & J. W. Senders (Eds.), *Eye movements and psychological processes*, Hillsdale, New Jersey: Erlbaum.

MacKay, D. M. (1973). Visual stability and voluntary eye movements. In R. Jung (Ed.), *Handbook of sensory physiology* (Vol. 7). New York: Springer–Verlag.

Mason, M. (1980). Reading ability and the encoding of item and location information. *Journal of Experimental Psychology: Human Perception and Performance, 6*, 89–98.

Nodine, C. F., Carmody, D. P., & Kundel, H. L. (1978). Searching for Nina. In J. W. Senders, D. F. Fisher, & R. A. Monty (Eds.), *Eye movements and the higher psychological functions*, Hillsdale, New Jersey: Erlbaum.

Noton, D., & Stark, L. (1971). Scanpaths in saccadic eye movements while viewing and recognizing patterns. *Vision Research, 11*, 929–942.

O'Regan, J. K. (1980). The control of saccade size and fixation duration in reading: The limits of linguistic control. *Perception & Psychophysics, 28,* 112–117.

Parker, R. E. (1978). Picture processing during recognition. *Journal of Experimental Psychology: Human Perception & Performance, 4,* 284–293.

Posner, M. I. (1980). Orienting of attention. *Quarterly Journal of Experimental Psychology 32,* 3–25.

Ranklin, J. E., & Barber, P. J. (1978). *Peripheral visual cues during reading.* Paper presented to British Psychological Society Annual Conference, York.

Rayner, K. (1975). The perceptual span and peripheral cues in reading. *Cognitive Psychology, 7,* 65–81.

Rayner, K. (1978). Eye movements in reading and information processing. *Psychological Bulletin 85,* 618–660.

Rosen, L. D. (1975). Memory influence during reprocessing. Unpublished doctoral thesis, University of California, San Diego.

Walker–Smith, G. J., Gale, A. G., & Findlay, J. M. (1977). Eye movement strategies involved in face perception. *Perception, 6,* 313–326.

Wanat, S. F. (1976). Relations between language and visual processing. In H. Singer & R. B. Ruddell (Eds.), *Theoretical models and processes of Reading.* Newark: International Reading Association.

Weiner, S. L., & Ehrlichman, M. (1976). Ocular motility and cognitive processes. *Cognition, 4,* 31–43.

Yarbus, A. (1967). *Eye movements and vision.* New York: Plenum.

Kate Ehrlich

# 15

# Eye Movements in Pronoun Assignment: A Study of Sentence Integration[1]

## I.   Introduction

When people read a text, they use a number of cognitive operations to translate from the printed words on the page to some internal representation that corresponds to their understanding of the text. One set of operations leads to the intake and subsequent encoding of perceptual information. Another set of operations leads to comprehension of the text. These operations progress from the stage where the words receive their initial encoding through the syntactic and semantic processes that form part of the core of comprehension, to the complex processes that tie together the parts of the text into a single coherent representation. This chapter explores those integrative processes that are part of pronoun assignment. It reports a study in which eye movements of subjects were tracked as they read short paragraphs that contained pronouns. The study determined when assignment takes place and whether readers assign referents to pronouns by initiating a regression back to the antecedent phrase in the text. The study also addressed some assumptions underlying the use of eye movement data to investigate language processes.

[1]The work in this chapter was supported by a postdoctoral grant from the Sloan Foundation and by NSF grant BNS 79-17600.

The author thanks Keith Rayner for his help and advice in running the experiment, and Charles E. Clifton, Jr. for his comments on an earlier draft of the chapter.

EYE MOVEMENTS IN READING:
PERCEPTUAL AND LANGUAGE PROCESSES

## II.  Eye Movements and Comprehension

Most of the operations that mediate between printed words and the mental representation of the text are carried out automatically by skilled readers. The very features that make reading proceed so smoothly for the reader also make the study of reading difficult for the researcher, for these operations are expertly executed and are neither visible nor amenable to introspection. However, recent theoretical and technological advances in the use of eye movement recording have considerably enhanced the study of the cognitive process in reading (see Rayner, 1978 for a review of the field). This technique can provide a moment by moment record of where a reader is looking and for how long, in a way that does not intrude or disrupt natural reading habits. Considerable progress has been made in mapping out many of the cognitive operations in reading using this technique.

As the reader progresses through the many perceptual and cognitive stages of reading, it becomes increasingly difficult to isolate the particular process of interest to the researcher without eliminating other contributing processes by imposing artificial constraints on the reader. Eye movement recordings have the potential of being extremely useful in this regard because they provide much fine-grain data while minimizing any artificiality.

Even with this technique, serious problems can emerge in the analysis and interpretation of the data. For example, the record of eye movements can show where the eye was directed but cannot indicate unambiguously what part of the text the reader actually saw. More critically, there is a problem in knowing on which fixation a particular word was encountered and which fixation should be taken as reflecting the process of interest. For example, if there is a delay in accessing the meaning of a word, the fixation on which lexical access is reflected may not be the fixation on which the visual characteristics were encoded. This problem has been termed the eye–mind lag problem. So far, there is little evidence that resolves the problem. Some researchers have argued that semantic processing lags behind the perceptual encoding of a word (e.g., Bouma & de Voogd, 1974; Kolers, 1976; Morton, 1964). Others, however, argue that cognitive processes are synchronous with fixations (e.g., Rayner & McConkie, 1976). According to this latter view, the extra processing required to, say, retrieve the meaning of an unusual word should be evident in a longer fixation duration on the critical word. Evidence supporting this prediction has been furnished by Just and Carpenter (1980). They found that the gaze duration on unusual words such as *thermoluminescence* was 2431 msec,. This time reflects not only the infrequency of this word but also its length. These researchers (see also, Carpenter & Daneman, 1981; Carpenter & Just, 1977) are perhaps among the strongest protagonists of the view that processing does not lag behind fixations. They make an even stronger immediacy assumption: Not only is there no lag but also a word is processed at all levels as soon as it is encountered. Just and Carpenter (1980), however, agree that the integration of material may be distributed across fixations, rather than being restricted to a single fixation.

## A.  Integration Processes

There are a number of reasons for readers to integrate material. At one level, sentence integration can help the reader to select the appropriate meaning of a word. At another level, integration is necessary for readers to determine the relation between the events described by the text. For instance on reading a text such as:

*John pushed the button. The light came on.*

the two events are understood not to be separate but to be causally linked. Integration is also part of the process of selecting and assigning a referent to a pronoun. All processes of integration may be considered to have in common, the retrieval and use of information from some previous part of the text to aid in the comprehension of current material. Nevertheless, integration processes vary in difficulty and for that reason it is possible that the main locus of the process will also vary. For instance, in a very neat experiment, S. Ehrlich (Chapter 11 in this volume) has shown that readers are more likely to fixate words that are less consistent with the previous text than words that are highly consistent. This result suggests that contextual information is available at the encoding of an incoming word. In contrast, Carpenter and Just (1977) have shown that for lexically based inferences, the locus of the effect is on the critical word and at the end of the sentence. They also found that readers spent more time reading the sentence when there was additional material intervening between the sentence and the opening sentence.

## B.  Pronoun Assignment

One way of using eye movements to examine some of these more complex processes of reading is to focus on pronoun assignment. Pronouns are short words that occur with a high frequency in English. They are understood by reference to an entity that has typically been mentioned some time previously in the text. For instance, in the following short passage

*The woman went to the store. She had lots of groceries to buy.*

the pronoun, *she* refers to the woman who was mentioned in the previous sentence. Pronoun assignment has two features that make it an appropriate topic for the use of eye movements to study language processing.

1. The pronoun itself provides a source point for an analysis of the data.
2. Pronoun assignment reflects the integration of information from separate sources rather than the ease of accessing information from a single source.

Pronoun assignment can roughly be described as resulting from the interplay between processes that help a reader to select a referent from among the entities mentioned in the text and processes that help a reader to recover some representation of the referent which is then assigned to the pronoun. The selection processes make use of information from a variety of sources, ranging from linguistic constraints such as those that cover number and gender agreement, to complex inferences that are drawn from general knowledge. Many of these factors have been shown to influence the choice of referent and the speed with which that choice is made (e.g., Caramazza, Grober, Garvey, & Yates, 1977; Ehrlich, 1980; Garrod & Sanford, 1977). Of more interest for the current project, however, is the general finding that the speed of pronoun assignment varies according to the amount of text that intervenes between the pronoun and its antecedent phrase; as the distance increases, the time taken to read a sentence containing a pronoun increases (e.g., Clark & Sengul, 1979).

## III.   Eye Movements and Pronoun Assignment

Although it is important to understand how people reach decisions about referents, it is equally important to understand when these decisions are made. A critical issue in pronoun assignment is whether some initial decision about assignment is made as soon as the pronoun is encountered, even though the decision may turn out to be wrong, or whether assignment is delayed until some suitable point after the pronoun. A possible decision point may be at the end of the clause or at the end of the sentence. Ehrlich (1978) argued that in sentences such as the following:

*John lent his car to Bill because he needed it.*
*John lent his car to Bill because he was generous.*

there is inadequate information prior to the pronoun to choose between John and Bill at the point when the pronoun is first encountered. However, it has also been argued that decisions about reference are made much earlier, probably by the time the pronoun is encountered (e.g., Caramazza *et al.*, 1977). The notion that processing decisions are made early has also been put forward in the context of parsing strategies (see Frazier, Chapter 13 in this volume) and is similar to the immediacy assumption of Just and Carpenter (1980). The claims concerning pronoun assignment are often based on techniques that do not directly measure the moment by moment processing that is possible with eye movement recordings. The study reported here was designed to examine the time-course of pronoun assignment in cases where there is sufficient information prior to the pronoun to make a decision.

The study was also designed to examine whether readers select referents by initiating a regression back to the antecedent phrase or whether they search their mental representations of the text. There are a number of reasons why readers might not look back to the antecedent when they encounter a pronoun. Mainly, it is suggested that regressions are a disruption in the normal left to right movement in reading. But pronouns occur frequently in English so it seems unlikely if their occurrence disrupts reading. There is also no evidence to suggest that people find pronouns harder to understand in spoken discourse, when regressions are not possible, than in written discourse. Pronouns can also occur at arbitrarily long distances from their antecedents. Hence, for regressions to be the main mechanism for finding antecedents, it would be necessary for readers to remember the location of the antecedent in the text. Despite these intuitions, it has been claimed that readers do often initiate regressions back to the antecedent. In a recent study, Carpenter and Just (1977) found that readers would initiate a regression back to the antecedent phrase on the previous line, nearly 50% of the time. Moreover, the frequency of regressions hardly altered when there was some ambiguity over the choice of referent. In that experiment, subjects were given the task of deciding for each line of the text whether it was consistent or inconsistent with the text. That this task encourages readers to initiate regressions cannot be ruled out as being the main factor responsible for the large proportion of regressions.

## A.  Method

In the study reported here, pronouns were embedded in short passages. The antecedent phrases denoted professions in which there was a majority of male members. If it can be assumed that the feature "male" will be attached to the antecedent phrase by default, then use of the unexpected pronoun *she* to refer to that person should evoke some surprise reaction at the point when the assignment takes place. Thus, it should be possible, by varying the pronoun between *he* and *she,* to localize when a referent is assigned to a pronoun. In case the assumption was not warranted and as a comparison for the experimental passages, two extra passages were constructed in which the pronoun blatantly violated the explicit gender of the antecedent. Two neutral passages from the filler material were also analyzed. In these passages, the pronoun naturally occurred in subject position, making the passages suitable for comparison with the experimental passages. Examples of the experimental, disruptive, and neutral passages are shown in the Appendix to this chapter.

A more direct test of pronoun assignment was also provided by varying the distance between the pronoun and its antecedent phrase. The antecedent was either at the beginning of the preceding sentence, or there were one or two sentences intervening between pronoun and antecedent. In addition, a case was included where the antecedent appeared at the end of the preceding sentence and immediately before the pronoun. In this case it is possible that the visual characteristics of both the antecedent and the pronoun are being seen in the same fixation. The average length of a saccade is between 8 and 10 characters. Evidence from McConkie & Rayner (1975) and Rayner (1975) suggests that readers can pick up information over this range within a single fixation, with more information being acquired to the right than to the left of fixation point. Hence, if readers fixate on the antecedent, then it should be possible for them to also pick up the visual characteristics of the pronoun. This case is an important one because it is the only instance in the experiment when information about the antecedent can be picked up through direct visual encoding, after the pronoun has been encountered. For the other three levels of distance, information about the antecedent can only be accessed indirectly from the mental representation of the text. In those cases, readers could only access the antecedent visually by initiating a regression back to the antecedent. However, Carpenter and Just's (1977) data notwithstanding, it seems unlikely that readers do initiate regressions back to the antecedent in the normal course of reading.

## B.    Issues

The design of the experiment permits a number of issues to be tested directly. The first issue concerns the eye–mind lag problem. According to many researchers, there is no appreciable lag between fixating a word and completing the semantic processing derived from that word. A stronger version of this claim is that readers will maintain fixation on a word until the processing is complete. According to these claims, readers should, on encountering a pronoun, remain at that fixation until they have found the antecedent and assigned it to the pronoun. According to these claims, any effect due to how recently the antecedent was mentioned will be reflected in an increased latency when the pronoun is encountered. An alternative claim is based on the observation that unlike ambiguous words, the meaning of a pronoun cannot be accessed from an internal mental lexicon but can only be accessed from wherever information about the text is stored. It is further claimed that information about the antecedent is not necessarily retrieved immediately the pronoun is encountered, but that assignment may take place after a reader has moved on to fixate a later portion of the text, particularly when the antecedent is far back in the text. To test these claims it will be assumed that the longest fixation duration in the vicinity of the pronoun will represent the locus of pronoun assignment.

One additional issue concerns the function and purpose of regressions. It has been argued that regressions may be the way in which readers determine the referents of pronouns. Other research suggests that readers initiate a regressive eye movement when they have overshot a target or when they need to check that a word or phrase was encoded correctly. Moreover, regressions are generally initiated when readers have a good idea of where to direct the regression. Frazier and Rayner (1982) found that readers who encounter a structural ambiguity, often initiate a regression directly back to the source of the ambiguity. Similarly, Carpenter and Daneman (1981) report that readers examine the text selectively rather than reread the entire portion of the text. These claims can be examined in the present experiment. As the distance between the pronoun and its antecedent increases, readers are less likely to retain information about the specific location of the antecedent in the text. Hence, if they do initiate regressions back to the antecedent, say, to resolve possible misassignments, these regressions should be less likely to occur as the distance increases. Alternatively, readers may initiate more regressions as the distance increases and pronoun assignment gets harder. It is also of interest to examine whether the pattern of regressions varies between the experimental passages and the disruptive passages where there was an explicit violation in the gender agreement between the pronoun and its antecedent.

A third issue concerns the probability of fixating the pronoun. There is evidence to suggest that short words are fixated less often than long words (e.g., Rayner & McConkie, 1976) and that function words, such as *the*, are fixated less often than content words. Rayner (1977) found that the mean number of fixations on sentence initial *the* was 10.5 per subject, whereas there was a mean of 47.2 fixations per subject on the main verb of the sentence. Pronouns may be fixated with the same frequency as other function words or at a rate that is closer to that of short content words. Readers are more likely to fixate a word when it is less predictable from the context or when the word contains a spelling error (see S. Ehrlich, Chapter 11 in this volume). In the disruptive passages in the present study, the use of the pronoun *she* to refer to someone male (and vice versa) can be considered either as unpredictable or as a spelling error. In either case, readers should fixate the pronoun more often than in the other passages.

The data were analyzed to show local processing effects, (effects that occur in the vicinity of the pronoun) and global processing effects (effects that persist throughout the sentence). In addition, regressions and the locus of fixations were analyzed.

## C.  Local Effects

To determine the time course of pronoun assignment, three fixations were used in the analysis. These were: the fixation nearest the pronoun; the fixation before; and the fixation after. Ambiguities over the nearest fixation were resolved in favor of the fixation to the right of the pronoun, so long as that fixation was within six characters of the pronoun. The main reason for adopting this criterion was to make the fixation before the pronoun the one on which the visual characteristics of the pronoun could first be encountered. The fixation before was, on average, between six and eight characters to the left of the pronoun. The nearest fixation to the pronoun was generally within two to three characters.

The mean durations of these three fixations are shown in Table 15.1 and are further illustrated in Figure 15.1. The data indicate that the locus of the longest fixation, and hence the assumed locus of pronoun assignment, does vary as a function of the distance between the pronoun and its antecedent: As the distance increases, the locus of the longest fixation is further from the pronoun. The data in Table 15.1 also suggest that pronoun assignment may be completed later for the pronoun *she* than for the pronoun *he*.

It is interesting to note that the data for the neutral passages is very similar to that for the intermediate condition in the experimental passages. In both cases,

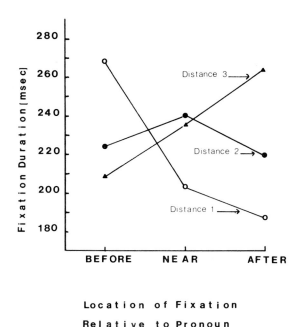

FIGURE 15.1. *The mean fixation durations at varying distances between pronoun and antecedent as a function of fixation location.*

the antecedent occurred at the beginning of the sentence prior to the pronoun. Since most antecedents do occur within two sentences of the pronoun (Hobbs, 1978), we can conjecture from these data that pronoun assignment will generally be completed within two fixations, or approximately 450 msec, of when the pronoun is encountered.

Subjects spent longer reading the beginning of the critical sentence when the antecedent was not mentioned recently. The mean reading time for the nearest fixation to the pronoun and the one after was 195 msec when the antecedent was near, 229 msec. when the antecedent was at an intermediate distance, and 249 msec when the antecedent was far. This result is consistent with previous research that has shown that reading time for a sentence increases as the distance to the antecedent increases (e.g., Clark & Sengul, 1979). Previous research has generally used the technique of measuring reading time over the whole sentence, thus making it difficult to localize the effect of distance. The present result adds to previous research by showing that some effects of distance may occur early in the sentence.

These results suggest that there is no single place in the text at which pronoun assignment always occurs. Rather, the effect of increasing the distance between the pronoun and the antecedent is to shift the locus of assignment to a later point. Thus it seems that readers do not remain at a particular fixation until they have

**TABLE 15.1**

**Mean Fixation Durations (msec) as a Function of Pronoun Gender and the Distance Between Pronoun and Antecedent**

Fixation durations (msec)

| | Distance 1 (Near) | | | Distance 2 (Intermediate) | | | Distance 3 (Far) | | | Distance 4 (Very Far) | | |
|---|---|---|---|---|---|---|---|---|---|---|---|---|
| | Before | Nearest | After | Before | Nearest | After | Before | Nearest | After | Before | Nearest | After |
| He | 293 | 191 | 170 | 247 | 277 | 203 | 231 | 258 | 248 | 171 | 259 | 230 |
| She | 243 | 215 | 204 | 202 | 203 | 235 | 186 | 212 | 278 | 248 | 208 | 236 |
| Mean | 268 | 203 | 187 | 224 | 240 | 219 | 208 | 235 | 263 | 209 | 233 | 233 |

| | Disruptive | | | Neutral | | |
|---|---|---|---|---|---|---|
| | Before | Nearest | After | Before | Nearest | After |
| "Tom" | 257 | 222 | 230 | 202 | 241 | 200 |
| "Sarah" | 219 | 216 | 220 | | | |

recovered the antecedent, but they keep reading, perhaps pausing, when the antecedent has been accessed, causing a momentary increase in processing.

## D.  Global Effects

It is important, if we are to get a complete picture of language processes, to examine processing in the vicinity of a critical item and over a longer duration. In the present study, the local effects of varying the distance between pronoun and antecedent probably reflect some temporary delays in processing. Thus, it was shown that assignment occurred later and that there was an increase in reading time as the distance increased. In comparison, effects that persist over the whole sentence are more likely to reflect processing load. Two measures were used to reflect processing over the whole sentence. These measures were the average time spent per character (latency per character) and the average distance between fixations (saccade length). As processing load increases, it is expected that the latency per character should increase, to reflect the greater time spent on process- ing. Similarly, saccade length should decrease, to reflect the reduced capacity in short-term memory for holding the incoming information.

The latency per character and the saccade length for each level of distance are shown in Table 15.2. The data indicate an increase in processing load for the longer distances with the effect being apparent earlier for *she* than for *he*. Where there was one intervening sentence between the pronoun and the antecedent, at distance 3, subjects were experiencing difficulties when *she* was used to refer to the antecedent. Subjects spent 34.7 msec per character reading the sentence as compared with a reading rate of 25.3 msec per character when the antecedent immediately preceded the pronoun. Subjects also took in information less often; saccade length decreased from 8.6 characters to 6.6 characters for the near and far distances. Subjects seemed to experience very few long-term difficulties in re- trieving the antecedent when the pronoun was *he*. However, in the very far

TABLE 15.2
Mean Latency/Character and Saccade Length as a Function of Pronoun Gender and Distance

|  | Distance | | | | |
|---|---|---|---|---|---|
|  | 1 (Near) | 2 (Inter.) | 3 (Far) | 4 (Very Far) | Neutral |
| Latency–character (msec) |  |  |  |  |  |
| He | 28.9 | 28.9 | 27.3 | 33.1 | 25.9 |
| She | 25.3 | 26.0 | 34.7 | 28.4 | |
| Saccade length (msec) |  |  |  |  |  |
| He | 7.8 | 8.2 | 8.1 | 7.3 | 9.1 |
| She | 8.6 | 8.7 | 6.6 | 7.5 | |

condition, where two sentence intervened between pronoun and antecedent, subjects seemed to have some difficulty even for *he*.

Perhaps the most important point about these data is that they show that effects on processing can persist beyond a purely local level. The data are also consistent with the notion that these global measures reflect differences in the ease of accessing the antecedent, a process that is likely to vary in processing load.

## E.    Regressions and the Probability of Fixating the Pronoun

The data showing the number of regressions and the probability of fixating the pronoun are in Table 15.3. The main thing to notice about the data is that there are many more instances of regressive eye movements for the disruptive passages than for the experimental passages. For one passage in particular, the one in which the main protagonist was Tom Norman, readers would generally initiate the regression just prior to the pronoun, fixate an earlier portion of the sentence, and then move back through the text, in what seemed to be a clear goal of finding the antecedent phrase. In contrast, there were no instances when readers would look back in the text to find the antecedent and only a few cases where readers initiated a regression back to the antecedent on the same line as the pronoun. However, one or two readers did adopt the strategy of rereading the passage after they had completed one pass through. In these cases, they would often spend some time fixating the antecedent expression. Thus, these data suggest that readers do not, in general, look back in the text to find referents for pronouns. They will, however, look back in the text to check that they encoded the word or phrase correctly, even though these regressive movements may disrupt reading. There is also a considerable difference in the way the experimental passages and the disruptive passages are processed. The data in Table 15.3 show that the probability of fixating the pronoun is greater when the pronoun violates expectation, as in the disruptive passages, than when the pronoun is merely inconsistent with expectation, as in the experimental passages. There is a very low probability of fixating the pronoun in the neutral passages.

TABLE 15.3
Number of Regressions and the Probability of Fixating the Pronoun

|  | Experimental | | Disruptive | | |
|---|---|---|---|---|---|
|  | He | She | Tom | Sarah | Neutral |
| Mean number of regressions per condition initiated in a region from the pronoun to the end of the following line | 5.75 | 6.00 | 23.00 | 10.00 | 4.5 |
| Probability of fixating the pronoun | .10 | .16 | .50 | .25 | .00 |

# IV.   General Discussion

Two main topics have been covered in this chapter. One topic concerns the comprehension of text. The other topic concerns the use of eye movements as a method for investigating language processes. An experiment examined pronoun assignment as an example of an integrative process that serves to unite material from separate sentences. The results of the study showed that the assumed locus of pronoun assignment occurs increasingly later in the text as a function of how recently the antecedent has been mentioned. This result suggests that although there is a correspondence between fixating an item and processing it, it cannot be assumed that language processes are strictly synchronous with fixations. In general, pronoun assignment will probably occur on the fixation nearest the pronoun, at least in those cases where there is only one potential antecedent. It is an open question whether assignment occurs near the pronoun when there is more than one potential antecedent and the disambiguating information occurs after the pronoun. The study establishes the important point that pronoun assignment, and perhaps other integrative processes, need not invariably occur at the earliest possible fixation.

The process of reading and understanding a text utilizes a number of different and often highly complex processes. These processes make use of perceptual information, stored lexical information, material from the text, as well as linguistic and general knowledge. Moreover, the processes themselves are interdependent in that initiation of one process, say integration, may depend on the completion of another, say, perceptual encoding. There might be a temptation in using eye movements to examine language processes to view these processes as discrete and occurring at a single point. However, it is possible that a particular process extends over some period of time and affects the duration of more than one fixation. Moreover, the fixation duration itself may reflect simply that a process is occurring, or that there is a momentary increase in memory load, or that some other component of processing is occurring. Indeed, in the present study it was found that some processes of pronoun assignment could be clearly evident at a local level, whereas other processes associated with pronoun assignment persisted over a longer stretch of the text. All of these points bring attention to some possible dangers in relying on a simple analysis of eye movements to draw conclusions about language processes.

When readers encounter a pronoun, their goal is to find the referent as quickly as possible. When there is little ambiguity in the choice of referent, readers seem to be able to accomplish the task rapidly. It is therefore natural to wonder what the basis is for the speedy selection of a referent. Certainly it is clear that whatever the mechanism, it is not mediated by a regressive eye movement back to the antecedent in the text. Even when the gender of the pronoun is contrary to culturally based expectations, readers seem not to regress to the antecedent but to adjust their reading and perhaps their representation of the referent accordingly. The function of regressions seems therefore not to be to access information.

Rather, regressions are used to check on the source of information when there is some unresolvable inconsistency, for instance, when the pronoun of one gender is used to refer to a person who is unambiguously of the other gender.

If readers do not select referents by looking back in the text then they must select them from their representation of the text. As people read a story, they keep track of what the current topic is. The topic can change many times in a story, for instance, as the scene or time frame of the story changes, as new people get introduced, or as others are no longer mentioned. These dynamic changes in the representation of the text could easily form the basis on which referents are selected, such that entities that form part of the current topic are preferred as referents. Indeed, the felicitous production of a pronoun may demand that the referent be part of the current topic so as to be easily accessible by the reader, or that there is compensatory marking of the probable location of the referent. Readers, do seem to be able to detect very early when a pronoun has been used infelicitously. Data from the study showed that subjects were more likely to fixate the pronoun in the disruptive passages that exemplify the infelicitous occurrence of a pronoun. Since the pronouns were identical in all three kinds of material, subjects must have made some initial decisions about the use of the pronoun prior to their fixation. There is also evidence that readers are sensitive to the dynamic changes in the time or scene where the events described in the text take place. Sanford and Garrod (1981) reported a series of studies in which a time change is mentioned between the initial introduction of an entity and subsequent reference back to the same entity. As the time change increases, readers take longer to complete pronoun assignment.

Pronouns occur frequently in texts and cause no problems for comprehension. In fact, people are able to assimilate them easily in the course of reading and comprehending a text. The function of pronouns may be simply to reduce the repetition of words or phrases by replacing the name or phrase denoting an entity with a simple two or three letter pronoun denoting its number and gender. However, if the presence of a pronoun really does enhance the accessibility of those entities that are represented in the current topic of the text, then it may be that a pronoun is not only sufficient to denote entities, but that the use of a name or phrase instead, would be inappropriate. In this way, pronouns may make an important contribution to the smooth flow of reading.

### A Set of Experimental Passages
**(The pronouns are underlined here for expository purposes but were not underlined in the experiment)**

1. Distance = 1 (Near Condition)

THE LIGHTS HAD BEEN TURNED ON IN STUDIO
ONE FOR THE TAPING OF THE NEXT EPISODE OF
THE SERIES. SOME LAST MINUTE DETAILS WERE
BEING CHECKED BY THE PRODUCER. HE WANTED

(*continued*)

THE SESSION TO BE A SHORT ONE. THE SERIES
WAS ALREADY WELL BEHIND SCHEDULE. THE
MANAGEMENT WAS THREATENING TO CUT THE
BUDGET OF NEW SERIES IF THEIR SCHEDULES
WERE NOT MET.

2. Distance = 2 (Intermediate Condition)

THE LIGHTS HAD BEEN TURNED ON IN STUDIO
ONE FOR THE TAPING OF THE NEXT EPISODE OF
THE SERIES. THE PRODUCER WAS CHECKING
SOME LAST MINUTE DETAILS. HE WANTED
THE SESSION TO BE A SHORT ONE. THE SERIES
WAS ALREADY WELL BEHIND SCHEDULE. THE
MANAGEMENT WAS THREATENING TO CUT THE
BUDGET OF NEW SERIES IF THEIR SCHEDULES
WERE NOT MET.

3. Distance = 3 (Far Condition)

THE LIGHTS HAD BEEN TURNED ON IN STUDIO
ONE FOR THE TAPING OF THE NEXT EPISODE OF
THE SERIES. SOME LAST MINUTE DETAILS WERE
BEING CHECKED BY THE PRODUCER. THE SERIES
WAS ALREADY WELL BEHIND SCHEDULE. HE
WANTED THE SESSION TO BE A SHORT ONE. THE
MANAGEMENT WAS THREATENING TO CUT THE
BUDGET OF NEW SERIES IF THEIR SCHEDULES
WERE NOT MET.

4. Distance = 4 (Very Far Condition)

THE LIGHTS HAD BEEN TURNED ON IN STUDIO
ONE FOR THE TAPING OF THE NEXT EPISODE OF
THE SERIES. SOME LAST MINUTE DETAILS WERE
BEING CHECKED BY THE PRODUCER. THE SERIES
WAS ALREADY WELL BEHIND SCHEDULE. THE
MANAGEMENT WAS THREATENING TO CUT THE
BUDGET OF NEW SERIES IF THEIR SCHEDULES
WERE NOT MET. HE WANTED THE SESSION TO
BE A SHORT ONE.

Disruptive passages

THE WORST THAT ANYONE COULD FIND TO SAY
ABOUT TOM NORMAN WAS THAT HE COULD BE A
BIT OF A ROGUE AND A RASCAL, BUT NEVER
LESS THAN AN ENGAGING ONE AND ALWAYS A
POSITIVELY ROUGH DIAMOND. SHE COULD BE
DISARMING, EVEN CHARMING, IN SELF-
CRITICISM. HE REMEMBERED AS AN OLD MAN
THE VERY FLASH APPEARANCE WHICH HE HAD
CULTIVATED IN HIS YOUTH.

IT WAS DARK. A COLD AND GUSTY WIND HAD
COME UP AND IT WHISTLED ACROSS THE BIG
PARKING LOT. SARAH'S LONG HAIR STREAMED
OUT BEHIND HER. LATER WHEN HE GOT HOME,
SHE WOULD FIND A CRISP YELLOW LEAF CAUGHT
IN IT. THE THREE OF THEM WAITED ANOTHER
HOUR AND THEN LEFT.

Neutral passages

JIM SAW THE BLACK FIN SLICE THROUGH THE
WATER AND THE IMAGE OF SHARKS' TEETH
CAME TO HIS MIND. HE TURNED QUICKLY
TOWARD THE SHORE AND SWAM FOR HIS LIFE.
THE COAST GUARD HAD WARNED THAT SOMEONE
HAD SEEN A SHARK OFF THE NORTH SHORE OF
THE ISLAND. AS USUAL, NOT EVERYONE
LISTENED TO THE WARNING.

TODAY WAS HELEN'S FIRST DAY ON THE JOB
AT THE BAKERY. IT WAS A COLD AND DREARY
DAY AND SHE HAD TO WAKE UP QUITE EARLY.
SHE WANTED TO LOOK HER BEST, SO AFTER SHE
GOT HER COAT FROM THE HALL, SHE CHECKED
HER HAIR IN THE MIRROR. SHE WAS A LITTLE
FRIGHTENED BY THE WHOLE THING.

# References

Bouma, H., & de Voogd, A. H. (1974). On the control of eye saccades in reading. *Vision Research 14*, 273–284.

Caramazza, A., Grober, E., Garvey, E., & Yates, J. (1977). Comprehension of anaphoric pronouns. *Journal of Verbal Behavior and Verbal Learning 16*, 601–609.

Carpenter, P. A., & Daneman, M. (1981). Lexical retrieval and error recovery in reading: A model based on eye fixations. *Journal of Verbal Learning and Verbal Behavior 20*, 137–160.

Carpenter, P. A., & Just, M. A. (1977). Reading comprehension as eyes see it. In M. A. Just & P. A. Carpenter (Eds.), *Cognitive processes in comprehension*. Hillsdale, New Jersey: Erlbaum.

Clark, H. H., & Sengul, C. J. (1979). In search of referents for nouns and pronouns. *Memory and Cognition 7*, 35–41.

Ehrlich, K. (1979). *Comprehension and anaphora*. Unpublished doctoral dissertation, Sussex University,

Ehrlich, K. (1980). Comprehension of pronouns. *Quarterly Journal of Experimental Psychology 32*, 247–255.

Frazier, L., & Rayner, K. (1982). Making and correcting errors during sentence comprehension: Eye movements in the analysis of structurally ambiguous sentences. *Cognitive Psychology, 14*, 178–210.

Garrod, S., & Sanford, A. J. (1977). Interpreting anaphoric relations: The integration of semantic information while reading. *Journal of Verbal Learning and Verbal Behavior 16*, 77–90.

Hobbs, J. R. (1978). Resolving pronoun references. *Lingua 44*, 311–338.

Just, M. A., & Carpenter, P. A. (1980). A theory of reading: From eye fixations to comprehension. *Psychology Review 87*, 329–354.

Kolers, P. A. (1976). Buswell's discoveries. In R. A. Monty & J.W. Senders (Eds.), *Eye movements and psychological processes*. Hillsdale, New Jersey: Erlbaum.

McConkie, G. W., & Rayner, K. (1975). The span of the effective stimulus during a fixation in reading. *Perception & Psychophysics, 17*, 578–586.

Morton, J. (1964). The effects of context upon speed of reading, eye movements and eye–voice span. *Quarterly Journal of Experimental Psychology, 16*, 340–354.

Rayner, K. (1975). The perceptual span and peripheral cues in reading. *Cognitive Psychology 7*, 65–81.

Rayner, K. (1977) Visual attention in reading: Eye movements reflect cognitive processes. *Memory & Cognition 4*, 443–448.

Rayner, K. (1978) Eye movements in reading and information processing. *Psychological Bulletin 85*, 618–660.

Rayner, K., & McConkie, G. W. (1976). What guides a reader's eye movements? *Vision Research 16*, 829–837.

Sanford, A. J., & Garrod, S. (1981). *Understanding written language: Explorations in comprehension beyond the sentence*. New York: Wiley, 1981.

Charles Clifton, Jr.

# 16

# Psycholinguistic Factors Reflected in the Eye

I find it marvelous that one could trace the steps of understanding sentences by observing the behavior of the eye. A naive observer of the field of eye movement control gathers that a reader's eye has a period averaging 50–100 msec during which it can pick up information from text and decide to move on, and, perhaps, decide where to move. The reader has the next 150 or 200 msec to mull over the information picked up, but cannot use the products of this reflection to decide where to go next. At best, it seems, the reader can decide to abort a planned move and tarry a while. The reader can even decide, perhaps during the first 50 msec, perhaps later, to move the eye back to a position it left earlier. How in the world can the duration of the initial portion of these fixations, a portion whose average may be as little as 50 msec in duration, possibly reflect the elaborate and structured use of information that Frazier, Kennedy, and Ehrlich suggest it reflects? Regressive eye movements pose a different kind of problem. Unlike decisions about when to move one's eye, decisions to make regressive eye movements seem, at least upon occasion, to be open to consciousness. One's introspections about them indicate that they are due to a wide variety of causes, including the failure to remember some word or phrase, the need to concentrate one's attention on a particular item, and the realization that one's mind has drifted off and one has lost track of what one was reading. How can subtle effects show up through such a potpourri of powerful variables?

But the proof of the pudding is in the eating. The authors of the chapters in this section have used the eye movement measurement technique to uncover a variety of surprising and most interesting effects. Things cannot be so bad as I have made them out to be. One point I had not heard discussed before is that it

EYE MOVEMENTS IN READING:
PERCEPTUAL AND LANGUAGE PROCESSES

may not be relevant that the mean duration of fixations prior to the initiation of eye movement is short. What is relevant is the variability of this duration. I suspect that much of the variability in fixation durations can be traced to that portion of a fixation prior to issuing the instruction that the eye is to move. If this variability is large—relative, perhaps, to the more constant time taken to initiate an eye movement in response to a simple event—then one can legitimately expect substantial effects of processing variables to show up in fixation durations. Are fixation durations sufficiently variable? In a related vein, it seems just possible that all the immediate-processing effects that have been reported can be traced to abortions of planned eye movements in the period between the issuing of a movement command and the execution of the command. Perhaps the only decision relevant to initial fixation durations (aside, I suppose, from perceptual considerations) is the decision that something has gone awry. This is, I think, a slightly exaggerated version of a point made by McConkie (Chapter 5 of this volume). Is it possible? Could one check it by examining the distribution of fixation durations? If it is true, then one might have an easy time making up an explanation of why subtle linguistic processing variables seem to affect fixation duration but not fixation position, as Frazier has suggested. What about regressive eye movements? Maybe there really are different types, and the ones of which we are consciously aware constitute a small (if interesting) minority of them. Perhaps regressions are not determined by such a mixed bag of factors as introspection suggests. Perhaps the kinds of regressions that occur during fluent reading have a lighter burden of potential causes, and are free to reflect factors that operate in normal sentence processing.

Let me make a few more specific remarks about the chapters in this part. Kennedy's illustrations of the value of maintaining spatial representations of what one has just read are convincing, but only, I think, within the realm of problem solving. I suspect that the regressive eye movements that occur during syllogistic reasoning are consciously controlled, or at least accessible to consciousness. I suspect that Kennedy is quite correct in his suggestions that they are memory aids, or, perhaps, aids to attention. The phenomenon that used to be called redintegration, in which presentation of some attributes of an event call to mind the other attributes of the event, may well be instanced in a reader's looking at the position where a critical element of a syllogism has occurred. But I wonder what would happen to eye movements if subjects were trained in some visual strategy for solving problems, perhaps constructing mental Euler circles as they read. Would this change the pattern of regressive movements? If so, I would think that the regressive movements Kennedy studies have more to do with visual problem-solving processes than with sentence comprehension.

The regressions that Ehrlich thought might occur during the determination of pronoun antecedents should be different in kind from these. Note, though, that Ehrlich did not find them in any abundance. The only frequent regressive movements she found seem likely to be the kind of which we are painfully aware—when we find a pronoun that has no imaginable antecedent in memory. These are surely "second-cycle" regressions, in Kennedy's terms. What Ehrlich did find was an indication in fixation durations of when pronouns were being assigned to antecedents. Her data seem to show a particularly interesting effect of the one factor that clearly must have an effect in pronoun interpretation, namely, distance of the antecedent from the pronoun. At the risk of overinterpretation, it does appear as if the search for an antecedent goes on independently of eye movements, but when an antecedent is found, an eye fixation is lengthened while the pronoun assignment is made. This happens later when the antecedent is far away than when it is near, and later when the antecedent is less appropriate for the pronoun. If this analysis is correct, we would have an instance of a nonimmediate but interpretable effect of language processing on eye movements. It would also be an instance of using eye movements as a general measure of processing load, rather than a specific measure of how one is processing what one is looking at. These speculations, however, must be taken with a grain of salt, especially as there are some ambiguities in Ehrlich's data. One would be more comfortable had a fixation duration peak appeared in the case where two sentences intervened between antecedent and pronoun (distance 4 in Table 15.1; not shown in Figure 15.1). Perhaps the peak occurred at fixations subsequent to those Ehrlich analyzed, as is suggested by the data in Table 15.2; but one would like to know for certain.

Frazier's chapter is an ambitious and exciting attempt to argue for a coherent and highly structured analysis of language processing. I am persuaded by her arguments—several of them novel—that one must compute a detailed structural analysis, based upon syntactic rules of substantial scope and generality, in comprehending a sentence. I am also attracted by her arguments that this structural analysis is done very quickly, perhaps quickly enough to show up as an immediate effect in eye fixations. If she is right, eye movements in what Kennedy refers to as first-cycle inspection are influenced by far more subtle factors than the perceptual and lexical-access factors he suggested. Perhaps the effects of these factors are not immediate in all cases; perhaps the impact of a word for structural revision is not realized until a word or two downstream. Frazier's finding, though, that fixation durations were lengthened for the very first word that could tell a reader that he or she had gone down a garden path, does seem to be a good argument for immediacy. Can one really maintain that the word in question, the first word in a disambiguating region (typically a verb, I believe), is fixated longer because it was picked up on the previous fixation, and the implications for structural analysis are being worked out one fixation downstream? I doubt it.

Frazier's data about regressive eye movements highlight an interesting problem suggested by Kennedy's analysis: Are the entries in a spatial map of a sentence specific individual words, or are they positions occupied by structurally defined variables? When one regresses after reading Kennedy's sentence *The drunken captain crossed the deck to the mate*, does one look for the occurrence of the word *skipper*, or does one look for the subject noun, whatever it was? I think Frazier thinks in terms of the latter, but I am not certain.

One final point. Perhaps the single most central question in experimental psycholinguistics concerns what kinds of linguistic information are used, when, in understanding a sentence. The evidence from eye movement data presented in the chapters by Frazier, Kennedy, and Ehrlich and elsewhere (c.f., Frazier & Rayner, 1982; Holmes & O'Regan, 1981; Rayner, 1978) is by far the most illuminating evidence available concerning this question. I find it marvelous that a technique that could, in principle, fail in so many ways, should prove to be the first good source of evidence about this question.

# References

Frazier, L., & Rayner, K. (1982). Making and correcting errors during sentence comprehension: Eye movements in the analysis of structurally ambiguous sentences. *Cognitive Psychology, 14,* 178–210.

Holmes, V. M., & O'Regan, J. K. (1981). Eye fixation patterns during the reading of relative-clause sentence. *Journal of Verbal Learning and Verbal Behavior, 20,* 417–430.

Rayner, K. (1978). Eye movements in reading and information processing. *Psychological Bulletin, 85,* 618–660.

# V
# Eye Movements and Language Processes II

Patricia A. Carpenter and Marcel Adam Just

# 17

# What Your Eyes Do
# while Your Mind Is Reading[1]

## I. Introduction

*The apprehensive student perused the gallimaufry of people in the lecture hall and saw that the only remaining place to sit was in front of the lectern. Resignedly, the student sat down before the avuncular professor in the rumpled suit entered. He was anxious to begin the test, but the student asked for additional time to prepare. After a minute but rapid examination of the book, he signalled the professor to begin.*

The paragraph above was intended to make some reading processes especially difficult. For example, the unusual words, like *gallimaufry* (meaning hodgepodge), *avuncular*, and *perused*, made it more difficult to recognize words and determine their meaning. Syntactic analysis was made difficult by inducing the interpretion of *before* in line 4 as a locative preposition rather than a temporal conjunction, so that the verb *entered* at the end of the sentence was left without a subject. Another anomaly was induced by the phrase *After a minute*, since the more frequent "60 second" interpretation (rather than the correct "detailed" interpretation) made the subsequent phrase *rapid examination* nonsensical. Finally, there were cues that would initially mislead the reader about the correct referent of the pronoun *He* in the phrase *He was anxious to begin.*

The eye fixations of a person reading the opening paragraph would reflect many of these processes. The reader would spend more time fixating on longer words,

[1]This research was partially supported by Grant G-79-0119 from the National Institute of Education and Grant MH-29617 from the National Institute of Mental Health.

EYE MOVEMENTS IN READING:
PERCEPTUAL AND LANGUAGE PROCESSES

such as *apprehensive* and *resignedly*, and on unfamiliar words, like *perused, avuncular*, and *gallimaufry*. The words *before, minute*, and *He* would not cause difficulty initially, but later words would not make sense and the reader would spend extra time fixating the mutually inconsistent parts while resolving the inconsistencies.

The fact that these inconsistencies are noticed just as soon as they arise supports **the immediacy assumption**—the assumption that a reader (or, listener) tries to interpret each word of a text immediately on encountering it, rather than waiting to make an interpretation until a number of words have been encountered (Just & Carpenter, 1980). *Interpret* refers to several levels of cognitive processing, such as encoding the word, accessing a meaning, assigning it to its referent, and determining its status in the sentence and the discourse.

We all know that it is often easier to interpret a word when the context that follows is known. Because of this, many accounts of natural language processing suggest that there is an invariant delay of a fixed number of words before interpretation is executed (see Kimball, 1973; Marcus, 1980). Such buffering schemes allow the interpretive processes to make use of some aspects of the context that follows a word. The immediacy assumption does not deny the use of context, but it proposes that interpretation is not invariably postponed until the succeeding context is known. Readers and listeners try to interpret each word as they encounter it, before knowing exactly what will follow. The fact that they are sometimes surprised by what follows, as in the opening paragraph, indicates that an initial interpretation has already been made. Attempts at immediate interpretation of each word of a text may be unsuccessful or produce an erroneous interpretation that later has to be revised. But the attempt is made, as our data show.

A second assumption discussed in our chapter is the *eye–mind assumption*. The assumption is that the reader continues to fixate a word until all the cognitive processes initiated by that word have been completed to some criterion. The eye–mind assumption does not require that the cognitive system consider only the word that is currently being fixated. Obviously, concepts from previous knowledge and from previously fixated words are available without any change in eye position.

In this chapter, we show how eye fixations can be used to determine when encoding, lexical access, parsing, and integration processes are executed, and how they are affected by various properties of the text. First, we discuss some global features of eye fixations in reading—some of which run counter to common conceptions of reading. These features also provide support for the immediacy and eye–mind assumptions. Second, we describe a general model of language comprehension based on a computer simulation that has been developed to account for the eye fixation results. The simulation was developed both to formalize our models of specific processes and to make the processes function collaboratively in an interactive system. Third, we discuss our research on specific comprehension processes, including encoding, lexical access, syntactic parsing, and integrative processes. Our final discussion evaluates the approach and suggests some possible sources of the next generation of improvements.

## II.  Eye Fixations during Normal Reading

Many readers believe that when they read normally, they fixate only two or three places on a line and rely on extrafoveal vision to encode the rest of the words around where they fixate. However, these intuitions are not correct; normal readers sample the text very frequently, usually fixating adjacent words or skipping no more than one word. Moreover, the time that a reader spends on a word reflects processes initiated by that word.

The support for these claims comes from an analysis of the eye fixations of 14 college students who read 15 short (130-word) texts, excerpted from *Newsweek* and *Time* magazines, that described scientific discoveries and technological developments. We asked the students to read normally, not to memorize or study the text, and to recall what they could of each paragraph after they had finished it (see Just & Carpenter, 1980, for the details of the method). The readers appeared to follow our directions. Their reading rates averaged 225 words per minute (wpm), a typical rate for normal reading, and they made very few regressions to previously read parts of the text. Fixations on interword spaces were attributed to the word to the right and blinks that were bounded by fixations on the same location were attributed to that location. Other blinks, the durations of saccades, and regressions to reread earlier parts of the text were not included in the analyzed data. We computed the time each reader spent on each word for the passages in which the tracker maintained better than 1° accuracy (three character spaces), an average of 14 passages per reader.

### A.  Gaze Duration

The mean time on a word was 239 msec, but there was considerable variation among the times on different words. We will argue that these times reflect several kinds of comprehension processes: encoding the word, accessing it, and performing syntactic, semantic, and discourse level processes. To quantify these effects, we used linear regression techniques to analyze two dependent variables. The first was the *mean gaze duration,* the average time spent looking at a word, irrespective of the number of individual fixations and averaged over all subjects (a 0 msec observation was entered if the reader did not fixate a word) (Just & Carpenter, 1980). The second was a *conditionalized mean gaze duration,* the time on a word averaged over only those readers who fixated the word for at least 50 msec. (This cutoff eliminates spurious observations of 16 or 33 msec caused by measurement noise or measurement during a saccade.) This second measure removes the variation due to the probability of fixating a word and analyzes only variation due to the gaze durations on the word. The two analyses yield fairly similar results for the types of words that almost all readers fixated, namely, the content words.

The analyses of both variables revealed several word level and sentence level effects. For example, readers spent more time on infrequent words and less time on modified nouns whose referent could be easily inferred. This variation can be seen in the gaze durations of a single reader. Table 17.1 presents a typical protocol

TABLE 17.1
The Gaze Durations of a Typical Reader

| | | | | | | |
|---|---|---|---|---|---|---|

384     267             884         300     333     333                 517

Another answer to the ever-intriguing question of pyramid construction has been suggested.

267         283         200    350 283 283 733         333 266     183     467     200

The Egyptian Engineer of 5,000 years ago may have used a simple wooden device called a

1201         333             367 1151     583     568             417   267 183   217

weightarm for handling the 2½ to 7 ton pyramid blocks. The weightarm is like a lever or beam

600  167 200 617         383             300     550 234  217     200         650     117

pivoting on a fulcrum. Hundreds of weightarms may have been needed for each pyramid.

267         367         250   283         234  384     216  350             267     250  433

Weightarms may have been used to lift the blocks off the barges which came from the upriver

899     300         400         217  217  633   83   383             634         350     333

quarries. Also, they would be needed to transfer the blocks to skid roads leading to the base and for

333     267   267   550             317         350  100   350   317             367   333

lifting the blocks onto sledges. The sledges were hauled up greased tracks to the working levels.

267         766         350     350 217     333     300         333     333     350   400

Again, weightarms were used to pick up the blocks from the sledges and put them on skidways

316         437     2150

where workers pulled them to their placements.

---

(chosen because the proportion of words that the reader fixated overall approximated the mean across the 14 readers). Even in this small sample, one can see that the reader paused longer on harder and more important words, such as *weightarm* in line 3, *fulcrum* in line 5, and *quarries* in line 7. The analysis of the average gaze durations across readers indicated considerable systematicity. Eleven independent variables accounted for 79% of the variation in the mean gaze durations on words and 60% of the variance in the conditionalized mean gaze durations. The systematic relations between the gaze durations and the properties of the text provide support for the eye–mind assumption, and hence, for the immediacy assumption.

## B.  The Pattern of Fixation

Simple inspection of the pattern of gazes in Table 17.1 makes it clear that this reader sampled the text very densely. To quantify this observation for the entire data base, we analyzed the distribution of successive unfixated words, focusing on the length of the run of unfixated words. The number of unfixated words is zero if the reader successively fixates two adjacent words. The length of the run is one if the reader skips exactly one word between successive fixations, and so on. Figure 17.1 shows the average number of runs of each length for each 1000 words of text.

When readers move their eyes forward in the text from one word to some other word, most of the time (93%) they fixate the very next word or skip over only one word. For every 1000 words of text, the mean number of words fixated at least once was 678. On average, these 678 fixated words were distributed as follows: The gazes were on adjacent words in 410 cases, involved one skipped word between consecutive gazes in 221 cases, two skipped words in 43 cases, three skipped words in 3.6 cases, and almost never involved more than three skipped

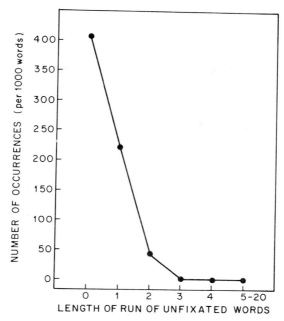

**FIGURE 17.1.** *The length of the run of unfixated words between successive fixations, conditionalized on a passage of 140 words.*

words. As the protocol in Table 17.1 suggests, the words that were likely to be skipped were short, function words, like *a, of, the, to,* and so on. Overall, readers fixated only 38% of the function words (conjunctions; articles; prepositions; modal, auxiliary, and copula verbs). By contrast, they fixated 83% of the content words (adjectives, adverbs, nouns, verbs, pronouns), and longer words were more likely to be fixated than shorter ones.

## C.  Support for the Immediacy and Eye–Mind Assumptions

The clearest support for the immediacy and eye–mind assumptions is the copious evidence that the time spent looking at a word is strongly influenced by the characteristics of that word (e.g., Just & Carpenter, 1980). Additional tests of the immediacy and eye–mind assumptions can be made by determining whether the gaze duration on a given word is influenced by the characteristics of the preceding word. If the eye were exactly one word ahead of the mind, then the semantic processing of word $N-1$ would occur during the gaze on word $N$. In one set of analyses, the dependent variable was the conditionalized mean gaze duration on word $N$, given that the reader fixated both word $N-1$ and word $N$. In another set of analyses, the dependent variable was the gaze duration on word $N$, given that the reader fixated word $N$ but skipped word $N-1$. Each dependent variable was analyzed with three regressions that used as independent variables the length and frequency of (1) word $N$ alone; (2) words $N$ and $N - 1$; and (3) word $N - 1$ alone. Length and frequency were used as independent variables because these two variables are assumed to affect encoding and lexical access and their large effects should be detected easily. We restricted the analysis to words that were not at the beginning or end of a line, and not sentence initial or terminal, since such words tend to be processed differently (Just & Carpenter, 1980; Rayner, 1977, 1979).

The major result, shown in Table 17.2, is that the gaze duration on word $N$ is not affected by the length or frequency of the preceding word. The account of the variance in gaze durations on word $N$ is not significantly improved by considering the characteristics of word $N - 1$. This result holds regardless of whether the reader did or did not fixate word $N - 1$. These results suggest that the reader generally has finished encoding and accessing the preceding word before fixating the next. This finding provides strong support for the eye–mind and immediacy assumptions. Word length and frequency presumably affect encoding and lexical access. Consequently, these analyses suggest that these processes, at least, begin on the word that enables them, as immediacy posits, and that they tend to be completed before the next word is fixated, as the eye–mind assumption posits.

The analyses above do not indicate whether the immediacy and eye–mind assumptions are equally supported for higher level processes or processes that require more extended computations. Experiments reported later in the paper suggest that many processes do conform to the immediacy assumption. One boundary condition is that readers postpone some integrative processes until sentence boundaries, so these are sometimes not computed immediately. In addition, we have isolated a boundary condition on the eye–mind assumption. For more difficult inferences, some readers do not complete the computation on the word that enabled it and they may continue the computation while fixating on an adjacent word. The study which showed this examined the eye fixations of readers making verb based inferences (Just & Carpenter, 1978). For example, in one passage, a person was described as having been *murdered* and a latter sentence mentioned a *killer*. In another version of the passage, the person was described as *dead* and then the latter sentence introduced the concept of *killer*. As immediacy would predict, readers spent more time on *killer* in the second case, 105 msec. In addition, there was a small increment in the gaze duration on the word following *killer*, approximately 55 msec, suggesting that some readers may have continued to compute the inference while moving onto the next word. Thus, the eye–mind assumption may have to take into account the possibility of some spillover of processing onto the gaze on the next word when the computation is extremely demanding.

The characteristics of the word to the right also have a negligible influence on the time spent on the fixated word. If the reader usually semantically processed word $N + 1$ while fixating word $N$, the length and frequency of word $N + 1$ should influence the time on word $N$. To test this, we separately analyzed those cases in which the readers fixated both word $N$ and $N + 1$, and those in which they fixated word $N$ and skipped word $N + 1$. As Table 17.2 shows, the length and frequency of word $N + 1$ have no appreciable effect on the gaze duration on word $N$, even when word $N + 1$ is skipped. This suggests that readers usually do not encode and access words to the right of the word that they are fixating, suggesting that the span of semantic processing is fairly small. In cases in which the next word is encoded and accessed, the processing takes either a small amount of time or a constant amount, relative to the processes associated with the currently fixated word.

Although the span of semantic processing is small, there are some cases in which the reader encodes and accesses a word during the fixation on a preceding word. We hypothesized that this was most likely to have occurred in those cases in which the reader had fixated a function word and then skipped over an immediately following content word. The conjecture was that the content word was encoded parafoveally and processed during the gaze on the function word. We analyzed this subset of the data and found that the length and frequency of the skipped content word accounted for 6% of the variance in the gaze duration on the function word. The length and frequency of the function word accounted for only 1% of this variance. These cases are relatively infrequent; only 3.5% of the gazes were on function words adjacent to a skipped content word (at locations that were not at the beginning or end of a line or sentence).

## 1. SKIPPING FUNCTION WORDS

There was additional evidence that readers could sometimes semantically process words adjacent to the word they were fixating. The evidence was that readers were somewhat selective about which words they skipped. When word length is

**TABLE 17.2**
**Variance in the Conditionalized Mean Gaze Duration
on Word $N$ Accounted for by Regression[a]**

| Independent variables: length and frequency of | Reader fixated word $N-1$ (%) | Reader did not fixate word $N-1$ (%) |
|---|---|---|
| Word $N$ | 23.8 | 25.1 |
| Word $N$ and $N-1$ | 24.0 | 25.6 |
| Word $N-1$ | 0.4 | 0.2 |
| | Reader fixated word $N+1$ (%) | Reader did not fixate word $N+1$ (%) |
| Word $N$ | 24.2 | 18.1 |
| Word $N$ and $N+1$ | 24.7 | 19.9 |
| Word $N+1$ | 0.4 | 0.5 |

[a] The total variance accounted for by these analyses is reduced from that of the original analysis because the mean gaze durations are based on less than half the number of observations in the original analysis and because there are fewer independent variables.

held constant by considering only three-letter words, three-letter function words still have a significantly lower probability of fixation (.40) than do three-letter content words (.57), $F(1, 265) = 45.37$, $p < .01$. This analysis was restricted to 267 three-letter words in the text that neither began nor ended a line or a sentence. The probability of fixation was .29 for 37 occurrences of *and*, .40 for 122 occurrences of *the*, .47 for 47 other three-letter function words (such as *was*, *may, can, but, for, off, has*), and .57 for 61 three-letter content words (such as *act*, *red, use, ant, run, two, not*). This result replicates O'Regan (1979), who found readers were less likely to fixate *the* than three-letter verbs. The result suggests that readers sometimes encode at least some aspects of a word without directly fixating it and that this occurs more frequently for short, predictable function words.

It should not be assumed that all unfixated words are completely visually encoded, in the sense that their constituent letters enter into the recognition process. In some cases, the context plus some minimal visual information such as word length and shape may be sufficient cues for lexical access. This may be particularly true for common function words (like *a, the,* and *and*). Some unfixated words may be inferred on the basis of prior and subsequent context. Finally, some words may not be processed at all. We have all had the experience of reading something that just did not make sense and rereading it to discover that we had missed a word. In skimming, many words are not encoded, semantically processed, or inferred (Just, Carpenter, & Masson, 1981), and some of the skipped words in normal reading may fall into this category as well.

## D.    The Role of Parafoveal Encoding

Research on perceptual processes has shown that different information is available at different distances from the locus of fixation. Rayner (1975) found that gross word shape and word length information are available perhaps as far away as 12 character spaces. However, semantic interpretation may only occur for a word that is directly fixated or immediately adjacent. Rayner's (1975) study found that when a nonword was embedded in a text, the fixation duration was considerably elevated if the reader directly fixated the nonword; the duration was much less elevated if the reader fixated on the last two letters of the adjacent word to the left; and it was not elevated at all if the reader fixated farther to the left of the nonword, suggesting a very small span of semantic processing.

The analysis of our eye fixation results and the results reported by Rayner (1975) allow us to outline in more detail how parafoveal encoding processes may interface with cognitive processes. Our approach must deal with the possibility that a reader is processing some word proximal to the one he or she is fixating, and must attempt to estimate the probability of such events and the extent (i.e., depth) of the processing when they do occur.

There are several ways to obtain evidence that a reader is processing some word other than the one he or she is fixating. One way is to change the word at some point between the time when the word could be processed extrafoveally and the time when it is directly fixated, and then measure some aspect of performance that indicates that the subject noticed the change. This is a paradigm that Rayner (1975) used, and an elevation in the fixation duration following the change was an indication that the reader noticed the information that had been present prior to the change. Since there was a reliable elevation if the reader had fixated close enough to the changed word on the preceding fixation, it can be concluded that on some proportion of the trials, some proportion of the readers had encoded the word before having fixated it. However, this result does not permit us to estimate the frequency of occurrence of such encodings.

Another way to obtain evidence that a word adjacent to the fixated one is being processed is to find that the gaze duration on a given word is influenced by the properties of the neighboring words. We reported that in general the gaze duration on word $N$ is unaffected by the length and frequency of word $N - 1$ or word $N + 1$, with two exceptions. One exception is Rayner's (1975) result, described earlier, in which a fixation within three character spaces to the left of a nonword was somewhat elevated. A second exception is the occasional gazes on a function word followed by a skipped content word. The gaze duration on the fixated function word is modestly influenced by the length and frequency of the skipped content word, accounting for 6% of the variance.

A third index of the processing of words that are not fixated is the systematic skipping of certain classes of words, which could occur only if some discriminative property of the words (their position in the sentence, length, shape, constituent letters, and so on) is encoded before they are fixated. The analyses of three-letter words suggests that on some occasions they receive some processing while the reader is on the adjacent word. But we do not know how often this occurs, nor do we know what kind of information is being encoded. It is possible to recognize a great proportion of the three-letter function words on the basis of the prior syntactic context and the length and shape of the two words *the* and *and*.

The conclusion from all these results is that there is some probability of encoding sufficient information from a word adjacent to the fixated word so that it can be accessed. This is more likely to occur for short function words. When it does occur, the gaze duration on the fixated word generally is not influenced.

The general pattern of results above can be explained as follows. The reader encodes and accesses the word fixated, in keeping with the immediacy and eye–mind assumptions. In addition, the reader can encode the initial letters of an immediately adjacent word, but only in those cases where the locus of fixation happens to be very close to the boundary of the currently fixated word.[2] First

---

[2]We have described the encoding process as though only the word to the right can be processed and not the word to the left. Evidence suggests that such a bias is present in readers of English, at least for content words.

consider the case in which the immediately adjacent letters constitute a short function word (*the*) or phrase (*and the*). These may be encoded and accessed concurrently with the processing of the fixated word. Such function words and phrases are short, frequent, relatively predictable, and semantically impoverished and so would contribute little to the processing duration of the current word. In some contexts, a short content word may be sufficiently frequent, predictable, and impoverished, and hence, be more likely to be skipped. If the processing of an unfixated word is completed before the fixated word is entirely processed (as would generally be the case if the unfixated word were a short frequent word), then the next saccade tends to be longer, to skip over the adjacent word that has been processed without fixation. If the unfixated word requires processing time beyond that required by the fixated word, then the next saccade is targeted at the unfixated word that was not processed to completion. The fact that not all short inferrable words and phrases are skipped may partially reflect the fact that readers' fixations are not always close to the beginning of the next word. In this scheme, many short function words are skipped because they have been processed.

Now consider the case where the adjacent word is long, less predictable, less frequent, or semantically richer—a description that is true of most content words and some function words (e.g., *however*). The adjacent word generally cannot be encoded or accessed before the currently fixated word has been processed to completion. The current word is processed and a saccade is programmed to bring the word on the right into foveal position. Thus, the word on the right will have almost no influence on the duration of the currently fixated word, although, it may influence the decision about where to fixate next.

The decision of where to fixate next is not entirely a function of the information received in the current fixation. It is also influenced by more global factors, such as the readers' attentiveness, whether they are reading carefully, carelessly, or skimming. As we mentioned earlier, not all skipped words are necessarily semantically processed in normal reading. In addition, the decision of where to fixate may also be influenced by the local difficulty and importance of the segment (see Just *et al.*, 1981). If the exact same words occur in a more difficult context or at a point where the information is cued as important, readers appear to fixate more densely. The decision about where to fixate may also be influenced by word length and shape information, which is available farther into the periphery. Finally, it also appears to be influenced by individual and developmental differences among readers (Daneman & Carpenter, 1981; Jackson & McClelland, 1975).

We have proposed a detailed account of the processing of unfixated words that is consistent with the available evidence. The skipping phenomenon seems to be an integral part of reading an orthography like English. However, we also stress that content words in these passages are generally fixated, and in any case, words that are skipped have little effect on the gaze durations on fixated words. The next sections show how the gaze durations on fixated words can be used to examine specific processes and the influence of the text on their duration.

# III.  A General Theory and a Specific Reading Model

A central characteristic of reading, and of most complex cognitive tasks, is that it requires collaboration among a variety of processes. Consequently, any general theory of reading must provide a structured forum for the interaction of processes, as well as mechanisms to account for the specific computations that are based on word, sentence, and text-level information. In this section, we describe both components. The first is a theory of human processing that has general properties that are applicable to more than reading. The second component is a specific computer model of reading, called READER, that operates within the general theory and was developed to account for the time course and content of reading. The reading simulation was motivated by the human experimental work (Just & Carpenter, 1980), and it is described in more detail elsewhere (Thibadeau, Just, & Carpenter, 1982).

## A.  CAPS

The general theory is a Collaborative Activation-based Production System (CAPS). Production systems are formalisms in which the procedural knowledge is embodied in a set of condition–action rules (Newell, 1980). The condition part specifies what element(s) should be present in (or absent from) working memory to enable the action. For example, one parsing production in READER specifies that if an article (*the, an,* or *a*) has been encoded (condition), a slot for a noun phrase should be established (action).

Productions are executed in recognize–act cycles. On each cycle, the contents of working memory are assessed and all productions whose conditions are satisfied are executed concurrently, modifying the contents of working memory. Then the new contents of working memory are assessed and another cycle occurs, and so on. This processing mode corresponds to the immediacy assumption in that a process is executed as soon as the enabling conditions are present. READER, for example, does not routinely buffer information; a production will execute as soon as working memory contains sufficient information to initiate it.

CAPS allows several productions to fire at the same time, meaning that several computations may occur concurrently. For example, having encoded *hammer* and accessed the concept, the reader can simultaneously compute that it is used as a noun, that it is an instrument, and that it may be coreferential with a previously mentioned hammer. The fact that several computations may go on concurrently allows different processes to influence each other, not only by feeding the results of one computation into another, but also by being exposed to (and potentially influenced by) each other's partial results in working memory.

READER's knowledge base consists of propositions in the form of concept–relation–concept triplets, constituting a semantic network. Every proposition has an associated numerical activation level or confidence value that can be modified (incremented or decremented) by the productions. The modification is often linearly related to the activation level of one of the production's condition elements. Thus, a production can direct activation to a given proposition, with the size of the modification determined by the activation level of another proposition. It is possible for several different productions to collaboratively increase READ-ER's belief in a particular piece of information to some threshold level, where one production alone would have failed to do so. If there are two or more alternative interpretations of some proposition, each interpretation may accumulate support-ing evidence until one of their activation levels reaches threshold and becomes the accepted interpretation. For example, in the reading simulation, the word–concept *before* might be retrieved with two associated interpretations; the temporal interpretation would have a certain activation level (say .5), and the locative interpretation would have a lower activation level (say .3), reflecting their relative frequencies in American English. However, a preceding context concern-ing location could increase the activation of the locative hypothesis and bring it to threshold, thus ending the subthreshold debate.

## B.  READER

READER works within the CAPS framework, using concurrent productions, directed activation, and subthreshold debate. READER consists of 225 produc-tions that embody the lexical, syntactic, semantic, and schema-level knowledge necessary to read one passage and construct a representation of the information. Each traditional "stage" of reading such as encoding, lexical access, parsing, and so on, is realized as a number of productions in its long-term procedural knowl-edge base. Currently, READER has a vocabulary sufficient to read only one passage. However, as we show, many of READER's mechanisms are quite general and can be used to explain a variety of processes we have found in human reading. Like human readers, READER identifies and accesses individual word concepts. It determines how word meanings combine to produce the meaning representation of a sentence by doing something resembling a conceptual dependency analysis (Schank, 1972). It checks for noun–verb agreement, assigns case roles, and iden-tifies referents of described objects. In addition, READER possesses a schema of a scientific text that specifies the general categories of information to expect, such as the mechanism's name, purpose, operating principles, applications, examples, and so on. The schema guides the inference processes during reading and orga-nizes the subsequent recall.

The structure of CAPS and READER allow both quantitative and qualitative comparisons between READER's performance and human reading data. The number of cycles READER requires to interpret various words and phrases can be compared to human gaze durations. In addition, READER constructs a represen-tation of the text and uses it to recall the text so that the content of what READER recalls can be compared to what human readers recall. We have found that READER provides a good account of both reading times and recall

(Thibadeau *et al.*, 1982). In the next sections, we describe the mechanisms and their empirical underpinning in more detail.

## IV.   The Mechanisms of Reading

### A.   Encoding and Accessing Processes

The first mechanisms that we discuss are those that encode words from their written form into an internal representation of the word percept. The major results are from the experiment described earlier, in which undergraduate students read scientific passages. One very striking result from the analysis of the reading times is that gaze duration increased linearly with word length, whether length was measured in number of letters or number of syllables. Figure 17.2 shows both the mean gaze duration and the conditionalized mean gaze duration on a word as a function of its length (measured in number of characters) and the logarithm of its normative frequency. Although number of letters accounted for slightly more of the total variance than did number of syllables, there were clear syllable effects. For example, digits consistently took longer than would be predicted on the basis of the number of characters (see also Pynte, 1974). The most likely resolution is that both letters and syllables are functional units in reading. The word length effects are extremely robust. Not only have they been found with these scientific texts, but similar effects were found in another study involving long narratives (2000 words) taken from *Reader's Digest* and long expository passages from *Scientific American* (Just *et al.*, 1981).

The proposed mechanism to account for the word length effects is that word encoding processes operate on successive parts of a word, such that the duration of the encoding process is sensitive to subword orthographic length. There is a strong bias in favor of processing the units from left to right. The subword units could be syllables or letters, but READER currently uses letters.

There exists an alternative but less satisfactory account of the word length effect that does not depend entirely on a sequential encoding process. The alternative account is that long words are difficult to see with sufficient acuity within a single eye fixation, so that longer words are more likely to require more fixations. For example, a reader fixating near the beginning of a long word might be more likely to require a second fixation to bring the letters at the end of the word into clear vision. Two sources of evidence suggest that this alternative account is not satisfactory. The first is that word length effects are present even for very short words having less than five characters. As Figure 17.2 shows, two-letter words take less time than three-letter words, and these take less time than four-letter words, and so forth. This is true even for the conditionalized mean gaze durations, where the dependent variable does not include differential probabilities of fixation. Words that are two, three, four, or five letters long are within the span of apprehension, and there should be little need for a second fixation to make all the

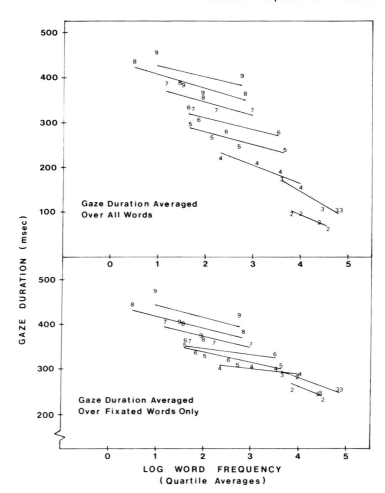

FIGURE 17.2. *(Top) The mean gaze duration on a word as a function of the logarithm of its frequency and its length in number of characters (the parameter on the curves). Each point represents the mean of a quartile of the words of that length. (Bottom). The same function except that the dependent measure is the conditionalized mean gaze duration.*

letters visually perceptible. The encoding hypothesis easily accounts for this word length effect, whereas the acuity hypothesis does not.

The second data that are difficult to reconcile with an acuity explanation come from an experiment with a different mode of presenting the text, one that did not require the reader to make eye movements to read the text. Instead, successive words were presented one word at a time, centered on the screen and the reader pressed a button to terminate the presentation of the word and to begin the presentation of the next word (Just, Carpenter, & Woolley, 1982). The time between successive button presses reflects the duration of processes operating on the displayed word. Even in this condition, in which eye movements play a minimal role, the time readers spent on a word was linearly related to its length. The effect was present for even short words, two, three and four characters long. Both results suggest that the source of the length effect is best explained by a sequential constituent encoding process.

READER generates word length effects because it encodes a word letter by letter, forming chunks and looking for subword units and then for word units. When a word has more letters or syllables, READER has more encoding cycles and may form more chunks. Hence, the time that READER spends on a word tends to increase with the length of the word, similar to what is observed in the human reading times. Some very short and frequent words, like *the* and *and* might be coded as a single chunk; but overall, frequency has effects that are independent of length.

### 1. LEXICAL ACCESS MECHANISMS

As Figure 17.2 illustrates, over the entire range of lengths, less frequent words were fixated for a longer duration. This was true for both the unconditionalized and conditionalized gaze duration. The effect followed a log function; that is, small differences among infrequent words had comparable effects to large differences among frequent words. The effect of frequency, like that of word length, is robust. A very similar function was found in the button pressing paradigm described earlier and in the eye fixation experiment with long narrative and expository texts.

Length and frequency effects are additive, suggesting that they may arise from different processes. The locus of the frequency effect for READER is in lexical access, retrieving a word's meaning. In READER, lexical access is direct access, rather than search through a dictionary. The access mechanism is based on the idea of self-activation. Each concept in READER's lexicon has a base level of activation that is linearly related to the normative frequency of the corresponding word. When a word is encoded, the word percept directs activation to the underlying concept. The concept then starts activating itself over successive cycles, such that the added activation is proportional to the immediately preceding level of activation. So, if the base level activation were .6, after one cycle of self-activation the level would be $(.6 + .6y)$, where $y$ is some constant. This continues until the concept reaches a fixed threshold that is the same for all words. In this scheme, the number of cycles of self-activation necessary to reach threshold is a log function of a word's normative frequency.

### 2. THE EFFECT SIZE ISSUE

Word length and frequency account for a relatively high proportion of the variation in the mean gaze duration on words. In the experiment involving scientific texts, the two variables alone account for 69% of the variance, the other variables alone account for 37%, and all 11 variables together account for 79%.

The other variables coded whether the word introduced a topic, began a line, was at the end of a sentence or paragraph, was totally new, was a digit, a modified noun, an inferrable function word, or the first content word in the passage. For the conditionalized mean gaze duration, length and frequency alone account for 40%, the other 9 variables alone account for 39%, and all 11 variables account for 60%. (The variances accounted for are not additive because some variables are intercorrelated).

There is a temptation to equate proportion of variance accounted for by a variable with the theoretical importance of the underlying process, but such an inference is unwarranted for at least three reasons (see Sechrest & Yeaton, 1979, for a discussion of "effect size" issues). First, the variance accounted for by a factor is not an inherent property of the factor; it depends on the variation of that factor relative to other factors in the task. The current texts involved words of widely varying lengths and frequencies. If a text were constructed of words of a small range of lengths and frequencies, then word length and frequency would account for a much lower proportion of the variance. Second, these variables may account for a relatively high proportion of the variance because we know how to measure them; as the metrics improve for describing higher-level factors, they may account for more of the variance. Finally, it is clear that encoding and accessing words are not sufficient processes for reading; it is also necessary to interrelate concepts to form the meanings of phrases, clauses, sentences, the text, and the referential domain.

In spite of these caveats, there is a theoretically interesting implication of the finding that length and frequency effects are generally more robust than the effects of the other variables. The processes influenced by length and frequency appear to be more uniform across readers and texts; a given word is encoded and accessed relatively similarly by all readers. In contrast, the higher-level processes may be more variable across readers in several aspects, such as their time of enablement, their duration, and their content. One way to reduce the variability is to experimentally manipulate when a higher-level process is executed or to make it especially difficult, so that almost every reader will take extra time. Later sections of this chapter describe experiments that manipulate the difficulty of higher-level syntactic and semantic analyses and examine the effects on the pattern and duration of eye fixations.

### 3. THE INTERPRETATION OF REGRESSION WEIGHTS

The way a regression weight is interpreted depends on whether the theory specifies that the process operates concurrently with other processes or sequentially. If it is believed that two processes are executed sequentially, the interpretation of the regression weights is straightforward; the regression weight indicates the amount of extra processing time per stimulus unit. For example, a regression weight of 32 msec associated with word length is interpreted as an extra 32 msec of encoding time per letter. However, a regression weight is given a different interpretation if the underlying process is assumed to be executed concurrently with other processes. In that case, the regression weight indicates the increase (or decrease) in the total processing time when that process is executed; the weight does not indicate the total duration of the process. For example, if the regression weight for sentence-final words is 100 msec, we can infer that these words are associated with extra processing that extends 100 msec longer than the other concurrent processes, although the absolute duration is unknown.

### 4. NOVEL WORDS

Some words in the scientific passages, such as *staphylococci* and *thermoluminescence*, were probably entirely new to the readers. These words were fixated for an especially long time, 802 msec beyond what would be predicted by their infrequency and their length. We hypothesized that when such a word is encountered, the reader tries to infer its meaning and construct a dictionary entry with information that includes its orthographic, phonological, syntactic, and semantic properties (as far as they can be determined). This entry will help the reader identify the word if it is encountered again later in the text, and the entry will aid the reader in later recalling the word.

READER also spends extra cycles on entirely novel words. If the word is not in its lexicon, READER tries first to identify the word by segmenting out subwords, prefixes, and affixes. Thus, READER can identify the plural of a noun or the past tense of a verb even if it never saw that particular variant before. But if these processes fail, READER creates a new word–concept, taking considerable additional time, just as in the case of human readers.

If the additional time on a novel word results because the reader is creating a new lexical entry, then the next time the reader sees this word the time should be less. The human reading data support this. Processing a novel word the second time is much faster. We also found a more general repetition effect; certain other words were also fixated for less time on the second and subsequent occurrences (Thibadeau *et al.*, 1982). Interestingly, the repetition effect was limited to topical words, like *red fire ant, fluorocarbons, radioisotopes, vitreous humor, Pteranodon, glial cells.* Nontopical words did not show repetition effects. This suggests that the repetition effect is not due entirely to faster encoding, but in part, may be due to relating topical words to a schema.

## B. Immediacy in Lexical Access

Frequency alone does not determine the time course and outcome of the lexical access process. It also depends on the preceding context. One of our eye fixation studies examined how context interacts with frequency to determine which meaning is chosen as the interpretation of an ambiguous word. The second focus of the study was inconsistency detection—when does a reader detect an inconsistency and how does he or she recover from it (Carpenter & Daneman, 1981).

We will describe the experimental paradigm in some detail because it is used in a number of experiments. Our subjects read "garden-path" passages, such as the following:

> *The young man turned his back on the rock concert stage and looked across the resort lake. Tomorrow was the annual, one-day fishing contest and fishermen would invade the place. Some of the best bass guitarists in the country would come to this spot. The usual routine of the fishing resort would be disrupted by the festivities.*

If asked to read this passage aloud, most people initially give *bass* in line 3 the pronunciation corresponding to the "fish" meaning, the meaning primed by the earlier references to fishing. But the "fish" interpretation is inconsistent with the subsequent disambiguating word, *guitarists,* and a resolution requires the reinterpretation of *bass* to mean "a low music note." These processes, the initial interpretation, the detection of the inconsistency, and its resolution can be seen in a reader's pattern of eye fixations.

## 1. A PROTOCOL

A typical reader's eye fixations, shown in Figure 17.3, illustrate the major processes. The subject read the target sentence (indicated in large print) embedded in the paragraph given above. The reader's oral protocol, indicated in small print, gives both his initial interpretation and subsequent reinterpretation of the ambiguous word. The sequence of eye fixations is denoted by the numbers above and below the words in the sentence. The fixation duration is indicated in milliseconds below the sequence number. The reader made a series of forward fixations until he came to the word *guitarists,* then he reread the word *bass* (fixations 6 and 7) and finished the sentence (fixations 8 to 12).

We have interpreted the gaze duration on the ambiguous word as the time that it takes to encode the word, retrieve an interpretation, and integrate it with the representation of the text. The long duration on the disambiguating word (fixation 5) is interpreted as reflecting the reader's attempt to integrate the word *guitarist* and his discovery of the inconsistency. At that point he regressed to the word *bass,* indicating that he had found a source of inconsistency. The oral reading indicates that this reader successfully recovered by discovering and integrating the alternative meaning.

One interesting point in this protocol is that it illustrates the delay between eye and voice, and the relative lack of delay between eye and mind. The voice lags behind the eye, giving rise to the typical eye–voice span. It also indicates that the eye–mind span is short. The reader typically detects the inconsistency when he or she fixates the first word that is inconsistent; that word is usually verbalized at a later time. Thus the eye and mind are close together in time, whereas the voice lags behind both of them.

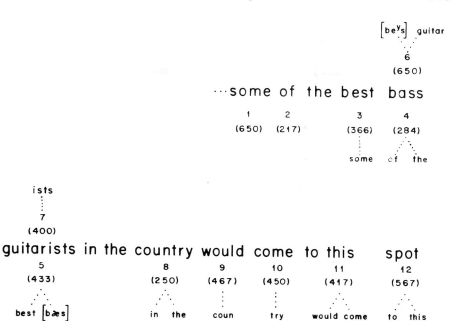

FIGURE 17.3. *The* bass *target sentence with a reader's eye fixations and read aloud protocol in small print. The numbers 1–12 indicate the sequence of fixations; the forward fixations are indicated by the numbers below the fixated word, and the regressive fixations are indicated by the numbers above the fixated word. The numbers in parentheses indicate the gaze duration (in msec). The read aloud protocol shows that* bass *was initially interpreted as [b ae s], meaning "fish," and then revised to [be Y s], meaning "music note." [From Carpenter & Daneman, 1981.]*

## 2.  ACCESSING CONCEPTS

As we described in the section on lexical access, retrieving a concept is not an all or none process. There is a subthreshold state in which more than one candidate interpretation may receive at least some activation. The first one to reach threshold becomes the accepted interpretation. There are two major sources of activation that determine which concepts reach threshold. One is the prior context, which includes structures in working memory derived from information in the prior text and from previous knowledge about the topic. For example, the context in the sample paragraph in the last section included references to fishermen and a fishing resort. These help to partially activate the "fish" concept before the word *bass* is fixated.

As the study with scientific texts indicated, a second determinant of activation is a word's frequency. However, in the case of polysemous words, activation of alternative meanings depends on the relative frequencies of each meaning. The effect is striking with ambiguous words that have one very common interpretation and one uncommon interpretation, such as the "drain" and "tailor" interpretation of *sewer*. In the phrase *There is also one sewer near our house*, most readers interpret *sewer* to mean "drain" rather than "tailor," because the "drain" interpretation is more frequent. In the READER model this also occurs because the interpretation with the higher base activation level will reach threshold sooner.

### 3. THE ORAL INTERPRETATION RESULTS

To study how these processes influence lexical access, we developed passages like the one above, using ambiguous words such as *bass*, *sewer*, *tears*, and *wind* and had 20 college students read them aloud while we monitored their eye fixations. As we predicted, readers generally gave the ambiguous word the pronunciation that was consistent with the context. However, the relative frequencies of the two interpretations also had an influence. For words like *sewer*, readers chose the infrequent meaning only 5% of the time in paragraphs that primed the infrequent meaning. In contrast, when the context primed a meaning with a moderate or high frequency, it was given 80% of the time. The fact that the very infrequent meanings are seldom chosen reflects the strong bias that readers have toward common interpretations; even context effects cannot entirely compensate for this bias. This result suggests that context may play a different role in helping to select one interpretation of a polysemous word, depending on whether or not the various interpretations are approximately equally likely. If the two meanings have similar frequencies, both meanings may be retrieved, with context selecting the more appropriate one (Swinney, 1979). But if the two meanings have very different frequencies, the less common meaning may not be retrieved at all and a strong context is necessary to bring it to threshold (see also Simpson, 1981).

The time readers take to encode, access, and integrate the ambiguous word should be less if the retrieved interpretation has a high frequency and matches the preceding context. These processes should be reflected in the time readers spend on the ambiguous word. The results clearly confirmed the predictions. Readers spent less time on the ambiguous word when the interpretation they chose (as indicated by the oral protocol) was the higher frequency interpretation and was consistent with the context. The fact that both context and a concept's frequency affect the time readers spent on the ambiguous word provides further support for the immediacy and eye–mind assumptions—readers are encoding the word, selecting a meaning, and trying to integrate it while fixating the word itself.

## C. Detecting Inconsistencies and Revising Interpretations

To recover from having previously chosen the wrong interpretation of a word, a reader must realize that some inconsistency exists, determine that the problem resides with an earlier word, and then revise that earlier interpretation. For example, readers who interpreted *sewer* as "drain" would find *who* anomalous in the sentence *There is also one sewer near our house who makes terrific suits*. The source of the inconsistency between *sewer* and *who* resides in the interpretation of *sewer.* Detecting the inconsistency and attempting to recover should take extra processing time, reflected in longer gazes. If readers detect the inconsistency on the disambiguating word, there should be longer gazes on that word and more regressions after it is fixated. The results supported the hypothesis. Readers spent more time on the first disambiguating word and on the entire disambiguating phrase when it was inconsistent, and they were more likely to regress to the previous ambiguous word.

Readers had relatively little difficulty recovering from inconsistencies if the interpretation they had incorrectly rejected was relatively frequent, as in the *bass* example. They had much more difficulty and often did not recover if the incorrectly rejected interpretation was very infrequent, such as in the case of *sewer, minute, buffet,* and *row.* These cases are also interesting because the patterns of eye fixation reveal different recovery processes.

A protocol for one sentence can be used to illustrate the general results. Figure

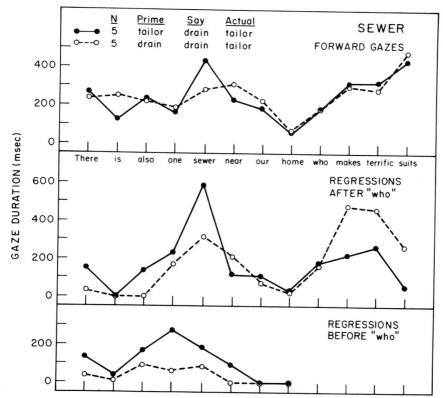

**FIGURE 17.4.** *The mean gaze duration on each word of the* sewer *target sentence for readers in the two context conditions. All 10 subjects initially read* sewer *as meaning "drain." The top panel shows the forward gazes; the middle panel shows regressions after readers fixated* who; *the bottom panel shows regressions before readers fixated* who. *[From Carpenter & Daneman, 1981.]*

17.4 shows the time on each word of the sentence *There is also one sewer near our home who makes terrific suits* for two groups of readers. One was primed to interpret *sewer* as "drain," and the other, as "tailor." The three panels in Figure 17.4 show three different gaze duration measures. The top panel is the mean gaze duration on each word, composed of forward fixations and averaged across readers, counting 0 msec for a reader who did not fixate the word. The second panel shows the average time spent in regressions after readers encountered the first disambiguating word, *who*. The bottom panel shows the duration of regressions before the disambiguating word was fixated.

Irrespective of the context, everyone initially pronounced *sewer* according to the more frequent "drain" meaning. Readers who had the "tailor" context had more difficulty in accessing and integrating "drain," as reflected in the longer time in forward fixations on the word *sewer* (the top panel) and the greater time spent in regressions (the bottom panel). Both groups had difficulty with the phrase *who makes terrific suits*, because it was inconsistent with their prior interpretation. The difficulty is reflected in the longer forward gazes on this phrase (the top panel) and the long times spent in regressions (the middle panel).

Readers who initially had problems integrating their interpretation of the ambiguous word were more likely to recover. (Recovery was assessed from their oral reading and by questions asked after the passage was read, such as *Who made terrific suits?*) The eye fixation protocol shows that these readers spent more time on *sewer* after the disambiguation. The readers who had less trouble initially accessing and integrating *sewer*, because they had been primed to interpret it as "drain," spent less time on *sewer* after encountering the inconsistency, spent more time on the disambiguating phrase, and were less likely to recover. This suggests that error recovery processes focus on places that contain a trace of earlier difficulties.

## D. Individual Differences

Recently, we have explored how individual differences in reading skill interact with the text to determine whether a reader recovers from a misinterpretation (Daneman & Carpenter, 1981b). Our proposal is that the functional capacity of working memory plays an important role in reading comprehension performance. Traditional tests of short-term memory, such as digit-span and word-span tests, do not correlate with reading comprehension performance. The reason for the low correlation may be that such tests are primarily tests of passive storage capacity. For example, in a digit-span test, the subject must recognize and encode very familiar digits and try to maintain some record of their order of occurrence. This traditional test reflects a view of short-term memory as primarily a storage place with a fixed number of slots, with the number varying among individuals. In contrast, current conceptions of working memory view it as having both processes and storage components (Baddeley, & Hitch, 1974; Hunt, 1978). What is needed to test the proposal regarding functional capacity was a task that requires more taxing processes, especially processes that are related to reading itself.

We developed a reading span test that includes both processing and storage components (Daneman & Carpenter, 1980). In the test, the subject reads a set of sentences and at the end of the set recalls the final word of each sentence. The subject's reading span is the number of sentences for which he or she can success-fully recall the final words. We have found that among college students, the range of reading spans is usually 2 to 5.5 sentences. Unlike the traditional digit span and word span tests, reading span does correlate with global reading comprehension test scores; a correlation typically lies between .45 and .6 (Daneman & Carpen-ter, 1981b). The correlation between reading span and comprehension is even higher (.7–.9) if the comprehension test taps specific comprehension abilities, such as the ability to answer a question about a fact mentioned in the passage or the ability to relate a pronoun to a distant prior referent (Daneman & Carpenter, 1980).

Reading span also correlates with the ability to recover from inconsistencies in garden-path passages. Readers with low spans recover less often than do readers with intermediate or high spans. Poorer readers have particular difficulty if a sentence boundary intervenes between the ambiguous word and the subsequent inconsistency. For example, these poorer readers have more difficulty with *There is also one sewer near our home. He makes terrific suits* than with *There is also one sewer near our home who makes terrific suits.* The explanation is that ends of sentences are often places where readers do additional wrap-up processes that may tax working memory and purge it of at least part of the verbatim representation (Jarvella, 1971; Just & Carpenter, 1980). The processing of a sentence boundary taxes the readers with a small working-memory capacity, making it less likely that they recover from an inconsistency whose resolution requires information from a preceding sentence.

## E.  Parsing Processes

A central aspect of comprehension is the parsing process—determining the syntactic and semantic roles and boundaries of sentence constituents. One major approach to parsing has been a syntactically oriented one, in which determining the syntactic roles of the words in a sentence constituted the core of comprehen-sion (see Fodor, Bever, & Garrett, 1974; Kimball, 1973; Marcus, 1980). This approach often focuses on function words, suggesting that these words narrow the range of possible roles that an upcoming content word may play. At the other extreme is the semantic approach which emphasizes how the semantic properties of the major constituents plus schematic and pragmatic knowledge will often determine the roles of the constituents in a sentence (Schank, 1972). For exam-ple, a reader can infer the roles of *boy*, *apple*, and *ate* without the benefit of syntactic information. However, neither the syntactic nor the semantic approach alone is entirely satisfactory. Our research on parsing suggests that syntactic cues, semantic relations, and referential interpretation all play a role in computing the role of a constituent in a clause or sentence and determining the boundary.

## 1.  PARSING AMBIGUOUS PHRASES

Detection of constituent boundaries depends in part on the ability to find a referent for the candidate constituent. This point is illustrated very clearly in a study that examined parsing processes in a translation task (McDonald & Carpenter, 1981). Bilingual translators read passages in English and translated them into spoken German as quickly as possible as they read. Embedded in the passages were idioms such as *kick the bucket* and *hit the nail right on the head*. Such phrases are of interest because they have different parsings and different interpretations depending on whether they are used idiomatically or literally. If interpreted idiomatically, each such phrase is a single constituent; if interpreted literally, each phrase has more than one constituent, such as *(((hit) (the nail)) (right (on (the (head)))))*. We constructed passages that primed either one interpretation or the other, and found that translators produced very different patterns of eye fixations in the two cases, reflecting the different constituent boundaries of the two types of interpretations. Translators visually scanned each major constituent of a sentence twice. During the first pass, which presumably reflected English comprehension, the translators read at normal speed and paused at the constituent boundary. Then, the gaze returned to the beginning of the constituent for a second, much slower pass during which the translator output the German equivalent. The place at which the translator stopped between the first and second passes indicated how he or she parsed a segment of text.

A typical passage, one that primed a literal translation of *hit the nail right on the head*, described a man, David, who was having problems building a bookshelf and asked his friend, Mike, to help him: *Mike picked up the hammer to show David some basic woodworking techniques. Mike hit the nail right on the head . . . .* During the first pass, the translators scanned to the end of *Mike hit the nail*, stopped, and returned to the beginning of the sentence to translate it. They parsed this as a clause. However, when the context primed an idiomatic meaning, the individual words did not have plausible literal referents. In those cases, the translators did not stop and translate idioms at an internal phrase boundary; they continued until they reached the end of the idiom. The differential parsing pattern reflected in the eye fixations predicted whether the oral translation would be literal or idiomatic. The study suggests that the interpretaton of such ambiguous phrases is determined as the phrase is read, as part of the reader's attempt to integrate the currently processed information with the preceding representation.

## 2.  SPECIFIC HEURISTICS

We are currently exploring the interaction of syntactic and semantic information in some specific parsing heuristics (Carpenter & McDonald, 1981). Our initial research has focused on the words *before* and *after*, which can be prepositions or conjunctions. As a preposition, *before* introduces a phrase that modifies the immediately preceding verb phrase (e.g., *He stood before the jury*). The prepositional phrase is "right-attached" to the verb phrase in a tree structure diagram. As a conjunction, *before* introduces a new clause (e.g., *He stood before the jury entered*). According to one parsing theory, the right-attachment interpretation is preferred, because it results in a simpler structure (Frazier & Fodor, 1978; Kimball, 1973). However, according to the READER model, the preceding context should interact with this syntactic bias to determine which interpretation is chosen.

The experiment that examined the parsing processes used the garden-path procedure, priming one interpretation of an ambiguous word and later presenting confirming or inconsistent information. The stimulus set is illustrated by the sentence in the opening passage of this chapter, which discussed where the student would sit, *Resignedly the student sat before the avunular professor in the rumpled suit entered.* A reader who made the preposition interpretation should spend more time on *entered* than one who made a conjunction interpretation. The subjects read texts using the button-pressing paradigm described earlier. This paradigm provides a measure of processing time for a word or phrase. It also forces the reader to rely exclusively on working memory to recover from an inconsistency, because the previous words are not visually available. We assessed the readers' ultimate interpretation by asking comprehension questions about the target sentence after the passage had been read.

Both the reading times and question–answering data showed that readers had a strong bias to interpret words in accordance with the principle of right attachment but that contextual and semantic cues could modify the interpretation. In addition, the effects were found early in the inconsistent phrase, suggesting that the syntactic analysis does not lag behind the word being fixated.

## 3.   AN OVERVIEW OF PARSING EFFECTS

Parsing difficulties have a large effect on performance in experiments that intentionally make the syntactic assignments difficult. They are also reliably found in normal texts, such as the scientific texts. However, the parsing effects in naturally occurring texts are generally small and account for much less of the variance than do the variables that affect encoding and lexical access. This suggests that parsing processes are concurrent with other processes that are longer or more variable in duration, so that parsing effects are not visible under most circumstances. Nevertheless, an analysis of certain systematic parsing effects has revealed some parsing procedures and suggested that they differ from a popular syntactically based parser, the Augmented Transition Network (ATN).

One parsing effect in the scientific texts was that readers spent less time on nouns that contained multiple modifiers, such as *red fire ant*. On the first occurrence, readers spent a relatively long time on *ant*; however, on subsequent occurrences, the average gaze duration was considerably shortened. One explanation is that the reader could begin constructing a referent for the noun phrase as soon as one or two modifiers were read, such as the words *red fire*, and it was not necessary to wait for the entire phrase. This strategy differentiates human parsing schemes from those proposed by ATNs. As an ATN grammar processes a constituent, it puts the components on a push-down stack until the end of the constituent is reached, at which point it "pops" the stack and processes the entire constituent. This model would suggest that, if anything, nouns that are modified would take longer, since the reader would process the noun and its modifiers after encountering the noun. However, the reading time data suggest that this hypothesis is incorrect and that readers attempt to process constituents as soon as possible, sometimes before the last part of the noun phrase is fixated.

Other parsing effects were found if a phrase caused some momentary difficulty. For example, in the phrase *Flywheels are one. . . ,* readers pause longer than would be expected on *one,* presumably because it is inconsistent in number with the plural subject and verb.

READER's parsing processes were developed to simulate the human reading data (Thibadeau *et al.,* 1982). READER attempts to parse constituents, interpret them, and assign them to referents as soon as possible. It has about 130 productions that constitute the parsing routines for the passage. About 30 of these productions are a "core parser" that is robust over passages. The semantic productions do a conceptual dependency analysis (Schank, 1972), whereas the syntactic productions analyze the sequential aspects of the surface structure. Although READER does not have a complete parser for English, we see no inherent obstacles to expanding READER while maintaining the qualitative features of its design.

## F.  End of Sentence Processing

Although it is clear that readers attempt to interpret words as they are encountered, there also is evidence that some processes are executed at ends of sentences. We have labeled this the sentence wrap-up effect. One source of evidence came from a study in which the texts elicited verb based inferences (Just & Carpenter, 1978). For example, one set of readers received a text that described the discovery of the body of a millionaire who had *died.* Another group read that he had been *killed.* Both groups read a later sentence that described the search for *the murderer.* The first group of readers took longer to read the sentence involving *murderer,* because they had to make a more difficult inference to relate *died* and *murderer.* Part of the longer reading time for the later sentence was localized to the word *murderer* itself, agreeing with the immediacy assumption. However, part of the extra reading time was spent at the end of the sentence. End of sentence effects were also evident in the processing of garden-path sentences with ambiguous words like *sewer* and *bass* (Carpenter & Daneman, 1981). Readers sometimes initiated regressions after the first inconsistent word, but at other times, not until the end of the sentence. In some instances, they may have expected that the rest of the sentence would resolve the difficulty. We also found end of sentence effects in the scientific passages (Just & Carpenter, 1980). Finally, end of sentence effects were found in a study involving narrative texts, but only in those sentences that involved a switch in surface topic from the preceding sentence (Dee–Lucas, Just, Carpenter, & Danemann, in press).

All the evidence cited above for wrap-up processes at ends of sentences has come from correlational studies, in which the effects of other variables such as normative word frequency and word length were statistically controlled using multiple linear regression. Recently, we have also assessed end of sentence effects in an experimental study (Daneman & Carpenter, 1981b). The experiment used texts that were identical up to the sentence boundary. For example, one text was *He found a bat. It was very large and* and the comparison text was *He found a bat that was very large and.* In one set of conditions, the target word was ambiguous (such as *bat*); in another set of texts, the target was an unambiguous control word, but one that constituted a topic switch (like *bird*). The sentences were presented word by word in the button-pressing paradigm described earlier. There was a significant increase in the time on a word that occurred at the end of a sentence, compared to the time on the same word when it was not sentence terminal. The size of the effect was 150 and 200 msec in the silent reading condition and oral reading condition, respectively. Thus, sentence wrap-up effects can be relatively large.

End of sentence effects appear to occur if a sentence contains an extra processing burden. In the scientific passages, the additional processing was caused by the large proportion of novel and important concepts. In the narrative passages, additional processing was required when a sentence introduced a new topic. In the garden-path experiments, the extra processing was caused by the ambiguity and the error recovery. By contrast, we have examined other texts and tasks in which readers do not spend extra time at the end of sentences. The texts had a relatively low proportion of novel concepts and described very predictable events (Just, *et al.*, 1981). This contrast suggests that ends of sentences themselves do not necessarily require additional processes and that they may only be places to finish up integrative processes that could not be completed in mid-sentence. Furthermore, task requirements and individual differences in functional working memory capacity may also affect the probability of some wrap-up processes being held over until the end of the sentence.

## G. Schemas and Inferential Processes

Comprehension depends only in part on the information provided by the text itself; the reader also uses his or her knowledge of the topic. READER makes use of a schema, a frame and slot structure, to organize the information from the scientific texts. Since READER has been developed to comprehend a scientific exposition, READER's schema is specific to this domain. Nevertheless, the general principles of what kind of information is stored and how it is used may be more widely applicable.

To read a passage, READER uses a schema called the Mechanism schema, which specifies the kinds of information a reader expects to find about artificially made devices and biological mechanisms as they are used by human or animal agents. The schema consists of slots that specify the general types of information to be expected, and the slots are filled in the course of comprehension. For example, one slot is that of the mechanism's *name*. Another slot is its *goals*, which specify the end state that the mechanism is used to achieve. A third slot is for the *principles* that relate the mechanism's physical properties and actions to its goals. Another slot is the *exemplar* slot, which contains specific instances of the mechanism.

READER attempts to match what it is reading with the schema slots. One way this is done is by making inferences on the basis of the sentence level representations. For example, if a sentence describes something as a purpose or goal, READER can relate this information to its goals slot. In other cases, READER must make inferences based on probable categories of information and specific cues in the text. Finally, some slots may be filled with default values; if the text does not specify some particular piece of information, READER will assume a likely filler.

Human readers tend to spend different amounts of time on different kinds of information in a schema. For example, we found that readers spend extra time on relatively important pieces of information, like names and goals, relative to exemplars. This is time above and beyond that accounted for by the word level variables (Just & Carpenter, 1980). The explanation is that readers use this additional time to ensure that such information is correctly encoded and will be accessible in memory for later recall.

READER mimics this aspect of human reading. As successive words of a text are encountered, they are evaluated as a potential basis for action by all the productions, including those that attempt to fit the new information into schema slots. The schema level integration actions are actually evoked as soon as enough of the sentence has been processed to indicate how it fits into the schema. The place where the schema production will be evoked depends on the sentence wording and structure. Sometimes an entire clause or sentence must be read to determine its relation to the schema. At other times an arbitrary word within the sentence structure will evoke the production. This is consistent with the results reviewed earlier that integrative processes sometimes occur at the end of the sentence and at other times within the sentence itself (Carpenter & Just, 1977; Dee–Lucas *et al.*, in press).

## V.   Conclusions

The general characteristics of human reading are compatible with the overall theory of the processing architecture embodied in CAPS, and the specific results we have obtained can be accounted for by the READER model. The immediate, collaborative nature of the processes in READER captures important features of human reading. The scope of the model, from perceptual to schema level processes is sufficiently broad to accommodate many other temporal properties of human reading. The specific mechanisms of encoding, lexical access, parsing, and integration are compatible with a variety of detailed empirical results. The research also illustrates the advantage of using eye fixations to study the conceptual aspects of reading, in addition to the more commonly studied perceptual and motor aspects. In this section we discuss some of the issues that arise in using our research approach and suggest directions for the next generation of improvements.

## A. The Gaze Duration Measure

The main dependent variable in the studies we have discussed is mean gaze duration on each word. This measure is appropriate to the grain of the theory. The theory focuses on the comprehension processes that operate at a conceptual level that roughly corresponds to the word, although the theory also involves processing units at levels corresponding to letters, subword units, phrases, clauses, sentences, and schemas. But it is at the level of the word that the main semantic information is indexed. Measuring the processing time on each word simplifies the analysis of effects presumed to affect word level processes. Previous efforts to relate cognitive processes to smaller units of behavior such as individual fixations have been far less successful (e.g., Gaarder, 1975). Moreover, processing times on larger units can easily be derived from word gaze durations simply by aggregating over durations on individual words. In general, the compatibility between the theory and the performance measure in their unit of analysis is probably a major determinant of the success of a detailed modeling enterprise.

## B. Immediacy and Eye–Mind Revisited

The immediacy and eye–mind assumptions address two issues that have been important to reading theories. The first issue concerns the possible delay between the perceptual and cognitive systems. Some theorists have argued that because of saccadic suppression and the necessity for programming subsequent fixations, the cognitive system probably does not operate on the input of the perceptual system soon enough to influence either the duration of the current fixation or the location of the next. Our own research shows that this is not true; the currently fixated word does influence the time spent on that word, either by increasing the fixation duration or by influencing where the next fixation is made (on the same word or on other words).

The second issue concerns the processing of information in units larger than words, which we will refer to as bins. By binning we mean collecting input from several words before processing any one of them. When a bin is filled, either all its constituents are processed, or in a moving bin strategy, only some of the earliest constituents are processed. At the perceptual level, words could be binned by being visually chunked or grouped before being encoded. At the cognitive level, word concepts could be grouped or binned before being interpreted. Positions related to each of these levels have been espoused by various researchers.

One example of a cognitive binning strategy is the "look ahead" strategy of

Kimball (1973) and Marcus (1980), who have proposed that readers look one or two words ahead before deciding the syntactic status of a given word. Looking N words ahead of the word at issue means using a moving bin of size $N+1$. Kimball's scheme has another level of bins as well. Once a word's syntactic status is determined, it is held in a buffer (bin) until the current phrase is complete, at which time it along with the other constituents of the phrase are shunted off for semantic processing. Similarly, it has been suggested that clauses are the functional unit in language processing and that clause boundaries are important enabling conditions for syntactic and semantic analyses (Fodor et al., 1974). Buffering the words of a phrase or clause before analyzing them is an instance of using a variable size stationary bin.

Bouma and deVoogd (1974) have argued for both perceptual and cognitive bins on the grounds of empirical evidence they have collected. They found that readers' self-reported ability to comprehend a text was unaffected by a wide range of variation in the spatial and temporal arrangement of the words. They presented a few words of a text at a time, varying both the number of words per display and the duration of the display. Bouma and DeVoogd concluded that the processing was impervious to the temporal distribution of the input because the words were being buffered before being cognitively processed. One binning mechanism might be an iconic store that allows the cognitive system to lag behind the perceptual system by about two words. Another binning mechanism might be a store in which activated word meanings are held until a lagging syntactic or semantic analysis operates on them. One problem with the results of this experiment is that although subjects reported being able to comprehend the text, they were unable to do so if they expected a comprehension test at the conclusion of the reading. This suggests that the comprehension was unusual, at best, and grossly below normal, at worst. Thus, it is very unclear that the critical criterion of actually being able to comprehend was satisfied in this experiment.

The immediacy of the effects (i.e., the gaze duration response occurs on the very word that provides the stimulus) in our data suggests that mandatory binning does not occur. Interpretive processes of all levels occur as soon as they are enabled. Lower level processes are usually enabled as soon as the word is encoded. However, the point at which higher level integrative processes are enabled is unpredictable. But if the higher level processes are possible to execute immediately (i.e., without the benefit of information to follow), then they *are* executed immediately. This finding clearly shows that binning is not mandatory or fixed.

Contextual influences on immediacy can be illustrated with any word whose interpretation partially depends on another word which has not yet occurred. For example, the extensive meaning of the adjective *large* cannot be computed without knowing what concept it modifies, (e.g., *large insect* versus *large house*). A reader might have to wait until reading the head of the noun phrase to know what *large* modifies, in which case the extensive interpretation would not be immediate. Alternatively, a reader could guess the referent on the basis of the previous context. If a passage repeatedly referred to a *large house*, even the extensive meaning of *large* might be computed immediately on fixating the word *large*. The immediacy assumption states that the interpretation of the current word is computed as soon as possible, rather than routinely waiting until all possibly relevant information from succeeding words has been collected.

What the various bin theories have failed to recognize is that very often the interpretation of a word can be computed immediately. By focusing on sentences out of context, these theories have failed to appreciate that the semantic and pragmatic context, plus biases constructed over years of a person's language use, make the reader's interpretations correct much more often than incorrect. By focusing on infrequent sentence types, they have failed to discover the default strategy of immediate interpretation that succeeds on most sentence types.

## C.    Mental Chronometry in Comprehension

The studies reported in this chapter have shown that analyses of the temporal characteristics of comprehension are useful in modeling the underlying processes. Chronometric techniques, including the study of gaze durations and word and sentence reading times in subject-paced presentations, allow for monitoring the comprehension processes as they occur, rather than making inferences about comprehension on the basis of memory based measures, such as recall, recognition, or question answering. But the primary limitation of chronometric techniques is that they do not reveal the content of the comprehension processes. That must come from another source, either another methodology (such as computer simulation) or the intuitions of the researcher. The content of comprehension refers to what inference the reader made, what interpretation he or she gave an ambiguous word, what information he or she took to be the topic, and so forth. The methodologies that give the most insight into these involve qualitative measures, such as oral reading, recall, recognition, and question answering performance. The weaknesses of each methodology can be partially compensated for by using the methodology in concert with other methods with complementary properties and converging results. Thus, it is important not only to trace the eye movements of a reader, but also to determine what is understood, and what can be remembered or reconstructed. A theory of reading should account for both the time course of the on-line processes and the products of those processes.

### ACKNOWLEDGMENTS

Meredyth Daneman, Diana Dee-Lucas, Janet McDonald, and Robert Thibadeau collaborated in many aspects of the research reported here and their contributions are gratefully acknowledged.

# References

Baddeley, A. D., & Hitch, G. (1974). Working memory. In G. H. Bower (Ed.), *The psychology of learning and motivation* (Vol. 8). New York: Academic Press.

Bouma, H., & deVoogd, A. H. (1974). On the control of eye saccades in reading. *Vision Research*, 14, 273–284.

Carpenter, P. A., & Daneman, M. (1981). Lexical retrieval and error recovery in reading: A model based on eye fixations. *Journal of Verbal Learning and Verbal Behavior, 20,* 137–160.

Carpenter, P. A., & Just, M. A. (1977). Reading comprehension as eyes see it. In M. A. Just & P. A. Carpenter (Eds.), *Cognitive processes in comprehension.* Hillsdale, New Jersey: Erlbaum.

Carpenter, P. A., & McDonald, J. L. (1981). *Syntactic and semantic influences in parsing ambiguous phrases.* Pittsburgh: Carnegie–Mellon University, 1981.

Daneman, M., & Carpenter, P. A. (1980). Individual differences in working memory and reading. *Journal of Verbal Learning and Verbal Behavior,* 1980, **19,** 450–466.

Daneman, M., & Carpenter, P. A. (1981). *Developmental differences in reading and detecting semantic inconsistencies.* Pittsburgh: Carnegie–Mellon University. (a)

Daneman, M., & Carpenter, P.A. (1981). *The functional role of working memory in recovering from semantic inconsistencies.* Pittsburgh: Carnegie–Mellon University. (b)

Dee–Lucas, D., Just, M. A., Carpenter, P. A., & Daneman, M. What eye fixations tell us about the time course of text integration. In R. Groner & P. Fraisse (Eds.), *Cognition and eye movements.* Amsterdam: North Holland and Berlin: Deutscher Verlag der Wissenschaften, in press.

Fodor, J. A., Bever, T. G., & Garrett, M. F. (1974). *The psychology of language: An introduction to psycholinguistics and generative grammar.* New York: McGraw–Hill.

Frazier, L., & Fodor, J. D. (1978). The sausage machine: A new two-stage parsing model. *Cognition.* 6, 291–325.

Gaarder, K. R. (1975). *Eye movements, vision and behavior.* Washington, D.C.: Hemisphere Publishing Corporation.

Hunt, E. (1978). Mechanics of verbal ability. *Psychological Review,* 1978, 85, 109–130.

Jackson, M. D., & McClelland, J. L. (1975). Sensory and cognitive determinants of reading speed. *Journal of Verbal Learning and Verbal Behavior.* 14, 565–574.

Jarvella, R. J. (1971). Syntactic processing of connected speech. *Journal of Verbal Learning and Verbal Behavior.* 10, 409–416.

Just, M. A., & Carpenter, P. A. (1978). Inference processes during reading: Reflections from eye fixations. In J. W. Senders, D. F. Fisher, & R. A. Monty (Eds.), *Eye movements and the higher psychological functions.* Hillsdale, New Jersey: Erlbaum.

Just, M. A., & Carpenter, P. A. (1980). A theory of reading: From eye fixations to comprehension. *Psychological Review.* 87, 329–354.

Just, M. A., Carpenter, P. A., & Masson, M. (1981). *Eye fixations and cognitive processing during rapid reading.* Pittsburgh: Carnegie–Mellon University.

Just, M. A., Carpenter, P. A., & Woolley, J. D. (1982). Paradigms and processes in reading comprehension. *Journal of Experimental Psychology: General, 111,* 228–238.

Kimball, J. P. (1973). Seven principles of surface structure parsing in natural language. *Cognition, 2,* 15–47.

Marcus, M. P. (1980). *A theory of syntactic recognition for natural language.* Cambridge, Massachusetts: MIT Press.

McDonald, J. L., & Carpenter, P. A. (1981). Simultaneous translation: Idiom interpretation and parsing heuristics. *Journal of Verbal Learning and Verbal Behavior, 20,* 231–247.

Newell, A. (1980). Harpy, productions systems and human cognition. In R. Cole (Ed.), *Perception and production of fluent speech.* Hillsdale, New Jersey: Erlbaum.

O'Regan, K. (1979). Moment to moment control of eye saccades as a function of textual parameters in reading. In P. A. Kolers, M. E. Wrolstad, & H. Bouma (Eds.), *Processing of visible language* (Vol. 1). New York: Plenum Press.

Pynte, J. (1974). Readiness for pronunciation during the reading process. *Perception & Psychophysics, 16,* 110–112.

Rayner, K. (1975). The perceptual span and peripheral cues in reading. *Cognitive Psychology, 7,* 65–81.

Rayner, K. (1977). Visual attention in reading: Eye movements reflect cognitive processes. *Memory & Cognition,* 5, 443–448.

Rayner, K. (1979). Eye movements in reading: Eye guidance and integration. In P.A. Kolers, M. E. Wrolstad, & H. Bouma (Eds.), *Processing of visible language* (Vol. 1), New York: Plenum Press.

Schank, R. C. (1972). Conceptual dependency: A theory of natural language understanding. *Cognitive Psychology, 3*, 552–631.

Sechrest, L., & Yeaton, W. E. (1979). *Estimating magnitudes of experimental effects.* Unpublished manuscript, Florida State University.

Simpson, G. B. (1981). Meaning dominance and semantic context in the processing of lexical ambiquity. *Journal of Verbal Learning and Verbal Behavior, 20*, 120–136.

Swinney, D. A. (1979). Lexical access during sentence comprehension: (Re)consideration of context effects. *Journal of Verbal Learning and Verbal Behavior, 18*, 645–659.

Thibadeau, R., Just, M. A., & Carpenter, P. A. (1982). A model of the time course and content of human reading. *Cognitive Science*, 6, 101–155.

Thomas W. Hogaboam

# 18

# Reading Patterns
# in Eye Movement Data

## I.   Introduction

There is a very general hypothesis, which is sometimes explicitly stated and sometimes left unstated, that fixation duration measures cognitive processing time. This hypothesis, in a general form, has been investigated in several studies (cf. Rayner, 1978). If true, this hypothesis would have many implications. A continuous on-line measure of processing time obtained during normal reading would represent a methodological breakthrough in the study of reading.

There are arguments in the literature contending that the individual fixation duration cannot be taken as a measure of the processing time allocated to a particular piece of text. There are two general forms this argument takes. The first presents time estimates for various processes that are hypothesized to be a part of each fixation, and when these times are added up there is no time left over for language processing (Russo, 1978). This argument is often advanced as counter to direct cognitive control models of eye guidance. Although the status of this argument is questionable to begin with and counter arguments have been presented (McConkie, Chapter 5 in this volume), at issue is a basic empirical question. Either we can identify factors related to higher cognitive processes that predict individual fixation durations, or else we cannot identify such factors. If such factors are found, this argument becomes difficult to maintain.

A second line of argument advanced against the hypothesis is more subtle. Carpenter and Just (1978), citing results of Walker (1933), have pointed out that it may be the case that a reader may trade off number of fixations and fixation duration. Thus, for example, when a word requires more processing time, the

EYE MOVEMENTS IN READING:
PERCEPTUAL AND LANGUAGE PROCESSES

reader will sometimes devote one long fixation and sometimes two shorter ones to the word. Thus, they contend, the measure of processing time is to be found by combining fixation duration and number of fixations into gaze durations. This is not, however, a necessary conclusion. First, it rests on the assumption that readers frequently trade off number of fixations for fixation duration, and it is not clear that this claim is currently supported, although it could be true. It does not follow that this type of trade-off is a common within subject event simply because some readers have larger average fixation durations with fewer fixations whereas others have more fixations that are shorter on average. Second, in constructing gaze durations one is needlessly throwing away information. If some variables influence gaze duration, then certainly these variables will influence fixation duration, or number of fixations, or both. Multivariate techniques could be used to determine the nature of these effects and, in fact, to document any trade-off if it is occurring.

Additionally, the method of combining information used to construct gaze durations introduces several sources of systematic bias into the measure (Hogaboam & McConkie, 1981; Kliegl, Olsen, & Davidson,). It is unclear whether it is possible to construct any measure of this type that does not introduce systematic bias (but see Hogaboam & McConkie, 1981, for an alternative approach). In these types of measures, any text factor that correlates with probability of fixation will show up as causing variation in processing time. Thus, for example, short words that tend to receive fewer fixations will, of necessity, show up as having shorter processing time (Hogaboam & McConkie, 1981). This might be appropriate if a very precise trade-off could be documented. This seems unlikely, however, because of the overhead involved in each fixation. That is, a fixation will last a certain amount of time even if no processing takes place. At a minimum, an adjustment for this overhead must be made whenever comparing words having unequal numbers of fixations.

An additional problem is that more than one word may be read during some fixations. Whenever this occurs, the interpretation of gaze durations becomes a problem. It is clear that before reasonable methods of aggregating fixation durations can be used with confidence it will be necessary to know more about what influences individual fixation durations.

## II.   What Influences a Fixation Duration?

There may well be a multitude of factors that contribute time to each fixation. Certainly there are low-level perceptual processes that require some minimum amount of time and certainly the eye stays fixated for some amount of time after a "go" signal has been issued. It seems unlikely, however, that the variance in fixation durations during normal reading, with a typical Standard Deviation around 100 msec, will be explained by these types of factors. Rather, it seems likely that text, reader, and strategic characteristics will account for this variance

(Gibson & Levin, 1975). For present purposes the focus will be on text characteristics, although it is still unclear where the lion's share of the variance will be found.

The question becomes, then, What text characteristics influence fixation durations? In answering this question, several approaches can be taken. The method to be presented here is in the tradition of dust bowl empiricism. It invokes one general premise: If a word is being processed during a particular fixation, then some characteristic of that work should predict the fixation duration. The analyses to be presented represent an attempt to determine which characteristics of which word predict fixation duration. In all of these analyses, the pattern of fixations will always be considered.

## A.  Why Should Pattern Matter?

Although the evidence will not be reviewed here, there is reason to suspect that the notion of a fixed perceptual span is inappropriate. Earlier work on perceptual span seems to support a notion that the information from a fixed amount of text is picked up on each fixation (McConkie & Rayner, 1975). More recent work (Hogaboam, 1979; Rayner, Well, & Pollatsek, 1980) suggests that the amount of information picked up during a fixation, as indexed by character positions, varies from fixation to fixation. Let us suppose for the moment that this is indeed the case, and consider the implications for the use of eye movement records to measure processing time attributable to psycholinguistic processes. The situation initially seems rather grim. If the fixation location cannot be used to reliably indicate what information was picked up during a fixation, there is no way to know when the processing of any particular unit was initiated.

This problem can be avoided if there is some information in the records, other than fixation location, that can be used to indicate what textual information was picked up during the fixation. One possibility is the pattern of fixations. If the eye guidance system works to successively place the eye in a manner sensitive to the information picked up on prior fixations then the resulting pattern of fixations can be used to indicate what was picked up on each fixation. The trick, of course, is to discover the exact manner in which pattern indexes the extent of prior information pickup. The analyses that follow attempt to unravel this relationship.

## B.  Pattern Definition

In defining what is meant by pattern, three separate aspects of every fixation were considered: direction of preceding saccade, direction of following saccade, and the extent of the following saccade. Saccade extent is measured in terms of number of words. That is, a saccade of length zero occurs whenever two successive fixations fall on the same word. If two successive fixations are on two consecutive words, the saccade length is one. This is in contrast to the more usual method of measuring saccade length in characters or degrees of arc. When saccade length is measured only in characters, however, word boundary information is ignored and, as will be argued latter, this may be critical information. Ideally, one should simultaneously consider both sources of information, but this requires additional data.

Figure 18.1 shows an example of the type of pattern that results from considering the information just discussed. In this figure the solid straight lines represent words. The fixation under consideration is called F0. This is the defining fixation as the pattern is defined with respect to it. The word that the defining fixation F0 falls on is designated W0, the word immediately to the right is W1, the word immediately to the left is W−1, etc.. In the same fashion, the fixation following the F0 fixation is designated the F1 fixation.

Each fixation was coded according to the pattern it fell into. That is, every fixation can be preceded by either a forward or regressive saccade, followed by a forward or regressive saccade, and the following saccade can be of length −2, −1, 0, 1, etc.

In addition to this pattern information, other aspects that were coded included whether the fixation was the first or last on the line, whether it was the rightmost or leftmost, and whether this was the first time through the text or whether the text was being "reread."

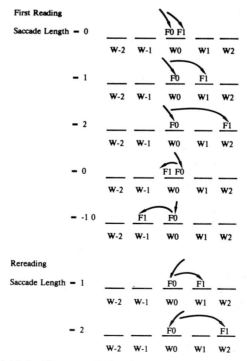

FIGURE 18.1. *Illustration of selected patterns. See text for explanation.*

It should be noted that there is nothing magical about the characteristics that might have been used to define pattern. Additional information might also be considered. For instance, the saccade length of the preceding saccade could also be coded. If this had been done, however, there would have been, roughly, four times as many different patterns to consider and each pattern would have, on average, one-fourth as many instances. Hence, as the number of factors entering into the pattern definition increases, the statistical power of tests on each pattern decreases, for a given data set. The solution, ultimately, is to collect enough data to examine as many factors as is deemed useful. For present purposes, the factors were restricted to those already mentioned as they were felt to be most critical.

The analyses that follow were taken from a study where 30 college students read a 417-word passage about the history of Alaska. They were instructed to read for comprehension and a short answer test was administered after reading. All subjects had previously participated in eye movement studies with similar procedures.

The text was presented one line at a time on a cathode-ray tube (CRT) located 19 in. from the eyes, with three letters to a degree. The subjects pressed a button to bring the next line of text to the screen, which appeared within .1 sec. Eye movements were monitored using a limbic reflective technique described in McConkie, Zola, Wolverton, and Burns (1978). Eye position was sampled every millisecond and for the reported data was accurate to within 2.5 character positions (worst case) to .5 character positions (best case).

## III.   Characterizing Eye Movement Patterns: How Often Do Various Patterns Occur?

Table 18.1 presents the relative frequency of occurrence for many of the patterns that occur most frequently, along with mean fixation duration and standard deviations. In the classification scheme used here, 10.4% of the fixations were excluded because of data disturbances or unclassifiable patterns—almost all were blinks. All the remaining fixations were classified as falling into one of the defined patterns and the patterns that occur more frequently are presented in Table 18.1.

A number of analyses could be done on data of this type. For present purposes there are a few points worth noting. First, by a factor of over four to one, the most common pattern is a forward move followed by a forward move. This in itself is not a surprise. What may come as a surprise to those unfamiliar with eye movements is that the pattern occurred slightly less than half the time—42.4% in the present sample. Yet descriptions of eye movements during reading often lead one to believe that this pattern is much more common. Certainly an "eyeball" examination of eye movement records leaves the impression that this pattern is much more common.

Even more surprises emerge when saccade length of the following saccade is considered. Eye movements during skilled reading have been characterized (Just

TABLE 18.1
Mean, Standard Deviation, and Frequency
of Selected Patterns

| Pattern | Mean Fixation Duration | Standard Deviation | Relative Frequency |
|---|---|---|---|
| **First Reading** | | | |
| **Forward-Forward** | | | |
| Sac Length — 0 | 269 | 116 | .055 |
| 1 | 244 | 103 | .227 |
| 2 | 247 | 101 | .124 |
| 3 | 254 | 117 | .017 |
| ≥4 | 284 | 76 | .001 |
| **Forward-Regression** | | | |
| Sac Length — 0 | 242 | 105 | .028 |
| -1 | 246 | 112 | .038 |
| -2 | 257 | 120 | .010 |
| -3 | 273 | 150 | .003 |
| ≤4 | 249 | 116 | .003 |
| **Rereading** | | | |
| **Regression-Forward** | | | |
| Sac Length — 0 | 300 | 122 | .008 |
| 1 | 245 | 123 | .034 |
| 2 | 225 | 108 | .030 |
| 3 | 203 | 119 | .012 |
| ≥4 | 227 | 91 | .005 |

& Carpenter, 1980) as largely consisting of fixations on almost every word followed by saccades that take the eye forward to the next word. Although it is true that this pattern was the single most prevalent pattern, it occurred only 22.7% of the time! Models of reading assuming this characterization of eye movements might be disregarding over three-fourths of the normal eye movement data.

The second single most common pattern, occurring on 12.4% of the fixations, is a forward movement followed by a forward movement that skips exactly one word. The interpretation of these percentages deserves a word of caution. These are percentages of the total number of fixations (or movements). It cannot be concluded, for instance, that if $X\%$ of the movements skip a word that $X\%$ of the words were skipped. In fact, in the present study about 40% of the words were skipped even though the percentage of movements skipping words was considerably less.

The next most common patterns are forward moves followed by regressions, and regressions followed by forward moves, each occurring about 8% of the time. The remaining fixations fall into a rather large number of different kinds of patterns, each occurring fairly infrequently, but collectively accounting for a large proportion of the data. The point to be taken from this is that it is inaccurate to characterize skilled reading as a process of moving ones eyes forward from one word to the next with occasional regressions. There are a large number of different patterns occurring, many infrequently, and none with sufficient frequency to allow characterization of a dominant pattern. Much of the remainder of this chapter will be concerned with the patterns that occur most frequently. However, it is important to remember the diversity of pattern.

There are a few additional points worth noting about the mean fixation durations of the fixations in each pattern. First, it has been reported that the fixations preceding regressions tend to be shorter than normal (Hawley, Stern, & Chen, 1974). In this study, this was only true for fixations that are both preceded and followed by regressions, averaging 230 msec when this sequence is initiated from the middle of a line and only 150 msec for the short fixations that are often seen after a return sweep. If the preceding saccade was a forward movement, the fixation duration is not effected by the direction of the following saccade.

Another interesting comparison involves cases where a word receives two fixations. The first fixation is abnormally long if the following saccade goes forward, but not if the following saccade is regressive. It is possible that these two patterns represent qualitatively different processes. This suggestion will be supported by latter analyses.

## A.    Under What Conditions Do Various Patterns Occur?

There are a number of ways to glean information about language processes from pattern information. One way, illustrated earlier, is to examine the frequency with which various patterns occur and average fixation durations.

A second approach is to examine the conditions under which various patterns occur. If the pattern of fixations is indeed sensitive to text characteristics, then one should expect different patterns to be associated with different text characteristics. An example of this type of approach is present in Table 18.2. For each of six patterns, the average log printed frequency of various words was found. Thus, for example, when a fixation is preceded and followed by a forward saccade but

TABLE 18.2
Mean Log Printed Frequency of Words in Various Locations

| Pattern | Word Location | | | | | |
|---|---|---|---|---|---|---|
| | W-2 | W-1 | W0 | W1 | W2 | W3 |
| **Forward-Forward** | | | | | | |
| Saccade Length = 0 | 2.32 | 3.21 | 1.28 | 2.58 | 2.61 | 2.57 |
| = 1 | 2.53 | 2.72 | 2.14 | 2.07 | 2.74 | 2.56 |
| = 2 | 2.36 | 2.52 | 2.07 | 3.51 | 2.04 | 2.48 |
| = 3 | 3.16 | 2.43 | 3.16 | 3.42 | 3.79 | 1.71 |
| **Forward-Regression** | | | | | | |
| Saccade Length = 0 | 2.37 | 2.66 | 1.31 | 2.41 | 2.54 | 2.53 |
| = -1 | 2.50 | 2.36 | 1.99 | 2.63 | 2.52 | 2.48 |

remains within the same word (saccade length = 0), the frequency of that word tends to be low and the frequency of the preceding word very high. Also, when words are skipped (saccades of two or three words) the skipped words tend to be high frequency. These are not surprising results. More interesting is the finding that when a regression occurs to a previous word, the frequency of that word is about average. When a regression occurs within a word, however, that word tends to be a low-frequency word.

A third approach, which will be the concern of the remainder of this chapter, is to examine each pattern separately and determine what text characteristics influence the fixation durations for that pattern. With this approach, one is asking the question, Given that a pattern has occurred, what influences the fixation duration?

## IV. Simple Breakdowns

Table 18.3 presents the first step in this type of analysis. For each pattern, the fixation duration of F0 is found separately for high and low printed frequency words. Note there are three hypotheses that seem to be supported by this breakdown:

1. During a fixation you usually process the word you are fixating.
2. Printed frequency influences processing time.
3. The pattern of fixations can indicate which words are read on which fixations.

The reasons these data support the first two hypotheses are obvious. This type of data represents the traditional bootstrapping of a psychological measure. It is hypothesized that frequency influences processing time and that fixation duration measures processing time. Finding effects of frequency on fixation duration is then taken as simultaneous support for both hypotheses. The third hypothesis is supported because an effect of frequency is observed in all instances except when a fixation is preceded by a forward move and followed by a regression of one word.

But, of course, one would not expect an effect if the word was not being processed on that fixation. The results from the other patterns seem to persuasively argue that if a word is processed during a fixation, printed frequency affects the fixation duration. Therefore it can be concluded that when there is no effect of frequency, the word was not processed during that fixation.

Rayner (1978) has reviewed several studies using this type of analysis to support direct cognitive control models of eye guidance. After all, how could variables

TABLE 18.3

Mean Fixation Duration of F0 Broken Down by Pattern and Characteristics of Word Fixated on F0, W0

| Pattern | Printed Frequency | | Number of Syllables | | |
|---|---|---|---|---|---|
| | Low($\leqslant$10) | High($>$10) | One | Two | Three |
| **First Reading** | | | | | |
| **Forward-Forward** | | | | | |
| __ F0 __ __ | 287 | 256 | 248 | 273 | 264 |
| __ F0 __ __ | 268 | 235 | 235 | 244 | 254 |
| __ F0 __ __ | 272 | 238 | 238 | 251 | 258 |
| **Forward-Regression** | | | | | |
| __ F0 __ | 260 | 226 | 233 | 242 | 236 |
| __ F0 __ | 244 | 247 | 240 | 249 | 260 |

like the printed frequency of the fixated word influence fixation durations if the mind could not immediately control the length of the fixation?

Unfortunately, there are several ways this could happen, hence there are potential problems with this type of argument. First, there is the traditional problem that the effects that are attributed to printed frequency may not really be due to printed frequency, per se, but to some correlate of printed frequency. An example of this is number of syllables, which in this sample correlated .29 with printed frequency. The breakdown by number of syllables is also presented in Table 18.3. If there is particular interest in sorting out these two factors, additional experiments can be run or other types of analyses can be attempted. In any case, it is clear that on the basis of this evidence alone we cannot immediately conclude that printed frequency is affecting processing time.

However, it is tempting to at least conclude that processing of the fixated word occurred when it was fixated, because we did observe an effect. It is just unclear at the moment whether this effect is due to printed frequency or to some correlate. Unfortunately, this argument also has problems. To understand the nature of this problem, imagine that people never process the word they are fixating during that fixation, but instead always process the right adjacent word. Further, suppose that printed frequency does influence processing time. In this situation an effect of the printed frequency of the fixated word is still observed because there is a correlation between the printed frequency of the fixated word and the printed frequency of the right adjacent word! In this particular study the correlation was $r = .21$, $p < .05$. Thus, we cannot even be sure that a word is being processed on a particular fixation simply because some characteristic of that word predicts the fixation duration. We must first eliminate the alternative possibility that sequential correlations of word characteristics in natural language are accounting for the observed effects.

To make matters worse, these first two problems combine orthogonally. It is possible that effects attributed to the printed frequency of the fixated word are in fact due to the number of syllables of the right adjacent word. Or even the sentence position of the left adjacent word or any other word. There is little known, in general, about these types of correlation in natural language. How often, for example, does a high frequency word follow a low frequency word, or a two syllable word? It is this correlational structure of language that must be taken into account in interpreting eye movement records.

As an illustration of these problems, Table 18.4 presents a breakdown of the fixation durations of the fixations on word W0 by the printed frequency and number of syllables in words at various locations. There are several points to note here. First, when the F0 fixation durations are broken down by the frequencies of the fixated word, W0 one indeed sees a significant frequency effect. When this same set of data is broken down by the number of syllables in the preceding word, W−1, there is no frequency effect. Thus the frequency of the left adjacent word appears not to influence F0. When the same set of data is broken down by the frequency of the right adjacent word W1 significant frequency effects (t tests,

TABLE 18.4

Mean Fixation Duration of F0, in Milliseconds, Broken Down by Printed Frequency of Words W-1 through W2

| Printed Frequency | Location of Word with Respect to Location of F0 | | | |
|---|---|---|---|---|
| | W-1 | WO | W1 | W2 |
| | — | F0 | — | — |
| Low | 269 | 287 | 275 | 283 |
| High | 269 | 256 | 263 | 258 |
| | — | F0 | | — |
| Low | 244 | 268 | 254 | 245 |
| High | 244 | 235 | 241 | 242 |
| | — | F0 | — | |
| Low | 253 | 272 | 282 | 249 |
| High | 245 | 238 | 243 | 246 |

$p < .05$) appear for saccade sizes 1 and 2. One is tempted to conclude that the frequency of the right adjacent word influences the F0 fixation duration. However, in this breakdown, many of the data points that were in the low-frequency category were also in the low-frequency category of the W0 breakdown. Thus it is not clear how much of the effect is due to the fixated word and how much is due to the right adjacent word. The same problem arises for any other comparisons of this type.

## V. Multiple Regression Approaches

There are at least three general solutions to these problems. First, one can attempt to construct text that allows orthogonal comparisons of different word characteristics; that is, to conduct a true experiment. This involves constructing text with particular locations that accept different words that vary in the characteristics under consideration. One of the major problems with this approach is cost; these are low yielding–high cost experiments. Second, one can take the approach illustrated by Kliegl, Olson, and Davidson (Chapter 19 in this volume).

One simply samples to obtain orthogonal comparisons on the factors of interest. This is a low cost–high yield procedure, but it has at least two well-known problems. First, depending upon the covariance structure involved, one can often only look at a small number of variables at any one time. It becomes harder and harder to find a full set of comparisons as the number of factors increases. Second, the range of all variables can get attenuated and the representativeness of the samples becomes a major concern.

The third solution is to apply multiple regression models. This is perhaps the best solution, but requires that the investigator invoke a model of some sort. The model used in the present analysis is very general. It divides reading comprehension into only two parts. The first part includes all processes that occur from word onset up to and including the mobilization of semantic resources associated with a lexical entry. These are word decoding processes. The second part includes all other processes necessary to arrive at a coherent interpretation of the word in context. These are word integration processes.

This division of the processes involved in comprehension is not to be taken as a complete model. Rather, it is a simple heuristic decomposition of comprehension processes into two time dependent components. It proposes that there are lower level, early occurring processes involved with word recognition and lexical access and other higher level latter occurring processes involved with more integrative aspects of comprehension. No assumptions are made about whether these processes are arrayed serially or in parallel or in some other fashion with the exception that decoding processes involving a particular word occur prior to integrative processes involving that same word. Thus, both decoding and integration operations may be going on in parallel, but in any given slice of real time no integrative processes will involve a word that has not been decoded.

This decomposition does not preclude (or necessitate) any particular contextual effects on decoding. Context may help or hinder decoding processes and certainly decoding processes help or hinder integrative processes. This decomposition does exclude the radical forms of contextual interactions where a word is decoded without the benefit of visual information. This general model, then, is neither theoretically restrictive nor very new.

## A.  Decoding Processes

To measure the effects of decoding processes, three variables were selected: printed frequency, average spatial frequency, and number of syllables. The printed frequencies were taken from Kucera and Francis (1967) and the average spatial frequencies were calculated from tables provided by Mayzner and Tresselt (1965). These variables were always treated as a set. That is, it is proposed that these variables together will tap variance due to decoding processes and not variance due to integrative processes. No attempt is presently made to determine which of these variables or even what particular combination of these variables is

# TABLE 18.5
Results of Regressing Decoding Characteristics of Various Words on FO Fixation Durations[a]

| Pattern | Location of Word with Respect to Word Fixated on Fixation FO | | | |
| --- | --- | --- | --- | --- |
| | W-1 | WO | W1 | W2 |
| **First Reading** | | | | |
| Forward-Forward | | | | |
| *(pattern diagram)* | 0 | * | * | * |
| *(pattern diagram)* | 0 | * | * | * |
| *(pattern diagram)* | 0 | * | * | 0 |
| Forward-Regression | | | | |
| *(pattern diagram)* | 0 | 0 | 0 | 0 |
| *(pattern diagram)* | 0 | 0 | 0 | 0 |
| **Rereading** | | | | |
| Regression-Forward | | | | |
| *(pattern diagram)* | 0 | 0 | 0 | * |
| *(pattern diagram)* | 0 | 0 | 0 | 0 |

[a] Log printed frequency, average spatial frequency, and number of syllables of each word were used in separate analysis to predict FO durations.

* Indicates a significant multiple $R^2$, $p = .05$

most effective in predicting fixation durations. There are, of course, many studies in which these variables have been found to be sensitive to word level processes.

Table 18.5 presents the results of an analysis where the decoding variables were used to predict the fixation duration of the defining fixation, F0. In column W0, the word characteristics of the fixated word are used to predict F0, in column 1 the word characteristics of the right adjacent word are used to predict F0, etc.. The cell entry is an asterisk if the multiple $R^2$ was significant at $p < .05$, and a zero otherwise.

The character of the table is fairly easy to summarize. The decoding characteristics of the left adjacent word have no influence on the fixation duration, and if you are rereading or about to regress, the decoding characteristics of the surrounding words do not seem to matter. Presumably in these cases you are doing something other than decoding. When a fixation is preceded and followed by a forward saccade, however, the decoding characteristics of the fixated word affect the fixation duration. If the subsequent saccade is going to leave the eye within the same word, only the characteristics of the fixated word matter. If the subsequent saccade is one or two words long, decoding characteristics of words to the right of the fixated word influence the fixation duration.

Again, it is tempting to conclude that a particular word was being decoded whenever the decoding characteristics of that word influence a fixation duration. However, it is still possible that the observed effects are due to correlations of decoding characteristics of consecutive words.

Table 18.6 presents the results of stepwise multiple regressions where the F0 fixation duration is the dependent variable. For the patterns where there are two consecutive forward saccades, the decoding characteristics of the fixated word were entered on the first step, followed by the decoding characteristics of the first word to the right, then the second, and so forth. For all patterns the order of entry is indicated by the number in parentheses.

Again it is evident that the decoding characteristics of all the surrounding words do not seem to predict fixation duration when you are rereading or when you are going to regress on the next saccade. Presumably other nondecoding processes are taking place.

When a fixation is preceded and followed by a forward saccade, however, an interesting pattern emerges. When the following saccade takes the eye to the right adjacent word, only the characteristics of the fixated word matter. If the eye is going to skip the right adjacent word, the decoding characteristics of both the fixated word and the right adjacent word, that will be skipped significantly influence the fixation duration. This seems to indicate that when you have only decoded the fixated word you move forward to the next word. If you have decoded both the fixated word and the right adjacent word, the subsequent saccade skips the decoded right adjacent word. This is in agreement with the breakdowns in Table 18.4.

It is worth emphasizing that in the other patterns the decoding characteristics of the word falling directly on the fovea had no influence on the fixation duration.

TABLE 18.6

## Results of Stepwise Regression Predicting F0 Fixation Duration with Decoding Characteristics of Various Words[a]

| Pattern | W-1 | W0 | W1 | W2 |
|---|---|---|---|---|
| **First Reading** | | | | |
| Forward-Forward | | | | |
| *(pattern diagram)* | | *[b](1) | 0(2) | 0(3) |
| *(pattern diagram)* | | *(1) | 0(2) | 0(3) |
| *(pattern diagram)* | | *(1) | *(2) | 0(3) |
| Forward-Regression | | | | |
| *(pattern diagram)* | 0(3) | 0(1) | 0(2) | |
| *(pattern diagram)* | 0(3) | 0(1) | 0(2) | |
| **Rereading** | | | | |
| Regression-Forward | | | | |
| *(pattern diagram)* | | 0(1) | 0(2) | 0(3) |
| *(pattern diagram)* | | 0(1) | 0(2) | 0(3) |

Column header spanning W-1, W0, W1, W2: *Location of Word with Respect to Word Fixated on Fixation F0*

[a] An "*" indicates a significant increase in multiple $R^2$ when the characteristics of the corresponding word are entered. The number in parentheses indicates the order of entry.

[b] $p = .068$

Thus we have examples of two phenomena: (*a*) cases where the fixated word and words other than the fixated word are influencing the fixation duration; and (*b*) cases where the fixated word is not influencing the fixation duration. These different cases are marked by the pattern of fixations. In analyzing fixation durations for effects of language variables, it is critical that the pattern of fixations be taken into account. In this sample, failing to consider pattern would have washed out the effects noted above.

It is also interesting in comparing Table 18.6 with Table 18.5 that for a forward move followed by a forward move of exactly one word, the apparent effects of the decoding characteristics of the right adjacent word in Table 5 were apparently due to sequential correlations of word characteristics. When the effects of the characteristics of the fixated word are removed the decoding characteristics of the right adjacent word have no effects.

## B.    Higher Level Variables

It is difficult to motivate a selection of one or a number of variables that would be expected to tap higher level integrative processes. Theories of word recognition are much more well developed than theories of meaning integration. Although not very satisfactory, an old fashioned syntactic category coding was used to classify each word into 1 of 11 different categories such as noun, verb, adverb, quantifier, number, proposition, and so forth. It was felt that these were aspects of words that would have their effects, if any, because they serve different semantic roles in integrating the meaning of a message.

Table 18.7 presents the results of a stepwise regression using syntactic category as the independent variable. Dummy codes were used for each syntactic category, generating 11 variables, 1 for each syntactic category.

These results are similar to the results from the decoding analysis with a few exceptions. First of all, although not reaching traditional levels of significance, there is at least a hint that syntactic category may, on rereading, be influencing the fixation durations. The argument cannot be supported statistically at this time, but it may be the case that on rereading decoding variables do not have an influence but higher level integrative factors do.

When a fixation is preceded and followed by a forward saccade, there are a couple of interesting differences. First, when the second fixation is going to be on the same word, there is no effect of syntactic category on the duration of FO but there was an effect of decoding variables. Perhaps in these cases the second fixation is required to complete the integrative processes. This explanation would predict that the duration of the second fixation will be predicted by syntactic category and, as will be discussed, this is indeed the case.

The remaining difference comes in the case where the following forward saccade moves exactly one word. In this case the syntactic category of the following word predicts the F0 fixation duration, even after the syntactic category of the

## TABLE 18.7
### Results of Stepwise Regression Predicting FO Fixation Duration with Syntactic Category of Various Words[a]

| Pattern | | W-1 | W0 | W1 | W2 |
|---|---|---|---|---|---|
| | **Location of Word with Respect to Word Fixated on Fixation FO** | | | | |
| **First Reading** | | | | | |
| **Forward-Forward** | | | | | |
| (pattern) | | | 0(1) | 0(2) | 0(3) |
| (pattern) | | | *(1) | *(2) | 0(3) |
| (pattern) | | | *(1) | *(2) | 0(3) |
| **Forward-Regression** | | | | | |
| (pattern) | | 0(2) | 0(1) | | |
| (pattern) | | 0(2) | 0(1) | | |
| **Rereading** | | | | | |
| **Regression-Forward** | | | | | |
| (pattern) | | | $0^b$(1) | 0(2) | *(3) |
| (pattern) | | | $0^c$(1) | 0(2) | 0(3) |

[a] An "*" indicates a significant increase in multiple $R^2$ when the characteristics of the corresponding word are entered. The number in parentheses indicates the order of entry.

[b] p = .13

[c] p = .07

fixated word has been entered into the model. This was not true for decoding variables, where the decoding characteristics of the following word did not affect the F0 fixation duration. This remains an unexplained result.

## VI.   Lagged Effects

One of the problems involved in attributing mental processing time to textual units on the basis of fixation durations is the possibility of eye–mind lag (Hogaboam & McConkie, 1981). The basic question is whether the time due to a particular unit is spread over several fixations. Just and Carpenter (1980) have made the simplifying assumption that processing of a unit is complete before a new saccade is initiated. In fact, whenever anyone examines the durations of single fixations as a processing time measure, this assumption is implicitly involved.

For those wishing to use eye movement records to study language processes, this question is of considerable importance. If lagged effects are present, using eye movement records to study language processes becomes an even more complex problem; somehow the extent of lag and variance in the lag, if any, must be measurable.

With the type of analysis presented above, there is a straightforward way to check for lagged effects and the conditions under which they occur. It is only necessary to repeat the analyses using the F1 fixation as the dependent variable. Table 18.8 presents the results of using the decoding characteristics of various words to predict the duration of the F1 fixation and Table 18.9 presents the results of using syntactic category to predict F1 fixation durations. Evidence for lag effects would be present whenever the characteristics of a word that predicted F0 also predict F1. As a comparison of Tables 18.7 and 18.5 shows, this was never the case for decoding characteristics. Only the decoding characteristics of the word fixated on F1 predict the duration of F1. Thus there is no evidence from this analysis that decoding operations are carried over to succeeding fixations.

An interesting implication of this result is that the eye guidance system may be particularly sensitive to the status of decoding processes and advance the eye contingent upon the status of some aspect of these operations.

There are two other points worth mentioning about this analysis. The first concerns the cases where there are two successive fixations on a word. When the first fixation is followed by a regression, decoding characteristics of the word predict the duration of the second fixation, but not the first. When the first fixation is followed by a forward move, the decoding characteristics predict the first fixation but not the second. The implication is that if decoding processes take place on the first fixation, the eye is sent forward. If they do not, for whatever reason, the eye is sent back a few spaces and at this point both decoding characteristics and syntactic category influence the duration.

When there are two fixations on a word with an intervening forward move,

## TABLE 18.8
### Results of Stepwise Regression Predicting F1 Fixation Duration with Decoding Characteristics of Various Words[a]

| Pattern | W-1 | WO | W1 | W2 |
|---|---|---|---|---|
| **First Reading** | | | | |
| **Forward-Forward** | | | | |
| | | 0(1) | 0(2) | 0(3) |
| | | 0(1) | *(2) | $0^b$(3) |
| | | 0(1) | 0(2) | *(3) |
| **Forward-Regression** | | | | |
| | 0(2) | *(1) | | |
| | $0^c$(2) | 0(1) | | |
| **Rereading** | | | | |
| **Regression-Forward** | | | | |
| | | 0(1) | 0(2) | 0(3) |
| | | 0(1) | 0(2) | 0(3) |

Location of Word with Respect to Word Fixated on Fixation FO

[a] An "*" indicates a significant increase in multiple $R^2$ when the characteristics of the corresponding word are entered. The number in parentheses indicates the order of entry.

[b] $p = .10$

[c] $p = .08$

## TABLE 18.9
### Results of Stepwise Regression Predicting F1 Fixation Duration with Syntactic Category of Various Words[a]

| Pattern | | Location of Word with Respect to Word Fixated on Fixation FO | | |
|---|---|---|---|---|
| | W-1 | WO | W1 | W2 |
| **First Reading** | | | | |
| Forward-Forward | | | | |
| | | *(1) | 0(2) | 0(3) |
| | | *(1) | *(2) | *(3) |
| | | *(1) | 0(2) | *(3) |
| Forward-Regression | | | | |
| | 0(2) | *(1) | | |
| | *(2) | 0(1) | | |
| **Rereading** | | | | |
| Regression-Forward | | | | |
| | | 0(1) | *(2) | 0(3) |
| | | 0(1) | 0(2) | 0(3) |

[a] An "*" indicates a significant increase in multiple $R^2$ when the characteristics of the corresponding word are entered. The number in parentheses indicates the order of entry.

only decoding characteristics influence the first fixation and only syntactic category influences the second. This could be taken as evidence for a particular type of lagged effect. Even stronger evidence for lagged effects comes from the W0 column in Table 18.9. In all three cases where a forward move is followed by a forward move, the syntactic category of the word fixated on F0 is influencing the duration of the following fixation!

One problem with the above arguments is that under some real time models of exactly when lagged processes have their effects, this analysis could be viewed as biased toward finding lagged effects. This is because the syntactic category of the previously fixated word is entered first in the regression analysis. This was originally done on the assumption that any operations left over from the previous fixation would be expected to occur first on the following fixation. This may, however, not be the case. The more conservative approach is to enter the syntactic category of the subsequently fixated word first and then work backward to the previously fixated word. This analysis is presented in Table 18.10. Here there are still strong lagged effects when the eye advances zero or one word, but not when a word is skipped. Thus, when a word is skipped, the decoding characteristics and syntactic category of the fixated word and the skipped word have effects on F0,

TABLE 18.10

Results of Reverse Order Stepwise Regression Predicting F1 Fixation Durations from Syntactic Category of Various Words[a]

|  | Location of Word with Respect to Word Fixated on Fixation FO | | | |
|  | | | | |
| Pattern | W-1 | WO | W1 | W2 |
| **First Reading** | | | | |
| **Forward-Forward** | | | | |
| | | *(1) | | |
| | | *(2) | *(1) | |
| | | 0(3) | 0(2) | *(1) |

[a] An "*" indicates a significant increase in multiple $R^2$ when the characteristics of the corresponding words are entered. The number in parentheses indicates the order of entry.

but there are no carry-over effects to F1. When the eye only advances to the next word, there are effects of decoding characteristics and syntactic category on F0 and there are carry-over effects of syntactic category to fixation F1.

These analyses thus demonstrate two additional phenomena. First, there are decoding characteristics of words that appear to have no lagged or carry-over effects. Presumably the processes affected by these word characteristics are largely completed before a saccade is initiated. Second, there are cases where the processes licensed or required by a word decoded on one fixation are still having their effects during the next fixation. There are also cases where this does not happen, and the pattern of fixations is useful in differentiating these cases.

## VII.  Process Interpretations of Lagged Effects

Given that syntactic category shows lagged effects, it is likely that there are other variables as well that will show lagged effects. There are, however, two different explanations for these effects, which have very different implications.

### A.  The Pipeline Model

The first explanation is the simplest and perhaps the most parsimonious. Under this explanation after a word is decoded it is integrated with the prior context, but the eye does not always wait until this process is finished. It sometimes proceeds to the next fixation. At this point the mind continues its previous work and the eye pauses until the previous work is caught up. Note that it is necessary to postulate that the eye does, in fact, often wait for previous work to be completed rather than go on. Otherwise the lagged effects on F1 could never be observed. Under this explanation the processing of prior information is not completed when a fixation ends, or at any fixed interval measured from the end of the fixation.

### B.  The Integration Model

Under this explanation, processing of prior text is completed before the eye proceeds. Lagged statistical effects are attributed to systematic variability in the difficulty of integrating one word with the prior word. For example, suppose the phrase *green grass* appears in a text and that each word gets one fixation. Suppose further that the processing of *green* is completed to its highest level before the eye moves. During subsequent processing the word *grass* will need to be integrated with the word *green*. This may be easier or harder to do than if the sequence had been *the grass*. In general, different sequences of words may differ in their ease of integration. This would create carry-over effects when there was no real time processing lag. At the present time it is not possible to empirically differentiate these explanations using the eye movement records.

# VIII.   Summary

A number of specific results of these analyses contribute to the body of facts that a real time model of reading must account for.

First, there is a wide diversity of patterns of fixations with no one pattern accounting for a majority of instances. Second, if fixations are preceded and followed by forward going saccades, decoding operations appear to be carried out during that fixation, with no carry-over effects into the next fixation. If the following fixation is on the next word, integration processes appear to take place on the first fixation and also appear to carry over into the following fixation.

Third, if the right adjacent word is subsequently skipped, the decoding of the skipped word occurs on the prior fixation. In fact, when a word is skipped the decoding and integration of both the fixated and skipped words occur on the prior fixation. There is no carry-over effect of the decoding processes and possibly no carry-over of integration processes.

Four, when a fixation is followed by a regression to another word the characteristics of the fixated word do not influence the fixation duration. This perhaps represents a decoding failure. The fixation following the regression, however, is influenced by the integrative properties of the word subsequently fixated, and possibly the decoding characteristics. A possible explanation is that the word regressed to was not fully decoded when the eye moved on. Hence a return was necessary to complete decoding and integration.

Fifth, there are two cases where a word receives two consecutive fixations. When a forward move intervenes, the first fixation is only influenced by decoding variables and the second is only influenced by integration factors. When a regression intervenes, nothing predicts the first fixation, and both decoding and integration factors appear to occur on the second fixation. Again the regression appears to signal a decoding breakdown and not an integration breakdown. If the regressions did signal an integration breakdown, effects of decoding variables on the first fixation would still be expected, but none were found.

On a more general level, it is apparent that the pattern of fixations is sensitive to the types of mental processes occurring during reading. There are two major implications of this result. First, it appears that the eye guidance system is indeed quite sensitive to the operation of various language understanding processes during reading. The pattern of fixations that results from the operation of this system are thus indicants of the nature of the processes that occurred. Failure to take account of these patterns would lead to measures that were aggregated over different types of situations. Depending upon the particular pattern involved, there are instances of

1. Fixated words influencing the fixation duration.
2. Fixated words not influencing fixation duration.
3. Nonfixated words that are skipped influencing fixation duration.
4. Words that were fixated on prior fixations influencing current fixation durations.

Clearly, pattern information is critical to the analysis of eye movement records during normal reading.

Finally, the duration of the individual fixation seems to be a viable index of processing time if pattern is simultaneously taken into account. Examining fixation durations without taking account of pattern may give misleading results. It is likely that there are other aspects of pattern information that will prove to be useful indicants, as well as other variables that predict fixation durations. In particular, variables that index more critical aspects of meaning integration need to be identified. The present research presents a useful analytical approach to using fixation durations to measure processing time.

## References

Carpenter, P. A., & Just, M. A. (1978). Inference processes during reading: Reflections from eye fixations. In J. W. Senders, D. F. Fisher, & R. A. Monty (Eds.), *Eye movements and higher psychological functions*. Hillsdale, New Jersey: Erlbaum.

Gibson, E. J., & Levin, H. (1975). *The psychology of reading*. Cambridge, Massachusetts: MIT Press.

Hawley, T. T., Stern, J. A., & Chen, S. C. (1974). Computer analysis of eye movements during reading. *Reading World, 13*, 307–317.

Hogaboam, T. W. (1979). *The relationship of word identification and eye movements during normal reading*. Paper presented at the meeting of the Psychonomics Society, Phoenix, November.

Hogaboam, T. W., & McConkie, G. W. (1981). *The rocky road from eye fixations to comprehension*. (Tech. Rep. 207). University of Illinois, Center for the Study of Reading, Urbana, Illinois.

Just, M. A., & Carpenter, P. A. (1980). A theory of reading: From eye fixations to comprehension. *Psychological Review, 87*, 329–354.

Kucera, H., & Francis, W. N. (1967). *Computational analysis of present-day English*. Providence: Brown University Press.

Mayzner, M. S., & Tresselt, M. E. (1965) Tables of single-letter and diagram frequency counts of various word-lengths and letter position combinations. *Psychonomic Monograph Supplements R*, (1, Whole No. 2).

McConkie, G. W., & Rayner, K. (1975). The span of the effective stimulus during a fixation in reading. *Perception & Psychophysics, 17*, 578–586.

McConkie, G. W., Zola, D., Wolverton, G. S., & Burns, D. D. (1978). Eye movement contingent display control in studying reading. *Behavior Research Methods & Instrumentation*, Vol. 10 (2), 154–156.

Rayner, K. (1978). Eye movements in reading and information processing. *Psychological Bulletin, 85*, 618–660.

Rayner, K., Well, A. D., & Pollatsek, A. (1980). Asymmetry of the effective visual field in reading. *Perception & Psychophysics, 27*, 537–544.

Russo, J. E. (1978). Adaptation of cognitive processes to the eye movement system. In J. W. Senders, D. F. Fisher, & R. A. Monty (Eds.), *Eye movements and the higher psychological functions*. Hillsdale, New Jersey: Erlbaum.

Walker, R. Y. (1933). The eye movements of good readers. *Psychological Monographs, 44*, 95–117.

Reinhold Kliegl, Richard K. Olson, and Brian J. Davidson

# 19

# On Problems of Unconfounding Perceptual and Language Processes

## I.   Introduction

Over the past decade we have witnessed a major revival of research on eye fixations in reading. In contrast to earlier work (e.g., Tinker, 1958), which was concerned with questions of average fixation duration and frequency, most recent studies have focused on factors influencing the durations and locations of individual fixations, and on the amount of information available during a single fixation (cf. McConkie, 1979; O'Regan, 1979; Rayner, 1979b). Although the influence of psycholinguistic variables has been demonstrated in some of these studies, more attention has been directed toward perceptual factors associated with acuity limitations in eye guidance. One could conclude from this research that acuity limitations play a dominant role in length of saccades and placement of fixations on words.

Just and Carpenter (1980) evaluated eye fixation data from a very different perspective. They examined the influence of psycholinguistic variables on eye fixations, and perceptual variables were not considered. Word length, which would play a dominant role from a perceptual point of view, was coded by number of syllables in their psycholinguistic model. Kliegl, Olson, and Davidson (1982) demonstrated that some of Just and Carpenter's (1980) psycholinguistically relevant variables, such as number of syllables, number of letters, and word frequency, are highly correlated with each other in natural text. Hierarchical regression analyses of our data showed that the amount of variance in fixation time explained independently by these variables is small compared to the amount of variance they share. When word length in letters rather than syllables was entered in the analyses, the fit of the model improved. Moreover, the independent contribution

EYE MOVEMENTS IN READING:
PERCEPTUAL AND LANGUAGE PROCESSES

of syllable length was nonexistent, and the independent contribution of word frequency decreased from 12 to 3%. If one were to interpret word length in number of letters as a perceptual indicator and word length in number of syllables as a psycholinguistic process indicator, this result would lend support to the relevance of perceptual processing.

The use of eye fixation data for theory development in reading will require a better separation of perceptual and psycholinguistic influences. In natural text, variables that may be theoretically related to psycholinguistic and perceptual processes, like word length and word frequency, are highly correlated or—as is the case for word length—may be claimed for both types of processes. Consequently, multiple regression analyses employing these indicators will not provide much insight into the relative importance of the underlying processes.

One way to avoid correlations in natural text is via traditional experimental designs. The advantage of the experimental approach lies in the strict orthogonality of the factors. The cost of the clean design is the artificiality of the experimental material. Further, since experimental conditions are usually conceptualized as fixed factors, ANOVA designs cannot provide process parameters; they only allow us to ascertain that a certain factor is significantly related to the dependent measure. Nevertheless, it seems important to assess the presence of these effects in natural text. Therefore, we have adopted an alternative data-analytic approach that introduces orthogonality post hoc by selective sampling in the data base. This approach isolated different perceptual and psycholinguistic influences by holding one variable constant in the sample and noting fixation time variance with the other.

The data used in the following analysis included various subsets of the data used for the global regression analysis reported by Kliegl (1981b). In this experiment six skilled adult readers carefully read the beginning pages (1260 words) of Camus's novel *The Plague* (1947/1948). Eye fixations were monitored with an Applied Sciences Eye View Monitor Model 1996. This is a video based system with a sampling rate of 60 Hz and an accuracy of about $\frac{1}{2}°$ of visual angle. Character position accuracy was within one character to the right or left of the fixated character at least 90% of the time (see Davidson, 1981; Kliegl, 1981a; Kliegl & Olson, 1981 for technical details).

Two sets of analyses were performed to test for the influence of perceptual and psycholinguistic processes on the number, duration, and placement of fixations on a word. The first set separated the effects of syllable- and letter-length of words and their frequency. To this end, words were selected to conform to an orthogonal design with syllable length (SL) and letter length (LL) as independent factors. The second set replicated previous experimental findings on fixation durations and positions of fixations. The analyses were carried out separately for words that received one fixation and words that received two fixations. The two-fixation cases were also analyzed for differences between regressive sequences and progressive sequences of fixations within words.

## II.   Word Length and Word Frequency

One of the issues central to the development of an eye fixation based process theory of reading is how to disentangle the influence of perceptual and psycholinguistic factors. The regression analyses performed by Kliegl *et al.*, (1982) suggested a further examination of the relation between word length and word frequency, as these were the parameters contributing most to the fit of the model. Variance contributed by word frequency can be taken to reflect psycholinguistic processing demands. The length of the word might be taken to reflect psycholinguistic factors from the point of view of syllables (Just & Carpenter, 1980; Pynte, 1974), and eye guidance, peripheral acuity, or letter processing from the perspective of number of letters. In the hierarchical regression analyses discussed earlier, number of syllables did not contribute to fixation time independently of number of letters, and the independent contribution of word frequency was small. However, the type of data entered in those models might have buried independent contributions of these two parameters. The data were gaze durations, that is, the total time spent on a word (cf. Just & Carpenter, 1980). Gaze duration reflects the number of fixations on a word as well as fixation duration per se. To illustrate, suppose that a given word is fixated only 50% of the time, but when it is fixated the durations are 250 msec (approximately the average fixation time). Gaze duration for that word would be 125 msec. Similarly, consider a word that receives two fixations half of the time, and one fixation the other half. If each fixation again lasts 250 msec, the gaze duration would be 375 msec, even though for a given subject the total fixation time would be either 250 or 500 msec. Thus, gaze duration cannot disentangle the number of fixations on a word from fixation durations per se. In fact, a large amount of the variance in our earlier analyses was due to words that were not fixated or that were fixated more than once. Skipped words tended to be short and of high frequency, and multiple fixation words tended to be long and of low frequency.

To unconfound the number of fixations from fixation duration, we focused on words that received only a single fixation. Words were selected from the text to conform to a post-hoc orthogonalized design. Only words 5–11 letters long were selected. This restriction ensured that there were enough words in the central cells of the letters (5,11) by syllables (1,4) matrix. Also, an upper cutoff of 500 msec was used to remove some outliers.

The average fixation durations for the various letter-syllable combinations, standard deviations, and number of observations are shown in Table 19.1. The rightmost column will be discussed later. There was no significant influence of either letter length or syllable length on the fixation durations. Thus, when a word receives a single fixation, the fixation duration is essentially unrelated to word length. Notice that all letters of these words would be well within the span of perceptual acuity. One might expect double fixations on longer words, because of acuity limitations. From a psycholinguistic perspective, however, this result

TABLE 19.1
Descriptive Statistics for One-Fixation Case (OFC)[a]

| Number of letters | | Number of syllables | | | | Letter position of fixation |
|---|---|---|---|---|---|---|
| | | 1 | 2 | 3 | 4 | |
| 5 | FT | 250 | 235 | — | — | 2.8 |
| | (s) | (75) | (80) | — | — | (1.6) |
| | N | 318 | 91 | — | — | 409 |
| 6 | FT | 245 | 257 | — | — | 3.0 |
| | (s) | (73) | (85) | — | — | (1.8) |
| | N | 79 | 226 | — | — | 305 |
| 7 | FT | — | 255 | 235 | — | 3.3 |
| | (s) | — | (77) | (87) | — | (2.0) |
| | N | — | 186 | 47 | — | 233 |
| 8 | FT | — | 260 | 253 | — | 3.6 |
| | (s) | — | (95) | (78) | — | (2.1) |
| | N | — | 56 | 91 | — | 147 |
| 9 | FT | — | 287 | 248 | — | 4.4 |
| | (s) | — | (93) | (85) | — | (2.3) |
| | N | — | 30 | 49 | — | 79 |
| 10 | FT | — | — | 235 | 247 | 4.2 |
| | (s) | — | — | (97) | (90) | (2.6) |
| | N | — | — | 18 | 20 | 38 |
| 11 | FT | — | — | 257 | 223 | 4.2 |
| | (s) | — | — | (118) | (92) | (2.9) |
| | N | — | — | 12 | 9 | 21 |

[a]FT is fixation time (msec); s is standard deviation (msec); N is number of data points.

calls into question any assumption of serial processing of subword units based on number of letters or syllables (Gough, 1972; Just & Carpenter, 1980) and favors a whole-word processing hypothesis (Cattell, 1885; McClelland & Rumelhart, 1981).

Given that word length showed no relation to fixation duration, we then explored the influence of word frequency. The critical correlation, based on the same data set, was significant but rather low at .11.

The conclusion from the above analyses is that a substantial portion of the variance in gaze duration is attributable to the number of fixations on a word, rather than to fixation duration per se. In view of these results, the assumption that gaze duration reflects processing time seems unwarranted. However, it is possible that some words receive two fixations because they are more difficult to process. The following analyses, therefore, attempted to separate perceptual and psycholinguistic influences on fixation frequency.

# III. Preferred and Convenient Viewing Position

Strong support for the relevance of eye guidance for process theories of reading comes from the finding that fixations tend to be located slightly to the left of the middle of the word (Rayner, 1979a). For this to occur, some peripheral pre-processing must take place. Once the eye obtains this preferred viewing position, the whole word can be better apprehended within a single fixation. The right column in Table 19.1 gives the average letter position for words varying from 5 to 11 letters in length. Note that with increasing word length, the average fixation position moves further toward the right, confirming Rayner's results.

Recently, O'Regan (1980, 1981) demonstrated that under conditions of nonoptimal positioning of the eye, that is, close to the beginning or the end of the word, distributed processing is likely to occur. That is, a second fixation tends to be placed at the other end of the word. In this case, the normally preferred position is not taken. These findings can be tested in a post-hoc fashion with the present data. The question is whether fixation positions in the word differ significantly given one or two fixations.

We have examined all double- and single-fixation words five to nine letters long in our sample of text. Pooling across subjects and the selection criteria made statistical tests problematic. The same word could possibly appear in different categories. Other words might show up only once, or the same word might show up a different number of times in different categories. Analyses were made under the assumption that the words in the one-fixation case, in the progressive sequence, and in the regressive sequence form independent groups. The average fixation duration for the one-fixation case (OFC) was 253 msec. For the two-fixation case (TFC), the first fixation in a progressive sequence (PS) was 248 msec. The first fixation in a regressive sequence (RS) averaged 214 msec. The respective second fixations lasted 223 msec and 237 msec on the average. The left half of Table 19.2 displays these values and the corresponding number of observations and standard deviations. The OFC resulted in significantly longer fixation durations; fixation durations for PS and RS were not statistically different. Note that the values for PS and RS were based on the averages of two fixations occuring in these patterns. These results confirm, in continuous text, O'Regan's finding that single fixations on a word are typically longer than each of two fixations in the two-fixation case. Notice, however, that a gaze measure, such as the sum of the single fixation durations, would yield almost twice as much processing time under TFC.

The right half of Table 19.2 also shows the letter positions at which the various fixations occurred. The space in front of a word was interpreted as the 0-letter position. The following order describes the positions of the fixations across the different conditions: first fixation of PS, second fixation of RS, fixation of OFC,

TABLE 19.2
Mean (Standard Deviation) of Fixation Duration and Letter Position
for One and Two Fixation Case

| Case | Duration | | Position | |
|---|---|---|---|---|
| | First fixation | Last fixation | First fixation | Last fixation |
| One fixation case | 253 | — | 3.5 | — |
| (N = 1116) | (82) | — | (1.7) | — |
| Two fixation cases | | | | |
| Progressive sequence | 248 | 223 | 1.3 | 5.5 |
| (N = 166) | (93) | (87) | (1.3) | (2.0) |
| Regressive sequence | 214 | 237 | 5.0 | 2.1 |
| (N = 102) | (79) | (100) | (1.8) | (1.5) |

first fixation of RS, second fixation of PS. With the exception of the two fixations at the word end, all these positions were significantly different from each other (see Kliegl, 1981b, for details). Thus, during a PS the fixations are closer to the beginning of a word than during a RS. Also, the position of the fixation in the OFC is between the first and last fixation of the TFC.

The distinction between a progressive and a regressive sequence in the two-fixation case revealed differences that are plausible in the context of an asymmetry of processing in the visual field. Recent research shows this field to extend up to 15 characters to the right (O'Regan, 1979; Rayner & Bertera, 1979; Rayner, Inhoff, Morrison, Slowiaczek, & Bertera, 1981; Rayner, McConkie, & Ehrlich, 1978) and about 4 letters to the left (Rayner, McConkie, & Zola, 1980; Rayner, Well, & Pollatsek, 1980). The positions of the fixations and their variation with word length indicate that with a fixation at the beginning of a word, most letters will be processed from this location. The few remaining peripheral letters cause the second fixation to fall close to the end of the word and allow for a shorter fixation at this location.

The data summarized in Table 19.2 were obtained from words ranging from five to nine letters in length. It was shown earlier that word length had no effect on fixation time for words receiving a single fixation. The same result was obtained for the two-fixation condition. However, the relevance of word length for eye-guidance factors could be demonstrated if there were a dependence between fixation *position* and word length. Fixations too close to either end of a word may necessitate a second fixation, thereby nearly doubling the total fixation time. Several polynomial analyses were executed for the letter positions of the various fixations. Significant linear trends were found for the position of the last fixation in a progressive sequence, for both the fixations in a regressive sequence, and for the one-fixation condition. With the exception of the first fixation in a progressive sequence, fixation positions tended to shift toward the right as word length increased.

The two fixation conditions are certainly in agreement with what one would expect under peripheral acuity limitations. However, there is the possibility that the tendency to make a second fixation is related to psycholinguistic processing demands of the word. To test this hypothesis, the average word frequency was calculated as a function of number of fixations for each of the three submatrices indicated in Table 19.1. In all three tests word frequency was lower when two fixations occured, but the difference was significant only for the words 10 and 11 letters long. Thus, we again find some evidence for the effect of word frequency on eye movements.

## IV.   Influences across Words

So far we presented the problem of perceptual acuity limitations and language processing as a problem to identify what proportion of fixation duration variance is allocated to either of them. Our data provide relatively weak evidence for the relevance of language processes. Summing fixations on a word into a gaze measure and interpreting this time merely as a reflection of psycholinguistic processes as Just and Carpenter (1980) propose, seems not warranted in the light of our analysis on convenient viewing. If a second fixation occurs for perceptual reasons, a large proportion of the second fixation reflects the time it takes to generate a second saccade and determine its ballistic properties. Nevertheless, there might be a subtle interaction between achieving a convenient position on a word and the demands for psycholinguistic processing resources preceding this word. That is, perceptual acuity limitations might arise due to psycholinguistic processing demands. If a portion of the text requires intensive psycholinguistic processing, the quality of peripheral preprocessing might suffer and lead to saccades that are less than optimal in positioning the next fixation. We are presently designing experiments that will test the influence of cognitive processing demands on the accuracy of the saccade generating system.

An alternative explanation for the occurrence of two fixations due to inconvenient viewing position is the saccade generating system itself. We will test two possible hypotheses related to this explanation. First, inconvenient viewing positions might arise due to serial dependencies in the saccade and fixation duration series. Second, there might be a lack of resilience to make very long or very short saccades. Under situations where this would be required to obtain the convenient position, an undershoot or overshoot might result.

### A.   Serial Dependencies

As eye movements and fixations form a time series, an obvious question to ask from these data is whether subsequent fixation durations and saccade sizes show an autocorrelational structure. Further, one wonders whether there are any cross-correlations between these two parameters. If the length of a saccade were dependent on the length of preceding saccades, or on the duration of previous fixations, this would lead to inaccurate placements of fixations on a word. For example, if saccade N was long, saccade N + 1 might be short. These dependencies could theoretically exist independent of word and text characteristics and override the preprocessing abilities of the saccade calculating system.

There have been several studies looking for a correlation between and within the eye movement parameters. Rayner and McConkie (1976) came to the conclusion that saccade size and fixation duration are two factors that must be accounted for separately. Their basis for this is the lack of correlation between successive fixation durations, between successive saccade sizes, and between the size of a saccade and the preceding and following fixation time, respectively. Poor correlations among similar variables have been reported by Andriessen and de Voogd (1973). Further, Just and Carpenter (1980) did not find significant autocorrelations for the residuals of their data.

It is worth pointing out that all the studies reviewed only calculated the lag-one autocorrelation. Thus, it is not clear whether there are some higher order relations. To provide both a replication and an extension of the previous reports the complete autocorrelation functions were calculated. The results indicated that neither for fixation time, that is, the sum of the fixations on a word, nor the first fixation durations, nor for the saccade sizes out of a word were there significant correlations at any lag. Taking the sequence of fixations as the series—instead of the sequence of words—yielded similar results. Thus, at a global level, these results are in agreement with previous research and yield similar results for higher order correlations. They also do not support the hypothesis that serial dependencies might be a reason for inconvenient viewing positions.

## B.  Lack of Saccadic Resilience

The analysis of the one-fixation words showed that there was a strong tendency to fixate close to the center of a word. In regression terminology, word length was a good predictor of the fixation position on the word. Since saccades are ballistic movements, this is strong support for preprocessing of peripheral information. However, word length of the fixated word does not explain all of the fixation position variance. The position of a fixation might also be determined by the position on and the length of the previous word. For example, given a fixation at the end of a word, one could expect the next fixation to be also close to the end of the word. Or, given a long word and a middle fixation position, one might expect the following fixation position to be closer to the beginning of the word. Basically, it is assumed that saccade size lacks the required resilience to counteract any misplacements that might arise because of the partly stochastic nature of the saccade generating system. Consequently, nonoptimal positions might be obtained because of characteristics of word and position during the previous fixation. To test for the influence of the previous word length and previous fixation position, we calculated multiple correlations between the fixation position and length of the

TABLE 19.3
Multiple Correlation of Fixation Position with Length of Previous Word
and Position of Previous Fixation

| Subject | 1 | 2 | 3 | 4 | 5 | 6 |
|---------|-----|-----|-----|-----|-----|-----|
| $R^a$ | .20 | .35 | .10 | .32 | .20 | .24 |
| $N^b$ | 125 | 231 | 256 | 172 | 127 | 193 |

[a] $R$ is the multiple correlation between position of fixation and length of and position of fixation on previous word (length of present word partialed out).
[b] $N$ is the number of observations.

previous word, and the fixation position on the current word. We first partialed out the length of the current word. The only data included were word pairs that were next to each other in the text for which the eye progressed from the first to second word. The results are given in Table 19.3. The incremental $R$'s are significant for all but the third subject. The correlations confirm our expectations that the current fixation position is dependent on both the length of the previously fixated word and the fixation position of that word. The results suggest that the saccade generating system occasionally cannot generate the very short or very long saccades that are sometimes required to achieve an optimal viewing position. Fixations following long words tend to be at the beginning of the word; fixations following short words tend to be toward the end.

# V. Conclusion

This chapter presented some thought and data about the possibilities of unconfounding perceptual and language processes. In the first set of analyses on single-fixation words, length was not related to fixation duration for words ranging from 5 to 11 letters and one to four syllables. These results are inconsistent with the syllable-unit processing proposed by Just and Carpenter (1980) and Gough's (1972) serial letter-scanning model. The lack of a word-length effect on single fixation durations is consistent with word–unit and parallel letter processing models (cf. Cattell, 1885; McClelland & Rumelhart, 1981). It also is in accord with research on semantic classification and lexical decision. For example, Terry, Samuels, and LaBerge (1976) found that in a semantic classification task, word length had no effect on decision time. However, the lack of word length effects has only been shown for reasonably well-known words in a semantic context. Infrequent and novel words, beginning readers, and poor readers might yield different results.

In the second set of analyses, previous experimental results by Rayner (1979a) and O'Regan (1980, 1981) on the "preferred" and "convenient" position of fixations were replicated. The number of fixations on a word were interpreted to be mostly due to perceptual factors. For long words, however, the frequency of words that received two fixations was lower than for words of the same length fixated once. This corresponds to a result from the analysis of single-fixation words wherein fixation duration correlated at .11 with word frequency. Thus, fixation time appeared to be influenced by perceptual factors related to acuity limits in eye guidance, but there was also evidence for the relevance of psycholinguistic variables.

Kliegl *et al.* (1982) demonstrated that multiple regression approaches as the one advanced by Just and Carpenter (1980) are critically dependent on multiple fixations of words. The analyses of two-fixation cases from the perspective of inconvenient viewing called into question the justification of summing fixations on a word into a measure of gaze. It seems necessary to explore the causes of inconvenient viewing that then lead to the potential doubling of fixations. Although O'Regan's (1980, 1981) experimental induction, that is, shifting a word during a saccade, was ideal for demonstrating the relevances of an inconvenient position on a word, the "origin" of inconvenient viewing positions under conditions of normal reading is still an open question. The final part of this chapter tested two possible causes that would result as consequences of properties assumed for the saccade generating system. The first hypothesis, serial dependencies of subsequent saccades, was not confirmed by the data. However, there was support for the second hypothesis: The position of the fixation in a word can be predicted to some degree by the length of the previous word and the position of the fixation on this word. The data were consistent with an assumption that saccades do not tend to be very short or very long, even if this were required to achieve the optimal viewing position within a word. Thus, the doubling of fixations may have its cause in an inconvenient positioning of a fixation on a previous word. In a sense, only an "aggregation of inconvenience" might lead to doubling up.

There is, of course, the possibility that psycholinguistic processing demands will cause the saccade generating system to operate less accurately. This hypothesis predicts that the doubling up of fixations would occur in regions of the text that generate greater cognitive demands. The more we can determine the influences of previous conditions on present ones, the closer we will come to an understanding of the dynamics of the reading process.

In conclusion, the results argue for the consideration of both perceptual and psycholinguistic processes in the evaluation of eye fixation data. Further, the more challenging tasks will lie in exploring the interaction of the saccade generating system with the cognitive processing demands during reading. This will considerably enhance the value of these data for developing a flexible process model of reading that accounts for variations in individuals, materials, and task demands.

# References

Andriessen, J. J., & de Voogd, A. H. (1973). Analysis of eye-movement patterns in silent reading. *IPO Annual Progress Report*, 8, 29–53.

Camus, H. (1948). *The plague* (transl. by S. Gilbert). New York: Random House. (Originally published 1947.)

Cattell, J. McK. (1885). Ueber die Zeit der Erkennung und Bennenung von Schriftzeichen, Bildern, und Farben. *Philosophische Studien, 2,* 635–650.

Davidson, B. J. (1981). A rotating buffer system for on-line collection of eye monitor data. *Behavioral Research Methods and Instrumentation, 13,* 112–114.

Gough, P. B. (1972). One second of reading. In J. F. Kavanaugh & I. G. Mattingly (Eds.), *Language by ear and by eye.* Cambridge, Massachusetts: MIT Press.

Just, M. A., & Carpenter, P. A. (1980). A theory of reading: From eye fixations to comprehension. *Psychological Review, 87,* 329–354.

Kliegl, R. (1981). Automated and interactive analysis of eye fixation data in reading. *Behavioral Research Methods and Instrumentation, 13,* 115–120. (a)

Kliegl, R. (1981). *Eye-movements in reading: An attempt to separate perceptual and psycholinguistic factors.* Unpublished master's thesis, University of Colorado. (b)

Kliegl, R., & Olson, R. K. (1981). Reduction and calibration of eye monitor data. *Behavioral Research Methods and Instrumentation, 13,* 107–111.

Kliegl, R., Olson, R. K., & Davidson, B. J. (1982). Regression analysis as a tool for studying reading processes: Comment on Just and Carpenter's eye fixation theory. *Memory & Cognition, 10,* 287–95.

McClelland, J. L. & Rumelhart, D. E. (1981). An interactive activation model of context effects in letter perception: Part 1. An account of basic findings. *Psychological Review, 88,* 375–407.

McConkie, G. W. (1979). On the role and control of eye movements in reading. In P. A. Kolers, M. E. Wrolstad, & H. Bouma (Eds.), *Processing of visible language.* New York: Plenum Press.

O'Regan, J. K. (1979). Saccade size control in reading: Evidence for the linguistic control hypothesis. *Perception & Psychophysics, 17,* 578–586.

O'Regan, J. K. (1980). The control of saccade size and fixation duration in reading: The limits of linguistic control. *Perception & Psychophysics, 28,* 112–117.

O'Regan, J. K. (1981). The "convenient viewing position" hypothesis. In D. F. Fisher, R. A. Monty, & J. W. Senders (Eds.), *Eye movements: Cognition and visual perception.* Hillsdale, New Jersey: Erlbaum.

Pynte, J. (1974). Readiness for pronunciation during the reading process. *Perception & Psychophysics, 16,* 487–504.

Rayner, K. (1979). Eye guidance in reading: Fixation locations within words. *Perception, 8,* 21–30. (a)

Rayner, K. (1979). Eye movements in reading: Eye guidance and integration. In P. A. Kolers, M. E. Wrolstad, & H. Bouma (Eds.), *Processing of visible language.* New York: Plenum Press. (b)

Rayner, K., & Bertera, J. H. (1979). Reading without a fovea. *Science, 206,* 468–469.

Rayner, K., Inhoff, A. W., Morrison, R. E., Slowiaczek, M. L., & Bertera, J. H. (1981). Masking of foveal and parafoveal vision during eye fixations in reading. *Journal of Experimental Psychology: Human Perception & Performance, 7,* 167–179.

Rayner, K., & McConkie, G. W. (1976). What guides a reader's eye movements? *Vision Research, 16,* 829–837.

Rayner, K., McConkie, G. W., & Ehrlich, S. (1978). Eye movements and integrating information across fixations. *Journal of Experimental Psychology: Human Perception & Performance, 4,* 529–544.

Rayner, K., McConkie, G. W., & Zola, D. (1980). Integrating information across eye movements. *Cognitive Psychology, 12,* 206–226.

Rayner, K., Well, A. D., & Pollatsek, A. (1980). Asymmetry of the effective visual field in reading. *Perception & Psychophysics, 27,* 537–544.

Terry, P., Samuels, S. J., & LaBerge, D. (1976). The effect of letter degradation and letter spacing on word recognition. *Journal of Verbal Learning and Verbal Behavior, 15,* 577–585.

Tinker, M. A. (1958). Recent studies of eye movements in reading. *Psychological Bulletin, 55,* 215–231.

Maria L. Slowiaczek

# 20

# What Does the Mind Do
# while the Eyes Are Gazing?

## I.   Introduction

In reading, the eyes move in a pattern that reflects properties of the text. Although this statement is undeniably true, it is largely uninformative without specifying which properties are affecting the eye movements. Properties of the text range from visual properties, such as the spacing and positioning of words on a page, to the more complex properties of meaning that the reader uses to infer how one sentence should be integrated with another.

Early theories suggested that text properties had little direct influence on fixation patterns. For example, Bouma and DeVoogd (1974) proposed that the eyes moved in a regular pattern that did not reflect local changes in processing difficulty. According to this model, visual information was accumulated on each fixation and stored in a buffer, so that processing could continue after the eyes had moved. Suppose that the eyes moved at a constant rate of 200 msec per fixation. If the visual information accumulated during fixation $N$ required 250 msec of processing time, processing would be completed on the buffered information during fixation $N + 1$. For simple text, some subsequent fixation, $N + k$, might require only 150 msec of processing time. Although cognitive processing would lag behind the eye movements at difficult parts of the text, the lag would not accumulate. For difficult text, however, more of the fixations would require additional processing time, so that the buffer would reach the limit of its capacity. To remedy this situation, the eyes would move at a slower rate so that processing could be completed before new visual information was accumulated. Thus, this model proposed

EYE MOVEMENTS IN READING:
PERCEPTUAL AND LANGUAGE PROCESSES

that the difficulty of the text would determine the average fixation duration, but that individual fixations would not reflect the local processing difficulty of the fixated word or phrase.

More recently, experiments that used changing displays that were controlled by eye movements have demonstrated that fixation patterns are affected by local visual characteristics of the text. In a series of "window" experiments (McConkie & Rayner, 1975; see Rayner, 1978, for a review), partial information was presented in the parafovea but a prespecified region that included the fovea contained complete information. This "window" of complete information moved through the text in synchrony with the eyes. Fixation patterns were affected by the size of the window and by visual information presented in the parafovea. Rayner and Pollatsek (1981) used a window that varied in size from fixation to fixation to show that the visual properties of the display have an immediate effect on the fixation pattern. The size of the window affected the extent of the next eye movement. They also demonstrated that fixation duration was influenced by information available on the current fixation.

Demonstrations of eye movement control based on visual characteristics of text have encouraged language researchers to use eye movements to study sentence processing. Most sentence processing tasks do not provide a direct measure of processing difficulty while the sentence is being understood. Usually, a response is measured at the end of a sentence, or a secondary task is used to measure processing load during sentence presentation. If fixation patterns are controlled by the cognitive processes used in reading, then eye movements can provide an on-line measure of processing difficulty. Furthermore, if these effects occur immediately, as the difficult part of the text is encountered, fixation time will reflect local changes in processing time.

The chapters in Parts IV and V, on language processing, reflect the initial burst of optimism in using eye movements to study language processing. Many of the chapters have warned of the difficulties, although all of them report some success in isolating higher level variables that influence eye movements. In Chapter 17, Carpenter and Just argued for a model of eye movement control that emphasizes the role of text characteristics. They measured gaze duration, the total time spent fixated on a word. They proposed that the gaze duration for each word reflects the difficulty of the full range of cognitive processes that integrate that word into the developing meaning representation of the passage. They reviewed evidence that is consistent with this view, and they presented a model of reading to explain the observed effects. Both of the other chapters in Part V focused on the problems that arise in trying to determine the processes used in reading by measuring eye movements. Hogaboam stressed that the pattern of fixations is important in measuring how much information is processed during each fixation. Kliegl, Davidson, and Olsen pointed out the weaknesses of using a multiple regression analysis to infer underlying processes, and suggested a selective sampling technique as an alternative.

This discussion is divided into three sections. In Section II, I review the problems discussed by Hogaboam and by Kleigl *et al.* In Section III, I discuss the role of multiple regression analyses in developing a theory of reading. In Section IV, I compare the theory presented by Carpenter and Just to an alternative class of theories and I review the evidence for each of these.

## II.  Problems in Measuring Processing Time

If each fixation duration is to provide a measure of processing time for the fixated part of the sentence, it is necessary to know which part of the sentence is being processed on each fixation. Three questions must be addressed in using fixation during or gaze duration as a measure of local processing difficulty: What part of the text provides information on each fixation? How completely is the information processed before the eyes move on? What characteristics of the text are responsible for variations in fixation time? I shall discuss each of these questions in turn.

### A.  What Part of the Text Provides Information on Each Fixation?

By measuring gaze duration, Carpenter and Just assume that only information from the fixated word is accumulated. One of the problems with this assumption is that the eyes do not fixate every word in a regular pattern from left to right. Words are often skipped, some words are fixated more than once, and some words are fixated only after a regressive eye movement, when the reader returns to a part of the text that has presumably already been read. If $W_1$ is fixated and $W_2$ is skipped, the fixation time for $W_1$ might reflect processing time for $W_2$ as well as $W_1$. If a word is fixated twice, the fixation time might be inflated by the additional time required to plan the second eye movement within the word. As Hogaboam suggested, the fixation time for $W_1$ will not provide an accurate measure of processing time for $W_1$ unless the surrounding pattern of fixations is considered. Carpenter and Just dismissed this problem by asserting that, by and large, readers do fixate every word. Despite this assertion, they reported that readers skip 18% of the content words and 62% of the function words in a sample they collected. If the skipped function words are being processed parafoveally, this processing could be contributing to the fixation time that is associated with the content words.

The extent to which a word can be processed parafoveally probably varies with the processing demands of the fixated word, as well as with the distance of the parafoveal word from the center of fixation. This distance will depend on the length of the fixated word, the position of the fixation within the word, and the length of the parafoveal word. As a consequence, the location of a fixation can affect both the fixation duration and the location of the next fixation.

## B.  How Completely Is the Information Processed before the Eyes Move On?

There is no strong justification for the assumption that the fixation time for a word directly mirrors the processing time for that word. Possibly, the eyes stay fixated on a word just long enough to complete some set of low-level processes, and higher level processes "lag" behind as new visual information is accumulated. Carpenter and Just have suggested that, if this is so, fixation time on $W_2$ should reflect the difficulty of the processes that were initiated at $W_1$. However, they found no effect of the word length and word frequency of $W_1$ on the gaze duration of $W_2$. Since they did find effects of the length and frequency of $W_2$, this result suggests that word recognition processes are completed while the word is fixated. However, it does not rule out a delay for other more complex language processes.

The structure of language requires that some processes be delayed, because the full meaning of a word or phrase can often be determined only when it is organized with other information that appears later in the sentence. Perhaps these processes, which organize words into constituents or determine the relations among concepts, are completed at constituent boundaries. If so, we would not expect extra processing time to be reflected a constant number of words from where the process was initiated, because constituent length will vary.

Auditory sentence processing experiments that use click localization and detection tasks (Fodor & Bever, 1965; Garrett, Bever, & Fodor, 1966; Holmes & Forster, 1970) have provided some evidence for the importance of constituent structure in sentence processing. Although these experiments do not demonstrate which processes are delayed, they do suggest that phrasal constituents function as processing units. Any theory of language that proposes constituent structure as the basis for processing units would predict some processes that were constrained by the completion of these units. Thus, the processes that integrated $W_1$ with other parts of the sentence or text would not occur until the eyes were fixated at some subsequent position in the text.

## C.  What Characteristics of the Text are Responsible for Variations in Fixation Time?

Since many of the properties of natural language are highly redundant, it is difficult to determine which property of the text is responsible for variations in fixation time. Even simple properties of individual words such as word length, number of syllables, and word frequency are not independent. This is especially a problem in studies that use natural text. Kleigl *et al.* (Chapter 19) recommend selective sampling from natural text in order to control for factors that are likely to be correlated. However, selective sampling limits the amount of data that can be considered from a given sample and might also introduce biases into the samples. Some researchers (K. Ehrlich, Chapter 15 in this volume; S. Ehrlich, Chapter 11 in this volume; Zola, 1982) have conducted controlled experiments in which subjects read passages instead of individual sentences. Experimental manipulations eliminate some of the problems created by correlated properties in natural text. However, these experiments are costly since often only one word or phrase is manipulated in an entire passage. Experimental manipulations in full passages might best be used as the final stage of a research program after an exploration of natural text suggests the initial hypotheses.

## III. The Role of Multiple Regression Analysis

Many researchers have chosen to use multiple regression analysis to determine which text factors predict fixation duration and to infer the component processes that these factors reflect. A multiple regression analysis is a valuable first step in trying to determine what factors might play a role in controlling eye movements. Specifying a set of variables that predict fixation duration can lead to interesting hypotheses about the component processes in reading. These hypotheses can then be tested in controlled experiments. Problems arise, however, when a multiple regression analysis is taken not as an exploratory first step but as conclusive support for the underlying processes. Factors used in the analysis might not be determinants of ongoing language processes. If these factors are correlated with other variables that actually do control cognitive processing, they will serve as effective predictors of reading behavior although they will be misleading as indicators of the underlying processes. This problem is largely avoided in the experimental approach by constructing sentences that are identical except for the manipulated factor.

Reports of multiple regression analyses of fixation time have focused too strongly on the proportion of variance accounted for as the criterion for accepting some text factor as an indicator of the processes used in reading. Ultimately, a collection of unrelated factors that are used in a regression analysis will not satisfy our criteria for an explanation of reading, even if 100% of the variance could be accounted for. In addition to finding an effect of these factors on fixation time, a satisfying explanation of reading must show how these factors are used in the processing system.

Let us consider some examples of variables that suggest plausible processing components of reading and some that do not. In the work reported in Section V, word length and word frequency have been isolated as two predictors of fixation durations. These both seem like good candidates for factors that truly affect processes in reading. A theory of the perceptual mechanism should include an explanation of word-length effects. Perhaps word length effects are a consequence of how easily visual information can be extracted from the fixated word. The convenient viewing hypothesis (O'Regan, 1980) and the preferred viewing hypothesis (Rayner, 1979) suggest that the reader will fixate the position in a word that allows an optimal amount of visual information to be extracted (usually to the left of the center of the word). Word length effects might result from nonoptimal positioning of the fixation in longer words.

The length of the fixated word might also affect the time needed to plan the next eye movement. If the third character of a seven-character word is fixated, the next word will begin six characters away from the center of fixation. Parafoveal processing time needed to determine the position of the next fixation might increase when the next word is further from the center of fixation. If so, word length effects might be explained by the mechanism that plans where the eyes move, rather than by the encoding process for the fixated word. These hypotheses propose interesting alternatives that need to be tested experimentally. Carpenter and Just suggest that word length effects are not caused by differences in acuity, since they are obtained even for short words that are within the foveal region. However, they have not looked at where the eye was positioned in the words or how much information was available from the previous fixation.

Word frequency presumably influences word identification processes. These processes have been studied extensively, and several theories (Broadbent, 1968; McClelland & Rumelhart, 1981; Morton, 1969) have tried to explain word frequency effects.

Other predictors are less likely to correspond to components in a processing system. For example, syntactic category might initially seem to be a good candidate as a predictor of a syntactic component in language processing. However, because of the redundant properties in natural language, finding an effect of syntactic category cannot even provide evidence for a syntactic component. Imagine two extreme theories of language processing. One theory claims that a structural representation is built, independent of semantic factors, before the sentence can be interpreted. The second theory claims that the sentence is immediately organized into a semantic representation of predicates and arguments without any intermediate syntactic structuring. Finding an effect of syntactic category cannot even distinguish between these two extreme theories, because words that are distinct in syntactic category will often be distinct in semantic category as well.

On closer consideration, what intrinsic property of a syntactic category would lead us to expect longer or shorter fixations on any given category? Only by developing a specific theory do we have any reason to expect fixation duration to vary as a function of syntactic category.

An interest in syntactic category suggests an implicit theory. The theory proposes that phrases are important, since syntax is a way of describing how words are joined together in phrases. But once this theory is made explicit, it predicts that fixation duration should be affected by the function of a word in the structure of a phrase, not by its syntactic category alone. For example, in the following sentence

*The friendly old man who owns the hardware store down the street sells kite string in the spring.*

the word *man* and the word *street* are both nouns, but *man* is the head noun in the subject noun phrase, and *street* is the noun in a prepositional phrase embedded in a relative clause. The roles that these two nouns play in the syntactic structure of this sentence are very different. In addition, the noun *street* is the last word in the complex noun phrase subject which includes both the head noun and the relative clause. A theory that proposed a component in the processer that organized phrases into syntactic constituents might predict longer fixation times on *street* since this word marks the boundary of a major syntactic constituent. By simply looking at syntactic category without developing a specific theory, important distinctions such as this would be overlooked.

Carpenter and Just have used a multiple regression analysis of gaze duration as support for their theory of reading. Regrettably, the analysis they report primarily provides support for word recognition variables: 69% of the variance can be explained by word length and word frequency effects alone. Adding another 11 predictors can account for only an additional 10% of the variance. Not only are these additional predictors weakly supported by the data, but they also do not suggest interesting hypotheses about the underlying mechanisms. For example, words are coded for variables such as the first word in the line, the last word in a sentence or paragraph, and the first content word in a passage. These variables probably correspond to different component processes (e.g., the position in a line affects word perception and the position in a sentence affects sentence organization). However, describing these variables as predictors of fixation time does not specify the components or how they are used in a complete processing system.

## IV.  Toward a Theory of Reading

Carpenter and Just propose a general theory and a specific model of reading in the form of a computer simulation. Although a computer simulation has the necessary detail to lead to interesting claims about normal reading, it must be sufficiently constrained so that theoretical claims can be tested.

The model proposed by Carpenter and Just is a production system with the rules about language structure and world knowledge represented as condition–action pairs. As new information is added to working memory, all of the productions that are enabled (i.e., all those whose conditions are satisfied) are executed. The conditions for one production can be satisfied by information that is accumulated by another production within the same execution cycle.

The following important theoretical claims are implicit in this model:

1. All of the knowledge about language and the world that can be used in understanding a sentence is represented in the same format, with no distinction made between syntactic knowledge, semantic knowledge, and pragmatic knowledge. Thus, within this system a production that states an abstract rule such as "expect a noun after a determiner" functions in exactly the same way as a produc-

tion that states a specific fact about the world such as "people become concerned with plumbing problems and sewers when they buy a house."

2. One meaning representation is developed as the outcome of applying these productions to the input string. This representation includes the inferences that connect the sentence to the discourse, as well as the representation of the semantic relations within the sentence. There is no intermediate level of organization that allows words to be grouped into constituents before the full implications of their meanings are understood.

3. A direct consequence of having one representation is that all of the processes that integrate a word into the representation are completed immediately. There are no buffers to hold information for later stages of processing.

4. All of the productions are completely interactive. The output of any production can be used to satisfy the input of another. This is a very strong claim about the role of context in reading. The recognition and organization of each fixated word will be influenced by all aspects of the meaning of the prior discourse up to and including the word that is being recognized.

Carpenter and Just have used three kinds of evidence to support the immediate processing claim (3), and the interactive processing claim (4).

1. They have developed a computer simulation model that conforms to these properties. This computer model is successful in reading one scientific passage about flywheels. However, 130 production rules were written to accomplish this feat, and only 30 of these rules are general enough to apply to other passages. More critically, there are no constraints on the enabling conditions for each production, so that the model has the flexibility to be consistent with any pattern of fixation time data. For example, (3) states that all processing of a word is completed immediately. However, in this model, the productions can only be executed when the enabling conditions are satisfied. The system can mimic delayed processing by using enabling conditions that are not satisfied until later in the sentence. Although productions are not differentiated by stages of processing, enabling conditions that delay processing can be introduced whenever the reading time data suggest delayed processes. This flexibility makes the immediate processing claim untestable in this model.

2. A multiple regression analysis on gaze duration in normal reading has been presented as support for immediate processing. As mentioned earlier, these analyses primarily provide support for word perception and recognition processes and not for the processes that combine words into sentences.

3. Experiments that show effects of context and parsing rules in understanding sentences were presented as evidence for immediate processing and interactive processing. These experiments fall into two categories. In the first, subjects were presented with one word at a time, and they pressed a button to indicate that they were ready to read the next word. Reading time for each word was measured from one button press to the next. Reading time was longer on the disambiguating word for misleading garden-path sentences, than for sentences that followed the pre-

ferred interpretation. Although this technique may provide some insight into what the preferred interpretation of a sentence might be, it does not demonstrate immediate organization of the sentence as the eyes move across the text. Reading speed is considerably slower in this task than in natural reading. Manipulations that affect reading time for the disambiguating word in this task might not be evident until a later fixation, under normal reading conditions, when fixation time was shorter.

The other set of experiments provides more convincing evidence for the immediate processing claim. These experiments have manipulated text factors while recording eye movements. Carpenter and Daneman (1981) used homographs such as *bass*, in a context which primed either the fish or the guitar pronunciation of the word. They found that readers used both word frequency and the prior context in choosing a pronunciation for the homograph. If their pronunciation was inconsistent with the preceding context, fixation time on the homograph was longer. However, the pronunciation of the word was much more strongly influenced by the frequency of the meaning than by the priming context. When the context primed the low frequency pronunciation of the word, the high frequency pronunciation was still used 62% of the time. Given that sometimes the low frequency pronunciation was chosen spontaneously in a neutral context, this result does not demonstrate a strong influence of prior meaning on word recognition.

They also measured the fixation time on the disambiguating word. Readers fixated longer on the disambiguating word when it was inconsistent with the prior context. For example, readers fixated longer on *guitarists* in the phrase *bass guitarists* when the context primed "fishing," than when the context primed "music." This effect does support the interactive processing claim, in that fixation time can be influenced by prior semantic context. However, it does not provide support for the immediate processing claim. The immediate processing claim asserts that semantic processing is completed on each word as it is recognized. If the semantic interpretation of a word $W$ affected the fixation time for $W + 1$, then the semantic processing of $W$ must have been completed by fixation $W + 1$. Since the semantic context in this experiment was developed in several sentences prior to the test sentence, the context effect is not necessarily due to the semantic interpretation of the preceding word or phrase. The context provided by the prior sentence must be separated from the context given by the interpretation of the homograph. If the pronunciation of the immediately preceding ambiguous word affected fixation time on the disambiguating word in a neutral context, the immediate processing claim would be strongly supported.

In another experiment, Just and Carpenter (1978) found longer gaze durations for words that followed as indirect inferences from a prior sentence than for direct inferences. For example, a context sentence such as: *The millionaire had been murdered* (direct inference) or *The millionaire had died* (indirect inference) was presented. Gaze duration was longer on *killer* in the sentence *The killer left no clues for the police to trace* for the indirect inference case. Again, this effect provides evidence for interactive processing but not necessarily for the immediate processing claim. In this experiment, each sentence was presented individually and subjects were required to decide whether or not the sentence fit with the rest of the prior sentences, before reading the next sentence. Thus, they had the opportunity to complete the processing on one sentence before continuing to the next. This experiment demonstrates that inferences from one sentence can affect the reading time of the next, under conditions which probably allow enough processing time for the inferences to be complete. However, this does not necessarily show that inferences from one sentence are completed so that they can affect semantic decisions when sentences are read in a continuous passage.

These findings demonstrate that fixation times can be affected by properties of the text that go beyond the perceptual characteristics. However, these experiments only test fully developed semantic representations that are highly constrained, either by limited contextual domains or by the requirements of the experimental task. Many important questions remain unanswered. How much does this kind of contextual constraint exist in normal text? How much of the context that precedes a given word is normally processed fully enough to influence the fixation time of a given word? What aspect of the recognition and integration of the target word is being influenced by the context?

Other plausible theories of language processing are consistent with the present data. Consider one alternative class of theories which requires separate levels of representation. In these theories, words are initially recognized and grouped into some constituent organization by using some rules of syntax. This intermediate syntactic representation is used to group the words into their appropriate constituents and to provide the structure that allows them to be maintained in memory long enough for the full semantic representation to be developed. The processes that organize relations among words and integrate the meaning of one sentence with another would not be reflected immediately in the fixation time of each word. These processes would occur when processing units were complete, so that they would most likely affect fixation time at processing unit boundaries.

There are two arguments in favor of this class of theories. First, many sentences could not be understood without developing the constituent structure (see Frazier, Chapter 13 in this volume). Second, some sentences are long and complex, and the full meaning cannot be fully appreciated immediately as the words are encoded. Since human readers are assumed to have capacity limits, the information must be structured so that it can be maintained in memory. The syntactic structure helps to maintain the sentence in memory so that the complex semantic interpretation can be completed.

The experiments reported in support of the immediate processing and interactive processing claims are also consistent with this alternative class of models. These alternative models predict delayed processing because constituents are organized in a syntactic structure before the semantic interpretation is developed. However, context effects can still occur if the semantic information comes from an earlier processing unit that has already been completed.

Carpenter and Just have found that fixation duration is longer at the end of a sentence, even when the effects of word category are factored out. This result is consistent with theories that propose a delay for some processes until a major constituent boundary is determined. However, this result is difficult to explain within the model proposed by Carpenter and Just.

The language processing system, no doubt, uses some information immediately and relies on constituent structure to determine the interpretation for other information. Only by carefully specifying detailed theories of the mechanisms in the language processing system can we ever hope to eliminate even the most broadly contrasting sets of theories. Platt (1964) has proposed that science be conducted according to the principle of strong inference, whereby each experiment contrasts two or more specific hypotheses. Thus, each experimental finding will eliminate one hypothesis and support another. Without this kind of deliberate effort to contrast alternatives, we will be faced with hundreds of demonstrations of both immediate processing and delayed processing without any critical tests that will distinguish the two.

What of using eye movements to study language processing? Carpenter and Just have been extremely influential in taking the first steps to demonstrate cognitive control of eye movements. Others have followed, and these language processing chapters have demonstrated that we have reason to be hopeful. However, we must take advantage of the techniques provided by the advanced eye movement recording technology in carefully accounting for what information is being processed during each fixation. Much of the early exciting work that used multiple regression analyses of reading time for natural text has provided the initial impetus for rigorous controlled experimentation that will help us to understand the complex mechanisms underlying reading.

## ACKNOWLEDGMENTS

I thank Patrick Carroll, Jim Johnston, David Krantz, and Saul Sternberg for helpful comments on an earlier draft of this chapter.

# References

Bouma, H., & de Voogd, A. H. (1974). On the control of eye saccades in reading. *Vision Research, 14*, 273–284.

Broadbent, D. E. (1968). The word frequency effect and response bias. In R. Haber (Ed.), *Contemporary theory and research in visual perception*. New York: Holt, Rinehart & Winston.

Carpenter, P., & Daneman, M. (1981). Lexical retrieval and error recovery in reading: A model based on eye fixations. *Journal of Verbal Learning and Verbal Behavior, 20*, 137–160.

Fodor, J. A., & Bever, T. G. (1965). The psychological reality of linguistic segments. *Journal of Verbal Learning and Verbal Behavior, 4*, 414–420.

Garrett, M., Bever, T., & Fodor, J. (1966). The active use of grammar in speech perception. *Perception & Psychophysics, 1*, 30–32.

Holmes, V., & Forster, K. T. (1970). Selection of extraneous signals during sentence recognition. *Perception & Psychophysics, 7*, 207–301.

Just, M. A., & Carpenter, P. A. (1978). Inference processes during reading: Reflections from eye fixations. In J. W. Senders, D. F. Fisher, & R. A. Monty (Eds.), *Eye movements and the higher psychological functions.* Hillsdale, New Jersey: Erlbaum.

McClelland, J., & Rumelhart, D. (1981). An interactive activation model of context effects in letter perception: Part 1, An account of basic findings. *Psychological Review, 885,* 375–407.

McConkie, G., & Rayner, K. (1975). The span of the effective stimulus during a fixation in reading. *Perception & Psychophysics, 17,* 578–586.

Morton, J. (1969). Interaction of information in word recognition. *Psychological Review, 76,* 165–178.

O'Regan, K. (1980). The control of saccade size and fixation duration in reading: The limits of linguistic control. *Perception & Psychophysics, 28,* 112–117.

Platt, J. R. (1964). Strong Inference. *Science, 146,* 347–353.

Rayner, K. (1978). Eye movements in reading and information processing. *Psychological Bulletin, 85*(3), 618–660.

Rayner, K. (1979). Eye guidance in reading: Fixation location in words. *Perception, 8,* 21–30.

Rayner, K., & Pollatsek, A. (1981). Eye movement control during reading: evidence for direct control. *Quarterly Journal of Experimental Psychology, 33A,* 351–373.

Zola, D. (In press). The effect of redundancy on the perception of words in reading. *Perception & Psychophysics.*

# VI
## Eye Movements in Picture Processing and Visual Search

Geoffrey R. Loftus

# 21

# Eye Fixations on Text and Scenes[1]

## I.   Introduction

Everyday visual behavior in human beings can roughly be divided into two quite different types: processing "natural information"—that is, looking at normal scenes—and processing "artificial information"—principally reading text. Eye movement research over the past 50 years or so has reflected the general belief that eye fixation patterns can tell us something about the perceptual and cognitive processes underlying the processing of both scenes and text. The major question that I address in this chapter is: To what degree can investigation of eye movement patterns tell us similar kinds of things about these two quite different kinds of visual behavior? This question, in turn, involves four interrelated subquestions.

1. What are the goals of an observer reading text versus the goals of an observer looking at a natural scene?
2. What are the similarities and differences in the structure of physical information comprising text versus natural scenes?
3. What are the corresponding similarities and differences in eye movement patterns, particularly fixation locations and fixation durations?
4. What types of perceptual and postperceptual processing occur within a single eye fixation on text versus a single eye fixation on a scene?

[1]This chapter was supported by National Science Foundation grant BNS79-06522 to the author.

EYE MOVEMENTS IN READING:
PERCEPTUAL AND LANGUAGE PROCESSES

## II.  Goals of the Observer

Everyday reading of text is carried out for a variety of purposes. One may read primarily to comprehend, as when reading a story or a newspaper editorial. Another important goal may be to subsequently remember the material as when one studies a textbook in preparation for an exam or memorizes the script of a play. As a rule, however, an important characteristic of reading is that the reader is typically processing new information. Reading text that one has read before is done occasionally, but it is the exception rather than the rule.

With respect to scene processing, quite the reverse is true. Unless one is an explorer or is engaged in one of a few other equally exotic occupations, the majority of looking experiences involve scenes that one has observed many times before. We see the same face in the mirror when we brush our teeth, the same scenery when we travel to work, and the same office when we arrive there. Processing familiar scenes is the rule whereas processing of novel scenes is, by comparison, infrequent.

In order for the comparison of text processing and scene processing to be meaningful in terms of eye movements or anything else, it is important to equate, at least roughly, the goals of the observer. Laboratory research that does this explicitly is exceedingly rare and therefore any conclusions stemming from a retrospective comparison of text and scene processing have rather severe built-in limitations. In terms of the literature I discuss, I will try to equate picture and text processing as follows. Under the assumption that reading usually involves the continual acquisition of new information, I will generally restrict my discussion of scene processing to situations in which the observer is similarly attempting to acquire new information from the scene. I will always discuss studies in which an observer is being shown novel scenes, and I will usually discuss studies in which the observer is looking at the scene in anticipation of some type of memory test.

## III.  Physical Structure of Information in Text and Pictures

It does not require a great deal of insight to notice that there are rather substantial differences between the structure of text and the structure of a scene. However, I believe that it may be fruitful to classify the nature of these differences along some of their most obvious dimensions.

### A.  Microstructure of the Informational Array

The most fundamental difference between text and scenes occurs with respect to the elementary objects that constitute the informational array. Text is for the most part made up of the 80 or so alphanumeric symbols that appear on a typewriter keyboard. These symbols, as well as their ordering into words, are highly overlearned, and the symbols are very densely packed into the visual field.

Scenes, on the other hand, can be composed of a literal representation or a caricature of virtually anything that appears in the visual world. The elements that make up scenes are of varying sizes and discriminability and are relatively spread out in space.

## B.  Constraint of Element Order

As is well known, the structure of text involves a great deal of predictability or constraint. This constraint occurs at a variety of levels, ranging from the sequence of letters in a word (orthographic constraint) to the sequence of words in a sentence (syntactic constraint) to the sequence of sentences in a paragraph (logical and aesthetic constraint). There are also constraints in scenes (e.g., Biederman, Mezzanotte, & Rabinowitz, 1981; Mandler & Johnson, 1976), but substantially fewer than is the case with text. As an illustration, consider a street scene. A typical object in the scene such as an automobile is certainly constrained to some degree by the rest of the scene. For example, the automobile would be unlikely to be floating in midair; nor would it be larger than a building. Nonetheless, there is still a large amount of freedom with respect to the relationship between the automobile and the rest of the scene. A related issue is that text is structured hierarchically and, at least at some levels, any given component of text can be unambiguously defined as belonging to one particular level of the hierarchy. For instance, a string of letters can be classified as a word or not a word and a string of words can be classified as a sentence or not a sentence. Although scenes may in principle be thought of as being structured hierarchically (cf. Palmer, 1977), the assignment of particular components of the scene to particular levels of the hierarchy is somewhat arbitrary.

It is important to note that a good deal of the constraint in language is captured by linguistic theories (e.g., Chomsky, 1965, 1968). In contrast, analogous theories that capture the constraints in natural scenes are, where they exist at all, exceedingly primitive and are applicable to only a small variety of rather contrived stimuli.

## C.  Semantics

At the level of the semantics—the level of what is "meant" by the physical information—text and scenes may be somewhat more similar. One could, for example, write a description of a scene such that the description contained much the same information as the scene depicted. However, the relatively meager amount of research comparing the memorial representation of scenes versus "equivalent" verbal descriptions has indicated that the representations in memory are probably somewhat different (e.g., Dallett & Wilcox, 1968; Nelson, Metzler, & Reed, 1974).

In short, the differences between the physical structure of pictures and the physical structure of text becomes less salient as we progress from the level of physical elements to the level of interelement constraint to the level of semantics.

As we shall see, these differences and similarities will lead to rather predictable consequences in terms of eye movement patterns that are observed on text versus pictures and in terms of what we can infer from such eye movement patterns about the psychological mechanisms that underlie the processing of these two different types of information.

## IV.   Differences in Eye Movement Patterns

A variety of different characteristics of eye movement patterns are used as bases for inferring underlying psychological processes. Some of the principal characteristics are (a) the perceptual span, that is, the useful field of view within each fixation; (b) fixation location; and (c) fixation duration. These characteristics are no doubt interrelated to some degree. However, for ease of discourse I will first discuss them separately.

### A.   The Useful Field of View

It is quite well known that the structure of the retina is such that visual acuity is best in the fovea which subtends only about 2° of visual angle. Acuity then falls off rapidly into the periphery of the retina. An important consequence of this anatomical arrangement is that during an eye fixation, detailed processing can be carried out only on information falling within a small region around the point of fixation.

Visual information falling on the retinal periphery can be seen and can be useful in a variety of situations. Text processing, however, does not appear to be one of these situations. The small size of the alphanumeric symbols constituting text (there are typically three or four such symbols per degree of visual angle) means that substantial acuity is required to distinguish these symbols from one another. This in turn means that very little peripheral processing should be possible with text.

Scenes, on the other hand, do not necessarily share this property. The physical features that comprise a scene are also subject to acuity limitations, but these features can be and often are large enough to allow identification of objects and relationships among objects in the visual periphery. These considerations lead to three identifiable consequences with respect to the useful field of view while viewing scenes versus text and the effects of this useful visual field on the eye movement pattern.

#### 1.   DETERMINATION OF FIXATION LOCATIONS

An issue that is currently the focus of a good deal of research concerns the mechanisms by which the locations of eye fixations are determined. It is almost certainly true that when viewing a scene, part of any given fixation is spent determining where subsequent fixations will fall (Gould, 1969). This determination is probably based both on the physical structure of the scene and on the information that is acquired during the current fixation. In any event, information that falls relatively far into the visual periphery can be used to determine the location of subsequent fixations. A demonstration of this assertion is provided in an experiment reported by Loftus and Mackworth (1978), the principal goal of which was to determine the "cognitive determinants of fixations locations on pictures." As will be discussed below, the major results of the experiment indicated that observers tended to fixate objects in pictures that were unusual with respect to the overall gist of the picture. The finding relevant to the present discussion, however, was that the average extent of a saccade preceding the first fixation on such an "unusual object" was about 7.4° of visual angle with a standard deviation of about 2.24°. This finding suggests that during any given fixation, information far into the visual periphery is potentially useable as a basis for determining the location of the next fixation.

With text the situation is somewhat different. First, the issue of whether peripheral information acquired during a given fixation is actually used to determine the location of subsequent fixations has been under debate (see Rayner, 1978, for a review). As things now stand, the resolution of this debate seems to be that such information is indeed used, although nobody knows exactly how this is done. But it does appear that any information that is used is only information that falls within about 4° of the current point of fixation (McConkie & Rayner, 1975; Rayner, 1975).

## 2. THE PERCEPTUAL SPAN: ACQUISITION OF USEFUL INFORMATION WITHIN A FIXATION

We can contrast two different types of information that are acquired within a fixation. The first, just discussed, is information used primarily for determining the location of subsequent fixations. The second type of information might be termed "substantive information." This is information that is used for comprehension and/or is stored away in memory for subsequent use. Walter Nelson and I have recently reported a series of experiments in which we have investigated this useful field of view with respect to acquisition of substantive information during picture viewing (Nelson & Loftus, 1980). In these experiments, a series of target pictures was initially presented to a subject in the study phase of a picture recognition paradigm, and subjects' fixation locations over the picture were monitored. In a subsequent test phase, the target pictures were presented in a two-alternative forced choice test in which a distractor differed from a target in that only one small "critical detail" was changed. For example, if the target picture was a scene of a backyard in which a beer can was sitting on a fence, the distractor picture would be identical except that the beer can was replaced by a pack of cigarettes. Thus, encoding of the critical detail at the time of the original study was necessary to discriminate the target in the recognition test at an above chance level. Of primary interest in this experiment was the probability of correct recognition as a function of the distance of the closest fixation to the critical detail at the time of original study. When this distance was zero (i.e., when a fixation had been made directly on the critical detail), recognition memory performance was quite high: around 85 or 90%, with guessing being 50%. As this distance increased, performance likewise decreased up to the point where recognition probability was about 60% at a distance of about 2° of visual angle. At greater distances, performance remained constant at around 60% which is low but clearly above chance. The conclusion was that whereas the majority of substantive information within a fixation is drawn from the area within about a 2° radius around the point of regard, some useful information was being acquired from quite far into the periphery.

Again with respect to text, the situation is somewhat different. An extensive series of experiments investigating this issue has been reported by McConkie, Rayner, and their associates. Earlier studies (e.g., Rayner, 1975) utilized a technique in which subjects read text that was displayed on a cathode-ray tube (CRT). The text was controlled by a computer that was simultaneously monitoring the subject's eye position. A major manipulation involved changing the meaning of some target word that fell at varying distances from the current point of regard. Semantic analysis was assumed to have been carried out on the target word if the eventual fixation duration on it increased relative to duration in a control condition. The results of these studies (summarized by Rayner, 1978) were quite straightforward: The only text analyzed for its semantic content was that falling in an area within about ±1° around the point of regard, that is, in the fovea or just outside the fovea. Using the somewhat more sensitive technique of obliterating the foveal region with a noise mask during reading, Rayner and Bertera (1979) found that a mask extending only about ±1.25° around the point of regard drove comprehension (as measured by a subsequent test) virtually to chance. In short, the conclusion is that substantive information is acquired from text from a considerably smaller region than is the case with scenes.

### 3.  HOMOGENEITY OF THE EYE MOVEMENT PATTERN

There is a good deal of evidence that the "gist" of a scene can be acquired fairly rapidly—probably within the first 100 msec or so following the onset of the scene (Biederman, 1972; Biederman, Rabinowitz, Glass, & Stacy, 1974). This means that the first fixation on a scene is very special since the gist of the scene is acquired during this fixation. Subsequent fixations on the picture can be and probably are guided in large part by the gist that is initially revealed.

A necessary condition for such gist acquisition is that a large amount of peripheral processing be possible—since the gist of a scene could not typically be acquired if only a very small window of the scene were available to the visual system. With text, the situation is quite different. Since only a small amount of text can be processed during a given fixation, the gist of the information in a block of text cannot be revealed during the first or even during the first few fixations on the text. It is perhaps noteworthy that a reader's inability to acquire the gist of a block of text within a single fixation has implications with respect to writing skills. Specifically, one of the skills required of a good writer is the ability to structure text such that the gist is revealed as quickly as possible; such structure is implemented via heading arrangements and the judicious placement of information within the first few sentences of the text. Conversely, one of the hallmarks of a poor writer is the failure to arrange the structure of text in this way. (We have probably all had the experience of reading text and never really figuring out its gist at all.)

However, no matter how cleverly the text is structured, the processing of at least a sentence or two—which will require several fixations—is required to get the gist. When reading text, there may be a shift in processing strategy after the first few fixations when the gist has been acquired, but this shift is nowhere near as marked as it is following the first fixation on a scene. Indeed, a good case can be made for the proposition that a substantial number of the thousand words that a picture is worth are those that are required to unveil the gist (Mandler & Johnson, 1976).

## B. Location of Fixations

The question of which locations are fixated in a scene or a block of text can be addressed in two somewhat different ways. The first involves sequential predictability; that is, given a current fixation location, where is the next fixation likely to be? The second question involves overall location predictability; that is, to what degree can we predict which locations will be fixated at one time or another during some fixation sequence?

### 1. SEQUENTIAL PREDICTABILITY

There are enormous and obvious differences in terms of predictability of the sequence of fixation locations on scenes versus text. Again these differences reflect, in a quite natural way, differences in the physical structure of the stimulus array. The general idea is that when looking at text, an observer shows relatively little variation with respect to the fixation sequence, which consists of a series of sequential fixations along the line of text followed by a return sweep to the beginning of the next line. The only real exception to this rule is seen in the occasional occurrence of regressions. (That regressions constitute the only real exception to the regular fixation pattern on text is probably the major reason that so much attention has been paid to the topic.)

With scenes, on the other hand, there is a large amount of uncertainty in terms of the sequence of fixation locations. Given that an observer is fixating on a given place in a picture, it is extremely difficult to predict where the next fixation will be. The only suggestion of even minimal predictability has been reported by Noton and Stark (1971) who reported a modest degree of correspondence with respect to sequential fixation locations when a specific observer views a specific picture on separate occasions. However, this correspondence vanishes in the case of (a) a given observer viewing different pictures; or (*b*) a given picture being viewed by different observers.

## 2. OVERALL PREDICTABILITY

With respect to overall predictability, a comparison of the fixation pattern on text versus scenes produces a somewhat different conclusion. Research on text processing has not been very revealing in terms of particular places that will be fixated (cf. Rayner, 1978). This is in part because the fixation pattern on text is so dense—average saccade length on text is only about 2°—that virtually all of a block of text is fixated foveally. With respect to scenes, however, it has been known since the work of Buswell (1935) that a large proportion of fixations are made on a relatively small proportion of the scene's area. A variety of subsequent studies has indicated that observers tend to fixate "informative areas" in pictures, where *informative* refers to the idea of nonredundancy or lack of predictability of a given area with respect to the rest of the scene. Subsumed under this definition is high spatial frequency (Antes, 1974; Mackworth & Morandi, 1967), irregularity of pattern (Berlyne, 1958), and what might be termed "cognitive irregularity" (Friedman, 1979; Goodman & Loftus, 1981; Loftus & Mackworth, 1978). I will discuss cognitive irregularity in more detail later, but for the time being, the term warrants some explanation. It refers to the fact that a feature in a scene may be defined as "informative" to the degree that the feature is improbable given the gist of the scene and given the observer's past history. One picture in the Goodman and Loftus study, for example, depicted a fishing scene. In one version, a fisherman was pulling a fish out of the water; whereas in another, the fisherman was pulling a portrait out of the water. The portrait attracted many more fixations than did the fish. This result indicates that fixations are drawn to areas in a scene that are determined not only by the physical structure of the scene but by features that can only be defined as informative by reference to the subject's schema for whatever the scene depicts.[2]

---

[2]A provocative analogy with respect to text processing has been reported by Scinto (1978). Scinto proposed that text be divided into words expressing "theme" (old information) versus words expressing "rheme" (new information). The theme–rheme dichotomy was not new in and of itself, being similar to the "given–new" dichotomy proposed by Clark and Haviland (1977). Scinto, however, claimed to show that eye fixations on rheme information were more numerous and of longer duration than fixations on theme information. If correct, this finding would indicate an important similarity between text and scene processing. However, there are some problems in interpreting Scinto's results. First, his subjects were, according to his report, "fully cognizant of the purpose of the experiment." If so, the subjects may have been behaving in such a way as to confirm the hypothesis. Second, eye fixation durations were abnormally short—the means were on the order of 100–170 msec—thereby raising doubts about the generalizability of data emerging from these particular subjects reading this particular passage. Third, and most important, there were serious confoundings that did not seem to be adequately controlled for. For example, Scinto pointed out that there were more rheme words relative to theme words to begin with, but he apparently did not control for this factor with respect to number of fixations on theme versus rheme.

## C.  Fixation Duration

Accounting for variance in fixation duration has been something of a Holy Grail for eye movement researchers. Unfortunately, this venture has not met with a good deal of success with respect to either text processing or scene processing. However, there are at least signs of progress in the area of text processing.

Earlier, I noted that a principal task of linguistics has been to characterize the structure of language in terms of grammatical rules. A concomitant task undertaken by psycholinguists has been to construct psychological theories whose purpose is to delineate the mechanisms by which this structure is processed by a human being while listening to or reading text. The principal link between these psycholinguistic theories and the data designed to test them is processing time. That is, various processes involved in comprehension (for example, the process of negation) are assumed to take specific amounts of time. In a typical psycholinguistic experiment, test sentences are constructed in such a way as to require the use of certain combinations of these hypothetical processes. The reaction times to comprehend the sentences can be predicted and the predictions can be tested using a standard, laboratory reaction time task. Data emerging from these reaction time paradigms have provided substantial success for theories (Carpenter & Just, 1975; Clark & Chase, 1972). More recently, principally through the efforts of Just and Carpenter and their associates, these theories have been tested using experiments in which something related to fixation, namely "gaze duration"—the sum of fixation durations on a particular word—has been substituted for reaction time as the dependent variable. This technique has been quite successful as applied both to the relatively simple task of sentence verification (e.g., Carpenter & Just, 1977; Just & Carpenter, 1976) and to the more complex task of reading and comprehending entire blocks of text (Carpenter & Daneman, 1981; Just & Carpenter, 1980). By "successful" I refer to the substantial portions of the variance in gaze durations on text that are accounted for by the models. This success does not, of course, bring us any closer to answering the question of what causes a reader to terminate one fixation on a string of text and begin another. But this should not be seen as a shortcoming of the research, since the research uses eye fixation measure as a tool to investigate psycholinguistic processes in real life situations and does not seek to investigate eye fixations in and of themselves.

Unfortunately, accounting for variation in eye fixation durations on scenes has not reached even this sort of modest plateau. It is well known that there is wide variation in such durations; in a recent unpublished study, for example, Steve Gillispie, Jane Messo, and I found fixation durations on pictures to have a standard deviation of 140 msec even when variance due to subjects and pictures was eliminated. However, theories to account for this variation have not been forthcoming. As suggested earlier, the problem stems in large part from the fact that theories of picture grammar, in contrast to theories of language grammar, are currently so primitive that they are virtually nonexistent. In the next three sections, I will describe three different methodologies for trying to account for fixation durations. None has so far produced any particularly enlightening results; but neither have any of the methodologies been thoroughly explored.

### 1. FIXATION DURATIONS DURING INITIAL EXPLORATION OF A PICTURE

As noted earlier, the gist of a picture is typically acquired early during the first fixation on the picture. What then are subsequent fixations used for? There is a growing consensus that one major purpose of subsequent fixations is to seek out unusual features in the picture. This makes sense from an a priori standpoint. If I am shown a picture and know 100 msec following its onset that it is a street scene, what else is there to know about the picture? A plausible answer is that I want to know what it is about this particular street scene that distinguishes it from all other street scenes. Thus, I will focus my attention on features of this street scene that would be least likely to appear in typical street scenes. Such features (described above in conjunction with the issue of fixation location) have been variously referred to as "low probable" (Friedman, 1979; Loftus & Bell, 1975), "unexpected" (Goodman & Loftus, 1981), "informative" (Loftus & Mackworth, 1978), "discriminanda" (Loftus, 1981a), and "surprising" (Yarbus, 1967).

Whatever one wishes to call these features, there is substantial evidence that to the degree that a feature in a scene is improbable, that feature will be fixated (*a*) earlier; (*b*) more often; and (*c*) with longer durations. This leads to the following hypothesis about a sequence of fixations on a picture: The first fixation will be the shortest, since all that usually occurs during the initial fixation is gist acquisition. Subsequent fixations are then directed to low probable features, with earlier fixations going to lower probability features. This hypothesis would predict a sequence of fixations in which the first fixation is relatively short, the second is longest, and duration decreases monotonically thereafter.

Figure 21.1 shows data from two experiments, depicting fixation duration as a function of ordinal fixation number on a picture. The two panels show data from somewhat different situations. The left panel shows data reported by Loftus (1971). In this experiment, subjects were shown a pair of pictures for a period of 3 sec in anticipation of a recognition test. The subjects were allowed to look back and forth between the two members of the pair; thus pictures differed in terms of how many fixations were made on them. The three curves are conditionalized on pictures that received three, four, or five fixations. The right panel (Loftus, Gillispie, & Messo, 1982) depicts data from an experiment in which subjects saw a single picture for 2 sec in a free-viewing situation. The data exclude the last fixation to be made, whose duration is undefined since the picture ended in the middle of it.

These functions provide some degree of support for the general hypothesis sketched earlier. The first fixation on a picture is shorter than subsequent fixations. Fixation duration is longest on the second or third fixation, which may

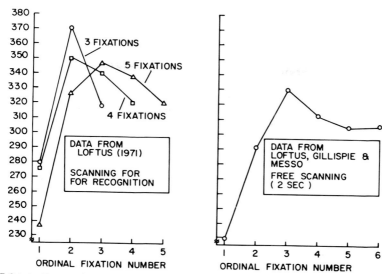

**FIGURE 21.1.** *Fixation duration as a function of ordinal fixation number on pictures. In the left panel, the data have been conditionalized on pictures that received exactly three, four, or five fixations. In the right panel data are unconditional.*

reflect the necessity of an occasional intervening fixation in order to find the lowest probability feature. From the fourth fixation on, fixation declines monotonically.[3]

Although this line of reasoning and the data shown in Figure 21.1 suggest some organizing principles to account for variation in fixation durations on scenes, it certainly cannot be characterized as a theory. A theory that might emerge from these principles must at least provide mechanisms to account for (a) how certain areas of the picture are deemed by the cognitive system to be low probable to begin with; and (b) more fundamentally, what it is about low probable features that causes processing of them to be longer.

[3]Antes (1974) has reported results from a picture-viewing experiment that superficially bear on this general issue. He found that rated informativeness of fixated areas conformed to the predicted pattern, being greatest on the second fixation and declining on subsequent fixations. Unfortunately, he also found that fixation duration appeared to increase monotonically. There are several problems, however, in relating Antes's results to the current problem. First, although rated informativeness was plotted against ordinal fixation number, duration was plotted against tenths of total fixations. Thus it was difficult to make the appropriate comparisons. Second, Antes's pictures were shown for quite long periods of time, and it is probable that after the first few fixations, the subject was no longer acquiring genuinely new information from the picture, and the exploration goals and strategy may well have shifted. Third, Antes used only one relatively naturalistic scene, the rest of his stimuli being TAT drawings. Finally, "informativeness" in Antes's study was defined by subject ratings, not by reference of the relative probability of a feature of the scene.

## 2. THE TIME COURSE OF INFORMATION PROCESSING WITHIN A FIXATION

Some years ago, I reported a series of experiments, the results of which indicated that recognition memory for pictures is critically determined by the number of fixations that had been made on the picture at the time of original study (Loftus, 1972). Consider, for example, pictures shown for 3 sec during the study phase of a recognition experiment. Subsequent memory performance was higher if a large number of short fixations were made on the picture during the 3 sec than if a smaller number of longer fixations were made. Moreover, a given number of fixations (e.g., 12 fixations) led to the same recognition performance whether those fixations were made during a long exposure time (e.g., 5 sec) or during a short exposure time (e.g., 3 sec). The conclusion was that number of fixations was critical in terms of determining recognition memory performance, whereas fixation duration was irrelevant.

More recently, however, I have reperformed this study using a paradigm in which numbers and durations of eye fixations on pictures at study were under stricter experimental control (Loftus, 1981b). This was done by showing each picture in the form of from one to four sequential, tachistoscopic flashes, the duration of each flash ranging from 50 to 400 msec, and each flash followed by a noise mask. The results of this study indicated that "fixation" duration was not at all irrelevant: Recognition memory performance increased monotonically for flash durations up to 400 msec.

To account for both sets of data—the Loftus (1972) and the Loftus (1981b) results—a model was proposed that attributed picture recognition performance to the interaction between the physical characteristics of a picture and the processing that is done on the picture. This model is embodied in the following four assumptions:

1. Any fixation on a picture is designed to encode some feature of the picture.
2. Features differ in the amount of time required to encode them.
3. A fixation lasts at least as long as needed to carry out encoding of the feature.
4. Recognition memory performance is a monotonically increasing function of the total number of features that are encoded.

To see how this model handles the data, let us see how it would be applied to the two sets of data that have just been described. Consider a typical condition in the Loftus (1972) exposure time experiment in which a subject has some fixed amount of time (e.g., 3 sec) to view a picture. If the picture being viewed contains easy to encode features, then many fixations will be made and recognition performance will be high. If, on the other hand, the features in the picture take long amounts of time to encode, then each fixation will have a long duration. Consequently, there will be fewer fixations on the picture, and subsequent recognition performance will be low.

Now consider the Loftus (1981b) multiple flash paradigm. The key characteristic of this paradigm is that the duration and number of fixations are controlled by the experimenter rather than by the subject. Thus, whenever the duration of a flash is decreased, there is some probability that processing of whatever feature is being encoded will be terminated prior to completion. It then follows that any shortening of flash duration will lead to a decrease in the expected number of encoded features from the pictures and hence to a decrease in subsequent recognition.

The model just described will have to be strengthened if it is to make any more specific predictions. For the present, it can be viewed as a foothold—a suggestion of how one might begin to characterize the structure of a picture and the psychological processes that might operate on this structure. In the next section, I will offer some suggestions about how the model might be fleshed out.

### 3.   WHAT ARE THESE FEATURES?

We are currently carrying out research designed to correlate specific physical features of pictures with eye movement patterns and with subsequent recognition memory. This work is predicated on the assumption that the relevant features in pictures with respect to recognition memory are those that, as discussed above, are unusual with respect to the gist of the picture. Using a rating procedure, we have assessed a set of 80 naturalistic scenes with respect to the number of such features (termed "discriminanda" by Loftus, 1981a). Separate groups of subjects were then shown the same pictures to gather recognition measures and eye fixation patterns. The number of discriminanda in a picture were found to have correlations (Pearson $r$'s) of .31 and −.50 respectively with hit and false-alarm rates on the picture.[4] However, the story becomes more complicated when eye fixation patterns are considered. First, the fixation rate (number of fixations per unit time) had an across-subjects, split-half reliability of only .20, indicating that there are large individual differences in terms of which pictures have easy to encode features and which have difficult to encode features. This low reliability in turn makes it difficult to assess the correlation between fixation rate and other measures of interest. However, when corrected for reliability, the correlation of fixation rate with hit rate was .40. In contrast, the correlation of fixation rate with number of discriminanda was .03. Taken as a whole, these data appear to warrant a cautious and tentative conclusion that number of discriminanda in and number of fixations on a picture provide independent contributions to the recognizability of a picture. That is, it appears that recognition performance on a particular picture will be high to the degree that there are many discriminanda in the picture to begin with and to the degree that these discriminanda can be encoded quickly.

---

[4]These correlations have been corrected for reliability. The uncorrected values are .20 and .33.

# V.   Perceptual and Postperceptual Processes within a Fixation

As noted, I spent several years arguing in favor of the hypothesis that fixation duration on a picture is irrelevant with respect to the acquisition of information germane to subsequent recognition memory (cf. Loftus, 1976).

A convenient way of characterizing this hypothesis is in terms of a hypothetical function relating amount of information acquired within a fixation to the duration of that fixation. I argued that the key property of this function was that it asymptoted; that is, information acquisition ceased after 100 msec or so following the onset of the fixation.

## A.   Asymptotic Processing of Letter Strings and Text

One of the reasons that I found this model so compelling is that it appeared to account for a variety of perceptual data as well as the picture memory data that originally prompted it. The Loftus (1981b) multiple-flash data described earlier has resulted in the demise of this model insofar as it is applicable to pictures; recall that these data indicated that perceptual processing occurs throughout the extent of a fixation on a picture. The perceptual data, however, are still worth considering, and I will briefly describe them here.

### 1.   TACHISTOSCOPIC FLASHES OF SYMBOL STRINGS

These data come from experiments that have been designed to mimic an eye fixation or a series of eye fixations on alphanumeric symbol strings, using a series of one or more tachistoscopic flashes. A prototype of such experiment was reported by Sperling (1963). In this experiment, an array of letters was presented to a subject for an exposure time ranging from 5 to 200 msec. A noise mask immediately followed presentation of the letter array, and the subject's task was to report as many letters as possible from the array. This experiment mimics a single eye fixation and is designed to reveal the time course of information acquisition within a fixation. Sperling reported his results in terms of number of letters correctly reported as a function of exposure time. This curve rose rapidly and then asymptoted after approximately 100 msec at an asymptotic value of four to five letters.

A possible conclusion of Sperling's finding is that the mechanisms within the brain that are responsible for processing the visual scene will operate only for a burst of 100 msec or so following a change in retinal stimulation. But an alternative explanation is that the result derives from short-term memory limitations, that is, that the asymptote derives from the fact that four or five items are all that the subject can fit into short-term memory prior to reporting them. Two subsequent experiments, however, cast doubt on this explanation. Allport (1968) repeated Sperling's experiment but added a second condition in which Landolt C's rather than letters were used as stimuli. Performance for both the letters and the

Landolt C's asymptoted after about 100 msec, but at different asymptotic levels. (The asymptote for the Landolt C's was lower.) Since short-term memory is typically found to be relatively constant in terms of the number of items it holds (Miller, 1956), it is difficult to attribute two different asymptotes to short-term memory limitations.

A second experiment reported by Sperling, Budiansky, Spivak, and Johnson (1971) used a task that eliminated the need for short-term memory altogether. In this experiment, a series of 25 letter arrays was presented in rapid succession on a CRT. Embedded in one location of one of the arrays was a digit and, following presentation of all 25 arrays, the subject attempted to report the location of the digit. The exposure time per array was varied from 5 to 320 msec. In this paradigm, the sequence of arrays mimics a series of eye fixations. There cannot be any short-term memory limitations since only detection is required. Again, performance was plotted as a function of the array presentation time, and again, performance asymptoted after about 100 msec of exposure time.

## 2. PROCESSING ASYMPTOTES WITHIN EYE FIXATIONS WHILE READING TEXT

A recent experiment reported by Rayner, Inhoff, Morrison, Slowiaczek, and Bertera (1981, Experiment 3) indicates that a similar perceptual processing asymptote occurs during the normal reading of text. In this experiment, subjects read text displayed under the control of a computer while the computer simultaneously monitored the subject's eye position. After varying periods of time following the onset of each fixation, the text, or some portion of it was replaced by a noise mask. Various indicants of reading difficulty could then be assessed as a function of the delay of the mask following the onset of the fixation. These measures, which included effective reading rate, fixation duration, number of fixations, and saccade length all showed a similar pattern which was that they asymptoted (at a normal level) when the mask was delayed about 50 msec. Accordingly, Rayner et al. (1981) concluded that most of the visual information necessary for reading can be obtained within the first 50 msec of a fixation and that the remaining portion of the fixation was used for determining the location of the next fixation and for the operation of nonperceptual processes.

This leads to the conclusion that eye fixations on scenes and text are quite different with respect to the sequence of processing within an eye fixation. A fixation on text—or on artificial symbols in general—can be viewed as being divided into two distinct phases. In the first or perceptual phase, the visual system is at work acquiring information from the physical stimulus. In the second, or postperceptual phase, the psycholinguistic processes such as those suggested by Just and Carpenter (1980) come into play. It is probably in this latter phase that the bulk of the variance in fixation duration occurs. (Or at least it is in this phase that the variance occurs that is accounted for by current psychological models.) With pictures, in contrast, perceptual processing occurs throughout the fixation, and if this processing is interrupted using a mask, processing suffers rather severely. As I have noted earlier, however, theories to account for exactly what is happening during an eye fixation on a picture are still in embryonic stages.

## VI.  Summary

Eye fixations on scenes differ from their counterparts on text in a number of ways. Empirically, we find that:

1. The useful field of view is substantially narrower on text than on scenes. This would be predicted from a consideration of the nature of the physical elements constituting scenes and text.
2. Sequential predictability of the fixation pattern is far greater for text relative to scenes. However, overall predictability appears to be greater for scenes relative to text.
3. The perceptual processing carried out during a fixation on text appears to be completed quite early in the fixation. The rest of the fixation is probably used in large part to carry out psycholinguistic processes of the sort proposed by a variety of psycholinguistic models. Much of the variability in fixation durations on text can be accounted for by such models.
4. Perceptual processing on scenes, in contrast, appears to continue throughout the extent of the fixation. However, models postulating exactly what this processing consists of and what causes processing time to vary are so far relatively primitive.

## References

Allport, D. A. (1968). The rate of assimilation of visual information. *Psychonomic Science, 12,* 231–232.

Antes, J. R. (1974). The time course of picture viewing. *Journal of Experimental Psychology, 103,* 62–70.

Berlyne, D. E. (1958). The influence of complexity and novelty in visual figures on orienting responses. *Journal of Experimental Psychology, 55,* 289–296.

Biederman, I. (1972). Perceiving real-world scenes. *Science, 177,* 77–80.

Biederman, I., Mezzanotte, R. J., & Rabinowitz, J. C. (1981). Detecting and judging scenes with incongruous contextual relations. *Cognitive Psychology, 14,* 143–177.

Biederman, I., Rabinowitz, J. C., Glass, A. L., & Stacy, E. W. (1974). On the information extracted from a glance at a scene. *Journal of Experimental Psychology, 103,* 597–600.

Buswell, G. T. (1935). *How people look at pictures.* Chicago: University of Chicago Press.

Carpenter, P. A., & Daneman, M. (1981). Lexical retrieval and error recovery in reading: A model based on eye fixations. *Journal of Verbal Learning and Verbal Behavior.*

Carpenter, P. A., & Just, M. A. (1975). Sentence comprehension: A psycholinguistic processing model of verification. *Psychological Review, 82,* 45–73.

Carpenter, P. A., & Just, M. A. (1977). Reading comprehension as the eyes see it. In P. A. Carpenter & M. A. Just (Eds.), *Cognitive processing in comprehension.* Hillsdale, New Jersey: Erlbaum.

Chomsky, N. (1965). *Aspects of the theory of syntax.* Cambridge, Massachusetts: M.I.T. Press.

Chomsky, N. (1968). *Language and mind.* New York: Harcourt Brace Jovanovich.

Clark, H. H., & Chase, W. G. (1972). On the process of comparing sentences against pictures. *Cognitive Psychology, 3,* 472–517.

Clark, H. H., & Haviland, S. E. (1977). Comprehension and the given-new contract. In R. O. Freedle (Ed.), *Discourse production and comprehension.* Norwood, New Jersey: Albex Publishing.

Dallett, K., & Wilcox, S. (1968). Remembering pictures vs. remembering descriptions. *Psychonomic Science, 11,* 139–140.

Friedman, A. (1979). Framing pictures: The role of knowledge in automatized encoding and memory for gist. *Journal of Experimental Psychology: General, 108,* 316–355.

Goodman, G. S., & Loftus, G. R. (1981). *The relevance of expectation.* Paper presented at the meeting of the APA, Los Angeles, August.

Gould, J. D. (1969). *Eye movements during visual search.* (Research report RC2680). Yorktown Heights: IBM Thomas J. Watson Research Center.

Just, M. A., & Carpenter, P. A. (1976). Eye fixations and cognitive processes. *Cognitive Psychology, 8,* 441–480.

Just, M. A., & Carpenter, P. A. (1980). A theory of reading: From eye fixations to comprehension. *Psychological Review, 87,* 329–354.

Loftus, G. R. (1971). *Eye fixations and recognition memory for pictures.* Unpublished doctoral dissertation, Stanford University.

Loftus, G. R. (1972). Eye fixations and recognition memory for pictures. *Cognitive Psychology, 3,* 525–551.

Loftus, G. R. (1976). A framework for a theory of picture memory. In J. W. Senders and R. Monty (Eds.), *Eye movements and psychological processes.* Hillsdale, New Jersey: Erlbaum.

Loftus, G. R. (1981). Models of picture memory. In R. Wu & S. Chipoman (Eds.), *Learning by eye.* (a)

Loftus, G. R. (1981). Tachistoscopic simulations of eye fixations on pictures. *Journal of Experimental Psychology: Human Learning & Memory, 7,* 369–376. (b)

Loftus, G. R., & Bell, S. M. (1975). Two types of information in picture memory. *Journal of Experimental Psychology: Human Learning & Memory, 104,* 103–113.

Loftus, G. R., Gillespie, S., & Messo, J. (1982). Unpublished data.

Loftus, G. R., & Mackworth, N. H. (1978). Cognitive determinants of fixation location during picture viewing. *Journal of Experimental Psychology: Human Perception & Performance, 4,* 565–572.

Mackworth, N. H., & Morandi, A. J. (1967). The gaze selects informative details within pictures. *Perception & Psychophysics, 2,* 547–552.

Mandler, J., & Johnson, W. (1976). Some of the thousand words a picture is worth. *Journal of Experimental Psychology: Human Learning & Memory, 2,* 529–540.

McConkie, G. W., & Rayner, K. (1975). The span of the effective stimulus during a fixation in reading. *Perception & Psychophysics, 17,* 578–586.

Miller, G. A. (1956). The magical number seven, plus or minus two. *Psychological Review, 63,* 81–97.

Nelson, T. O., Metzler, J., & Reed, D. A. (1974). Role of details in the long-term recognition of pictures and verbal description. *Journal of Experimental Psychology, 102,* 184–186.

Nelson, W. W., & Loftus, G. R. (1980). The functional visual field during picture viewing. *Journal of Experimental Psychology: Human Learning & Memory, 6,* 391–399.

Noton, D., & Stark, L. (1971). Scanpaths in eye movements during pattern perception. *Science, 171,* 305–311.

Palmer, S. (1977). Hierarchical structure in perceptual representation. *Cognitive Psychology, 9,* 441–475.

Rayner, K. (1975). The perceptual span and peripheral cues in reading. *Cognitive Psychology, 7,* 65–81.

Rayner, K. (1978). Eye movements in reading and information processing. *Psychological Bulletin, 85,* 618–660.

Rayner, K., & Bertera, J. H. (1979). Reading without a fovea. *Science, 206*, 468–469.

Rayner, K., Inhoff, A. W., Morrison, R. E., Slowiaczek, M. L., & Bertera, J. H. (1981). Masking of foveal and parafoveal vision during eye fixations in reading. *Journal of Experimental Psychology: Human Perception & Performance, 7*, 167–179.

Scinto, L. F. (1978). Relation of eye fixations to old–new information in text. In J. W. Senders, D. F. Fisher, & R. A. Monty (Eds.), *Eye movements and the higher psychological processes*. Hillsdale, New Jersey: Erlbaum.

Sperling, G. (1963). A model for visual memory tasks. *Human Factors, 5*, 19–31.

Sperling, G., Budiansky, J., Spivak, J., & Johnson, M. C. (1971). Extremely rapid visual search: The maximum rate of scanning letters for the presence of a numeral. *Science, 174*, 307–311.

Yarbus, A. L. (1967). *Eye movements and vision*. New York: Plenum Press.

# 22

# A Spatial Relational Logic behind Visual Differentiation: Gibsonian Constructivism?

## I.  Introduction

A number of years ago, together with a number of graduate students, I set out to study the development of perceptual–learning skills in beginning readers. In searching the literature I found an article by E. J. Gibson, "Learning to Read" (1965). I remember being impressed with Gibson's approach because of the way she tied learning to read to the fundamental skills of detecting distinctive features, decoding letters to sounds, and discovering patterns in the structure of written language. The particular aspect of Gibson's theory that appealed to me most was the visual differentiation of distinctive features of letters, that is, those visual elements that constitute a unique feature set when one symbol is contrasted with another. For example, *R* and *P* share straight line and curved line nondistinctive features, but *R* has an oblique line and *P* does not, and this unique contrast defines the distinctive-feature relationship for *R* versus *P*.

The abstraction of distinctive-feature relationships is a basic perceptual learning skill that can be studied developmentally using eye movement methods. I reasoned that researching this problem could help articulate Gibson's theory by identifying what features children fixate when differentiating symbol pairs, and whether children's eye movement strategies for selecting features reveals a developing logic in which distinctive-feature relationships play a central role.

From 1968 to 1974 my students and I studied what aspects of letter pairs children, spanning an age range from 3.5–9 years, looked at to decide whether they were the same or different. As I look back at the six studies that were published, there is little doubt that these eye movement studies were useful in

*EYE MOVEMENTS IN READING:*
*PERCEPTUAL AND LANGUAGE PROCESSES*

determining what features beginning readers fixated. As a result, at least in my mind, Jackie Gibson's distinctive features became a perceptual reality in a much more concrete sense than her late husband's real world counterparts, "formless invariants," from which distinctive features were derived (J. J. Gibson, 1973). But, knowing what readers look at does not tell one *how* they learn to read. Basically, in my zeal to pinpoint what it was that made one letter visually distinctive from another, I had overlooked the more fundamental question: *How* do children *use* the visual information they extract to make same–different judgments about letter pairs?

One naturally assumes that children's scanning patterns will reveal fundamental insights about how extracted information is translated into decisions about whether two letters are the same or different. However, the cognitive processes underlying scanning patterns are highly theoretical and speculative, as I will point out when I review some of our findings. The review will attempt to remedy some earlier shortcomings of my experiments by integrating the *what* question with the *how* question; focusing on extraction *and* utilization of visual information.

Looking back 7 years gives one a fresh perspective on the original research problem. The basic theoretical framework was, and still is, Gibsonian but, this framework has been tempered by Piaget, David Olson, and my own interests in children's art. Although it seems that Gibson and Piaget are far apart theoretically, and reading and drawing are far apart conceptually, I am going to argue that they are connected by a spatial relational logic that guides the child's thinking about how to test for differences, thus giving a broader meaning to the notion of distinctive features. I will develop my argument first by reviewing the evidence that suggests that beginning readers do not logically understand how to test graphic symbols for differences. Second, I will show why spatial relational logic is a necessary part of distinctive-feature testing. Finally, I will present evidence that suggests that the spatio–relational logic behind visual differentiation plays a significant role in determining how children perceive and represent real objects in drawings.

## II.   Are Two Letters the Same or Different?

Three types of graphic symbols were used in the tasks that we studied. Children were asked to differentiate either pairs of alphabet letters (Nodine & Steuerle, 1973), pairs of letterlike symbols (Nodine & Simmons, 1974), or pairs of pseudowords (Nodine & Evans, 1969; Nodine & Lang, 1971). To be brief, I have chosen to focus my discussion on the letterlike symbols used by Nodine and Simmons. Examples of these symbols are shown in Figure 22.1. Each example illustrates a different distinctive-feature contrast that served as the basis for differentiation. All but one set of letterlike symbols can be differentiated on the basis of a single feature contrast. Because the letterlike symbols were constructed from fewer stimulus dimensions they are experimentally "purer" than alphabet letters but require the same differentiation logic.

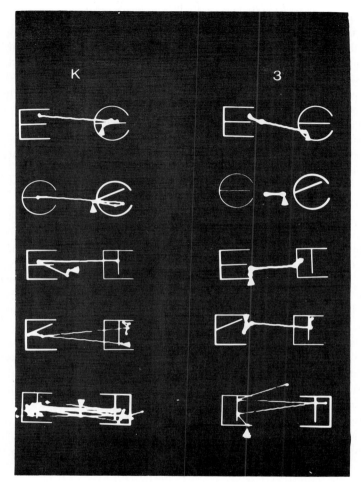

FIGURE 22.1. *Computer generated displays showing eye movement patterns of kindergarten children (left) and third-grade children (right) to letterlike symbols differing from top to bottom respectively in form, line, origin, line and origin, and orientation. (Arrow designates initial fixation.)*

In all of our studies the symbol pairs were large (12° for each letterlike symbol) so that children had to view them piecemeal. The large size of the symbols aided eye movement analysis, but undoubtedly reduced their ecological validity as reading stimuli.

Let us examine the logical basis for abstracting distinctive features from the total set shared by each of these letterlike symbols. To determine whether two symbols are the same or different the child must select a feature of one symbol and note whether the same feature is present or absent in the corresponding spatial position of the comparison symbol. Thus, testing symbols for differences logically demands of the child consideration of both form and spatial position of the feature dimension. This logical distinction depends on both feature presence–absence and, spatial relational correspondence. Because most letters of the alphabet can be differentiated on the basis of feature differences alone, the logical significance of maintaining spatial correspondence is often ignored. In fact, Gibson indicates that the filtering of nondistinctive or irrelevant information is an important part of perceptual learning (E. J. Gibson, 1969). The need to refer to spatial relational correspondences becomes critical only for a limited number of cases with the standard alphabet. These are the so-called mirror image cases such as *b* versus *d* and *p* versus *q*. The comparable cases for letterlike symbols involve the stimulus dimension labeled "orientation," and for pseudowords, reversals of letter order. (See Figure 22.1.)

## III.   The Experimental Findings

Although the stimuli in the series of experiments conducted between 1969 and 1974 shifted from pairs of letter strings (pseudowords) to pairs of letters or pairs of letterlike symbols, the aim of all of these experiments was essentially the same: to trace the development of perceptual–cognitive strategies used in testing differences between graphic stimuli by focusing on: (*a*) *what* features receive attention; and (*b*) *how* are these features are utilized in making same–different judgments.

In answer to the first question, all three studies showed that proportionally more fixations were directed to distinctive features as grade level of the children increased from kindergarten to third grade. Table 22.1 summarizes findings for pseudowords, letterlike symbols, and letters. Thus, the fixations of third-grade children showed more interest in those aspects of the graphic displays that carried information relevant to the question, Are the graphic units the same or different?

The second question was concerned with *how* the distinctive feature information was used to answer the same–different question. A reasonable strategy for answering this question is to systematically compare features between the two letters using the method of paired comparisons. The successful use of this method depends upon the comparison of letter features in equivalent spatial positions between letter pairs. Our findings indicate that not only do older children's fixations focus on relevant (distinctive) features, but they used paired-comparison strategies more logically and efficiently in making same–different judgments of

TABLE 22.1
Proportion of Fixations on Distinctive Features per Pair

| Grade level | Pseudowords | Letterlike words | Letters |
|---|---|---|---|
| Kindergarten | .56 | .36 | .24 |
| First | — | — | .27 |
| Third | .65 | .41 | .29 |

TABLE 22.2
Number of Paried Comparisons per Pair

| Grade level | Pseudowords | Letterlike symbols | Letters |
|---|---|---|---|
| Kindergarten | 6.04 | 2.5 | 3.1 |
| First | — | — | 2.2 |
| Third | 4.48 | 1.3 | 1.5 |

pseudowords, letterlike symbols, and letter pairs. This more effective use of visual attention was reflected, in part, by the number of paired-comparison eye movements required by third-grade children in making same–different judgements being less than that of younger children, as shown in Table 22.2.

The greater selectivity and economy in the use of eye fixations for making same–different judgments by third-grade children suggests a shift in scanning strategy from one that depends on an almost mechanical analysis of visual features of letter pairs to one in which feature contrasts confirm or disconfirm rulelike expressions that form the logical basis of same–different judgments. The large increase in the economy of the third grader's fixation strategies (shown in Figure 22.1) may signal a switch from a bottom–up to a top–down analysis of letter pairs. According to Piaget, a conceptually driven scanning strategy would not be possible until the child achieved the capacity of logico-mathematical or reflecting abstraction (Forman & Sigel, 1979) at around 9 years of age. The shift from perceptual to conceptual emphasis that occurs when the child's analysis moves from empirical extracting to reflecting abstraction is suggested by the decreasing use of multiple comparisons and the increasing use of single fixations and single comparisons displayed by third-grade children, as shown in Table 22.3.

These findings suggest that visual scanning becomes progressively more logical and systematic as the child exerts more cognitive control over his or her eye movements. This shift to a more logical strategy has been observed in the fixation patterns of older children performing same–different judgments not only with graphic symbols but with pictures (Day, 1975; Vurpillot, 1968) and with conservation problems (Boersma, O'Bryan, & Ryan, 1970; Boersma & Wilton, 1974; O'Bryan & Boersma, 1971).

TABLE 22.3
Proportion of Single Fixation and Single and Multiple Comparisons per Pair

| | Letterlike symbols | | | Letters | | |
|---|---|---|---|---|---|---|
| | | Comparisons | | | Comparisons | |
| Grade level | Single fixation | Single | Multiple | Single fixation | Single | Multiple |
| Kindergarten | .05 | .26 | .69 | .00 | .07 | .93 |
| First | — | — | — | .02 | .15 | .83 |
| Third | .25 | .37 | .37 | .01 | .24 | .75 |

## IV.   Theoretical Implications of Paired
Comparison Strategies

The stress on paired-comparison strategies in testing distinctive-feature relationships is significant for Piaget's theory as well as for Gibson's. The use of paired-comparison strategies for Piaget depends on the child's capacity to decenter in order to be able to coordinate contrasting perceptual features while holding their spatial positions constant.

The child must be able to represent the spatial position of the features of each symbol of the pair. This calls for a spatial references system in which point for point correspondences can be identified between symbols independent of their featural content. According to Piaget and Inhelder (1967), the child uses a crude referencing system for identifying the spatial location of objects at first, but eventually the child develops a system of horizontal and vertical coordinates for mapping objects in space.

Children make errors in differentiating lines on the basis of spatial orientation before they achieve a unified spatial referencing system of horizontal and vertical coordinates. They acquire this coordinate system around the end of the concrete-operations stage (e.g., 9 years of age) according to Olson (1970, 1975). Recently, Kershner (1975) demonstrated that lack of a stable spatial references system is linked to reading problems.

Distinctive features, according to Gibson, express rulelike relationships of the form: two letters are different if a feature is present in one letter but not the other; in other words a mismatch.

E. J. Gibson (1977) has characterized her theory as one of "seek and ye shall find." The objects of search are invariant properties of the *world*, of the *spatial layout*, which must have a stable and objective structure, of *objects*, with constant dimensions and reliable affordances that have survival value, and of *events*, which have order and predictability.

But reading is not concerned with real world perceptions. Rather, it is concerned with the world of graphic symbols (Gibson & Levin, 1975, p. 243). The invariant properties of this symbol world are graphic features and their spatial configurations. These graphic features which belong to the world of symbols are governed by arbitrary rule systems which the child must *learn*, and learning about the world of symbols, for Gibson, depends on differentiation of distinctive graphic features, *not* real world invariants. Visual differentiation is a process of abstracting contrasting relationships between distinctive graphic features so as to reduce uncertainty, rather than to adapt to the environment.

Gibson argues that young children do not understand certain types of graphic transformations. For example, E. J. Gibson, J. J. Gibson, Pick, & Osser (1962) showed that line-to-line curve and break-and-close transformations which did not involve spatial relations were easy for children to detect regardless of age. However, rotational and reversal transformations which involved spatial relationships were more difficult for young children (4–6 years) to detect; and, perspective transformations which reflect complex spatial relationships were practically "invisible" to children through 8 years.

The discovery of invariant relationships whether being of geometric, linguistic, or logico-mathematical origins is the key to understanding the meaning of a difference for both Gibson and Piaget. For Gibson, invariants are discovered by discrimination and differentiation of visual information expressed as perceptual rules. For Piaget, invariants are discovered by the interaction of visual data with conceptual schemata.

## V.   The Feature-Contrast Rule Restated

The studies that we have considered thus far, particularly Nodine and Simmons (1974), indicate that differentiation of certain feature dimensions was more difficult than differentiation of others. This was evidenced by the greater number of fixations and larger proportion of paired comparisons required to differentiate letterlike symbol pairs that depended on distinctive-feature contrasts based on line origin, line slant, and letter orientation (directionality of opening), rather than letter form or a combination of line slant and line origin. All of these former distinctive-feature relationships require consideration of both visual and spatial relationships. The earlier rule needs restating: Two letters are different if a feature is present in one letter but not in the other *in equivalent spatial locations.*

The scanning strategies of young children violated the new rule by typically centering on finding feature differences without attending to, and thus holding constant, spatial location. Piaget would say that our kindergarten children could not use the rule because their conception of space lacked the necessary referencing system needed to define *equivalent spatial locations.*

## VI.   Comparison Strategies in Solving Letter Puzzles

A study by Susan Back and I (Back & Nodine, 1972) examined the kinds of strategies used by children to differentiate letters (taken from Nodine & Simmons, 1974) when the letter pairs are covered by two 3 × 3 arrays of 1-in. blocks arranged to resemble a puzzle as illustrated in Figure 22.2. This puzzle task allowed us to observe the kinds of comparison strategies children used to test whether two letters were the same or different. In a sense we were trying to confirm our speculations about the use of paired-comparison strategies that we found in the eye movement studies. In particular, we were interested in whether children understood distinctive-feature relationships expressed by the restated rule that requires a feature contrast based on equivalent spatial locations.

The subjects were 14 kindergarten and 14 third-grade children. Sixteen letter pairs, 8 matched and 8 unmatched, were tested. Each letter pair was hidden under the puzzle-block array and the child was instructed to take the blocks away

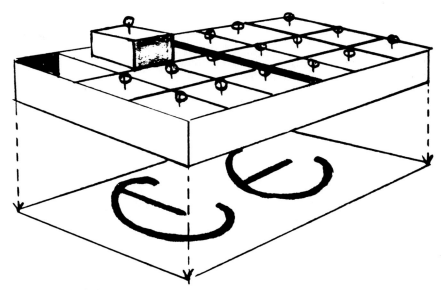

**FIGURE 22.2.** *Sketch of puzzle task used by Back and Nodine, 1972.*

one at a time and tell the experimenter as soon as he or she knew whether they were the same or different. A record of the order in which the children removed the blocks was recorded on graph paper, and the results were then scored by two judges who assigned to the removal sequences one of five strategies: feature for feature correspondence, row for row correspondence, letter for letter correspondence, random between letters, and, random within letters.

The feature for feature strategy was the most efficient one in determining whether the letters matched or were different. The removal of fewer blocks before a correct response' occurred for this strategy ($\bar{X} = 7.83$). All of the remaining strategies required nearly twice as many blocks to be removed before a correct response (all, $\bar{X} = 13.6$ or better), $F(5,218) = 31.43$ $p < .01$). Table 22.4 shows that third-grade children used the feature for feature strategy 79% of the time whereas kindergarten children used it only 33% of the time.

The evidence from this study coupled with eye movement data on comparison strategies in the differentiation of letters and pictures (e.g., Vurpillot, 1968) begin

**TABLE 22.4**
**Type of Strategy Used by Children to Perform Letter-Puzzle Task**

| Grade | Strategy (%) | | | | |
| --- | --- | --- | --- | --- | --- |
| | Feature for feature | Row for row | Letter for letter | Random across letters | Random within letters |
| Kindergarten | 33 | 09 | 17 | 09 | 32 |
| Third | 79 | 01 | 03 | 06 | 11 |

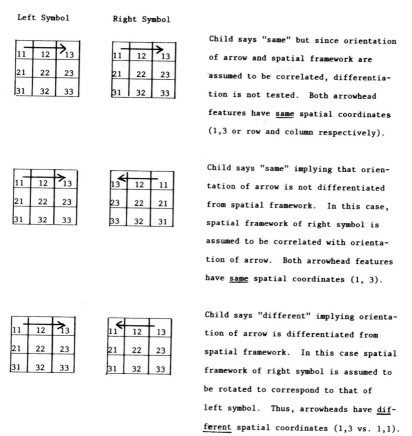

Left Symbol    Right Symbol

Child says "same" but since orientation of arrow and spatial framework are assumed to be correlated, differentiation is not tested. Both arrowhead features have **same** spatial coordinates (1,3 or row and column respectively).

Child says "same" implying that orientation of arrow is not differentiated from spatial framework. In this case, spatial framework of right symbol is assumed to be correlated with orientation of arrow. Both arrowhead features have **same** spatial coordinates (1, 3).

Child says "different" implying orientation of arrow is differentiated from spatial framework. In this case spatial framework of right symbol is assumed to be rotated to correspond to that of left symbol. Thus, arrowheads have **different** spatial coordinates (1,3 vs. 1,1).

FIGURE 22.3. *Diagram illustrating three possible relationships between orientation of left and right symbols (indicated by arrows) by framework (indicated by two-digit number designating row and column coordinates).*

to provide a developmental picture of how children utilize distinctive-feature relationships to test graphic symbols for differences. The increasing use of paired comparisons with age suggests that older children are beginning to understand the logic behind distinctive-feature testing.

The logic requires that the child differentiate distinctive features from equivalent locations in order to make accurate same–different judgments. The differentiation of distinctive-feature locations assumes understanding of a spatial coordinate system, such as the underlying grid system shown in Figure 22.3, which can be superimposed over the letter pair to identify distinctive-feature locations. Thus, the child must simultaneously coordinate two systems, one focused on feature contrasts, the other focused on spatial locations. Piaget would refer to this ability to coordinate perceptual and spatial conceptual systems as reflecting abstraction.

Braine (1978) distinguishes two types of orientation judgments: (1) judgments of "uprightness" based on a match–mismatch between stimulus input and natural coding processes of shape information that are rooted in perception of phenomenal verticality; and (2) judgments of the orientation of realistic shapes and letters that require relating the figure to a spatial framework. Braine speculates that errors in matching left–right mirror image orientations are due to the child relating one figure to another by not placing analogous parts close together (tops near tops, bottoms near bottoms). This interpretation is what would be predicted if the child failed to differentiate featural information from its spatial framework.

Differentiation based on discrimination of perceptual features works for single and multidimensional stimuli, but breaks down when spatial orientation becomes a relevant feature dimension. I think the problem here is that the spatial information has no perceptable features. Rather, the spatial tag that is required to carry out systematic paired comparisons between features of stimulus pair is derived from a conceptual mapping of the spatial coordinates onto the visual features.

The rule that defines a difference between symbols is more complex for contrasts that require *both* variance in features and invariance in spatial positions. This more complex rule applies to differences in line origin, line slant, and letter orientation in our set of letterlike symbols. Interestingly, the simpler version of the rule which requires only the detection of a feature difference between symbols works for most alphabetical letter pair contrasts. It is not surprising, therefore, that children encounter difficulty and confusion when they apply the feature difference only rule to such letter contrasts as *b* versus *d* and *p* versus *q* which are exceptions to the rule.

The absence of the repetitive paired-comparison eye movement strategies in third-grade children called upon to make visual discriminations of letterlike symbols (Nodine & Simmons, 1974) contrasted with their perference to use paired-comparisons strategies when visual discriminations are limited to a piecemeal analysis of the same symbols (Back & Nodine, 1972) suggests that construction of a spatial reference system is critical for testing and understanding contrasting relational correspondences between graphic stimuli.

## VII.   Spatial-Relational Logic and Drawing

Spatial relational logic also plays an important role in determining how children interpret and represent real world objects in drawings. Both interpretation and production aspects of representational art require an understanding of the relationship between the appearance of an object and its underlying reality. It is well documented that young children up to the age of 8–9 years lack an appreciation of the distinction between appearance and reality (e.g., Arnheim, 1969; Gardner & Wolfe, 1979). Unfortunately, much of the art instruction that children receive during elementary schooling (and beyond) exacerbates the problem by avoiding confrontations between appearance and reality. Art teachers tend to stress the imaginative basis rather than the perceptual–cognitive basis of drawing.

The relationship between appearance and reality is expressed in art by pictorial perspective. The development of pictorial perspective is a major theme in the history of art (Gombrich, 1972) and has received a great deal of attention recently by perceptual psychologists (e.g., J. J. Gibson, 1979; Hagen, 1980; Nodine & Fisher, 1979). From a developmental standpoint, the appearance of perspective representations of real world objects when children are asked to draw from a model signals a significant landmark for the Gibsons and for Piaget.

For both Gibson and Piaget, drawing from a real world model requires visual differentiation of the invariant or conceptual features of the model from its optical or perceptual features seen from a given perspective viewpoint. The problem confronting the young artist is the differentiation of reality from appearance. Both E. J. Gibson (1969) and Piaget (Piaget & Inhelder, 1967) have documented the difficulties children have discriminating the objects as such from their optical distortions as they undergo the perspective transformations required for mapping the three dimensional object onto a two dimensional surface. But, in addition to discriminating this constancy in change, the child must be able to correlate the changing appearance of objects with changes in perspective viewpoint.

The first step in drawing from a model is careful observational analysis of the unique distortions in the shape of individual objects and their relationships to one another from a given perspective. The second step is mapping of the distinctive features from this unique three dimensional perspective transformation of the model scene onto a flat two dimensional surface using graphic methods to produce lines that specify invariants: the features of objects, particularly their shape and the spatial arrangement (layout) of objects (J. J. Gibson, 1979).

The foregoing analysis assumes that visual discrimination and differentiation are fundamental for learning about both symbols and real world objects. But as I have already stressed, differentation involves more than discriminating distinctive or invariant features. It involves an analysis of feature relationships, which in turn depend on a spatial relational framework.

This spatial relational framework may evolve from treating stimuli, whether symbols or objects, as patterns, configurations, or perceptual wholes. These higher order units (E. J. Gibson, 1969) are assumed to have inherent structural organization in which features and spatial framework form a Gestalt whole. For Piaget (Piaget & Inhelder, 1969) higher order units evolve from schemata that act as a conceptual framework for organizing perceptual features within a spatial framework. Piaget refers to these higher order units as operative wholes, different from figurative wholes that lack perceptual–conceptual integration.

The child's conception of space can be understood by the way in which he or she depicts perspective relationships among real world objects. According to Piaget and Inhelder (1967), the child's drawings initially reflect naive spatial intuitions that progressively become more logical with the development of projective spatial concepts (e.g., left–right, above–below, before–behind). These concepts coordinate the different positions of objects relative to one another and adjust for variation in apparent size as seen from the child's viewing perspective.

The ultimate conceptualization of space is achieved by coordination of object positions within a unified spatial framework containing a metric reference system based on Euclidian geometry. The logical basis of such a system facilitates conservation of surfaces and objective distances (Laurendau & Pinard, 1970, p. 17) because it is no longer dependent on the relationship of one individual object to another. Whether spatial relational logic emerges from the perception of higher order structural units as Gestalt wholes or the evolution of Euclidian spatial knowledge, I believe it plays a key role in the differentiation of both symbols and objects. Drawing is a complex task because it requires both visual differentiation and experimentation with a nonnotational system (in the sense of Goodman, 1968) of marks on a paper for recording what one sees, or perhaps more accurately, what one believes to be the representational solution to a visual problem solving task.

We attempted to relate visual analysis and differentiation to graphic representation by designing a two part experiment. (Nodine, Kenney, & Nodine, 1981) In the first part of the experiment children from grades one through eight were asked to draw from a model during the regular weekly meeting of their art class. The model consisted of some familiar objects arranged on a checkerboard tablecloth. The children were carefully stationed around the model and their station points were coded on their drawings. Before starting, the children were told to walk around the model and examine it. The teacher emphasized that they were to draw only what they saw, pretending that their pencils were touching the objects as they drew them (after Nicolaides, 1969).

In the second part of the experiment, 10 children from each of grades one, four, six, and eight who had participated in the first part were randomly tested for their comprehension of pictorial perspective. This was accomplished by showing them four different sets of pictures. One set tested visual differentiation of perspective between pairs of pictures differing in the use of depth cues that included relative size, interposition, linear perspective, and blur (aerial perspective). A second set tested perspective taking by having children match photos to hypothetical viewpoints of a model taken 90° apart. A third set of pictures tested differentiation and utilization of two dimensional versus three dimensional perspective information. A final set assessed the basis for judging realism between pairs of postcard reproductions of paintings. The results of the picture comprehension tests, shown in Table 22.5, indicate that first-grade children experienced the greatest difficulty analyzing and utilizing perspective information to differentiate pictorial depth, distance, and size relationships. Performance improved significantly by grade four and continued to improve, but was by no means perfect, by grade eight.

Pictorial depth is created by producing a visual illusion in which graphic information on a flat two dimensional surface is treated by a viewer as if it existed in three dimensional space. Our test battery measured the child's sensitivity to perspective by obtaining both judgments of the presence or absence or magnitude of the illusion *and* the child's explanation of his or her reason for making that judgment. Our results indicate that first-grade children and to some extent fourth-grade children had difficulty in reading and comprehending perspective illusions.

TABLE 22.5
Results of Pictorial Comprehension Tests

| Task | Percentage correct[a] | | | |
|---|---|---|---|---|
| | Grade | | | |
| | First | Fourth | Sixth | Eighth |
| Understanding perspective in photos | 66 | 79 | 90 | 82 |
| Taking perspective by predicting appearance of model from different station points | 45 | 86 | 91 | 95 |
| Understanding perspective in drawings | | | | |
| Judgment of apparent size at a distance | 10 | 60 | 80 | 90 |
| Differentiation of apparent vs. real size | 0 | 30 | 20 | 20 |
| Identification of false perspective | 19 | 66 | 75 | 97 |
| Analysis of whole–part relations | 55 | 65 | 71 | 85 |
| Recognition of hidden figure | 40 | 80 | 100 | 100 |

[a] $N = 10$ per grade.

The problems that young children had reading perspective information can be clearly illustrated by their judgments and explanations of the size of the cylinders depicted against a perspective background shown in Figure 22.4. The cylinders in the picture on the left are depicted as decreasing in size, consistent with the perspective framework of the hallway. The cylinders remain constant in size against the perspective framework in the picture on the right.

Table 22.6 shows the children's judgments when asked whether the cylinder ("cans") were the same or different sizes in each picture. Because children's same–different judgments could be based on either apparent or actual size, they needed to be qualified by looking at the reasons behind each judgment.

Although all but one first grader failed to read the perspective relationship ("same" judgment) based on actual size between a cylinder size and background in the picture on the left, paradoxically all first graders were fooled ("different" judgment) by the illusion that the cylinders in the picture on the right increased in size, a judgment based on apparent size despite the fact that actual size remained constant. In both cases, the perspective background interacted with the cylinders to produce a size illusion; but the more compelling effect for first graders was inverse perspective which distorts the relationship between apparent size and apparent distance. Older children were less fooled by the inverse perspective case, and were more sensitive to perspective information in both cases as revealed by their increased use of spatial relational terms (e.g., "larger—near," "smaller—farther away") and/or their use of linear perspective size (e.g., using converging lines to judge size) to express rule-like apparent size, apparent distance relationships.

The problems that first-grade children had reading and understanding perspective in pictures were reflected in their drawings of the model. These drawings

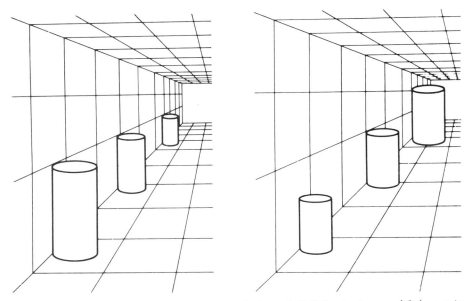

**FIGURE 22.4.** *Cylinders depicted against perspective background. Cylinders in picture on left decrease in size, consistent with hallway background. Cylinders in picture on right remain constant in size against hallway background producing size illusion. [From Haber & Hershenson, Figs. 12.9 and 12.10, 1973, pp. 289–292.]*

were scored for both representational accuracy (i.e., degree to which depicted objects were differentiated on the basis of distinctive features) and perspective accuracy (i.e., degree to which objects were depicted in correct spatial arrangement). Drawings were sorted by station point and compared against photographs of the model taken from equivalent station points in order to identify perspective errors.

The results of the analysis of the drawings is shown in Table 22.7. Accuracy in terms of both representational differentiation and perspective layout increased significantly from first to fourth grade. First graders scored low on perspective

TABLE 22.6
Judgments of Apparent Size of Cylinders in a Perspective Background

|  | Grade | | | |
|---|---|---|---|---|
|  | First | Fourth | Sixth | Eighth |
| Consistent perspective (% "same") | 10 | 60 | 80 | 70 |
| Inverse perspective (% "different") | 100 | 70 | 80 | 80 |
| % Use of relational terms | 25 | 35 | 65 | 25 |
| % Use of linear perspective | 05 | 15 | 15 | 55 |
| % Measurement | 30 | 30 | 20 | 10 |

TABLE 22.7
Analysis of Perspective Representation in Children's Drawings

| Task | Percentage response[a] | | | |
|---|---|---|---|---|
| | Grade | | | |
| | First | Fourth | Sixth | Eight |
| Perspective accuracy: Depiction of objects in correct spatial location | 37 | 83 | 78 | 91 |
| Errors of Depiction | | | | |
| Wrong spatial location | 23 | 6 | 8 | 1 |
| Invisible object | 14 | 3 | 2 | 0 |
| Failure to depict | 25 | 7 | 11 | 8 |
| Use of perspective devices: Overlap, linear perspective, modeling and texture | 17 | 39 | 43 | 59 |
| Type of perspective | | | | |
| Side view | 60 | 40 | 10 | 0 |
| Mixed view | 40 | 40 | 30 | 10 |
| Perspective view | 0 | 20 | 60 | 90 |

[a] $N = 10$ per grade.

accuracy because they either depicted objects in the wrong spatial location or they depicted objects that were invisible from their station point. This latter error suggests that younger children were having difficulty distinguishing between what they saw while drawing and what they saw during their exploration prior to the drawing task.

The failure to recognize the distinctive appearance of the model from a given viewing angle may have also accounted for the high incidence of spatial location errors in the first graders' drawings. Many of these drawings displayed a total lack of concern with spatial relations, or, for that matter, for surfaces to support the objects that they depicted. The most common drawing strategy focused on the enumeration of objects with no clear organizational framework. Not only did this drawing strategy result in spatial errors of commission, but also in a large percentage of errors of omission (i.e., failing to depict objects as shown in Figure 22.5).

By grade four, children had overcome many of the spatial relational problems expressed in the younger children's drawings. Not only did accuracy increase, but the focus of the drawings shifted from simply enumerating a collection of objects, to depicting relationships among objects, surfaces, and planes. This shift in focus from enumeration of objects to the depiction of object relationships was accompanied by an increase in the use of perspective devices designed explicitly to represent projective spatial relationships. The use of perspective devices in the older children's drawing strategies combined with the appearance of linguistic and perceptual rules for expressing perspective relationships resulted in more accurate

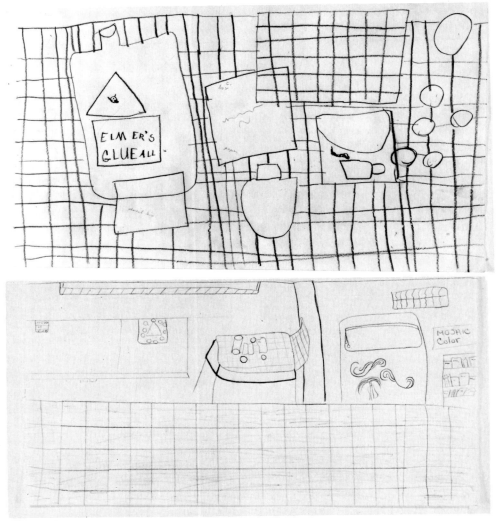

**FIGURE 22.5.** *Drawings of model by children of different grade levels. Top by a fourth-grade child, bottom by a sixth-grade child, facing top by a sixth-grade child, and facing bottom by an eighth-grade child.*

graphic representations. Pictorial comprehension scores correlated highly with drawing accuracy scores, $r = .80$, $p < .01$, and as the drawings became more accurate, they also displayed a greater concern for the space surrounding the objects depicted.

## VIII.   Conclusions

Reading, like drawing from a model (which is different from drawing from imagination), begins with visual differentiation of features of symbols or real world objects. Visual differentiation of features utilizes what I have referred to as the feature-contrast rule—look for a difference, contrast, or mismatch between features of the stimuli being compared. As I have shown, this rule works in differentiating most alphabet symbols and letterlike symbols except for those that are distinguished on the basis of spatial position or spatial orientation of line features (e.g., letterlike symbols differing on line origin, line slant, and opening

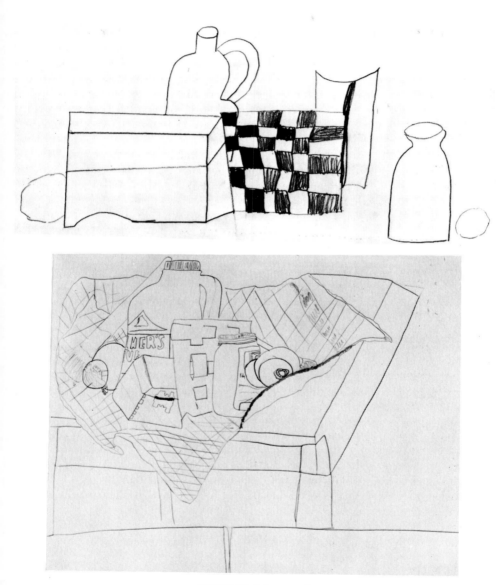

**FIGURE 22.5** (*continued*)

orientation, Nodine & Simmons, 1974). The feature-contrast rule also breaks down when applied to the task of drawing real world objects which requires the depiction of spatial mapping of real world objects within a unified perspective framework.

Errors caused by the overgeneralization of the feature-contrast rule lead to its reformulation. Visual differentiation calls for detection and analysis of both features and their spatial coordinates.

Gibson proposes that the reformulation of the feature-contrast rule comes about as the result of perceptual learning in which the focus of visual differentiation shifts from feature contrasts to contrasts involving more global perceptual units (e.g., patterns, grapheme–phoneme correspondences). The shift from analysis of features to analysis of higher order units is significant because patterns result from perceptual organization which links features to a unique spatial map. Thus for Gibson the problem of coordinating featural and spatial information is taken care of automatically by the chunking of features into higher order perceptual structures.

For Piaget, differentiation of letter orientation calls for the child to analyze differences between graphic features having equivalent spatial coordinates. This differentiation requires coordination of sensory information derived from a perceptual analysis of graphic features as the result of eye movements with nonsensory information derived from a conceptual scheme for mapping graphic features within a system of spatial coordinates.

The child's ability to coordinate visual features with the spatial positions they occupy within the stimulus configuration demands a form of reflecting abstraction which is illustrated by an example provided by my son who interrupted me at this point by calling out from his room where he was doing his homework. "Mom, Dad!" I answered, "Ricky what do you want?" His reply was, "How do you make a small *d*?" I thought to myself there must be some mental telepathy going on between us. Here I was struggling to find a final example that would show the importance of spatial relational logic in reading, and out of the mouth of my 11-year-old son comes the answer.

Taking advantage of this opportunity, I asked Ricky to come into my den and repeat his question.

Ricky:  "How do you make a small *d*?"
Dad:    "How do you think you make a small *d*?"
Ricky:  "I remember. This is a big *D* (drawing a big *D*). The little *d* is *opposite* of the big *D*. (Ricky draws little *d* and shows relation *D : d*).
Ricky:  "See the little *d faces* the big *D*" (Ricky uses arrow to show relationship *D ← d*).
Dad:    "Oh"
Ricky:  "Why do you want to know all about this? Don't you know how to make a small *d* either?"

Ricky's answer suggests that he was initially having difficulty differentiating *d* from its often confused mirror-image partner *b* at the grapheme–phoneme level. Somehow the inherent spatial code for "little *d*" got lost in Ricky's memory. His solution was to use "big *D*," which evidently carried a clearly differentiated spatial orientation code for him, as a "spatial anchor" for determining whether *d* or *b* was "little *d*." Gibson's notion that higher order perceptual units automatically carry their own spatial codes is partially supported (e.g., Ricky's reference to "big *D*'s" orientation).

But Ricky's answer does not end here. Ricky's explanation of *why* he picked *d* over *b* needs to be examined. The first reason was that *d* is *opposite D*. The second reason was that *d faces D* as his arrow from *d* to *D* clearly indicated. So, perceptual learning has been supplemented in this illustration by a spatial orientation framework constructed from coordinating a perceptual reference to spatial orientation contained in the "big *D*" with linguistic references to spatial orientation carried by the relational terms *opposite* and *faces*. Ricky's solution was generated by deriving spatial knowledge about the orientation of letters from the integration of perceptual and conceptual analyses of spatial relationships.

Solutions of this type which go beyond the analysis of empirical relationships are the result of what Piaget calls reflective abstraction. Such solutions imply that even basic beginning reading tasks like letter differentiation require the integration of both perceptual and conceptual sources of spatial knowledge. The spatial relational logic behind left–right and oblique orientations is not automatically picked up as a part of the distinctive feature information, but is constructed from the coordination of visual features with the child's growing awareness of the finite and logico-mathematical dimensions of space. If I am correct, then the theoretical differences between Gibson and Piaget are not as far apart epistemologically as one would think.

To support my point, I close with a quote from a loyal Gibson student, Margaret Hagen, who says that the creative or "generative" capacity of perception "provides one of the rarer solutions to the problem of meaning . . . by arguing with Helmholtz *or Piaget* and the Gibsonians that the meaning or structure of the perceptual experience resides not in the 'stimulus out there' nor 'in the head' but in the relation between the two [italics added, p. 44]."

# References

Arnheim, R. (1969). *Visual thinking*. Berkeley: University of California Press.
Back, S., & Nodine, C. F. (1972). *A study of the strategies used by kindergarten and third-grade children in a letter-like discrimination task*. Unpublished manuscript, Temple University.
Boersma, F. J., O'Bryan, K. G., & Ryan, B. (1970). Eye movements and horizontal decalage: Some preliminary findings. *Perceptual and Motor Skills, 3,* 386.
Boersma, F. J., & Wilton, K. M. (1974). Eye movements and conservation acceleration. *Journal of Experimental Child Psychology, 17,* 49–60.
Braine, L. G. (1978). A new slant on orientation perception. *American Psychologist, 33,* 10–22.

Day, M. C. (1975). Developmental trends in visual scanning. In H. W. Reese (Ed.), *Advances in child development and behavior* (Vol. 10). New York: Academic Press. Pp. 153–159.

Forman, G. E., & Sigel, I. E. (1979). *Cognitive development: A life-span view.* Monterey: Brooks/Cole.

Gardner, H., & Wolf, D. (1979). First drawings: Notes on the relationship between perception and production. In C. F. Nodine & D. F. Fisher (Eds.), *Perception and pictorial representation.* New York: Praeger. Pp. 361–387.

Gibson, E. J. (1965). Learning to read. *Science, 148,* 1066–1072.

Gibson, E. J. (1969). *Principles of perceptual learning and development.* New York: Appleton–Century–Crofts.

Gibson, E. J. (1973). *Trends in perceptual development: Implications for the reading process.* Paper presented at University of Minnesota Symposium, Minneapolis, April.

Gibson, E. J. (1977). How perception really develops: A view from outside the network. In D. LaBerge & S. J. Samuels (Eds.), *Basic processes in reading.* Hillsdale, New Jersey: Earlbaum. Pp. 155–173.

Gibson, E. J., Gibson, J. J., Pick, A. D., & Osser, H. (1962). A developmental study of the discrimination of letter-like forms. *Journal of Comparative & Physiological Psychology, 55,* 897–906.

Gibson, E. J., & Levin, H. (1975). *The psychology of reading.* Cambridge: MIT Press.

Gibson, J. J. (1973). On the concept of formless invariants in visual perception. *Leonardo, 6,* 43–45.

Gibson, J. J. (1979). *The ecological approach to visual perception.* Boston: Houghton–Mifflin.

Gombrich, E. H. (1972). *Art and illusion.* Princeton: Princeton University Press.

Goodman, N. (1968). *Languages of art: an approach to a theory of symbols.* Indianapolis: Bobbs-Merrill.

Haber, R. N., & Hershenson, M. (1973). *The psychology of visual perception.* New York: Holt, Rinehart & Winston.

Hagen, M. A. (Ed.). (1980). *The perception of pictures* (Vol. 1: Alberti's window). New York: Academic Press. (a)

Hagen, M. A. (Ed.). (1980). *The perception of pictures* (Vol. 2: Durer's devices). New York: Academic Press. (b)

Kersher, J. (1975). Visual-spatial organization and reading: Support for a cognitive developmental interpretation. *Journal of Learning Disabilities, 8,* 30–36.

Laurendeau, M., & Pinard, A. (1970). *The development of the concept of space in the child.* New York: International Universities Press.

Nicolaides, K. (1969). *The natural way to draw.* Boston: Houghton Mifflin.

Nodine, C. F., & Evans, J. D. (1969). Eye movements of prereaders to pseudowords containing letters of high and low confusability. *Perception & Psychophysics, 6,* 39–41.

Nodine, C. F., & Fisher, D. F. (1979). *Perception and pictorial representation.* New York: Praeger.

Nodine, C. F., Kenney, J. L., & Nodine, B. F. (1981). *Children's understanding of drawing as a perceptual–representational system.* Paper presented at Eastern Psychological Association meetings, New York, April.

Nodine, C. F., & Lang, N. J. (1971). The development of visual scanning strategies for differentiating words. *Developmental Psychology, 5,* 221–232.

Nodine, C. F., & Simmons, F. G. (1974). Processing distinctive features of letter-like symbols. *Journal of Experimental Psychology, 103,* 21–28.

Nodine, C. F., & Steuerle, N. L. (1973). Development of perceptual and cognitive strategies for differentiating graphemes. *Journal of Experimental Psychology, 5,* 221–232.

O'Bryan, K. G., & Boersma, F. J. (1971). Eye movements, perceptual activity and conservation development. *Journal of Experimental Child Psychology, 12,* 157–169.

Olson, D. R. (1970). *Cognitive development: The child's acquisition of diagonality.* New York: Academic Press.

Olson, D. R. (1975). On the relations between spatial and linguistic precesses. In J. Eliot & N. J. Salkind (Eds.), *Children's spatial development.* Springfield: C. C. Thomas.

Piaget, J., & Inhelder, B. (1967). *The Child's conception of space.* New York: W. W. Norton.

Piaget, J., & Inhelder, B. (1969). *The psychology of the child.* New York: Basic Books.

Vurpillot, E. (1968). The development of scanning strategies and their relationship to visual differentiation. *Journal of Experimental Child Psychology, 6,* 632–650.

Jonathan Vaughan

# 23

# Saccadic Reaction Time in Visual Search[1]

## I.   Introduction

The mechanisms that control the duration of the fixational pause of the eyes have been studied in many contexts: tracking of abruptly displaced targets, search for letters or symbols, and reading of prose for varying degrees of comprehension. This chapter attempts to bring together studies performed in different contexts that speak to the latency of the movement of the eyes and speculates on their common implications.

The control of fixation duration has been studied recently in a number of different contexts. Although the phenomena that are observed in one situation are not, of course, necessarily directly relevant to other situations, a pattern of similar results in psychophysical, visual search, and reading studies has appeared, so we may speculate on the importance of mechanisms that seem common to these different areas. This chapter will look at three approaches to the question of control of fixation duration, with particular reference to visual search situations. The first general approach is to set up an artificially restricted situation (to minimize the influence of extraneous variables) to determine the speed with which successive eye movements can be made, which normally limits the rate of acquisition of visual information. The second general approach is to determine the rate at which information can be processed in the absence of eye movements.

[1]The work reported here was supported by grant MH-26303 from the National Institute of Mental Health, and by the Hamilton College Faculty Research Fund.

*EYE MOVEMENTS IN READING:*
*PERCEPTUAL AND LANGUAGE PROCESSES*

Third, one may directly manipulate the stimuli that are presented within each fixation in a reading or search task, in order to determine how variation of the customary relationship between eye movements and visual information affects performance. Finally, some speculations about the implications of these experiments for theories of the control of fixation duration in reading and search will be presented.

## II.   Restricted Tasks

### A.   The Minimum Duration of Fixations

Studies of the reaction time of the oculomotor system can establish tentative time limits for the influence of visual information on the duration of the fixation in which it is viewed. If a theory for the control of fixation duration is to assume that the saccade that ends a fixation occurs in reaction to the stimulus viewed in that fixation, it must be shown that such a reaction time is physiologically possible; it would be instructive to show as well that manipulations that affect reaction time when a manual response is used also affect fixation duration in comparable situations.

The minimum time between successive saccadic movements ("corrective" saccades excluded) is as long as 200 msec. Arnold and Tinker (1939) first attempted to determine the shortest duration of a fixation under voluntary control. The subject fixated, successively, three points separated by 12° horizontally, attempting to make the middle fixation as short as possible. The fastest subject fixated the middle point for at least 116 msec, and the group average was 172 msec (157 msec when the middle dot was replaced by a letter). A recent replication by Salthouse and Ellis (1980) obtained similar results. The same time interval has been found in the saccadic tracking of suddenly displaced stimuli. The reaction time for a saccadic movement to the onset of a peripheral stimulus (4 or more degrees from the point of fixation) is about 180–210 msec (Becker, 1972; Saslow, 1967). These studies used very simple tasks which involved merely moving the eyes toward a peripheral stimulus when it appeared, and did not include any further cognitive processing (except deciding the distance and direction of the saccadic movement). Since the tasks used required minimal processing of the stimuli (compared to reading, for example) we might expect these laboratory situations to be most able to show optimum oculomotor performance. However, there are two reasons why this paradigm might differ in important respects from eye movements in reading or other complex tasks. First, the direction and perhaps the size of the next saccade is usually predictable for the reader, but they were not known to the subjects in the tracking tasks mentioned earlier. Second, despite the apparent simplicity of the saccadic tracking task, it produces saccadic latencies that may fall short of the optimum that might be obtained when suitable warning stimuli are used.

## B.   Saccadic Latency and Warning Intervals

It is well known that a warning stimulus before the presentation of a visual stimulus can facilitate reaction time in at least two independent ways. The warning stimulus may prime the perceptual apparatus if it presents information about the stimulus to be responded to or it may facilitate reaction time by permitting the preparation of the eventual response (Bertelson, 1967; Drazin, 1961; Posner & Boies, 1971). Two saccadic tracking studies in particular, those of Becker (1972) and of Saslow (1967), have extended this observation to the latency of saccadic eye movements. Both studies imposed a brief delay between the offset of a centrally located fixation point and the onset of the peripheral target; since the subject could not anticipate which side or position the stimulus would appear in, saccadic latency could not be reduced by a premature movement toward the target. In Saslow's study, the latency of the saccade to the peripheral target declined for one subject from 185 msec at simultaneous offset of the central fixation and onset of the target to about 125 msec when there was an interval of 300 msec between central fixation offset and peripheral target onset (Figure 23.1). Becker (1972) reports that a warning interval before stimulus onset lowered saccadic latency from 210 msec at zero delay to about 120 msec at a delay of 120 msec (Figure 23.1). Ross and Ross (1981) found facilitation of saccade latency by 30–50 msec with a warning interval of 100 msec, though the saccade latencies that they report are typically somewhat longer (about 260 msec at zero delay) than those of Becker (1972) and Saslow (1967). In a related paradigm, Becker and Jürgens (1979) have observed in a double-step tracking task that the size of a saccade may be affected by target movement as short as 80–100 msec before the saccade begins, when a

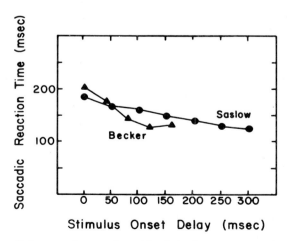

FIGURE 23.1.   *Saccadic latency to the onset of a peripheral stimulus at an uncertain location as a function of the interval between offset of a central fixation point and onset of the peripheral stimulus. [Data from Becker (1972) and Saslow (1967).]*

saccade had already been signaled by a prior target movement but had not yet occurred. When the direction of movement required is changed, however, or when a larger movement is called for than previously programmed, new information can affect the saccade only up to 200 msec prior to its occurrence (Becker & Jürgens, 1979). Given optimum response preparation, then, a saccade may be affected by information presented to the retina up to about 100 msec before the eyes move. If optimally prepared, a saccade may be elicited by a parafoveal cue with a minimum latency of about 120 msec; a previously initiated saccade may be modified with a latency of 80 msec. In the absence of such preparation, the saccadic reaction time seems to have a minimum of about 200 msec when elicited by a parafoveal stimulus change. Reaction time to make a saccade may generally be 100 msec longer than this when the movement is made in response to a cue not at the saccade target location, such as a left- or right-pointing arrow displayed at fixation (Remington, 1980; Klein, 1980).

To build a bridge between reaction time experiments and fixation duration experiments one might look for similar effects of warning intervals in the two situations. One impetus for doing so is that a model for the control of fixation durations that considered (unprepared) saccadic reaction time alone would seem to predict fixation durations that are too long when compared with what is actually observed in reading. A model that was built with the additional assumption that other processes could facilitate reaction time might prove to be more tenable.

## C.  The Maximum Rate of Processing Visual Information

A second major consideration in the control of fixation duration is the time required for processing of information that is presented sequentially to the same location on the retina. Stimuli may be presented so as to simulate the pattern of retinal excitation that occurs when the eye makes a series of saccades along a line of print; however, such stimulation differs in that (usually) there is absent the kind of peripheral information that is ordinarily available to the reader, and the duration of retinal stimulation is constant, rather than variable, from "fixation" to "fixation". If the subject must accurately and completely recall (rather than just recognize or detect) letters or words that are presented sequentially, the stimulus presentation time of each word that is required is a magnitude that is similar to the typical (unprepared) saccadic reaction time discussed earlier.

Bouma and deVoogd (1974), Eriksen and Eriksen (1971), Kolers and Katzman (1966), Kolers and Lewis (1972), Potter (1975), Potter, Kroll, and Harris (1980), and Travers (1973, 1975) have each investigated situations in which a series of stimuli is presented in a fixed temporal sequence at the same location on the retina, and have found that when the duration of each stimulus is sufficient (about 200–280 msec) performance is not impaired. For example, Kolers and Katzman (1966) observed that more than 250 msec presentation time per letter was necessary to permit correct report of English words, sequentially exposed one letter at a time at the same retinal location. Similarly, Eriksen and Eriksen (1971) demonstrated that a 200–250 msec interstimulus interval was required for the correct identification of three single-character test stimuli presented sequentially at the same retinal location. Massaro and Schmuller (1975) summarize a variety of experimental paradigms that indicate that this interval is the minimum during which effective perception and encoding of visual stimuli might occur.

Despite the variety of different tasks involved it is very clear that a duration of at least 150–200 msec is required for the encoding and complete processing of nonredundant visual stimuli that are presented as a series of visual stimuli (as are the retinal images resulting from the successive fixations made by a reader). Some exceptions to this generalization, which observed effective performance at higher presentation rates (Eriksen & Collins, 1969; Potter & Levy, 1969; Sperling, Budiansky, Spivak, & Johnson, 1971), required only detection of the presence of a known target, or recognition of a stimulus from the series after it had been presented, rather than recall of the stimuli. Finally, when the material is somewhat redundant, such as meaningful English sentences presented one word at a time to the same retinal location, effective comprehension is possible with a shorter exposure time of 83 msec per word (Potter *et al.*, 1980).

### III.   Control of Fixation Duration in Reading and Search

#### A.   Process Monitoring in the Control of Fixation Duration

The measurement of saccadic reaction time or the minimum time for which the eyes may be brought to rest suggests that the typical duration of a fixation in a task that involves the sequential processing of separate units of visual information each of which must be fixated (reading or search) ought to have minimum fixation durations of at least 200 msec, if we take this to be the sum of the time required to process the letters viewed in a fixation plus optimal reaction time (this conclusion has been drawn using similar logic by Russo, 1978, and by Salthouse & Ellis, 1981). Saccades in reading could not occur at a rate much faster than they do, because the eyes can move no more frequently in response to visual information. Some studies suggest that saccades in reading might also be limited because the visual system can not effectively process the high rate of information that would result, though this limit seems to vary with the task used.[2] Studies of the rapid presentation of information to the stationary eye may overestimate the minimum

---

[2]For the teleologist, there is perhaps no great mystery to the coincidence that about the same duration occurs at the optimum rate of stimulus presentation as is the minimum time for an eye movement to be initiated. If one constraint did not exist—for example, if the eyes could move so as to make 20 fixations per sec, rather than only 4 or 5—then there surely would have been, in evolutionary or individual development, some room for greater optimization of the other function, until they were more nearly equal.

time required for processing of information, because of the intentional exclusion of predictability of the stimuli. This predictability would ordinarily be provided by the redundancy of text, as the work of Potter *et al.* (1980) suggests.

Two general classes of models have been proposed for the control of fixation duration in reading and search, each of which shares its basic assumptions with the studies of oculomotor reaction time or the studies of rapid presentation of visual information, presented earlier. The first class of models, which Rayner (1978) has called "process monitoring" and which Just and Carpenter (1980) have recently developed as a part of a formal model of reading, the "eye–mind assumption" (see also McConkie, Hogaboam, Wolverton, Zola, & Lucas, 1979), is that the duration of fixation in reading or search corresponds precisely to the length of time required to process the stimulus seen in that fixation. The assumptions of the process monitoring model are simply that a stimulus is fixated until processing of it is completed; then the eye makes a saccade to a new stimulus. One line of evidence in favor of this is the demonstration that changing a stimulus within a fixation can affect the duration of that fixation (Rayner, 1975). Similarly, stimuli that require different lengths of time to process produce different durations of fixations in search. Gould (1973) has compared fixation durations in a search task that employed Sternberg's (1966) memory search paradigm. Fixation durations on comparison letters were 100 msec longer when the memory set was three characters than when it was one, which implies that each fixation duration is directly controlled by the visual information acquired during that fixation.

The process monitoring model in its many guises is at heart a reaction time model. The eye looks until the stimulus that is foveally visible has been processed, then it moves. The saccade is initiated only when processing is completed. This implies that a fixation duration represents two components: processing time and reaction time. Furthermore, any manipulation of a stimulus that can be shown to affect manual reaction time ought to have a similar effect on fixation duration (like Gould's 1973 memory search study, or the warning-interval studies discussed in section IIB).

## B.  Preprogramming of Fixation Duration

Preprogramming of fixation duration is an alternative to process monitoring which has been argued for by Bouma and deVoogd (1974), Shebilske (1975), and Vaughan (Vaughan, 1978; Vaughan & Graefe, 1977). The preprogramming class of models suggests that the eyes move so as to acquire visual information *before* the cognitive apparatus is completely finished processing prior information. In such a model, which we may refer to as a preprogramming model ("buffer," and "indirectly-regulated-scanning" model are the terms used by Bouma & deVoogd, 1974, and Shebilske, 1975, respectively), visual information would be acquired at a rate that was globally equal to the average rate of processing; but the strict identity of processing time of individual stimuli and fixation duration would not hold. The eye and mind would be in rough, rather than complete, synchrony. Evidence for this kind of model comes from the observation that comprehension is not completely impaired by conditions that prevent voluntary variation of individual fixation durations, such as the rapid serial presentation of words used by Bouma and deVoogd (1974) and Potter *et al.* (1980). A variation of preprogrammed control of fixation duration recognizes that some stimuli, at least, require an unanticipatedly long amount of processing time and that such a stimulus might cause a preprogrammed saccade to be canceled so that fixation duration could come under the control of the particular stimulus viewed. Such a model will be referred to as partial preprogramming.

Both process monitoring and preprogramming models seem to have serious problems which require some change from the simplest assumptions. Process monitoring would seem to predict fixation durations that are too long (when compared with actual observation of readers) or "waste time" in the reaction time of the eye. Preprogramming would seem to predict fixation durations that are homogeneous in duration and unaffected by the special characteristics of individual stimuli. But observed fixation durations in reading are variable rather than constant, and the stimulus viewed in a particular fixation may affect the duration of that fixation (Gould, 1973; Rayner, 1975); it is not possible to reconcile this with a preprogramming model that denies any role in determining fixation duration to the stimulus viewed.

## C. Recent Studies Using Stimulus Onset Delay

Let us now turn to some experiments in which subjects makes successive fixations in a reading or search task. Under normal conditions, there is a different stimulus presented to the eye during each fixation, which is visible from the beginning of the fixation until the eye next moves.[3] Experimentally, a computer that detects the occurrence of saccades could delay the presentation of each stimulus for a short or long time after the beginning of each fixation so that the subject would not be able to begin to process the information in that fixation right away. If strict process monitoring operated, fixation duration would have to increase in compensation of the delay; if preprogramming were used, fixation duration might remain constant. A combination of the two processes, or a more complicated variation of either, might give intermediate results.

### 1. STIMULUS ONSET DELAY IN VISUAL SEARCH

Some attempts to evaluate the preprogramming model by varying the delay of onset of a stimulus after the beginning of a fixation have produced data that are partially consistent with the pure model. If a short delay of stimulus onset is

---

[3] It is well known that there is a period of a few tens of msec of reduced visual sensitivity immediately after a saccade (Volkmann, 1962). Nevertheless, Rayner, Inhoff, Morrison, Slowiaczek, and Bertera (1981) have recently shown that reading is unimpaired if the stimulus is made visible only during the first 50 msec following each saccade.

imposed, the preprogramming model predicts no increase in fixation duration. Several studies (Vaughan, 1978; Vaughan, 1982, Experiment 1; Vaughan & Graefe, 1977) have shown essentially no effect on fixation duration of short stimulus onset delays in the range 0–60 msec. For instance, fixation duration at 0 msec stimulus onset delay was 371 msec, and at 60 msec it was 369 msec. This is consistent with preprogramming. (If fixation duration had been increased from the 0 delay value to compensate for the stimulus onset delay, it would have been 431 msec long—371 plus 60— at the 60-msec delay.) At longer delays (up to 300 msec), however, oculomotor latency was more nearly constant (i.e., fixation duration increased almost as much as the increase in delay). This is consistent with a shift from preprogramming (at short delays) to process monitoring (at longer delays), that is, partial preprogramming.

In a recent study, Salthouse, Ellis, Diener, and Somberg (1981) observed similar data in a detection task. The subjects were instructed to fixate (as briefly as possible) the middle of three asterisks separated by 10°. At a random time after the beginning of the fixation, that asterisk was replaced by one of two cues ("<" or ">") for 40 msec. When the delay of cue onset was 0, fixation duration on the middle asterisk was about 280 msec. When the delay was increased to 150 msec, fixation duration increased only to about 315 msec, not 430 msec.

As discussed in Section IIIC4, there is an alternative explanation for these data in which the stimulus onset delay is hypothesized to act as a warning interval to facilitate the saccadic reaction, which will be developed later.

## 2. STIMULUS ONSET DELAY IN READING

A similar pattern of results has been observed by Rayner and Pollatsek (1981) who imposed varying delays of stimulus presentation as subjects read sentences for a later recognition test. In their experimental condition most directly comparable to the search studies just discussed, at the beginning of each fixation the 17 letters of the sentence around the point of fixation were replaced by masking characters for 25–100 msec. Although fixation duration was increased somewhat at the shorter delays, the increase was not as much as the delay imposed, as would have been predicted by a process monitoring model; on the other hand, there was some increase in fixation duration, contrary to the prediction of the preprogramming model. The results of three search and reading studies are shown in Figure 23.2. Note that to facilitate comparison with the Saslow (1967) and Becker (1972) saccadic reaction time data, the dependent measure has been transformed from fixation duration to oculomotor latency (the time from stimulus onset to the saccade that ends that fixation) by subtracting the stimulus onset delay from each average duration. (Thus, the values of oculomotor latency at 0 and 60 msec delay corresponding to the fixation durations of 371 and 369 msec, discussed at the end of Section IIIC1, are 371 and 309 msec, that is, 369 minus 60 msec, respectively). If there were complete compensation for the stimulus onset delay, such that fixation duration were increased in direct proportion to the delay imposed, we would expect the oculomotor latency functions of Figure 23.2 to be horizontal; but all curves decline at the short delays.

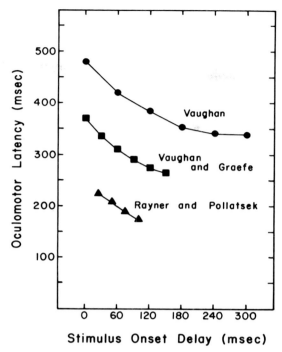

**FIGURE 23.2.** *Oculomotor latency (time from stimulus onset to the saccade that ends the fixation) as a function of the interval between the beginning of the fixation and stimulus onset in studies that have imposed a delay of stimulus onset after the saccade in search (Vaughan & Graefe, 1977; Vaughan, 1982) and in reading (Rayner & Pollatsek, 1981).*

### 3.    STIMULUS ONSET DELAY IN COMBINED VISUAL SEARCH AND MEMORY SEARCH

One way to differentiate process monitoring and stimulus onset delay in visual search would be to present a task in which the processing times of individual stimuli were variable. If the effect of stimulus onset delay on oculomotor latency represented partial preprogramming (i.e., a shift from preprogramming at short delays to process monitoring at longer delays) then oculomotor latency ought to be relatively insensitive to the processing time of different stimuli at the short delays, compared with the longer delays. The process monitoring hypothesis would predict uniform effects on fixation duration of different processing times at all stimulus onset delays. So, a further experiment was undertaken with a strong manipulation of the time required to process each stimulus. This was to use the Sternberg memory search paradigm (Sternberg, 1966), which Gould (1973) had shown to reliably affect fixation duration in search.

In the Sternberg memory search paradigm, a subject is given a small set of items, such as letters or numbers, to remember and is then asked whether a test letter is or is not a member of that memory set. The time the subject requires to make that decision, measured by traditional reaction time methods, varies with the number of letters in the memory set. When the memory set is small, just one letter, it takes less time than when the memory set is larger, say three or four letters. This implies that on each trial the subject performs a serial comparison of the target with each of the letters in the memory set. Typically, about 30–40 msec are added to reaction time for each additional letter in the memory set.

In a recent study (Vaughan, 1982) memory-set size was varied to affect the processing time of individual stimuli, and this manipulation was combined with stimulus onset delay to further explore the control mechanisms of fixation duration. Like Gould's (1973) study, fixation duration was measured as a function of memory-set size. At the same time, stimulus onset delay was varied from fixation to fixation. Memory-set size made a consistent difference of about 30 msec increase in oculomotor latency per item, as well as in reaction time (Figure 23.3). The result of the memory-set size manipulation was, then, consistent both qualitatively and quantitatively with that of Gould (1973). There was *no* statistically significant interaction between set size and stimulus onset delay. Thus, the overall effect of stimulus onset delay is similar to that of prior studies which were taken as evidence of partial preprogramming. The lack of an interaction, however, is not consistent with partial preprogramming. That is, despite the decline in

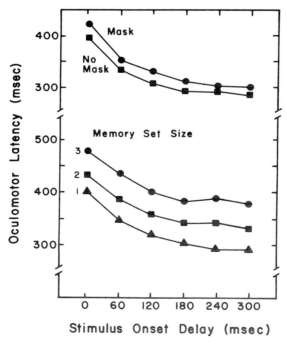

FIGURE 23.3. *Oculomotor latency as a function of stimulus onset delay when the processing time of individual stimuli is varied by the size of the memory set to which each stimulus must be compared (the three lower lines) or by presence or absence of a flanking mask (the two upper lines). [Data after Vaughan, 1982.]*

oculomotor latency with increased stimulus onset delay, the oculomotor latency very nicely increased by about 30 msec for each additional letter in the memory set, regardless of stimulus onset delay. From this, we may conclude that the stimulus onset delay effect (the decline in oculomotor latency) probably does *not* result from the partial preprogramming model discussed earlier, since such a model would predict a smaller memory-set size effect at the short delays (where preprogramming would presumably prevail) instead of the constant effect of memory-set size at all stimulus onset delays.

There is one way a preprogramming model could produce data such as these, but it requires what is, perhaps, an implausible assumption. Suppose the subject (who knows at the beginning of each trial the size of the memory set for that trial) preprogrammed a fixation duration that took into account the time required to process each stimulus plus the added time required if the memory-set size were greater than one. Then the effect of memory-set size could occur at all delays despite the use of preprogramming. This possibility was ruled out by a related study that used much the same paradigm as the memory-set study, except that the processing time of individual stimuli was varied by having each search stimulus flanked by a noise mask (Vaughan, 1982). The subject saw whether the mask was present only after the fixation had begun, the delay had expired, and the stimulus was presented. The results of this experiment also showed a main effect of the processing time manipulation that was constant across stimulus onset delays: Oculomotor latency was about 10 msec longer when the mask was present, and there was again no discernable interaction of that effect with the duration of the stimulus onset delay (Figure 23.3).

### 4. SUMMARY OF STIMULUS ONSET DELAY EFFECTS

Several recent studies in search and reading have shown main effects of stimulus onset delay on oculomotor latency that are consistent either with partial preprogramming or with process monitoring with warning interval effects. The absence of an interaction between stimulus processing time and stimulus onset delay is, however, consistent with only the second of these models—process monitoring with a warning interval effect. The interaction between stimulus onset delay and the processing time of individual stimuli that would have been expected if preprogramming were used at short delays and process monitoring at long delays was not observed.

Thus, the warning-interval explanation of stimulus onset delay effects at short delays would seem to be the most likely explanation at the present time. A variable stimulus onset delay before stimulus presentation seems to facilitate the saccadic response in reading or search in a manner similar to the effect of a warning stimulus in manual or saccadic reaction time. Presumably the period of stimulus onset delay produces nonspecific alerting or response preparation which makes the saccadic response to the stimulus faster.

To decide that the stimulus onset delay effect does not provide evidence for preprogramming in reading or search does not mean that the issue of the control of fixation duration in such tasks is settled in favor of process monitoring models. For one thing, the search experiments of Vaughan (Vaughan, 1982; Vaughan & Graefe, 1977) required subjects to inhibit movements away from the stimulus before the termination of the delay interval; the subjects' behavior was therefore constrained to minimize preprogramming, and it might still be a factor in other situations. In contrast to these search studies, for example, Rayner and Pollatsek (1981) did not impose such a constraint in their reading study. Subjects saw a masking stimulus during the period of stimulus onset delay, followed by the text to be read at the conclusion of the delay interval. In their Experiment 2, which used delays as long as 300 msec, on many fixations (18 and 43%, respectively, at delays of 200 and 300 msec) the subject initiated a saccade before the stimulus actually appeared. Since the text was not yet present to be viewed, those "anticipatory" saccades clearly represent some sort of preprogramming of saccades, at least in that experimental situation. At the 300 msec delay the subjects' eyes behaved as the mixed preprogramming model describes: sometimes (43% of fixations) the eyes moved early, and sometimes (57%) the preprogrammed saccade was aborted in favor of a fixation that was lengthened to compensate for the delay imposed. These percentages may in fact underestimate the proportion of anticipatory saccades, since (as we have seen in Section IIB) a saccade is not likely to be influenced by information present only during the last 100 msec of the fixation. As Rayner and Pollatsek argue, a saccade occurring during the 133 msec after the mask offset is probably not initiated or affected by what is seen in that fixation. Thus the percentage of anticipatory saccades at 200 and 300 msec could be estimated to be 53% and 66%, respectively. Similar anticipatory saccades may be inferred from Gould's (1973) study of different memory-set sizes in visual search. On 27% of trials, subjects refixated a target letter after having once fixated it. His subjects were twice as likely to make such a regressive saccade to a target when the memory-set size was three than when it was one. One interpretation of this difference is that in the smaller set size, memory search and related processing was more likely to have been completed before the occurrence of a prepro-grammed saccade.

## IV.    Implications of Stimulus Onset Delay Effects for Models of Reading

Although most of the data reported here are concerned primarily with visual search, it is of interest to note the relevance to models of fixation duration in reading. In normal reading peripherally acquired information (e.g., word size or shape) may well facilitate processing of the contents of some fixations through alerting or priming mechanisms. Such peripherally presented information has been shown to decrease naming latency (Rayner, McConkie, & Ehrlich, 1978), and might decrease oculomotor reaction time as well. Hochberg (1970) outlined a means whereby peripheral information might be used to control the spatial extent of saccades in reading, and O'Regan (1979) has confirmed experimentally that the size of saccades in reading may be affected by peripherally perceived word size. A similar mechanism might be proposed for the control of the duration of fixations which could use the fragmentary information (about word length, shape, etc.) that is available in peripheral vision as a warning stimulus, carrying information about (roughly) how long it might take to process the peripheral stimulus when it is later viewed foveally.

What evidence there is that such facilitation might operate in normal reading is at the present only indirect. Readers do extract some information from the near periphery. It has been shown that the attentional "fovea" is asymmetrical (Mc-Conkie & Rayner, 1976; Rayner, Well, & Pollatsek, 1980), by presenting text to subjects whose position of gaze is monitored so that words beyond the edge of a variable size region around the point of fixation may be degraded. If such degradation of a particular peripheral area does not disrupt reading, it may be assumed that no useful information is being extracted from that area. The useful range of peripheral vision is greater to the right for readers of English and to the left for readers of Hebrew, consistent with the direction (left to right or right to left) of the reader's saccadic eye movements in each language (Pollatsek, Bolozky, Well, & Rayner, 1981). Similarly, parafoveal information (peripheral presentation of a word to be named, before a saccade to it) facilitates word naming when it is on the side to which a saccade is about to be made but not when it is on the side opposite the eventual saccade (Rayner et al., 1978). If information extracted from the periphery in anticipation of an eye movement served to predict how long it would take to process the text seen in the next fixation, it might facilitate the reaction time of the oculomotor system. Further studies like that of Rayner and Pollatsek's (1981) experiment in which the presence of only foveal or only peripheral information was delayed might show whether stimulus onset delay and peripheral information facilitated saccadic reaction time using the same or different mechanisms.

### ACKNOWLEDGMENTS

I thank Kathryn Devereaux and Judi Diamond for assistance in conducting the experiments, and Keith Rayner for discussions of the problems addressed here. I appreciate the comments of Yoav Cohen, Douglas J. Herrmann, Michael I. Posner, and Douglas A. Weldon on drafts of this chapter.

# References

Arnold, D. C., & Tinker, M. A. (1939). The fixational pause of the eyes. *Journal of Experimental Psychology, 25,* 271–280.

Becker, W. (1972). The control of eye movements in the saccadic system. *Bibliotheca Ophthalmologica, 82,* 233–243.

Becker, W., & Jürgens, R. (1979). An analysis of the saccadic system by means of double step stimuli. *Vision Research, 19,* 967–983.

Bertelson, P. (1967). The time course of preparation. *Quarterly Journal of Experimental Psychology, 19,* 272–279.

Bouma, H., & deVoogd, A. H. (1974). On the control of eye saccades in reading. *Vision Research, 14,* 273–284.

Drazin, D. H. (1961). Effect of foreperiod, foreperiod variability, and probability of stimulus occurrence on simple reaction time. *Journal of Experimental Psychology, 62,* 43–50.

Eriksen, C. W., & Collins, J. F. (1969). Visual perceptual rate under two conditions of search. *Journal of Experimental Psychology, 80,* 489–492.

Eriksen, C. W., & Eriksen, B. A. (1971). Visual perceptual processing rates and backward and forward masking. *Journal of Experimental Psychology, 89,* 306–313.

Gould, J. D. (1973). Eye movements during visual search and memory search. *Journal of Experimental Psychology, 98,* 184–195.

Hochberg, J. (1970). Components of literacy: Speculations and exploratory research. In H. Levin & J. P. Williams (Eds.), *Basic studies in reading.* New York: Basic Books.

Just, M. A., & Carpenter, P. (1980). A theory of reading: From eye fixations to comprehension. *Psychological Review, 87,* 329–354.

Klein, R. (1980). Does oculomotor readiness mediate cognitive control of visual attention? *Attention and Performance (Vol. 8).* Hillsdale, New Jersey: Erlbaum.

Kolers, P. A., & Katzman, M. T. (1966). Naming sequentially presented letters and words. *Language and Speech, 9,* 84–95.

Kolers, P. A., & Lewis, C. L. (1972). Bounding of letter sequences and the integration of visually presented words. *Acta Psychologica, 36,* 112–114.

Massaro, D. W., & Schmuller, J. (1975). Visual features, preperceptual storage, and processing time in reading. In D. W. Massaro (Ed.), *Understanding language.* New York: Academic Press.

McConkie, G. W., Hogaboam, T. W., Wolverton, G. S., Zola, D., & Lucas, P. (1979). Towards the use of eye movements in the study of language processing. *Discourse Processes, 2,* 157–177.

McConkie, G. W., & Rayner, K. (1976). Asymmetry of the perceptual span in reading. *Bulletin of the Psychonomic Society, 8,* 365–368.

O'Regan, J. K. (1979). Moment to moment control of eye saccades as a function of textual parameters in reading. In P. A. Kolers, M. E. Wrolstad, & H. Bouma (Eds.), *Processing of visible language* (Vol. 1). New York: Plenum Press.

Pollatsek, A., Bolozky, S., Well, A. D., & Rayner, K. (1981). Asymmetries in the perceptual span for Israeli readers. *Brain and Language, 14,* 174–180.

Posner, M. I., & Boies, S. J. (1971). Components of attention. *Psychological Review, 78,* 391–408.

Potter, M. C. (1975). Meaning in visual search. *Science, 187,* 965–966.

Potter, M. C., Kroll, J. F., & Harris, C. (1980). Comprehension and memory in rapid sequential reading. In R. S. Nickerson (Ed.), *Attention and performance* (Vol. 8). Hillsdale, New Jersey: Erlbaum.

Potter, M. C., & Levy, E. I. (1969). Recognition memory for a rapid sequence of pictures. *Journal of Experimental Psychology, 81,* 10–15.

Rayner, K. (1975). The perceptual span and peripheral cues in reading. *Cognitive Psychology, 7,* 65–81.

Rayner, K. (1978). Eye movements in reading and information processing. *Psychological Bulletin, 85,* 618–660.

Rayner, K., Inhoff, A. W., Morrison, R. E., Slowiaczek, M. L., & Bertera, J. H. (1981). Masking of foveal and parafoveal vision during eye fixations in reading. *Journal of Experimental Psychology: Human Perception & Performance, 7,* 167–179.

Rayner, K., McConkie, G. W., & Ehrlich, S. (1978). Eye movements and integrating information across fixations. *Journal of Experimental Psychology: Human Perception & Performance, 4,* 529–544.

Rayner, K., & Pollatsek, A. (1981). Eye movement control during reading: Evidence for direct control. *Quarterly Journal of Experimental Psychology, 33A,* 351–373.

Rayner, K., Well, A. D., & Pollatsek, A. (1980). Asymmetry of the effective visual field in reading. *Perception & Psychophysics, 27,* 537–544.

Remington, R. W. (1980). Attention and saccadic eye movements. *Journal of Experimental Psychology: Human Perception & Performance, 6,* 726–744.

Ross, S. M., & Ross, L. E. (1981). Saccade latency and warning signals: Effects of auditory and visual stimulus onset and offset. *Perception & Psychophysics, 29,* 429–437.

Russo, J. E. (1978). Adaptation of cognitive processes to the eye movement system. In J. W. Senders, D. W. Fisher, & R. A. Monty (Eds.), *Eye Movements and the Higher Psychological Functions.* Hillsdale, New Jersey: Erlbaum.

Salthouse, T. A., & Ellis, C. L. (1980). Determinants of eye-fixation duration. *American Journal of Psychology, 93,* 207–234.

Salthouse, T. A., Ellis, C. L., Diener, D. C., & Somberg, B. L. (1981). Stimulus processing during eye fixations. *Journal of Experimental Psychology: Human Perception & Performance, 7,* 611–623.

Saslow, M. G. (1967). Effects of components of displacement-step stimuli upon latency for saccadic eye movement. *Journal of the Optical Society of America, 57,* 1024–1029.

Shebilske, W. (1975). Reading eye movements from an information-processing point of view. In D. W. Massaro (Ed.), *Understanding language.* New York: Academic Press.

Sperling, G., Budiansky, J., Spivak, J. G., & Johnson, M. C. (1971). Extremely rapid visual search: The maximum rate of scanning letters for the presence of a numeral. *Science, 174,* 307–311.

Sternberg, S. (1966). High-speed scanning in human memory. *Science, 153,* 652–654.

Travers, J. R. (1973). The effects of forced serial processing on identification of words and random letter strings. *Cognitive Psychology, 5,* 109–137.

Travers, J. R. (1975). Forced serial processing of words and letter strings: A reexamination. *Perception & Psychophysics, 18,* 447–452.

Vaughan, J. (1978). Control of visual fixation duration in search. In J. W. Senders, D. W. Fischer, & R. A. Monty (Eds.), *Eye movements and the higher psychological functions.* Hillsdale, New Jersey: Erlbaum.

Vaughan, J. (1982). Control of fixation duration in visual search and memory search: Another look. *Journal of Experimental Psychology: Human Perception and Performance, 8,* 709–723.

Vaughan, J., & Graefe, T. (1977). Delay of stimulus presentation after the saccade in visual search. *Perception & Psychophysics, 22,* 201–205.

Volkmann, F. C. (1962). Vision during voluntary saccadic eye movements. *Journal of the Optical Society of America, 52,* 571–578.

Mary C. Potter

# 24

# Representational Buffers: The Eye–Mind Hypothesis in Picture Perception, Reading, and Visual Search[1]

## I.  Buffers in Visual Processing and Eye Movement Control

A buffer, as the term is used here, is a memory device that maintains information at a particular stage of processing. During the time the information is maintained, it is available to later stages of processing. A familiar example is iconic memory, which is thought to maintain a sensory-like visual representation for a short period during which a later process such as identification can operate. The term "buffer" focuses on the transient nature of a given memory representation and the flexibility it gives to the timing of the next stage(s) of processing.

In the case of the control of eye movements in reading and the perception of scenes, there may be several levels of buffering. The significance of the buffers is that they permit some degree of decoupling of the eye and mind. The methodological implication is that buffers reduce the sensitivity of eye movements as immediate indicators of mental processing.

The relevant buffers for which there is at least some evidence include the following eight. It should be emphasized that the characterization of these buffers is tentative. I present some of the evidence for each buffer and discuss its functional significance for eye movements.

[1]This work was supported by Grant BNS80-15597 from the National Science Foundation.

*Input buffers* (vision)

1. Retinotopic icon or "visible persistence," localized in relation to the retinae.
2. Spatiotopic visual memory, localized in the visual world.
3. Reatopic visual memory, representing spatial relationships internal to some visual object or pattern ("res" is the Latin word for "thing," as in "real").

*Central buffers*

4. Acoustic/phonological/articulatory short-term memory (STM).
5. Conceptual very-short-term memory.
6. Working memory.

*Output buffers* (for eye movements)

7. Location of next saccade.
8. Timing of next saccade.

A visual event does not necessarily enter the buffers in the order given here. It is assumed that certain pairs of buffers are linked by processes that transform information from one to the other buffer. The relative timing and direction of flow of information is constrained by these links, which operate automatically or under central control. A diagram of possible connections among the buffers is given in Fig. 24.1 (Section III).

## A.    Buffer 1: Retinotopic Icon or "Visible Persistence"

Iconic memory has been extensively studied since Sperling revived the phenomenon in 1960. Most researchers have assumed that the subjective impression of continuing vision after the stimulus has stopped is what permits selective processing of some part of the array, in Sperling's partial-report paradigm. Recently, however, Coltheart (1980) has argued persuasively that visible persistence of the sort mediated by the photoreceptors (e.g., Sakitt, 1976) and probably also by some later stages in vision is *not* the basis for the poststimulus cuing effect in the partial-report paradigm, which is instead due to some later (more central) stage of processing (Buffer 3 or 5, in the present scheme).

It is worth looking briefly at Coltheart's argument, for it is a model of how one can dissociate buffers. His approach is to determine whether variables that affect persistence of vision also affect partial versus whole report in the Sperling task. He discusses seven different experimental procedures that seem on their face to measure *visible* persistence. Each of these compares some behavioral measure with the physical duration of the stimulus. The seven are: (*a*) judgment of synchrony between the visible offset of a target stimulus and the onset of a visual or auditory probe stimulus; (*b*) response latency to the onset and (apparent) offset of a stimulus; (*c*) stroboscopic illumination of a moving stimulus such as a single spoke; persistence is measured by the number of spokes reported to be seen simultaneously; (*d*) the moving-slit technique in which a stimulus is "painted" over the retina; (e) phenomenal continuity of an intermittent stimulus; (f) temporal integration of two incomplete figures; and (g) stereoscopic persistence, which can be distinguished from the persistence of the monocular input to the stereoscopic system and which is therefore cortical in locus. In most of these paradigms, visible persistence lasts from 0 to 150 msec; in the case of stereopsis, 300 msec.

Coltheart noted that all these measures of visible persistence indicate that within certain ranges, visible persistence is *inversely* related to luminance and to stimulus duration. In contrast, partial-report superiority is *unrelated* to luminance and stimulus duration, over the same range, provided that they are "adequate for legibility." Therefore, concludes Coltheart, visible persistence is not the basis for Sperling's iconic memory, which is measured by the persistence of information that is not necessarily in the form of a visible array (see Buffers 2–5). (Coltheart's conclusions have been questioned or qualified by Bowling & Lovegrove, 1982, and Long & Beaton, 1982.)

Coltheart also reviewed the possible neural basis of visible persistence and concluded there were several loci (in effect, several buffers of Type 1): Candidates are the photoreceptors (Sakitt, 1976) and the sustained cells of the ganglion cells, lateral geniculate nucleus, and the visual cortex. Stereoscopic effects also indicate central visual persistence.

From the point of view of eye movements, what is the significance of Buffer 1, visible persistence? I would argue that in normal perception it plays no role except perhaps to sustain vision during blinks and possibly during saccades, until the next fixation. (But even in these cases some later buffer is as likely to be the functional one.) Of course, the phenomenon of persistence reveals characteristics of the visual system that are functionally important, but their function is not to outlast the stimulus—that consequence is incidental, and becomes functional only in the laboratory tasks listed earlier. (Haber has commented that visible persistence would only be useful for reading in a lightning storm.) Thus, Buffer 1 is a possible source of artifacts or mistaken interpretations in experiments that study eye movements using interrupted stimuli. Otherwise, it has little significance as a buffer. Note that persistence is usually eliminated by a following stimulus, provided that the two stimuli are sufficiently different and have a stimulus onset asynchrony (SOA) of about 30 msec or more; otherwise there is integration, as in (f) above. Persistence would thus ordinarily be terminated by the next fixation.

## B.  Buffer 2: Spatiotopic Visual Memory

In perception, the retinally organized information from successive fixations is put together to produce the impression of a continuous, stable visual world. Several investigators have shown that this spatiotopic representation persists at least briefly after the stimulus has been removed (though for how long has yet to be investigated), that the representation can survive masking (at least if the subject attends to it), and that under some conditions the representation permits the visual integration of successive fixations. (For a related distinction between two visual buffers, see Mewhort, Campbell, Marchetti, & Campbell, 1981.)

Jonides, Irwin, and Yantis (1982) found that two stimuli presented in successive fixations can be seen as one figure, provided that they appear in the same
location in visual space (and hence in *different* retinal locations). Davidson, Fox,
and Dick (1973) showed something similar. A subject viewed a letter string on
fixation $N$, replaced on fixation $N + 1$ by a ring around the place where one of the
letters had been. The subjective appearance was of a ring surrounding the letter
that had been at that location in visual space, whereas the ring masked (blanked)
the letter that had been at the ring's *retinal* location. That is, subjects "saw" an
array of letters in which one letter was missing and another letter was visible but
surrounding by a ring. Metacontrast masking was retinotopic (Buffer 1), whereas
perceived overlap was spatiotopic (Buffer 2). (It should be noted that some laboratories have been unable to obtain the spatiotopic overlap reported by Jonides *et al.*
and by Davidson *et al.*; cf. Breitmeyer, Chapter 1 of this volume.)

Hallett and Lightstone (1976a, 1976b) obtained evidence for spatiotopically
controlled eye movements in an important set of experiments. The task was simply
to track a light spot in an otherwise dark environment. When the eyes were in
mid-saccade to one target position, the target was moved to a second position and
then extinguished. Thus, the only information about the second location was
obtained while the eyes were moving. In the dark that followed, the eyes were
immediately and accurately directed to the second position in space. This shows
that the oculomotor system had accurate information about the momentary position of the eyes relative to the stationary head, during the saccade, and could
combine that information with information about the retinal position of the target
to determine where to move the eyes next. (Incidentally, the experiments also
show that saccadic suppression is not absolute.) Experiments on monkeys in
which the superior colliculus was stimulated to produce an inappropriate eye
movement after the target had been removed (Mays & Sparks, 1980) gave a similar
outcome.

Whether it is appropriate to think of such eye movement control mechanisms as
making use of a "representation" of space is unclear. The neural computation may
result in appropriate targeting of the eyes without (for example) providing the kind
of general purpose map that could be used for reaching, or for reporting location.
Reported location is often erroneous under the conditions of the Hallett and
Lightstone experiments. Thus, it seems likely that the oculomotor system's spatiotopic performance is not invariably based on the representation I am calling
Buffer 2.

## 1.  SIGNIFICANCE OF BUFFER 2 FOR
## PERCEPTION WITH EYE MOVEMENTS

The purpose of some representation like that of Buffer 2 is to integrate successive views, taking into account head and eye movements. There have been no
studies to my knowledge that examine the duration of this form of memory, so it is
difficult to assess its importance as a buffer. One test of the duration of this type
of representation would be to discover whether information can be integrated over

three fixations. An additional question is what processes other than pattern recognition (e.g., Jonides *et al.*, 1982) and localization are based on the output of Buffer 2. One possibility is that the location of the next fixation (Buffer 7) is ordinarily determined at this level, in reading, based on the position of spaces and the lengths of words.

## C.  Buffer 3: Reatopic Visual Memory

Another form of short-term visual memory (STVM) in which the spatial or retinal location of successive views is less important than their overall similarity as patterns has been identified by some investigators. Phillips (1974), for example, showed subjects a matrix of 16 to 64 cells, half of them filled, and then a second matrix with no or one cell changed. He found evidence for a high capacity parallel store lasting about 100 msec (Buffer 1, presumably) and a second store that remained intact for some 600 msec and then decayed only slowly (if the subject was not distracted) over a period of 9 sec. This STVM for the pattern was distinguished from the brief sensory memory in that it exhibited limited capacity (larger matrices being less accurately remembered), was less sensitive to backward masking than the sensory store, and was tied neither to retinal nor to environmental location.

To demonstrate the latter, Phillips displaced the second matrix with respect to the first. That interfered markedly with sensory memory (i.e., when the interstimulus interval—ISI—was short) but minimally with STVM, as ISIs of 300 and 600 msec (the longest ISIs used). There was no control over eye movements during the ISI, so it is likely that subjects had made an eye movement during the longer intervals, the same intervals in which displacement of the stimulus had no negative effect. This indifference to precise spatial position contrasts with Buffer 2, where consistent alignment in space is evidently important. That indicates that Buffer 3 does not take input exclusively from Buffer 2, but also (or instead) takes it directly from Buffer 1. (Bear in mind that Buffer 1 is probably heterogeneous and includes cortical as well as peripheral stages.)

In research on eye movements during reading, O'Regan (1981) tried shifting the text three character-spaces to the left or right during a saccade. This turned out to be imperceptible to the reader (although it did lead to changes in subsequent eye movements that can be explained by the nonoptimal location of the shifted fixation). Insofar as the appearance of the text on two successive fixations was being integrated, the integration was based on a local form rather than on precise localization in visual space.

A major question is whether Buffers 2 and 3 are indeed independent representations that are space centered and object centered, respectively, or whether there is just one localization system. One possibility is that there is a single system that can be driven either by information from the eye—head system or by pattern information, whichever happens to dominate the system. If so, it should *not* be possible to integrate two successive views (or fixations) and at the same time to know whether the second had been displaced with respect to the first. There is at least one case when we can do both: apparent movement. Therefore, we can reject the either–or model.

The case of apparent (or real) movement is instructive, because it shows that the world centered and object centered representations must not only coexist but also interact, to produce the effect of a stable world with some moving objects (e.g., Rock & Ebenholtz, 1962). The phenomenon of induced movement (as for example when the moon appears to move behind clouds) demonstrates this interaction particularly vividly.

Another case in which retinal, spatial, and object-centered information seem to be independent has been discussed by Burr (1980). He asked the question why moving objects in the environment do not ordinarily look blurred or smeared across the scene. Since it is known that visual signals are summated over about 100 msec, objects in motion while the eyes were fixated might be expected to look blurred (as in a 1/10 sec photographic exposure). However, Burr found that as long as the objects moved for a long enough time to produce a sensation of motion (about 75 msec) there was virtually no smear: A clear object was seen as moving.

Since spatiotopic and reatopic representations are obliged to interact in interpreting movement, are the two representations part of a single buffer that represents both the stable world frame and pattern shifts (moving objects) within the stable world? That seems unlikely. The system that compares two temporally separated patterns and concludes that they are the same continuous object is logically separate from the system that corrects for head and eye movements to produce a visual world fixed in relation to the observer. A thorough discussion of these issues would take me too far afield; for examples of recent pertinent work, see Berbaum, Lenel, and Rosenbaum (1981) and Ullman (1979). Another reason for considering the reatopic representation to be distinct from the spatiotopic one is that in Phillips' experiments there was no apparent movement at the longer ISIs, just "knowledge" that the second pattern did or did not differ from the first.

There are three findings that raise the question of whether Buffer 3, which is object based, is visually "literal" or is somewhat more abstract. In apparent movement there is considerable tolerance for pattern changes, particularly if the second form is a possible rotation of the first form (Berbaum et al., 1981), and indeed Ullman demonstrates that such movement transformations can reveal three dimensional shape. Here, the abstraction is from a two to a three dimensional object. Another level of abstraction is to a conceptual equivalent, for example, *a* and *A*, or *r* and *R*. Two studies suggest that such an abstraction may take place at an early stage in perception. One is the observation (McConkie & Zola, 1979; Rayner, McConkie, & Zola, 1980) that readers neither notice nor are affected by a shift from (say) *aPpLe* to *ApPlE*, in successive fixations. The second is Friedman's finding (1980) that under near threshold conditions a reader reports the identity of letters such as *a* and *A* more accurately than their case (upper or lower). In both investigations the effect was immediate, not the consequence of forgetting in the ordinary sense.

The possibility that reatopic organization can be based on identification of an equivalence class of objects, not just on two dimensional shape as given on the retina, raises the question of its relation to later buffers that are clearly postidentification. An important related question is whether information from one or more other senses is combined with visual information at this level, as in the synchronization of a speaker's voice and face.

### 1.   BUFFER 3 AND EYE MOVEMENT CONTROL

The ability to retain information about a visual pattern for as much as several seconds (Phillips's STVM) despite visual masking suggests that it would be possible for the eyes to keep on reading or viewing a scene while the later perceptual system remained focused on an earlier glimpse. Note, however, that Phillips showed that viewers lost the contents of STVM if they attended to a subsequent visual stimulus or carried out mental arithmetic. Thus, in normal circumstances there is no reason to expect this buffer to decouple the mind and eye, for the eye is functionally blind as long as the buffer's old contents remain the focus of attention. Only in unusual circumstances (such as catching a fleeting glimpse of something of great importance) would this buffer be used to dissociate the focus of perceptual attention from the current focus of the eyes. Ordinarily, as the bulk of eye movement research shows, the eyes linger where the attention is focused.

## D.   Buffer 4: Acoustic/Phonological/Articulatory Short-Term Memory (STM)

I have characterized Buffers 4, 5, and 6 as central because they clearly entail learned recoding of visual stimuli. Since the same may be true of Buffer 3, the distinction between input and central buffers is somewhat arbitrary. If we were discussing auditory stimuli, Buffer 4 might be regarded as an input buffer roughly equivalent to Buffer 3 for vision.

The equivocation about the nature of the representation in Buffer 4—acoustic, phonological, or articulatory—respects a continuing theoretical dispute that I will not elaborate on here (cf. Baddeley & Lewis, 1981; Crowder, 1976, for reviews). The buffer is chiefly relevant for verbal material or the names of nonverbal material.

### 1.   READING AND THE PHONOLOGICAL BUFFER

The use of this buffer in reading, once regarded as the resort of beginning and slow readers, has undergone a rehabilitation in recent years and is now regarded by some theorists as important in skilled adult reading (e.g., Baddeley & Lewis, 1981; Schankweiler, Liberman, Mark, Fowler, & Fischer, 1979). Petrick and Potter (in preparation) showed that recoding into an "acoustic" form occurs even during very rapid reading: How far recoding lags behind the eye is not known, however. It seems quite possible that recoding is accomplished during the fixation on a given word; in fact, Just has reported (personal communication, Dec. 11,

1981) that gaze duration on a word in silent reading is strongly correlated with speaking time. The details of the way in which the acoustic representation is used in reading have not yet been worked out, but its potential role as a relatively durable buffer capable of retaining at least the last clause is clear.

## E.   Buffer 5: Conceptual Very-Short-Term Memory

Immediately after one has understood something—a word, picture, or whatever—there seems to be a very short interval during which the thought can be interrupted irretrievably by a second cognitive event, if that event commands attention. The relationship between the two events as well as their timing determines whether Event 2 masks Event 1 or enhances it. Because the interval of high susceptibility to cognitive masking is very brief (e.g., 1 sec or less), it is difficult to demonstrate unequivocally that there *was* transient understanding. That may be the reason that little attention has been paid to this buffer in comparison with the acoustic buffer (conventional short-term memory).

Evidence for the existence and the conceptual nature of very-short-term memory comes from work with meaningful pictures. Complex scenes presented rapidly in a sequence are unlikely to be remembered verbally, so Buffer 4 (acoustic STM) is not confounded with putative Buffer 5. The claim that one can momentarily understand but immediately forget such scenes (Potter, 1975, 1976; Potter & Levy, 1969) was made on the basis of the following argument and experimental results.

1. Detection of a semantically specified target picture (such as "a boat"), presented in a rapid sequence of diverse pictures, would only be possible if that picture were processed to a conceptual level, because the range of photographs meeting that semantic description is too broad to permit advance "physical" specification of the target.
2. If the target pictures are chosen randomly, then the detection rate is an index of the proportion of pictures in the sequence that were momentarily identified to a level that permitted matching to the semantic description. (This estimate is conservative, because the target-matching task might require cognitive resources that would otherwise be devoted to picture comprehension.)
3. In experiments of the kind described, semantic targets can be picked out more than 60% of the time when pictures are presented for 113 msec each, in a continuous sequence, and almost 90% of the time at 250 msec per picture (Potter, 1975, 1976).
4. If there is no very-short-term conceptual memory, then forgetting of "understood" pictures should follow the normal course of short-term forgetting of pictures, which many investigators have shown to be a slow decline—that is, pictures are ordinarily remembered remarkably well for days or weeks after viewing (Nickerson, 1965; Shepard, 1967; Standing, 1973). One

would therefore expect that subjects who simply viewed the sequence of pictures would remember almost all of the pictures they had understood, if they were given a recognition test right after viewing the sequence. Thus, if subjects in the detection task could detect 60% of the pictures at a given rate, subjects in the recognition memory task should recognize about the same proportion.

5. In a recognition memory experiment with the same sequences used in the detection experiment, subjects performed much more poorly than in the detection task: At 113 msec, they recognized only 11% of the pictures (compared with over 60% detected), and at 250 msec, only about 30% (compared with almost 90%). The pictures were easy to remember, however, if shown for 1 sec each, when over 80% were recognized, or 2 sec, when over 90% were recognized (Potter & Levy, 1969).

6. Results (3) and (5) are incompatible with the assumption that simply understanding a picture is enough to stabilize its memory, even for a short time. The disparity between understanding (which takes only about 100 msec for the average picture) and normal short-term retention (which takes 1 or 2 sec of processing to establish) implies that there is an intervening very-short-term conceptual memory that is readily disrupted by the following picture in a sequence.

7. This memory is not disrupted by a pattern mask. Since we know by (3) above that the picture was understood during viewing or very shortly thereafter, it is appropriate to call this transient postmask memory *conceptual* rather than *visual*.

In a series of recent studies, Intraub (e.g., 1980) has replicated and extended Potter's findings. She has shown that even a negative target ("not an animal") can be detected more readily than the same picture can be remembered immediately after viewing (1981). She has also shown that a following picture is only (or chiefly) disruptive *if the viewer attends to it*. This strengthens the evidence that the very-short-term memory involved is indeed conceptual and is to a large extent under the viewer's control.

### 1.  IS BUFFER 5 SPECIALIZED FOR MOMENTARY COMPREHENSION OF SCENES?

I speculated (Potter, 1976) on the basis of the evidence reviewed here that a viewer can understand each fixation, at the usual rates of eye movements, even if the fixation contains entirely unexpected information. (That, after all, is the most important kind of information.) This understanding allows appropriate control of subsequent fixations. It is not necessary, however, to retain the information in every fixation, so what chiefly gets remembered is a conceptual abstraction from the information in a series of fixations (e.g., Guenther, 1980). A recent experiment demonstrated that pictures in a short rapid sequence *can* be integrated, when they form a meaningful "story" (Inui & Miyamoto, 1981).

The same kind of short-term conceptual information might be important in other cognitive tasks such as reading. Forster (1975) argued that readers could momentarily understand words seen for only 63 msec in rapid sequential visual presentation (RSVP), although they could only retain about half of a seven-word sentence presented at that rate. Although the minimal time per word may not be as low as Forster claimed, other RSVP research supports Forster's claim for a marked disparity between understanding and retention, similar to that for pictures.

## 2. RELATION TO BUFFERS 1—4

Clearly Buffer 5 is not localized either retinally (Buffer 1) or spatially (Buffer 2), but its relation to Buffer 3 (reatopic short-term visual memory) is less clear. Simply on the basis of the logical distinction between visuospatial characteristics of a viewer-centered scene (a scene seen from a particular vantage point) and the conceptual significance of the scene (or an RSVP sentence), one might expect such a distinction to appear in processing. On the other hand, it could also be argued that the two kinds of information are represented in a single format (e.g., in propositions). The issue cannot be settled until it can be shown that the two putative buffers have different retention characteristics or respond differently to variables in a way that would not be expected if the propositional account is correct. (See Avons & Phillips, 1980, and Walker & Marshall, 1982, for some evidence of this kind.)

As for Buffers 4 (acoustic) and 5 (conceptual), there are obvious differences, both in what sort of information is represented and in time course. A scene's meaning can be represented in Buffer 5 without any corresponding representation in Buffer 4. Buffer 4 seems to remain available for at least 2 sec without attention, whereas Buffer 5 is transient, serving merely as a bridge into longer term memory.

## 3. BUFFER 5 AND EYE MOVEMENTS IN READING

Buffer 5, the first and perhaps the only "thinking" buffer, is at a level at which thoughts are separated from words. Since the conceptions expressed by sentences are represented by mental entities that do not stand in a perfect one-to-one relation to words, there is necessarily a level at which the serial intake of a sequence of words becomes partially dissociated from the conceptual structure being built. One might expect the eyes sometimes to lead and sometimes to lag behind the developing structure of thought, with the words accumulating in one of the earlier buffers in the former case, or skipped over briefly in the latter case (e.g., Ehrlich & Rayner, 1981).

If conceptual short-term "memory" is identified with active thought, then one can estimate the span of thought to be less than a second: That is, to influence each other, elements of thought must have been activated within that span. A possible evolutionary reason for the fragility of ideas in the first few hundred msec is to avoid cluttering longer term memories (such as working memory, next section) with all the momentary conjunctions of thought that "go nowhere." Only the more successful ideas (like the correct identity of a word or object, or an appropriate development of an embryonic thought, or the solution to any microproblem then active) last long enough to be stabilized in working memory.

The idea that thoughts may form and dissolve within a second may seem farfetched. Consider, however, the ability to read and understand an RSVP sentence presented at 12 words a second (to be discussed in Section VI). That is a rate of presentation at which only about three words from an unrelated list can be reported (unpublished experiments in my laboratory). The difference between unrelated words and sentences, at this rate, implies that conceptual operations occur very rapidly and determine what enters the more stable buffers, Buffers 4 and 6.

## F.   Buffer 6: Working Memory

If Buffer 5 is the active conceptual processor, how is it distinguished from working memory? (Note that the term "working memory" is sometimes used to encompass all forms of short-term memory, e.g., Buffers 3, 4, 5, and 6.) My basis for the distinction between Buffers 5 and 6 is the time course, which is very brief for Buffer 5 and longer (perhaps up to 10 sec) for Buffer 6. Our principal recent thoughts remain accessible for a time in working memory, available to be retrieved rapidly and reentered into Buffer 5 state. No cognitive work is carried out in working memory, however. This memory is clearly conceptual, not visual or acoustic. It seems probable that many of the classic studies of short-term memory and memory retrieval reflected a mixture of acoustic, visual, and conceptual representations, however.

## G.   Buffer 7: Location of the Next Saccade

Pollatsek and Rayner (1982) provide evidence that, in reading, the location of the next saccade is decided on the basis of the first 50 msec of the current fixation. This does not mean that, in real time, the decision is made by 50 msec, for by that time visual information has barely reached the striate cortex. Instead, it means that the next location is committed by the time the first 50 msec has been processed centrally (that *could* be as early as Buffer 2, the spatiotopic representation). Assuming that the movement is not initiated as soon as the location has been selected, there must be a buffer that holds the information until a triggering event occurs.

## H.   Buffer 8: Timing of the Next Saccade

Although under most conditions the timing of the next saccade is under at least partial control of information processed from the current fixation, there are some circumstances (such as those indicated by Vaughan, Chapter 23 in this volume) in which saccade timing is partially or entirely preprogrammed. Such preprogramming amounts to a timing buffer.

# III. Questions about Buffers

## A.  How Many Buffers?

As already indicated, it is not clear that all these buffers (forms of memory, levels of representation, processing stages) are distinct. Before rejecting this proliferation of buffers, however, one should note that physiology and anatomy suggest a much larger number of distinct levels, stages, or channels of processing. Which (if any) of these physiological stages serve as buffers in the present sense remains to be shown (only in the case of Buffer 1 are there any clear ideas). In any case, it must be emphasized again that the present list is only provisional.

One other buffer, long-term memory, has been omitted from the list because the focus is on buffers at the scale of eye movements. In principle, however, long-term memory serves the same functions as the other buffers, albeit on a much more extended scale: It holds information until called on by other processes. Long-term memories are probably associated with several of the buffers, not just Buffers 5 and 6 (the conceptual buffers). For example, object or word identification would require information of the kind represented in Buffers 1 and 3; memories of spatial layout, Buffer 2; and recognition of spoken words, Buffer 4. To what extent imagery (which draws on memory) employs one or another buffer is an active question (e.g., Baddeley & Lieberman, 1980).

The buffers are not arranged strictly in series. In the nature of such buffers, they operate in cascade, providing input continuously to the processors that link the buffers (McClelland, 1979). Moreover, the buffers are not strictly ordered. For example, information probably passes in parallel from visual to phonological and conceptual memory. Other examples have already been mentioned. The timing buffer (Buffer 8) may be filled either earlier or later than that for location (Buffer 7), according to Rayner and Pollatsek (1981); that is, Buffers 7 and 8 are independent. Some other buffers, however, are ordered more strictly: For example, Buffer 1 must precede all others, in vision.

## B.  Variability of Processing and the Role of Buffers

A stage of processing with a single impulse as its output cannot act as a buffer; a buffer implies a continuing output of roughly the same information over some period of time. (Equivalently, the information is "available" for that period of time; I make no distinction between information "continuously flowing" and information available to be called by another stage.) The potential for buffering will only be realized in practice if the timing of the input to a given buffer is not perfectly correlated with the timing of the process that follows the buffer. Although I have dwelt on the many stages at which buffers may allow such dissociations, it is still the case that the eye and mind are ordinarily correlated, as other contributors to this book show. What the system of buffers permits is some flexibility in the timing of processing, in particular after the point of no return for the next saccade. If processing is not quite complete by the time the eye begins to move, one or more of the buffers can maintain the information until processing has finished, without necessarily requiring a regressive eye movement.

## III.   The Buffers and Real Time Processing

Several attempts to estimate the time course of processing from the onset of a given fixation to the next saccade and fixation have been made (e.g., Becker & Jurgens, 1979; Carpenter, 1981; Russo, 1978; see also McConkie, Chapter 5 and Breitmeyer, Chapter 1 in this volume). Figure 24.1 gives an indication of the time course of the present buffers, in reading with fixations of 220 msec and saccades of 30 msec.

It takes approximately 60 msec for information to reach the cortex, and 40 msec elapse from initiation of a central motor command to initiation of the saccade. Thus, Buffers 2–8 have a maximum of 120 msec (i.e., the fixation duration minus 100) to process information from the *current* fixation before the next eye movement is irrevocably committed.

There are various pieces of evidence concerning the distribution of this 120-msec period over the intermediate buffers. Rayner and Pollatsek (1981) have evidence that the *location* of the next fixation is chosen after only the first 50 msec of the current fixation has been processed. The earliest buffer that *could* mediate the choice of location is Buffer 2 (spatiotopic). Adding 60 msec of Buffer 1 plus 50 msec of Buffer 2, the location (Buffer 7) is chosen 110 msec after the fixation, and delivers its message to the motor command system no later than 180 msec. Thus, the intended location is held in the buffer for 70 msec, when the total fixation duration is 220 msec. It is not clear whether location could be altered during that hypothetical wait, if the spacing of words to the right *changed* rather than disappeared after 50 msec. Since saccade timing is controlled independently of location, cancellation or delay of the saccade would presumably allow resetting of the intended location.

I have assumed that Buffers 2 and 3 take input directly from Buffer 1, at the same time, since I know of no evidence that specifies whether the spatial framework (Buffer 2) is computed before or after pattern identity is determined (Buffer 3). Insofar as the spatiotopic representation is based on motor commands to the head and eyes, that information could be available in advance of the current fixation, but insofar as the representation requires a retinal error signal, it depends on retinocortical information which is not available for about 60 msec (when it might also be available to Buffer 3). Since there is evidence (reviewed earlier) that Buffer 2 requires both sources of information, there is no basis for assuming a difference in onset of Buffers 2 and 3.

Buffer 8, the timing of the next saccade, is ordinarily bypassed in favor of

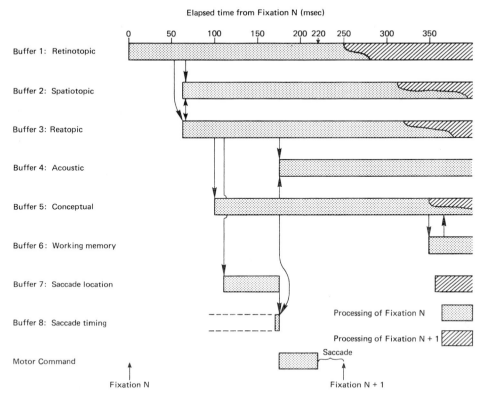

**FIGURE 24.1.** *A model of the temporal sequence of visual, cognitive, and response processes in eye movement control. Information from the following fixation, N + 1, is represented as merging with or replacing the information from fixation N, but arrows showing the flow of information are given only for N.*

"direct" central control of timing, presumably by Buffer 5, the thinking buffer in the present scheme. (In tasks simpler than reading, such as simple response to a light signal, the command might pass directly from Buffer 2 to the motor command system, bypassing Buffer 5 and the other central processors.) For control of timing that is based on the cognitive difficulty of the current word(s), Buffer 5 is required.

Various contributors to this book have presented evidence that the cognitive content of the last 140 msec of a fixation is incapable of influencing the duration of the fixation (that sounds as though it were a tautology, but the evidence is statistical). Using the same logic as before, 100 msec of that time would in any case be taken up with efferent (Buffer 1) and afferent (motor) processes, leaving by subtraction 40 msec for precognitive processing (processing that follows the 60 msec required to arrive at the cortex but precedes Buffer 5). Thus, we can estimate that it takes 40 msec to achieve an output from Buffers 2 and/or 3 to the conceptual level, Buffer 5: Buffer 5 thus begins processing the contents of the current fixation after a total of 100 msec. If Buffer 5 delivers the motor command directly (40 msec before the saccade begins), then there is about 80 msec of central (cognitive) processing before the next saccade is launched, in the case of a typical fixation of 220 msec. (In RSVP reading, 83 msec per word permits at least a shallow level of understanding; see Section VI.)

Buffer 6, working memory, takes input from Buffer 5 at the point that an item in conceptual short-term memory becomes stabilized, which can be estimated to be about 250 msec after arrival in Buffer 5 (i.e., 350 msec after stimulus presentation). This estimate comes both from the research with pictures described earlier and RSVP research referred to later. The time required for stabilization of material from Buffer 5 into working memory can be expected to be highly variable, however. It is appropriate to regard working memory as an inactive form of short-term conceptual memory that has no direct input into other processes, but whose contents may become further consolidated into long-term memory.

As for Buffer 4, acoustic short-term memory, a rough estimate of recoding time for visual words is 175 msec, based on a minimum word-naming latency of 400 msec and a simple articulation latency of about 225 msec, for a prepared response. Note that this would not allow any influence of exclusively acoustic–articulatory variables on the duration of the current fixation, only on the following fixation(s). One might be able to test this prediction by observing eye movements as a subject reads silently a sentence such as the following, with the instruction to look for sound similarities:

*The farmer explained that they use ewes rather than rams.*

## 1.    THE IMMEDIACY HYPOTHESIS

Contrary to the strongest version of the immediacy hypothesis, it is likely that the criterion for initiation of an eye movement is set lower than the completion of all relevant cognitive processing of the stimulus. It seems most unlikely that the system would have built into it a substantial dead time (the 140 msec after commitment to the next saccade), and in any case we know that processing does continue, as witnessed by spillover effects on the duration of the next fixation and other evidence (e.g., K. Ehrlich, Chapter 5, Hogaboam, Chapter 18, and Wolverton & Zola, Chapter 3 in this volume; Danks & Kurcz, 1981). What *is* completed prior to initiation of the eye movement is a shallow level of understanding sufficient to diagnose orthographic, lexical, semantic, or syntactic difficulties.

At times, however, one might expect processing difficulties to become apparent only after the next saccade is committed, as just mentioned. Then, the buffers may be resorted to, to reprocess or continue processing information from the previous fixation(s); if the problem is not immediately solved, a regression would be programmed. This whole buffering effect should rarely create a desynchronization greater than the average duration of a fixation; otherwise, an appropriate regression or refixation would be expected.

## IV.  Vaughan's Stimulus Delay Paradox: Can the Buffer System Explain It?

Vaughan's elegant experiments on eye movement latency in relatively simple tasks provide us with some puzzling facts:

1.  When the subject looks to point X and then to the left or right depending on a signal at X, delay of the directional signal after the eye has arrived at X has little effect on oculomotor latency provided the delay is no longer than 60–100 msec. Further delay adds more or less linearly to the latency (Vaughan, 1978; Vaughan & Graefe, 1977; Vaughan, Chapter 23 in this volume). Rayner and Pollatsek (1981) have a related result in reading: Imposition of a mask for the first part of a fixation is undercompensated for when the mask lasts for 50–100 msec. Again, with longer lasting masks, there is virtually complete compensation. These observations are readily explained by a model of eye movement control in which there is preprogramming of fixation duration, with cancellation of the programmed movement when stimulus delay is long but not when it is short. As Vaughan shows in (2) and (3) following, however, this explanation must be rejected.

2.  Vaughan adapted the Sternberg task in the following way. Subjects were given a variable memory set of letters and then they scanned alternately between two widely spaced letter locations, searching for any match between the visual letters and the memory set. Upon the eye's arrival at one of the locations, the onset of the test letter was delayed for a variable time, as in (1). Vaughan argued that preprogrammed durations should be insensitive to memory-set size, which is a factor affecting on-line processing. The preprocessing plus cancellation hypothesis would thus predict an interaction between stimulus delay and memory load, with little influence of memory load when delays were 100 msec or less and the preprogrammed saccade occurred.

But that is not what happened. Memory-set size added a constant time to oculomotor latency and did not interact with (1).

3.  Furthermore, adding a mask to the test stimulus in the Sternberg task produced a small increase in oculomotor latency, but again did not interact with (1) as the partial preprogramming hypothesis would predict.

4.  These facts become even more puzzling when an observation of Rayner, Inhoff, Morrison, Slowiaczek, and Bertera (1981) is added. Presenting the stimulus (text) for only the first 50 msec of a fixation, followed by a mask for the remainder of the fixation, causes virtually no change in oculomotor latency, the size of saccades, or reading accuracy. This result suggests that the first 50 msec of each fixation is all-important in reading, which is superficially at variance with (1) and with an experiment reported by Wolverton and Zola (Chapter 3 in this book).

To account for these results, the buffer model of Figure 24.1 might need to be modified. One possibility is that in a continuous task such as reading, conceptual processing (Buffer 5) sometimes runs behind perceptual uptake, so that perceptual information from the current fixation queues up briefly in one of the earlier buffers (2, 3, or even 4). As long as the delay of stimulus onset after fixation was no longer than the delay in entering Buffer 5 caused by the queue, the stimulus delay would have no effect on the duration of that fixation.

A different explanation of (1) was suggested by Rayner and Pollatsek. They proposed that the saccades in their experiment fell into two categories, those of normal latency as measured from the onset of the text (full compensation for the delay), and those initiated before any information from the text had been processed. The distribution of response time supported this hypothesis, not the queuing hypothesis.

Unfortunately, the superficially similar results reported by Vaughan and his colleagues cannot readily be explained in the same way. If the insensitivity to short delays was due to a subgroup of brief responses insensitive to the stimulus, then there would have been an interaction between delay and set size—see (2)—and between delay and visual degradation—see (3). There was not. Does the queuing hypothesis explain the Vaughan results? It is possible that there is a brief period of cognition preparation, after the eye arrives at the location of the upcoming stimulus, that delays the beginning of stimulus processing in Buffer 5. That would explain finding (1), albeit in a wholly ad hoc way.

The buffer model can readily explain finding (2). The larger the memory set, the longer the comparison process in Buffer 5. Finding (3), however, presents difficulties. Why should stimulus degradation have an effect on RT that is constant across delays? If the hypothesized queue occurs after initial visual processing, then the queue should absorb degradation at short stimulus delays. Possibly the degradation has an effect at the stimulus comparison stage, as has sometimes been reported in the Sternberg task.

Finally, according to (4), 50 msec at the beginning of a fixation (followed by a visual mask, for the balance of the fixation) is all that is needed to read perfectly normally. This result presents no difficulty; both Buffers 2 and 3 are posticonic, and 50 msec is presumably long enough to register written words in those buffers. (Note that the 60-msec cortical delivery time is irrelevant, because the mask also takes 60 msec to arrive; what matters is how long it takes for the retinal information to be fully encoded into Buffer 2 and/or 3, once it arrives there.)

### 1.   THE WARNING SIGNAL HYPOTHESIS

Vaughan accounts for the insensitivity of a reader's eye movements to short stimulus delays, point (1) above, by proposing that the delay interval has the effect of a warning signal, compensating for the delay. In effect, he proposes that in the delay range 0–60 msec, there is a precise trade-off between the advantage of a warning signal and the disadvantage of a delay in onset of processing. The claim is strengthened by previous evidence that a warning signal does reduce oculomotor latency; the size of the reduction and its time course are comparable to the present delay effect.

Although this explanation seems quite satisfactory for simple eye movement tasks, it seems much less satisfactory when applied to stimulus delays in reading

(Rayner *et al.*, 1981) or in Vaughan's Sternberg task. Why does a reader or scanner *need* a warning that information will appear during the current fixation? For these more continuous tasks, the cognitive queuing hypothesis gives a more plausible account. It is even possible that the effect of a true warning signal (in Becker and Saslow's experiments, cited by Vaughan) is to "clear the cognitive decks"—that is, reduce the delay in entering Buffer 5. If so, one effect of a warning signal should be to interrupt cognitive processing of prior material—a testable prediction.

## V.   Applying the Model to Picture Viewing

### A.   A Comparison with Loftus's Views

It is worth considering how the model of Figure 24.1 would account for some of Loftus's observations about picture processing. The cascade notion and the processing-time control over the duration of a fixation are both consistent with his views. The model's claim that there is poststimulus, postmask processing of visual information is not consistent, however: Loftus believes that one difference between reading and picture processing is that there is little postmask processing of pictures. He bases this conclusion on his own recent experiments (Loftus, 1981), showing that repeated brief exposures of a picture result in a recognition–memory performance that is at best equal to (and usually less than) the same exposure time presented continuously. If there were significant postmask processing, he argues, dividing the total time into several glimpses, each with postmask processing, should increase total processing time and thus improve performance. Since performance was not improved, Loftus concludes that there was not postmask processing.

There is, however, strong evidence from other studies that postmask processing of pictures does occur when the masking stimulus does not need to be attended to (Intraub, 1980; Lutz & Scheirer, 1974; Potter, 1976). Why do Loftus's experiments fail to show evidence for it? Loftus (1981) in fact gives a possible explanation: When a person views the *same* picture on successive occasions, he or she may automatically repeat the same initial steps of processing. Thus, information does not accumulate significantly over successive "glimpses" in Loftus's experiment unless the viewer happens to look at a different part of the picture. If Loftus is right about this, then his results do not contradict previous evidence for postmask processing.

An experiment that would usefully clarify this question would apply the masking techniques of Rayner *et al.* (1981) to picture viewing. The question would be whether the imposition of a mask during the latter part of each fixation would change the duration of the fixation and the extent of the subsequent saccade (as Loftus's hypothesis about continuous uptake would predict), or whether (as in reading) the mask would produce little interference as long as its onset was delayed for some minimal time after picture onset—say, 125 msec.

## B.  Comparisons between Pictures and Sentences

Loftus remarks that the gist of a text takes much longer to pick up than the gist of a scene. The only direct comparisons between scenes and equivalent descriptions that he mentions (Dallett & Wilcox, 1968; Nelson, Metzler, & Reed, 1974) were both concerned with memory, not initial processing. The same may be said of a number of more recent experiments addressing the question of the form of representation in memory of pictures and sentences (Baggett, 1975; Guenther, 1980; Pezdek, 1977; Rosenberg & Simon, 1977).

To discover how rapidly one extracts the gist of a picture or sentence, one needs a task that is immediate or almost immediate. In an experiment (Potter & Elliot, in preparation) comparing picture and sentence understanding, we obtained some indirect information on the relative times to extract the gist of pictures and sentences. Subjects in one group read a sentence and in a second group viewed a scene. The sentence or scene was immediately followed by a probe item (in the form of a line drawing or written word). The probe had not appeared in the scene or sentence, but was relevant to its meaning ("gist") on half the trials; the task was to decide whether the probe was relevant. For example, after the sentence *The tent is beside the lake,* the word *canoe* was the positive probe and *shoe* was negative.

The 5 to 12 word sentences were shown for 2 sec and the scenes were shown for 500 msec. The latency to respond to the probe was 171 msec longer following a sentence; that suggests that it took 2 sec + 171 msec to process the sentence to the same level as a pictured scene presented for 500 msec. This estimate is crude, but it does suggest that a picture is understood about four times faster than a comparable sentence. Incidentally, there was no difference between line drawings and single-word probes, either for sentences or for pictures. This supports the conclusion from other studies that the meanings of pictures and verbal materials are represented in a single underlying code, such as the conceptual code of Buffer 5.

## C.  Visual Buffers in Scene Perception

Is there perfect synchrony of the eye and mind in viewing a scene? If the model in Figure 24.1 holds for both reading and scene perception, then the input to higher level processing (Buffer 5, the mind) is from a visual buffer. If the buffer integrates successive fixations into a unified spatial representation of the visual world that is corrected for eye and head movements, then the mind would get information that is at least one step removed from the information in a given fixation. But the truth is likely to be more complicated than this, because we do have some awareness of the scene as given in a single fixation. Thus, all three visual buffers—one organized retinotopically, one that represents a unified visual world, and one that is organized by objects—may be able to be read directly by the mind.

## VI.   RSVP and the Buffer Model

Rapid serial visual presentation (RSVP) is a method in which word lists or sentences are presented one at a time at the same location, so that the viewer can read without having to move the eyes. The method permits the experimenter to control the duration of "fixations" and also the span of each fixation. Thus, it is complementary to eye fixation research in which those are the dependent variables. In RSVP, the dependent variables are latency to comprehend a sentence, accuracy of recall, latency and accuracy of target detection, and the like.

I will review briefly some results from RSVP research, discussing the relation of these results to the buffer model and to normal reading. A more detailed treatment may be found in Potter (1983).

1. College students can read and understand single sentences of 8–14 words (we have not tried longer ones) with considerable accuracy when they are presented one word at a time at 12 words per second (wps), that is, 720 words per minute (wpm) (Petrick & Potter, in preparation; Potter, Kroll, & Harris, 1980; Potter, Kroll, Yachzel, & Cohen, in preparation). These students would normally read only 300 wpm, although when pressed they can read the sentences (in normal format) at about 540 wpm. Thus RSVP seems to permit faster than normal reading, at least for single sentences.

I noted earlier that the presaccadic central processing time for the current fixation, in reading, may be as little as 80 msec: At that point, the reader seems to know just enough to carry on with the next fixation. At a steady state of 83 msec per word (with the word reaching the conceptual system—Buffer 5—about 100 msec after stimulus onset), the RSVP reader would pick up about the same amount as the presaccadic central processor, but would entirely miss the processing that occurs in normal reading between saccadic initiation and the central arrival of the next stimulus, which we estimated to be about 170 msec. (This calculation somewhat underestimates the time available for RSVP processing, because in normal reading the eye picks up fractionally more than one word per fixation.)

2. The rate limiting factor in RSVP reading seems to be memory storage, not initial comprehension (Frauenfelder, Dommergues, Mehler, & Segui, 1979; Potter et al., 1980). The same seems to be true in picture perception (Potter, 1976); that was taken as evidence for very-short-term conceptual memory (Buffer 5). These results are consistent with the importance of the processing that follows saccadic commitment, a claim that most of the authors of this book agree with.

3. There is phonological encoding (as well as semantic encoding) during RSVP reading at 12 wps that is as marked as at the more normal rate of 6 wps (Petrick &

Potter, in preparation). This finding is compatible with the present model, which assumes that there is input into Buffer 4 from Buffer 5 within about 65 msec.

4. When overall rate is equated, RSVP and conventional reading produce a similar level of understanding and retention (Juola, Ward, & McNamara, 1982; Masson, 1981; Potter 1983; Potter *et al.*, 1980; Potter *et al.*, in preparation). On the one hand, this finding offers support for the growing consensus that words outside the fovea receive little advance processing in normal reading, perhaps only that needed for eye movement guidance. On the other hand, the result suggests that the precise time the eyes dwell on a given word is not important, provided that the time is minimally sufficient for word recognition and the overall time across the sentence or text is adequate (Ward & Juola, 1982).

## A.  Rate and Memory Consolidation: The Conceptual Buffer

Several questions about eye movements arise from these observations. If it is *possible* to read at 12 wps, why do most people read only 4–5 wps? The possibility that "eye movements are a waste of time" (John Sender's phrase) can probably be rejected, for there is a marked reduction in what is remembered when people read RSVP paragraphs at faster than normal rates. If the rate limiting factor in reading is memory consolidation, however, the extra time must be required at a rather abstract conceptual level, not at the level of individual word recognition, since 83 msec (preceded and followed by a mask) is ample time for word recognition. But the abstract conceptual level does not map one-to-one onto individual words, which ought to weaken the correlation between gaze duration on an individual word and characteristics of that word. By including text–grammar variables in their regression analysis, Just and Carpenter (1980; Chapter 17 in this volume) account for some of the fixation duration variance due to such higher levels, but they cannot allocate the extra time to specific words within the affected sector of text. That is just as one would expect.

## B.  Speech Recoding and the Acoustic Buffer

A second factor that may free the mind from direct control by the eye is speech recoding. Speech recoding appears to be fast and automatic; if so, the speech code might conceivably replace the visual code in subsequent processing. As we know, the acoustic loop can hold several words, so the eyes could be dwelling on one word while the mind works on an earlier word or phrase.

## C.  Do the Buffers Decouple the Eye and Mind?

The speech code, the conceptual buffer (backed up by working memory), and the visual buffers constitute a system of buffers that permit the mind to be decoupled from the eyes. The ease of RSVP reading, in which each word is seen for a fixed and (in my work) equal time, is consistent with such partial decoupling. Nevertheless, the impressive success of models such as that of Just and Carpenter (as well as the work of Rayner, McConkie, and many others) shows that readers ordinarily do choose to look at the words most relevant to what they are thinking about. As Just acknowledges, however, the faster processes and those that cannot be readily allocated to single words (which would include most syntactic analyses) may not be revealed by analyses of eye movements. Other techniques, possibly including RSVP, may be necessary to study those processes (e.g., Forster, 1970; Forster & Ryder, 1971; Holmes & Forster, 1972; Holmes, 1973).

# VII.   Conclusion

In conclusion, the comparison of eye movements in reading, picture viewing, and visual search has shown that the obvious differences are accompanied by important similarities. I have focused here on one of these "similarities with a difference," the existence and nature of buffers or intermediate representations between the eye and the mind, and between the mind and the next eye movement. Further research could profitably address some of the open questions about the time course and character of such representational systems.

## ACKNOWLEDGMENTS

I thank Judith Kroll, David Rosenbaum, and Nancy Kanwisher for their comments.

# References

Avons, S. E., & Phillips, W. A. (1980). Visualization and memorization as a function of display time and poststimulus processing time. *Journal of Experimental Psychology: Human Learning & Memory, 6,* 407–420.

Baddeley, A. D., & Lewis, V. J. (1981). Inner active processes in reading: The inner voice, the inner ear, and the inner eye. In A. M. Lesgold & C. A. Perfetti (Eds.), *Interactive processes in reading.* Hillsdale, New Jersey: Erlbaum.

Baddeley, A. D., & Lieberman, K. (1980). Spatial working memory. In R. Nickerson (Ed.), *Attention and performance VIII*, Hillsdale, New Jersey: Erlbaum.

Baggett, P. (1975). Memory for explicit and implicit information in picture stories. *Journal of Verbal Learning and Verbal Behavior, 14,* 538–548.

Becker, W., & Jürgens, R. (1979). An analysis of the saccadic system by means of double step stimuli. *Vision Research, 19,* 967–983.

Berbaum, K., Lenel, J. C., & Rosenbaum, M. (1981). Dimensions of figural identity and apparent motion. *Journal of Experimental Psychology: Human Perception & Performance, 7,* 1312–1317.

Bowling, A., & Lovegrove, W. (1982) Iconic memory: Fallacies persist (?) *Perception and Psychophysics, 31,* 194–198.

Burr, D. (1980). Motion smear. *Nature, 284,* 164–165.

Carpenter, R. H. S. (1981). Oculomotor procrastination. In D. F. Fisher, R. A. Monty, & J. W. Senders (Eds.), *Eye movements: Cognition and visual perception*. Hillsdale, New Jersey: Erlbaum.

Coltheart, M. (1980). Iconic memory and visible persistence. *Perception & Psychophysics, 27*, 183–228.

Crowder, R. G. (1976). *Principles of learning and memory*. Hillsdale, New Jersey: Erlbaum.

Dallett, K., & Wilcox, S. (1968). Remembering pictures versus remembering descriptions. *Psychonomic Science, 11*, 139–140.

Danks, J. H., & Kurcz, I. (1981). *Reading comprehension processes in Polish and English*. Paper presented at the Psychonomic Society meetings, Philadelphia, November.

Davidson, M. L., Fox, M. J., & Dick, A. O. (1973). Effect of eye movements on backward masking and perceived location. *Perception & Psychophysics, 14*, 110–116.

Ehrlich, S. F., & Rayner, K. (1981). Contextual effects on word perception and eye movements during reading. *Journal of Verbal Learning and Verbal Behavior, 20*, 641–655.

Forster, K. I. (1970). Visual perception of rapidly presented word sequences of varying complexity. *Perception & Psychophysics, 8*, 215–221.

Forster, K. I. (1975). The role of semantic hypotheses in sentence processing. In F. Bresson & J. Mehler (Eds.), *Problemes actuels en psycholinguistique* (No. 206). Paris: Centre National de la Recherche Scientifique.

Forster, K. I., & Ryder, L. A. (1971). Perceiving the structure and meaning of sentences. *Journal of Verbal Learning and Verbal Behavior, 10*, 285–296.

Frauenfelder, U., Dommergues, J. Y., Mehler, J., & Segui, J. (1979). L'integration perceptive des phrases. *Bulletin de Psychologie, 32*, 893–902.

Friedman, R. B. (1980). Identity without form: Abstract representations of letters. *Perception & Psychophysics, 28*, 53–60.

Guenther, R. K. (1980). Conceptual memory for picture and prose episodes. *Memory & Cognition, 8*, 563–572.

Hallett, P. E., & Lightstone, A. D. (1976). Saccadic eye movements to flashed targets. *Vision Research, 16*, 107–114. (a)

Hallett, P. E., & Lightstone, A. D. (1976). Saccadic eye movements towards stimuli triggered by prior saccades. *Vision Research, 16*, 99–106. (b)

Holmes, V. M. (1973). Order of main and subordinate clauses in sentence perception. *Journal of Verbal Learning and Verbal Behavior, 12*, 285–293.

Holmes, V. M., & Forster, K. I. (1972). Perceptual complexity and underlying sentence structure. *Journal of Verbal Learning and Verbal Behavior, 11*, 148–156.

Intraub, H. (1980). Presentation rate and the representation of briefly glimpsed pictures in memory. *Journal of Experimental Psychology: Human Learning & Memory, 6*, 1–12.

Intraub, H. (1981). Identification and processing of briefly glimpsed visual scenes. In D. F. Fischer, R. A. Monty, & J. W. Senders (Eds.), *Eye movements: Cognition and visual perception*. Hillsdale, New Jersey: Erlbaum, 1981.

Inui, T., & Miyamoto, K. (1981). The time needed to judge the order of a meaningful string of pictures. *Journal of Experimental Psychology: Human Perception & Performance, 7*, 393–396.

Jonides, J., Irwin, D. E., & Yantis, S. (1982). Integrating visual information from successive fixations. *Science, 215*, 192–194.

Juola, J. F., Ward, N. J., & McNamara, T. (1982). Visual search and reading of rapid serial presentations of letter strings, words, and text. *Journal of Experimental Psychology: General, 111*, 208–227.

Just, M. A., & Carpenter, P. A. (1980). A theory of reading: From eye fixations to comprehension. *Psychological Review, 87*, 329–354.

Loftus, G. R. (1981). Tachistoscopic simulations of eye fixations on pictures. *Journal of Experimental Psychology: Human Learning & Memory, 3*, 369–376.

Long, G. M., & Beaton, R. J. (1982). The case for peripheral persistence: Effects of target and background luminance on a partial-report task. *Journal of Experimental Psychology: Human Perception and Performance, 8*, 383–391.

Lutz, W. J., & Scheirer, C. J. (1974). Coding processes for pictures and words. *Journal of Verbal Learning and Verbal Behavior, 13,* 316–320.

Masson, M. E. J. (1981). *Skimming and rapid sequential reading of text: Searching for and remembering information.* Paper presented at the Psychonomic Society Annual Meeting, Philadelphia, Pa.

Mays, L. E., & Sparks, D. L. (1980). Saccades are spatially, not retinocentrically, coded. *Science, 208,* 1163–1165.

McClelland, J. L. (1979). On the time relations of mental processes: An examination of systems of processes in cascade. *Psychological Review, 86,* 287–330.

McConkie, G. W., & Zola, D. (1979). Is visual information integrated across successive fixations in reading? *Perception & Psychophysics, 25,* 221–224.

Mewhort, D. J. K., Campbell, A. J., Marchetti, E. M., & Campbell, J. I. D. (1981). Identification, localization, and "iconic memory": An evaluation of the bar-probe task. *Memory & Cognition, 9,* 50–67.

Nelson, T. O., Metzler, J., & Reed, D. A. (1974). Role of details in the long-term recognition of pictures and verbal descriptions. *Journal of Experimental Psychology, 102,* 184–186.

Nickerson, R. S. (1965). Short-term memory for complex meaningful visual configurations: A demonstration of capacity. *Canadian Journal of Psychology, 19,* 155–160.

O'Regan, K. (1981). The "convenient viewing position" hypothesis. In D. F. Fisher, R. A. Monty, & J. W. Senders (Eds.), *Eye movements: Cognition and visual perception.* Hillsdale, New Jersey: Erlbaum.

Petrick, M. S., & Potter, M. C. (Manuscript in preparation). *Acoustic and semantic encoding during rapid reading.*

Pezdek, K. (1977). Cross-modality semantic integration of sentence and picture memory. *Journal of Experimental Psychology: Human Learning & Memory, 3,* 515–524.

Phillips, W. A. (1974). On the distinction between sensory storage and short-term visual memory. *Perception & Psychophysics, 16,* 283–290.

Pollatsek, A., & Rayner, K. (1982). Eye movement control in reading: The role of word boundaries. *The Journal of Experimental Psychology: Human Perception & Performance, 8,* 817–833.

Potter, M. C. (1975). Meaning in visual search. *Science, 187,* 965–966.

Potter, M. C. (1976). Short-term conceptual memory for pictures. *Journal of Experimental Psychology: Human Learning & Memory, 5,* 509–522.

Potter, M. C. (1983). Rapid serial visual presentation (RSVP): A method for studying language processing. In D. Kieras & M. Just (Eds.), *New methods in the study of immediate processes in reading comprehension.* Hillsdale, N.J.: Erlbaum, in press.

Potter, M. C., & Elliot, B. (Manuscript in preparation). *Probing the meaning of a scene or sentence.*

Potter, M. C., Kroll, J. F., & Harris, C. (1980). Comprehension and memory in rapid sequential reading. In R. Nickerson (Ed.), *Attention and performance VIII,* Hillsdale, New Jersey: Erlbaum.

Potter, M. C., Kroll, J. F., Yachzel, B., & Cohen, B. (Manuscript in preparation). *Pictures in sentences: Understanding without words.*

Potter, M. C., & Levy, E. I. (1969). Recognition memory for a rapid sequence of pictures. *Journal of Experimental Psychology, 81,* 10–15.

Rayner, K., Inhoff, A. W., Morrison, R. E., Slowiaczek, M. L., & Bertera, J. H. (1981). Masking of foveal and parafoveal vision during eye fixations in reading. *Journal of Experimental Psychology: Human Perception & Performance, 7,* 167–179.

Rayner, K., McConkie, G. W., & Zola, D. (1980). Integrating information across eye movements. *Cognitive Psychology, 12,* 206–226.

Rayner, K., & Pollatsek, A. (1981). Eye movement control during reading: Evidence for direct control. *Quarterly Journal of Experimental Psychology, 33A,* 351–373.

Rock, I., & Ebenholtz, S. (1962). Stroboscopic movement based on change of phenomenal rather than retinal location. *American Journal of Psychology, 75,* 193–207.

Rosenberg, S., & Simon, H. A. (1977). Modeling semantic memory: Effects of presenting semantic information in different modalities. *Cognitive Psychology, 9,* 293–325.

Russo, J. E. (1978). Adaptation of cognitive processes to the eye movement system. In J. W. Senders, D. F. Fisher, & R. A. Monty (Eds.), *Eye movements and the higher psychological functions.* Hillsdale, New Jersey: Erlbaum.

Sakitt, B. (1976). Iconic memory. *Psychological Review*, 83, 257–276.

Shankweiler, D., Liberman, I. Y., Mark, L. S., Fowler, C. A., & Fischer, F. W. (1979). The speech code and learning to read. *Journal of Experimental Psychology: Human Learning & Memory*, 5, 531–545.

Shepard, R. N. (1967). Recognition memory for words, sentences, and pictures. *Journal of Verbal Learning and Verbal Behavior*, 6, 156–163.

Sperling, G. (1960). The information available in brief visual presentations. *Psychological Monographs*, 74, 1–29.

Standing, L. (1973). Learning 10,000 pictures. *Quarterly Journal of Experimental Psychology*, 25, 207–222.

Ullman, S. (1979). *The interpretation of visual motion*. Cambridge: MIT Press.

Vaughan, J. (1978). Control of visual fixation duration in search. In J. W. Senders, D. W. Fischer, & R. A. Monty (Eds.), *Eye movements and the higher psychological functions*. Hillsdale, New Jersey: Erlbaum, 1978.

Vaughan, J., & Graefe, T. (1977). Delay of stimulus presentation after the saccade in visual search. *Perception & Psychophysics*, 22, 201–205.

Walker, P., & Marshall, E. (1982). Visual memory and stimulus repetition effects. *Journal of Experimental Psychology: General*, 111, 348–368.

Ward, N. J., & Juola, J. F. (1982). Reading with and without eye movements: Reply to Just, Carpenter, and Woolley. *Journal of Experimental Psychology: General*, 111, 239–241.

# VII
## Eye Movements and Dyslexia

George Th. Pavlidis

# 25

# The "Dyslexia Syndrome" and Its Objective Diagnosis by Erratic Eye Movements[1]

## I.   Introduction

Since its inception, research on eye movements has been intimately linked to the study of reading (Huey, 1908). The logic for this relationship is evident since eye movements provide a powerful source of data on human information processing mechanisms. Interestingly, most of this research has concentrated on the study of normal readers (McConkie & Rayner, 1975; Rayner, 1978; Tinker, 1958). However, little has been done in analyzing the eye movements of disabled readers. Given its proven value in uncovering the cognitive and perceptual skills of normal readers, it seems extremely useful to apply the ideas and technology of eye movement research to studying the behavior of disabled readers. This chapter is directed toward that goal. Specifically, it reviews some of the central work that has been conducted in reading disability and presents data that show how eye movements can be used to distinguish among different groups of reading disabled individuals.

### A.   Different Categories of Reading Failure

Before presenting the experimental paradigms and results, it is necessary to discuss some of the issues surrounding the definition of reading disability and the diagnostic criteria used for subject selection in both the psychological and educa-

[1]This work was supported by SSRC (England) research grants HR8pp31 and HR 6057 to the author and by U.S. Grant HD-12278-03.

441

tional literature (Rutter & Yule, 1975; Vernon, 1971). There has been a strong tendency to use behaviorally based test performance for diagnosing and selecting reading disabled subjects. That is, if a child is of normal intelligence and is reading 2 or more years below that expected for his chronological age, he or she is placed in the disabled group. Reliance on this chronological reading age discrepancy is, however, highly misleading since the discrepancy might be the result of a variety of causative factors. Should such a variety of factors exist, then one immediate and important consequence would be that different diagnostic and treatment procedures should be initiated for the various groups among the reading disabled.

Our knowledge to date suggests that at least two such groups exist. First, there is the group for whom the reading failure can be predicted on the basis of the known relationship between certain psychological and environmental factors and reading success or failure. These factors include intelligence, motivation, emotional stability, physical health, socioeconomic background, educational opportunities, language spoken at home, parent education, teacher quality, and culture (Downing & Thackray, 1975; Rutter & Yule, 1975; Vernon, 1971). If an individual has one or more problems associated with these factors, then reading problems are expected. The extent of the reading difficulty is determined by the specific factors and severity of impairment. This group for whom the reading disability can be predicted will in the remainder of this chapter be referred to as retarded readers. In line with my earlier comments, inclusion in this group necessitates that the minimum 2-year differential between chronological age and reading age (the commonly accepted criterion for reading disability) be associated with one or more unfavorable factors in the individual's psycho-environmental background.

In contrast to this group of retarded readers, there is a second group who must be identified. Although their degree of reading difficulty (chronological reading age discrepancy) may be of the same extent, the individuals in this group are marked by the fact that their reading failure is *unexpected* (Symmes and Rapoport, 1972); that is, all the psycho-environmental factors cited above are favorable and hence high reading skill ought to be observed. Nevertheless, reading difficulties are present and severe. These individuals have been identified by a variety of labels including "word-blindness," "specific developmental dyslexia," "reading disability," "specific reading disability," "learning disability," "strephosymbolia," "reading retardation," "primary reading retardation," "reading difficulty," "inferior reading," "inadequate reading," etc. (Farnham–Diggory, 1978; Fry, 1968). The most commonly used term and the one I will adopt is the Greek word dyslexia, which is composed of *dys* which means difficulty "with" and *lexis* which means word.

The fact that dyslexia represents unexpected reading failure has important, albeit negative, consequences for the conceptualization of this important syndrome. Implicit in the idea that the failure is unexpected is the idea that the psycho-environmental factors usually responsible for reading difficulty cannot be used to explain the problems of the dyslexic. Other factors responsible for the problem remain to be determined. Hence, at this point the aetiology of dyslexia is unknown.

The lack of knowledge about the causative factors in dyslexia has forced the adoption of a definition based on exclusionary criteria (Denckla, 1977); that is, dyslexia is diagnosed as severe reading difficulty that is *not* caused by the usual factors known to be associated with reading failure (Rudel, 1980). While the exclusionary definitions vary, they tend to be broadly similar to the frequently quoted ones adopted by the World Federation of Neurology (Critchley, 1970). This group defined specific developmental dyslexia as: "a disorder manifested by difficulty in learning to read despite conventional instruction, adequate intelligence and sociocultural opportunity. It is dependent upon fundamental cognitive disabilities which are frequently of constitutional origin." Critchley (1981) has further clarified the above definition of dyslexia, but it still remains an exclusionary definition.

For research purposes, for one to be diagnosed as dyslexic it must first be established that none of the factors known to cause reading failure is at work in that individual. Otherwise, one could reasonably be called a retarded reader, since the factors that have not been taken into account in the selection criteria, could have caused his or her reading problem. Any exclusionary diagnostic criteria of dyslexia have inherent limitations such as delayed identification of the problem, stemming from the fact that one has to fail in reading for 2 years before being diagnosed as dyslexic. But by that time it is likely that the child would have already developed an aversion to school and some psychological problems including lack of self confidence. Children who are from deprived socio-economic backgrounds, who lack adequate educational opportunities, or are of low intelligence, or are emotionally disturbed can not be unequivocally diagnosed as dyslexics with any exclusionary criteria. Of course, it is possible for one to be dyslexic and also be handicapped by socio-economic, educational, emotional, or intellectual problems, as well. But these factors can *not* cause dyslexia. If they could, dyslexia and reading retardation would then be describing the same population, and dyslexia would be a superfluous concept. Although it has long been established that the previously mentioned factors determine reading success or failure (Vernon, 1971; Downing and Thackray, 1975), researchers have often failed to carefully take each of them into account in the establishment of appropriate diagnostic criteria for dyslexia. Therefore, at present, an individual whose reading problems could be attributed to any of the factors known to cause reading retardation must be excluded. Such criteria, however, do not exclude the possibility that some dyslexics may slip into the retarded readers group (Pavlidis, 1981b).

A clear differentiation between dyslexics and retarded readers can contribute to the clarification of the aetiology of dyslexia. The use of incomplete diagnostic criteria for the selection of dyslexic subjects inevitably leads to the inclusion of an undetermined number of retarded readers in the dyslexic group. That, consequently, makes the results of such studies: (*a*) questionable, (*b*) confusing, (*c*) not specific either to reading retardation or to dyslexia, (*d*) impossible to compare, (*e*) unreliable indicators of the aetiology of dyslexia and (*f*) unreliable to subgroup dyslexics (Boder, 1971, 1973; Mattis, French, Rapin, 1975), because it is likely that these subgroups might instead reflect aetiological differences not of dyslexia *per se* but of reading disabilities, since various populations compose the mixed group of retarded readers and "dyslexics." I must make it clear, however, that it is worth searching for the possible existence of subgroups of dyslexics, as such a differentiation will greatly enhance the chances to discover appropriate methods of treatment. It is imperative, therefore, that the establishment of such subgroups should not be the result of a defective experimental design but rather the outcome of carefully designed and adequately controlled studies.

The absence of positive criteria, combined with such global, imprecise variables as "conventional instruction" and "sociocultural opportunity" has created difficulties in the application of the definition and consequently in subject identification. Cruikshank (1968) acknowledged these problems when he wrote that if the same child is diagnosed in one state in the United States and then moves to another state it is likely that in each state he will be given a different label. Similar confusion exists in Europe where selection criteria for dyslexia vary not only from country to country but also from one diagnostic research center to another even within the same country.

## B.   The Dyslexia Syndrome

The problems stemming from a definition based on exclusionary criteria could be overcome if we were able to arrive at a *positive definition* of the syndrome; that is, a definition that identifies the dyslexic on the basis of positive symptomatology (e.g., erratic eye movements) that reflects specific causative or pathogenic factors. At this point in our knowledge, such a definition is not possible. However, two independent lines of evidence exist that offer promising leads in guiding the development of a definition based on positive criteria. One source stems from clinical work that describes the symptomatology of the disorder; the other derives from experimental evidence on the deficits displayed by dyslexics. Although both converge in pinpointing a similar set of causative factors, for purposes of expositional clarity each will be discussed separately.

## C.   The Symptomatology

The symptoms of the "dyslexia syndrome" go beyond the unexpectedly wide discrepancy between a favorable psycho-environmental picture and a poor performance in reading and other related tasks. Dyslexics have difficulty performing "automated-sequential" tasks in which order is of crucial importance. For example, they have trouble reciting in order the days of the week, months of the year, letters of the alphabet, syllables in a long word and in tasks such as drawing a clock. Their performance deteriorates even further when they attempt the above tasks in reverse order. Particular problems are encountered in trying to perform these tasks quickly. If dyslexics are asked to report the correct order for the task they have failed they will probably succeed if they proceed slowly. This is especially so when associations can be used. The children's difficulties are best reflected in the problems they have with rote memory; that is, memorizing a series of stimuli without any attention to meaning. The performance of dyslexics also deteriorates far more than nondyslexics when they are under stress and thus their compensatory mechanisms cannot be employed effectively.

Other manifestations of their difficulties include frequent reversals in the ordering of letters (e.g., *was* for *saw*) which frequently persist beyond 8 or 9 years of age (at this age reversals by nondyslexic children are drastically reduced). Dyslexics also show transpositions (e.g., *left for felt*) and change the sequence of words within a sentence. When they write or read they can omit and/or repeat words. They often skip lines or find it difficult to keep their place on a line. Their oral reading often contains mispronunciations as well as monotonous intonation.

Along other dimensions, dyslexic children are sometimes clumsy and hyperactive. They may be accident prone and easily distractible. Some dyslexics, especially the severe cases, show problems in distinguishing left from right. Some are found not to have well-established laterality (Orton, 1937; Zangwill, 1981). It must be emphasized, however, that dyslexics as a group are not significantly different in laterality from other readers. Some dyslexics may never crawl and instead go straight from sitting to walking. Some of them may have coordination problems which make them less skillful in ball games. Also, low tolerance and frustration levels are characteristic.

Dyslexics often show delays in the development of language and when it does develop, it has syntactic errors comparable to the order problems they later exhibit in reading and writing. However, since their oral language problems are frequently subtle and conversation is not as constrained as written language, oral language difficulties may go undetected (Fine, 1982).

Dyslexia commonly runs in families. Up to 70–80% of dyslexics have other members of the immediate family with reading problems (Hermann, 1959; Owens, 1978). Although there is a "family" origin in many dyslexics, the actual mode of transmission from generation to generation is not yet clearly defined. Dyslexia is more common in boys than in girls with a reported ratio of about four to one.

Some of the symptoms just described in association with dyslexics may also be found in children who do not have reading or spelling problems. However, a child having most of these symptoms is likely to also have reading and spelling problems. The dyslexic's worst performance is usually in spelling, followed by reading and sometimes mathematics. A common and not unexpected characteristic among dyslexics is that they rarely read for pleasure. Some dyslexics find ways to compensate for their reading problems, but such individuals continue to be bad spellers, and somewhat less often have poor idiosyncractic handwriting characterized by unconnected, uneven letters, and a cramped, jagged style, such as that shown in Figure 25.1.

Although the symptoms just described are wide ranging, they seem to be subserved by a common core—specifically, regardless of the modality (linguistic, motoric, etc.) most of the tasks contain a multiplicity of stimuli that demand a combination of automated sequential–temporal–attentional skills. This common but subtle core of deficits, frequently goes undetected in the everyday setting. The children seem so normal that their unexpected failure at school is commonly and erroneously attributed, by the uninformed teacher and parent, to laziness and stupidity. This often leads to feelings of insecurity and worthlessness. Although the children frequently tend to believe these labels, it is vital to recognize that their intelligence and motivation are *not* usually in question.

### D.   Experimental Approaches

Along with the clinical picture, another line of evidence exists which provides promising information about the causative factors in dyslexia. In an effort to go beyond the limitations of the exclusionary definition, a number of investigators have put forth theories about possible causes of dyslexia. It is beyond the scope of this chapter to discuss in detail the various hypotheses that have been proposed, but some of the chief ones include cross-modal deficiencies, verbal labeling deficiencies, hemispheric dominance and oculomotor automated-sequential/attentional deficiencies (see Benton & Pearl, 1978; Pavlidis & Miles, 1981, for a review

```
I went on a sled    today with my school friend.    The
snow was very deep.  We hit a stone and went head
first.   Thankyou very much for my bubble bath.   Mum
and Dad took me to the pantomime.  We saw Dick Whittington
He had a cat.    His name was called Singer.
```

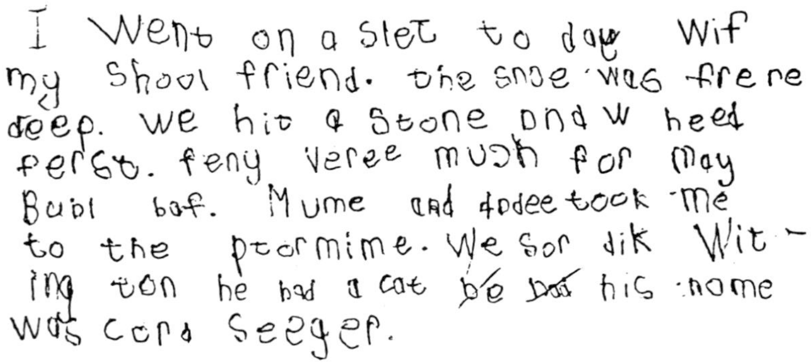

**FIGURE 25.1.** *Handwriting of an 8-year-old dyslexic boy with IQ of 120.*

of these topics). In all this work, a rich variety of behaviorally based experimental paradigms have been used. Despite their diversity, a central theme has emerged. Comparable to the descriptions of the symptomatology, dyslexics have great difficulty on experimental tasks demanding attentional and automated-sequential skills (Bakker, 1972; Bender, 1975; Birch & Belmont, 1964; Blank, 1978; Corkin, 1974; Doehring, 1968; Griffin, Walton, & Ives, 1974; Kinsbourne & Warrington, 1963a, 1963b; Naidoo, 1972; Pavlidis, 1983; Vernon, 1977).

The constellation of behavioral deficits has interesting and important consequences for understanding the syndrome of dyslexia. First, it indicates that the problems of the dyslexic are not confined to the written language system, but reflect a combination of subtle yet extensive impairments in important cognitive processes. Second, since by definition the impairments cannot be attributed to intellectual, emotional, or environmental factors, the only remaining cause is that of a constitutional nature that reflects a brain malfunction or disorder. In this regard, the recent cytoarchitechtonic analysis of the brain of a dyslexic by Galaburda & Kemper (1979) is important because it demonstrates that innate, but circumscribed malformations of the brain can exist and their existence can be manifested in the dyslexia syndrome. Further studies of dyslexic brains revealed similar malformations (Geschwind, 1982).

The relationship between behavioral deficits and brain malfunction in dyslexia makes this disorder an extremely profitable area for the application of eye movement research, because eye movements have been shown to be among the most sensitive indices of neurologically based behavioral disorders including schizophrenia (Holzman & Levy, 1977) and effects of alcohol (Aschoff, 1973). Furthermore, eye movements are potential indicators of the attentional–sequential deficits that the clinical and experimental work has suggested is of central importance in dyslexia. The remainder of this chapter will be concerned with research in eye movements. It will demonstrate how such research can be and has been applied to understanding the nature and causes of dyslexia.

### E.    Eye Movement Development and Reading

In order to interpret any eye movement behavior in dyslexics, it is necessary first to have information about the performance of normal readers so that meaningful comparisons can be carried out. Further, since the acquisition of reading skill takes place during periods of rapid developmental change, it is necessary to review the developmental changes in eye movement behavior that occur over the course of childhood.

Reading skills develop gradually, improving in precision and speed over the years. Evolving reading skills are clearly reflected in the pattern and characteristics of the reader's eye movements. Most of that development occurs during the first two to three years of schooling. About two–thirds of the total development of readers' eye movements, occuring between the first grade and college level, is achieved by the time that children are 9 years of age. The number of fixations is a better index of reading skill than the duration of fixations (Carmichael & Dearborn, 1948; Taylor, Franckenpohl, & Pette, 1960).

The developmental trends found in eye movements research are not unique to reading. Comparable findings have also been obtained during picture viewing and pattern recognition during which younger children usually have longer fixations and shorter saccades than adults (Lloyd & Pavlidis, 1977, 1978, 1983; Mackworth & Bruner, 1970; Spragins et al., 1976; Vurpillot, 1965; Zaporozhets, 1965). The overall emerging developmental pattern in terms of eye movements suggests that during both reading and visual search an inverse correlation exists between age and duration of fixation, at least until 9 or 10 years of age. On the basis of the existing knowledge it is difficult to assess how much of the decrease in the duration of fixation during reading and visual search is due to the maturation of the oculomotor control system and how much it is due to more effective information processing. As a result, developmental significance of the duration of eye fixation in cognition will be better understood only if we first understand the development of the saccadic latency which is its major component. Studies addressed to the above questions are much needed.

The developmental trends observed for duration and number of fixations during reading and scanning have also been found for perceptual span. Younger children do not seem to have the cognitive control over their eye movements that older children do. They also do not use peripheral vision to the same extent as older children. Another developmental change shows that the number of forward and regressive movements during reading drops by about 60% from first grade to college level (Gilbert, 1953; Taylor et al., 1960). Advanced, normal, and retarded readers make about 10–25 out of 100 regressions during reading. Regressions during reading are usually attributed to the problems that the reader has in comprehending the material (Bayle, 1942; Tinker, 1958). The relative frequency of regressions increase after large forward saccades (Anderson, 1937; Andriessen & DeVoogd, 1973). Just and Carpenter (1978) have considered regressions to be particularly susceptible to semantic control and to be corollaries of certain semantic processes, such as inference making. It is noteworthy that Pavlidis (1978, 1979, 1981a, 1981b) has found that the number and percentage of regressions in dyslexic readers is independent of the reading material as it also occurs in non-reading but reading related tasks.

Over and above developmental change, eye movement patterns and characteristics vary according to reading proficiency. Advanced and normal readers move their eyes from the beginning to the end of the line with saccades of similar size followed by fixations of similar durations. As shown in Figure 25.2, their overall pattern resembles the shape of a staircase. Retarded readers' eye movements are of the same nature as those of normal readers, but the size of their eye movements are smaller and the duration of fixations are longer and more variable. These characteristics presumably reflect the difficulties they experience with word recognitions and comprehension. Nevertheless, their overall pattern is similar to the staircase pattern shown by normal and advanced readers, although the pattern for each line is elongated (Figure 25.2).

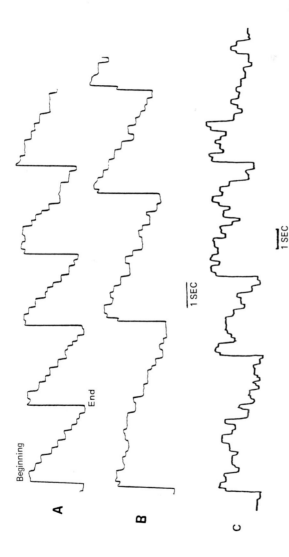

**FIGURE 25.2.** *Illustrative eye movement records of a normal and a retarded reader and of a dyslexic while they read. (a) Eye movements record of a normal reader during reading consists of successive similar eye movements and fixations that form a repetitive staircase pattern. The regressions are rare and they are invariably smaller in amplitude than the preceding forward saccade. The horizontal lines represent fixations. The vertical lines represent eye movements. (b) Retarded reader's eye movement record during reading. It is noteworthy that he makes more forward and regressive movements than normal readers, but the amplitude of their regressions is also smaller than the preceding forward saccades. His eye movements form a prolonged staircase pattern. (c) Dyslexic's "erratic" eye movement record. Every line has its own idiomorphic shape, unlike normal and backward readers' patterns which are consistent throughout. It is often difficult to distinguish the end of one line from the beginning of the next. Their regressions are not only very frequent but also often occur in clusters of two or more. Their amplitude is frequently bigger than that of the preceding forward saccade. These eye movement characteristics are unique to dyslexics.*

## F. Erratic Eye Movements in Dyslexia

In contrast to the characteristics and patterns shown by both normal and retarded readers, the eye movements of dyslexics are erratic and idiosyncratic.[2] The size of their eye movements and their durations of fixations are highly variable. Regressions often occur in clusters of two or more in succession whereas advanced, normal, and retarded readers make single regressions (Ciuffreda, Bahill, Kenyon, & Stark, 1976; Elterman, Ahel, Daroff, Dell'Osso, & Bornstein, 1980; Griffin et al., 1974; Heiman & Ross, 1974; Pavlidis, 1978, 1979, 1981a, b, 1982a, b; Pirozzolo & Rayner, 1978; Rubino & Minden, 1973; Zangwill & Blakemore, 1972). The dyslexics' erratic eye movements were first reported by Freeman in 1920 and attributed by Gray (1921) to a tendency to read in small units without proper attention to meaning. In 1959, Mosse and Daniels described a peculiar defect in the return sweep of dyslexics which was broken into many movements. They named the condition "linear dyslexia" and considered it responsible for difficulties in comprehension. Similar cases have been reported by Pavlidis (1978, 1981a) and Pirozzolo and Rayner (1978). The latter investigators associated the return sweep abnormalities with spatial orientation problems and suggested that the visual disorientation is caused by a congenital parietal lobe dysfunction.

The eye movement studies of dyslexics have usually been case studies with the exception of the work of Griffin et al. (1974), Lefton, Lahey, and Stagg (1978), Lesevre (1964), and Pavlidis (1978, 1981a, 1983). Lesevre tested 22 dyslexics and an equal number of normal controls in reading and nonreading tasks. She found that dyslexics exhibited more ocular instability, a greater number of short and long fixations than the controls, and irregular eye movement patterns. She concluded that the irregular eye movements of dyslexics could not be attributed to reading habits, poor teaching, or environmental factors.

One of the best known case studies of a dyslexic has been presented by Zangwill and Blakemore (1972). They recorded the eye movements of a 23-year-old dyslexic student while he tried to read and found that his oral reading was slow and marked by occasional self-corrected misreadings and verbal transpositions. His spelling was bizarre and included omissions of individual letters and homophones. When he was younger he was often reported to reverse words. His eye movements during reading were erratic with a strikingly large number of regressive movements. Sometimes, "he started from the right side of the line and made a perfect, fast series of flicks along the line from the right to left without a single 'regressive' movement in the correct direction." Zangwill and Blakemore thought

---

[2]The main characteristics of erratic eye movements are the excessive number of eye movements, particularly regressions which often occur two or more in succession. The sum of amplitudes or individual amplitudes of regressions can be larger than the proceeding forward saccade, unlike that of advanced, normal, and retarted readers who make singular regressions of the same or smaller size than the preceeding forward saccade. Other characteristics of erratic eye movements include a great variability in size and duration. The overall impression given by an erratic eye movement pattern is its irregularity, idiosyncratic shape and the lack of a consistent repetitive staircase pattern line after line.

that he had an "irrepressible tendency to move his eyes from right to left rather than left to right." Therefore, they explained his reversals and transposition in terms of his erratic eye movements. They further suggested that erratic eye movements "may not be a primary symptom in all dyslexic patients, but it may be in some, particularly those who show mixed laterality."

Pavlidis (1978) studied the eye movements of nine dyslexics and matched normal readers while they were silently reading material that was appropriate to their reading age. During this task in which they were instructed to read for comprehension, significant differences were found between the groups in their eye movement characteristics. The dyslexics' eye movements were erratic whereas the normal readers exhibited a systematic and consistent eye movement pattern. The differences between the two groups were of such a nature as to suggest a qualitative difference. The most striking difference was found in the number, size, and position of their regressions. For instance, normal readers' regressions were almost invariably smaller in size than the preceding forward saccade. This is in agreement with the results of similar studies by Tinker (1958) and O'Regan (1979). In contrast, the regressions of the dyslexics varied in size and sometimes were larger than the preceding forward movements. Further, unlike normal readers, their regressions occurred in clusters of two or more in succession. The dyslexics were unable to move their eyes accurately from the end of a line to the beginning of the next with only one saccade. Instead, they broke the return sweep into little saccades, giving the impression that they were scanning the text from right to left (Figure 25.2).

Although there is agreement that at least some dyslexics exhibit erratic eye movements, there is disagreement as to the nature of the relationship between erratic eye movements and dyslexia: Are the erratic eye movements only a reflection of the problems dyslexics have with reading material (Ellis & Miles, 1981; Goldberg & Arnott, 1970; Tinker, 1958); or are erratic eye movements and dyslexia the symptoms of one or more shared central deficits such as automated-sequential order disability or concentration or simultaneity problems (Pavlidis, 1981b, 1982a, 1982b); or is there an oculomotor disability that causes the erratic eye movements and then the erratic eye movements in turn cause the dyslexia (Griffin et al., 1974; Hildreth, 1963; Lesevre, 1964, 1968; Stockwell, Sherard, & Schuler, 1976; Zangwill & Blakemore, 1972)?

## II.  The Dyslexics' Erratic Eye Movements Are Independent of Their Reading Problems

The work to be reported in the material that follows is concerned with resolving the conflict between the first two questions just cited above.[3] If the dyslexics' erratic eye movements reflect the problems they have with reading material then the following should occur:

[3]Studies addressed to answering the third question are currently underway in our laboratory.

1. Dyslexics and retarded readers of the same reading and chronological ages should have similar eye movements since they have similar reading test performance.
2. When dyslexics read material easy for them, their eye movements should become normal because they will not have many problems reading the material. The normal readers' eye movements should become irregular or erratic as they read text that is difficult for them.

## A. The Issue of Subject Selection

In attempting to deal with these issues careful attention must be paid to the issue of subject selection. In most of the research cited, the erratic eye movements were not reported to be present uniformly in all subjects. In evaluating this information, it is important to return to an issue cited earlier; namely, the common failure to distinguish between dyslexics and retarded readers. Most of the studies did not provide sufficient information to assess whether subjects were dyslexics or not; even when information was given, the criteria used were insufficient to justify the classification of the subjects as dyslexics (for more detailed information on each of these studies, see Pavlidis, 1981b). Hence, it is not surprising to find a lack of uniformity in the results of the different studies. It is vital to differentiate between dyslexics and retarded readers if we are to avoid confusing and irreplicable results.

What can, at present, be used as the appropriate *research* diagnostic criteria for dyslexia? The word *research* has been emphasized since the criteria in experimental work must be extremely strict. Since dyslexia is of constitutional origin, in actual life, it is reasonable to expect that it be spread throughout the intellectual and socioeconomic spectrum. In selecting the research diagnostic criteria for dyslexia, however, we must exclude any factors that could be a primary cause of the reading problem. Another aim of such criteria should be the quantification of as many qualitative factors as possible (e.g., educational opportunities). Guided by these concepts, the following criteria were used in the selection of subjects:[4]

1. Performance or verbal IQ at least of an average level (90 or above)
2. At least 1.5 years retarded in reading below 10 years and at least 2 years retarded in reading above 10 years (with retardation assessed relative to chronological age)
3. Normal vision and hearing (people with nystagmus should be excluded)
4. Subjects should be of middle class socioeconomic background (with the language spoken at home being English). The establishment of the socioeconomic background should not depend only on the absolute income of the family but also on the per capita income.

[4]More precise criteria are used in our current studies.

5. have adequate motivation to read
6. have adequate educational opportunities, quantified according to the following two criteria. They should:
7. have had no more than two school changes (excluding normal transfer from nursery to primary to secondary school)
8. be absent not more than 2 weeks per term or not more than the average absenteeism occurring in the educational area from which the dyslexic and controls are drawn
9. have no overt physical handicaps that could account for their reading problems such as brain injury and/or tumor
10. have no overt emotional problems prior to beginning reading

It is necessary to have interviews with parents and teachers in order to establish the information needed for some of these criteria (e.g., criteria 4, 5, 6, 7, 8, 10). It is of vital importance for researchers studying dyslexia to adopt precisely the same diagnostic criteria for their subject selection. Only then will the replication of studies be meaningful and the comparison of results possible.

## B.  The Experimental Results

In the work to be reported here, of the 49 children referred to our laboratory as *diagnosed* dyslexics, only 14 fulfilled the above criteria. The eye movements of these dyslexics were compared with those of retarded readers, matched for both reading and chronological ages, and also with those of normal and advanced readers matched for chronological age. The exact criteria used for the selection for each of the groups as well as their ages, reading scores and statistical analysis of the data can be found in Pavlidis (1981b) and Pavlidis (1982a). The material in this chapter will concentrate on the comparison between dyslexics and matched retarded readers.

The horizontal and vertical eye movements of the children of our study were recorded using the photoelectric method modified by the author to suit the experimental requirements. The findings of a previous study were replicated (Pavlidis, 1979) in that most dyslexics were found to have erratic eye movements during reading whereas normal readers did not. Again, the most prominent characteristic of the dyslexics was their excessive number of regressions which frequently occurred in succession (see Figure 25.2). The dyslexics who did not exhibit erratic eye movement patterns had an excessive number of regressions.

In terms of the comparison between the dyslexics and the retarded readers, the following was found:

1. The eye movements (e.g., the number, size, and percentage of the forward and regressive eye movements) of the dyslexic and matched retarded readers were significantly different.
2. When dyslexics read easy text, a year below their reading age (which some-

times was almost 4 years 9 months below their chronological age), their eye
movements were not converted to the regular staircase patterns even though
their difficulty with the text was minimized.
3. Normal readers did not display erratic eye movements or an excessive number of regressions when they read difficult text (a year above their reading
level).
4. There were no significant differences in eye movement characteristics of
dyslexics when reading easy and difficult text.

These findings show that the dyslexics' erratic eye movements are not caused by
bad reading habits, poor teaching, other environmental factors, or even the difficulty of the text. Rather the findings support the view that although text difficulty
and comprehension requirements can exacerbate the dyslexics' eye movement
patterns and characteristics, they do *not* cause the erratic eye movements that
occur during reading.

The findings that dyslexics and retarded readers matched for both reading and
chronological ages have significantly different eye movement patterns and characteristics during reading reinforces the point that dyslexics are a category of readers
distinct from retarded readers. That eye movements during reading are a centrally
controlled function beyond conscious control make the above findings even more
important.

## C.   Erratic Eye Movements in Nonreading, but Reading Related Tasks

If the erratic eye movements in dyslexia are not caused by environmental
factors but by a central malfunction, then such a malfunction should manifest
itself not only in reading but also during nonreading but reading related nonverbal tasks (i.e., tasks that depend on skills that are fundamental to the reading
process). Further, the maintenance of the differential pattern of performance
between dyslexics and retarded readers on these nonreading tasks would add
support to the idea that these are distinct groups. One skill consistently found to
be involved in almost all stages of the reading process is that of sequential order
(Bakker, 1972; Doehring, 1968; Naidoo, 1972; Vernon, 1977). Further, as noted
earlier, this skill has also been consistently found by clinicians and researchers to
be one of the most fundamental deficiencies in dyslexia. Demands for "sequential
order" or "sequencing" in reading occur in such tasks as putting letters in the
right order to form a syllable; putting syllables together to form a word; putting
words in the correct order to make meaningful sentences (syntax); and moving
one's eyes in a properly timed correct sequential order from left to right to correctly transform the spatially arrayed visual sequences to temporally ordered language equivalents. Excluded from this list can be any sequential activity that is
not directly involved in reading and that does not require "automated-sequencing;" for example, the sequence of thoughts that are used to solve a problem.

Some sequential skills involving eye movements are present at birth. Gesell, Thompson, and Amatruda (1934) found that a 4-week-old child is able to fixate a number of points in succession. However, major developments occur over time and sequential order skills do not become accurate until at least the age of 7 (Gilbert, 1953; Kinsbourne & Warrington, 1963b; Lesevre, 1964, 1968; Vurpillot, 1976). A substantial relationship has been shown to exist between the eye movements during reading and during sequentially fixating digits (Gilbert, 1953).

Two series of experiments were performed to test the ocular–motor sequential performance of dyslexics and other readers in nonreading but reading related nonverbal tasks that involved sequentially presented stimuli. The stimuli were five small light emitting diodes (LED). The content-free nature of the stimuli allows them to serve as a universal cross-cultural stimulus and it permits the task to fulfill all the previously mentioned criteria for a critical test of dyslexia (i.e., eye movements and sequencing are both constituent components of the reading process and the task itself excludes all the main factors involved in reading such as memory, high-level information processing, emotional, and language factors, etc.). Not only is the task free of environmental and intellectual influences, but the eye movements that it evokes are a centrally controlled function beyond the awareness of the children. As a result, if dyslexics are found to be significantly different from normal, advanced, and retarded readers, then there would be direct evidence that dyslexics, unlike nondyslexic readers, have a unique handicap of central origin.

The first pilot study (Pavlidis, 1981a) involved a comparison of 12 dyslexics from 10–16 years (average age 12 years, 3 months) and 12 matched normal readers of the same age (average age 12 years, 1 month). The children's eye movements were recorded with the same photoelectric method used in the previous studies. The stimuli were five red LEDs, 5 min. of arc in diameter of matched luminance (2.0 log units above foveal threshold), spaced equidistantly (4°) in a horizontal array. Lights used as stimuli can substitute for words and "simulate" the oculomotor performance required during reading. The LEDS flashed one at a time; the lights at either end stayed on for 2 sec whereas the others stayed on for 1 sec. The sequence started at the extreme left and each LED was illuminated in turn. At the completion of the sequence, the reverse sequence was begun. The lights were lit up in this pattern three times in each direction to ensure that at least one "legible" record would always be clearly recorded. (In the analysis only the eye movements occurring during the first cycle [left to right and right to left runs of the LEDs] were analysed blind). Each child was asked to: "hold your eyes on the light which is on. Wait for it to move and then move your eyes to the new light as quickly and as accurately as you can. Although you might know where the light is going to move next, please do *not* move your eyes before the light moves."

In this task, dyslexics had significantly more fixations, both forward and regressive than other readers, but there was no significant difference in their left–right and right–left tracking. The differences found between dyslexics and other readers during reading tasks were therefore also present while following sequentially illuminated LEDs. When percentages are compared (instead of the absolute number of forward and regressive fixations), it is again found that dyslexics make a significantly higher percentage of regressions than the normal readers (Figure 25.3).

The results of this study, although encouraging, do not allow us to conclude that the dyslexics' erratic eye movements and number of regressions are independent of the psycho-environmental factors that are associated with the problems of retarded readers. Accordingly, a second study was carried out comparing dyslexics and retarded readers. Although both groups experience similar difficulties in reading, the causes are different: For dyslexics, the difficulties are constitutional, whereas for the retarded readers they are psycho-environmental (e.g., absenteeism, emotional instability, and adverse socioeconomic background). Hence, the two groups should not have shown similar behaviors on the eye movements task.

Our study was designed to fulfill two purposes: (a) to replicate the results of the first study using different groups of subjects, but still including normal, advanced, dyslexic, and retarded readers and (b) and most important, to make the vital comparison between dyslexics and retarded readers matched for reading and chronological age. The data analyses in this, as in all studies described in this chapter, were performed blind in that the research assistants had no knowledge of the groups to which the subjects belong. The results of the previous study comparing dyslexics and matched normal readers were replicated in this second study. As in reading, the most striking differences between dyslexics and all other groups of readers were found in the number of their regressions. Dyslexics and retarded

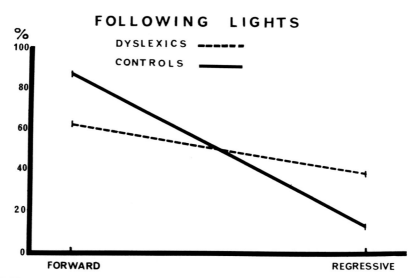

FIGURE 25.3. *Percentage of forward and regressive movements made by dyslexics and normal readers while following the lights moving from left to right. Dyslexics made more EM's (quantitative difference) but they also made a different kind of EM's (qualitative difference).*

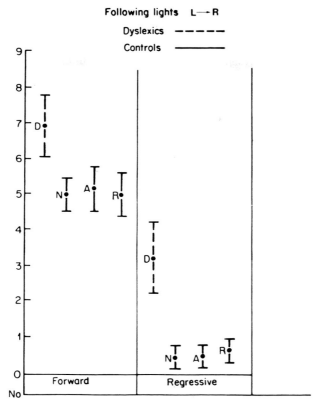

**FIGURE 25.4.** *Average and standard deviation of the number of eye movements made while children followed the lights from left to right. Note that no overlap exists between dyslexics and all other readers. (D = dyslexics, N = normal, A = advanced, and R = retarded), while all nondyslexics' performance was very similar indeed.*

readers had highly significant differences in almost all eye movement variables, whereas the performance of retarded readers was not significantly different from normal and advanced readers. As seen in Figure 25.4, there is little overlap between dyslexics and all other readers in the number of their regressions.

One could, however, ask the question, Do dyslexics have more regressions than other readers because they make more eye movements in general? This question can be answered by comparing the percentages of both forward and regressive fixations. Such a comparison yields interesting results. The "qualitative" differences found during reading between dyslexics and all other readers were also found when they followed the sequentially illuminated LEDs. The dyslexics still are clearly and significantly different in terms of percentages of regressions and forward eye movements from all other readers, whereas all differences between the nondyslexics disappear. Particularly noteworthy is the fact that dyslexics make almost the same percentage of regressions while following the sequentially illuminated LEDs as they do during reading the easy text (Table 25.1). On the other hand, the percentage of regressions for retarded, normal, and advanced readers drops significantly from reading to nonreading tasks because there is no high level information processing involved in the LEDs tasks (Table 25.1). A discriminant analysis using the number and percentage of eye movements while following the sequentially illuminated LEDs, shows that dyslexics can be accurately differentiated from all other readers on the basis of their eye movements. The data have also been analyzed to explore the maturational lag hypothesis (i.e., the hypothesis that the dyslexics are simply lagging in central nervous system development as opposed to qualitatively different components responsible for their behavior and thus dyslexics will never catch up in reading with their peers). The oldest dyslexics in the sample (mean age 11 years, 10 months) were compared to the youngest normal readers (mean age 8 years, 6 months)—a difference of 3 years, 4 months. The two groups were matched so that the dyslexics' reading age was comparable to that of the younger normal readers. The dyslexics' performance was still significantly worse than that of the matched younger normal readers. These findings suggest that a maturational lag cannot account for the dyslexics sequential oculomotor disability; rather the data favor the maturational deficit hypothesis. The combination of these findings suggest that the LED task might serve as an objective test of dyslexia. Since this task is independent of psycho–environmental factors, and it demands no reading, it could be applied to children prior to schooling to identify children at-risk for dyslexia. The task could also serve to clarify some of the problems associated with the exclusionary definition of dyslexia. In that definition, no child can be diagnosed as dyslexic if there is a psycho-environmental factor in the child's life that could account for the reading

TABLE 25.1

Average and Standard Deviation of Regressions During Reading Text One Year Below Reader's RA and During Following the Sequentially Illuminated LEDs[a]

| Groups of readers | Regressions during reading at RA—1 year (%) | Regressions during following LEDs (%) | Significance |
|---|---|---|---|
| Dyslexics | | | |
| $\bar{X}$ | 30.5 | 29.9 | t = −1.26, |
| Standard deviation | 7.3 | 8.1 | df = 9, P < .24 |
| Retarded readers | | | |
| $\bar{X}$ | 19.3 | 9.8 | t = −4.75, |
| Standard deviation | 7.1 | 10.0 | df = 15, P < .000 |
| Normal readers | | | |
| $\bar{X}$ | 21.0 | 6.8 | t = 4.49, |
| Standard deviation | 7.4 | 9.4 | df = 13, P < .001 |

[a] Dyslexics' percentage of regressions remained almost the same for both tasks. In contrast all other readers made 100% to 200% more regressions during reading than during the "information processing-free" task of the following the LEDs!

difficulty (e.g., poor schooling, poor social class background). As a result, children who are emotionally disturbed, who are of low intelligence, or who come from disadvantaged socio-economic environments *cannot* be diagnosed as dyslexic. This state of affairs, of course, does not reflect reality since brain malfunction does not reside only in well-educated, well-functioning middle class families. Rather the exclusion of all other groups is an artifact of the exclusionary definition to which we have been restricted up to this time. Since results of the author's test are not influenced by the psycho-environmental variables that might cause reading difficulties, it can now be proposed as a test to identify dyslexics throughout the total population.

## III.  Concluding Discussion

Since a number of diverse issues have been raised, it seems useful at this point to summarize the main findings. They encompass the following:

1. For the tasks involving reading, we have found that the dyslexics' erratic eye movements are *not* caused by the problems they have with the reading material;
2. The results of the nonreading but reading related non-verbal tasks further demonstrate that the dyslexics' erratic eye movement are basically independent of reading material in general.
3. The comparison of dyslexics and retarded readers shows that eye movement performance can differentiate among these two groups and that poor reading per se is not associated with erratic eye movements.

These findings are vital in allowing the diagnosis of dyslexia in children who come from deprived socio-educational environments, are of low intelligence, or have severe emotional problems.

A question that logically arises concerns the cause of the dyslexics' erratic eye movements, which can be attributed to at least five different factors: (*a*) a malfunctioning oculomotor control system, (*b*) an "automated sequencing" disability, (*c*) attentional/concentration problems, (*d*) an inability to anticipate the movement of the light and accurately synchronize their eye movements to it. An interaction between the above factors is also possible. The current studies do not allow us to distinguish amongst these alternatives, as erratic eye movements can be caused by one of these factors, several of them, or by an interaction among them. Although the information on each of these factors is scarce, it is worthwhile to consider them here at least briefly.

When oculomotor abnormalities are present, reading problems are likely to result. However, from the limited research to date it seems that the oculomotor control system is normal in many dyslexics(Adler–Grinberg & Stark, 1978; Zangwill & Blakemore, 1972). Well designed studies excluding the sequential element in a saccadic tracking task should be designed in order to assess the relative

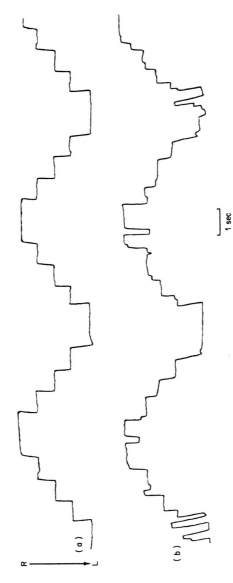

**FIGURE 25.5.** *Eye movement record of a normal reader (a) and a dyslexic (b) while following the sequentially illuminated LEDs: (a) Eye movement record of a normal reader 12 years, 6 months old, with average IQ while he follows sequentially illuminated LEDs as they proceed from left to right and right to left. (b) Eye movement record of a severely dyslexic boy 12 years, 6 months old with IQ 120 while he follows the sequentially illuminated LEDs as they proceed from left to right and vice versa. He makes many regressions and forward movements. This child's performance is better from right to left than from left to right. His erratic eye movements are "similar" to those he made while reading. It is noteworthy that the dyslexic, unlike the normal reader, is unable to hold his fixation when the light stayed on for 2 sec.*

R ——→ L

(a)

(b)

1 sec

contribution of the oculomotor control system to the dyslexics' erratic eye movements.

The presence of concentration problems is also quite likely. Both clinical and research evidence (Hornsby, 1980; Leary and Batho, 1981; Lefton et al., 1978; Pavlidis, 1982b) find that dyslexics have attentional/concentration problems. For example, Lefton *et al.* (1978) report that dyslexics' eye movements, unlike those of the control readers, become disorganized when they have to hold their attention for more than 5 sec. The dyslexics' inability to concentrate was observed among several of the subjects in our studies while they tried to fixate the LEDs during calibration in that their eyes wandered around the fixation point. As can be seen in Figure 25.5, when the light stayed on for 2 sec., the normal reader was able to hold the eyes and his attention; but in four out of five cases the dyslexic broke the fixation into shorter ones. These results indicate that the erratic eye movements found in dyslexics may partly be attributed to concentration problems or inability to correctly predict the movement of the next light and accurate fixate it.

The significance of order and temporally integrated actions has been emphasized by Lashley (1951) who wrote that "the problem of temporal integration . . . seems to me to be both the most important and the most neglected problem of cerebral physiology. Temporally integrated actions do occur even among insects, but they do not reach any degree of complexity until the appearance of the cerebral cortex. They are especially characteristic of human behavior and contribute as much as does any single factor to the superiority of human intelligence." Sequential order is involved in all stages of the reading process (Naidoo, 1972; Vernon, 1977) and it has consistently been found that the performance of inferior readers is significantly worse than that of normal readers on tasks involving sequential or temporal order. The above findings apply equally well to visual stimuli (Birch & Belmont, 1964; Bryden, 1972; Corkin, 1974; Doehring, 1968; Zurif & Carson, 1970), verbal stimuli (Corkin, 1974; Doehring, 1968), nonverbal stimuli (Corkin, 1974; Doehring, 1968; Zurif & Carson, 1970), and cross-modal stimuli (Bakker, 1972; Doehring, 1968; Zurif & Carson, 1970). The eye movement studies, in nonreading but reading related non-verbal tasks involving sequencing (Gilbert, 1953; Griffin et al., 1974; Lesevre, 1964, 1968; Pavlidis, 1979, 1981a, 1981b, 1983) are in agreement with those obtained in the non-eye-movement studies involving sequencing.

Recent neurological work is in accord with the above findings. Ojemann and Mateer (1979) using stimulation techniques have found that rapid nonverbal oral facial sequential movements and phoneme identification share the "same" portion of the language cortex. These data and the results from cytoarchitectonic analysis of a dyslexic brain (Galaburda & Kemper, 1979; Geschwind, 1980) support the view that the same parts of the brain are involved in language tasks (including reading) and in "automated-sequential" order tasks. Hence, when one function is disturbed, the other is expected to be affected as well. The results of both of our studies and the aforementioned neurological findings are in support of our view that language functions and "automated-sequencing" are closely linked.

For the diagnosis of dyslexia, it is irrelevant whether erratic eye movements are the cause of dyslexia or if erratic eye movements and dyslexia share a common cause. In both cases, though in different ways, the erratic eye movements will be linked to dyslexia. It must be emphasized that the knowledge of the relationship between eye movements and dyslexia can lead both to the objective diagnosis of dyslexia and also to the discovery of appropriate methods of treatment. At the very least this knowledge would indicate which methods we should not use for treatment of dyslexics. Currently, a new method for the treatment of dyslexia based on our work is being tested in the author's laboratory.

It is of vital importance to design well controlled experimental studies where each of the aforementioned four factors is systematically manipulated. By excluding or strengthening each of them in order to find out the relative contribution of each of those factors we may discover the causes of the dyslexics' erratic eye movements. Such knowledge would not only be of vital importance because it will lead to a better understanding of the causes of dyslexia, but it could even be a positive step toward a much needed *positive definition* of dyslexia. This in turn, could aid in the development of an appropriate method for treatment. Such studies are under way in my laboratory. A unequivocal diagnosis is one of the basic prerequisites for the discovery of an appropriate remedy. The possible prognostic capabilities of a diagnostic method enhance its usefulness.

The early diagnosis of dyslexia is useful for a number of reasons. On the one hand, the earlier the diagnosis the greater the possibility of ensuring maximum advantage of the plasticity of the brain by either energizing its "dormant" circuits or by forming new ones. On the other hand, early diagnosis will also increase the chances of ameliorating the consequent negative educational and psychosocial effects on the dyslexics' families, their schools, and, most important, the dyslexics themselves. Because the author's objective diagnostic test of dyslexia is independent of reading skills, it could be used even before reading age. The limits of its earliest possible diagnostic capabilities could be determined by the outcome of a developmental investigation into the development of oculomotor–sequential–attentional skills. It also provides the possibility of an early objective diagnosis of dyslexia that will benefit the family atmosphere, the child's psychological stability, and the teacher–child relationship. Indeed it may lead to both an adjustment of teaching strategies and to a more appropriate attitude toward the child.

The other advantage of the author's proposed test is that it takes only a few minutes. The screening of whole school population becomes feasable. It therefore becomes possible to screen large populations and to make known the exact percentage of the "dyslexia syndrone" in the general population. It is important that the recognition of the handicap of dyslexia should become neither a convenient excuse for the lazy child and the incompetent teacher, nor a socially accepted label used by "pushy" parents of "slow" children. The only way to prevent this is to make sure that objective and accurate criteria for the diagnosis of dyslexia are used. The author's potential test, once standardized, will provide a positive step in that direction.

## ACKNOWLEDGMENTS

I would like to thank my devoted assistants Elaine Baker, Lesley Dawson, Janet Gruber, Penny Harris, and Ida Michaelson for their most valuable help during the different stages of the research and especially for the data analysis. I would also like to thank George Noland for generously spending his time to finish the computerized data analysis, Dr. K. Hirsch-Pasek for commenting on the initial draft, and also Selma Aronowitz, Dorothy Caplan and Joan Hudock for typing this chapter. To the children of our studies I am particularly grateful for their warm cooperation, and for giving me the opportunity to play and feel like one of them once again.

# References

Adler–Grinberg, D., & Stark, L. (1978). Eye movements, scanpaths and dyslexia. *American J. of Optometry and Physiological Optics, 55,* 557–570.

Anderson, I. H. (1937). Studies in the eye movements of good and poor readers. *Psychology Monograph, 48,* 1–35.

Andriessen, J. J., & DeVoogd, A. H. (1973). Analysis of eye movement patterns in silent reading. *IPO Annual Progress Report, 8,* 30–35.

Aschoff, J. C. (1973). Eye movements as an indication of sensitivity. *Informa, 35,* 29–33.

Bakker, D. J. (1972). *Temporal order and disturbed reading.* Rotterdam: Rotterdam University Press.

Bayle, E. (1942). The nature of causes of regressive movements in reading. *Journal of Experimental Education, 11,* 16–36.

Bender, L. (1975). A fifty-year review of experiences with dyslexia. *Bulletin of the Orton Society,* 5–23.

Benton, A. L., & Pearl, D. (Eds.). (1978). *Dyslexia: An appraisal of current knowledge.* New York: Oxford University Press.

Birch, H. G., & Belmont, L. (1964). Auditory-visual integration in normal and retarded readers, *American Journal Orthopsychiatry, 34,* 852–861.

Blank, M. S. (1978). Review of Toward an understanding of dyslexia: Psychologial factors in specific reading disability. In A. L. Benton & D. Pearl (Eds.), *Dyslexia: An appraisal of current knowledge.* New York: Oxford University Press.

Boder, E. (1971). Developmental dyslexia: prevailing diagnostic concepts and a new diagnostic approach. In H. R. Myklebust (Ed.), *Progress in learning disabilities* (Vol. 2) New York: Grune and Stratton. Pp. 293–321.

Boder, E. (1973). Developmental dyslexia: A diagnostic approach based on three atypical reading-spelling patterns. *Developmental Medicine and Child Neurology, 15,* 663–687.

Bryden, M. P. (1972). Auditory, visual and sequential-spatial matching in relation to reading ability. *Child. Development, 43,* 824–832.

Carmichael, L., & Dearborn, W. F. (1948). *Reading and visual fatigue.* London: Harrap.

Ciuffreda, K. J., Bahill, A. T., Kenyon, R. V., & Stark, L. (1976). Eye movements during reading: Case reports. *American Journal of Optometry and Physiological Optics, 53,* 389–395.

Corkin, S. (1974). Serial-ordering deficits in inferior readers. *Neuropsychologia, 12,* 347–354.

Critchley, M. (1970). *The dyslexic child.* London: Heinemann.

Critchley, M. (1981). Dyslexia: An overview. In G. Th. Pavlidis & T. R. Miles (Eds.), *Dyslexia research and its application to education.* London: J. Wiley & Sons.

Cruickshank, W. M. (1968). The problems of delayed recognition and its correction. In A. H. Keeney & V. T. Keeney (Eds.), *Dyslexia: Diagnosis and treatment of reading disorders.* St. Louis: C. V. Mosby.

Denckla, M. B. (1977). Minimal brain dysfunction and dyslexia. In M. E. Blaw, I. Rapin, & M. Kinsbourne (Eds.), *Child Neurology.* New York: Spectrum. Pp. 243–261.

Doehring, D. G. (1968). *Patterns of impairment in specific reading disability.* Bloomington: Indiana University Press.

Downing, J., & Thackray, D. (1975). *Reading readiness.* London: Hodder and Stroughton.

Ellis, N., & Miles, T. R. (1981). A lexical encoding deficiency 1: Experimental evidence. In G. Th. Pavlidis & T. R. Miles (Eds.), *Dyslexia research and its applications to education*. London: J. Wiley & Sons.

Elterman, R. D., Abel, L. A., Daroff, R. B., Dell'Osso, L. F., & Bornstein, J. L. (1980). Eye movement patterns in dyslexic children. *Journal of Learning Disabilities, 13*, 16–21.

Farnham–Diggory, S. (1978). *Learning disabilities*. London: Open Books.

Fine, J. (1982). *Oral discourse skills in normal and dyslexic children*. Paper presented at the 27th Annual Convention of the International Reading Association, Chicago, April 26–30.

Freeman, F. N. (1920). Clinical study as a method in experimental education. *Journal of Applied Psychology, 4*, 126–141.

Fry, E. (1968). Do-it-yourself terminology generator. *Journal of Reading, 11*, 428.

Galaburda, A. M., & Kemper, T. L. (1979). Cytoarchitectonic abnormalities in developmental dyslexia: A case study. *Ann. Neurol., 6*, 94–100.

Geschwind, N. (1980). Brain "miswired" in dyslexics? *Medical News*, March 6.

Geschwind, N. (1982). *Biological foundations of dyslexia*. Paper presented at the British Psychological Society's International Conference on *Dyslexia*. Manchester, U.K., March 1–3.

Gesell, A., Thompson, H., & Amatruda, C. S. (1934). *Infant behaviour: Its genesis and growth*. New York: McGraw–Hill.

Gilbert, L. C. (1953). Functional motor efficiency of the eyes and its relation to reading. *University of California Publications in Education, 11*, 159–231.

Goldberg, H. K., & Arnott, W. (1970). Ocular motility in learning disabilities. *Journal Learning Disabilities, 3*, 160–162.

Gray, W. S. (1921). The diagnostic study of an individual case in reading. *Elementary School Journal, 21*, 577–594.

Griffin, D. C., Walton, H. N., & Ives, V. (1974). Saccades as related to reading disorders. *Journal of Learning Disabilities, 7*, 310–316.

Gruber, E. (1962). Reading ability, binocular co-ordination and the ophthalmograph. *Archives of Ophthalmology, 67*, 280–288.

Hieman, J. R., & Ross, A. O. (1974). Saccadic eye movements and reading difficulties. *Journal of Abnormal Child Psychology, 2*, 53–61.

Hermann, K. (1959). *Reading disability*. Copenhagen: Munkgaard.

Hildreth, G. H. (1963). Early writing as an aid to reading. *Elementary English, 40*, 15–20.

Holzman, P. S., & Levy, D. L. (1977). Smooth pursuit eye movements and functional psychosis: A review. *Schizoprenia Bulletin, 3*, 15–27.

Hornsby, B. (1980). *How can dyslexics be taught to read, write and spell?* Paper presented at the International Symposium on dyslexia research and its educational applications. Manchester, February 20–22.

Hue, E. B. (1908) *The psychology and pedagogy of reading*. New York: Macmillan.

Just, M. A., & Carpenter, P. A. (1978). Inference processes during reading: Reflections from eye fixations. In J. W. Senders, D. F. Fisher, & R. A. Monty (Eds.), *Eye movements and the higher psychological functions*. Hillsdale, New Jersey: Erlbaum.

Katz, P. A., & Deutch, M. (1964). Modality of stimulus presentations in serial learning for retarded and normal readers. *Perceptual and Motor Skills, 19*, 627–633.

Kinsbourne, M., & Warrington, E. K. (1963). The developmental Gerstmann Syndrome. *Archives of Neurology, 8*, 40–51. (a)

Kinsbourne, M., & Warrington, E. K. (1963). Development factors in reading and writing backwardness. *British Journal of Psychology, 54*, 145–156. (b)

Lashley, K. S. (1951). The problems of serial order in behaviour. In L. A. Jeffress (Ed.), *Cerebral mechanisms in behaviour*. New York: Wiley.

Leary, P. M., & Batho, K. (1981). The role of the EEG in the investigation of the child with learning disability. *South Africa Medical Journal*, 867–868.

Lefton, L. A., Lahey, B. B., & Stagg, D. I. (1978). Eye movements in reading disabled and normal children: A study of systems and strategies. *Journal of Learning Disabilities, 1*, 22–31.

Lesevré, N. (1964). Les Mouvements oculaires d'exploration: Etude electro-oculagraphique comparee d'enfants normaux et dyslexiques. These de 3 cycle (ronee).

Lesevré, N. (1968). L'organisation du regard chez des enfants d'age scolaire, lecteurs normaux et dyslexiques. *Review de Neuropsychiatry Infant, 16,* 323–349.

Liberman, I. Y., Liberman, A. M., Mattingly, I. G., & Shankweiler, D. (1980). Orthography and the beginning reader. In J. Kavanagh & R. Venezky (Eds.), *Orthography, reading and Dyslexia.* Baltimore: University Park Press.

Lloyd, P., & Pavlidis, G. Th. (1978). Child language and eye movements. The relative effects of sentence and situation on comprehension in young children. *Bulletin of British Psychological Society, 31,* 70–71.

Lloyd, P., & Pavlidis, G. Th. (1978). The relationship between child language and eye movements: A developmental study. *Neuroscience Letters Suppl., 1,* 248.

Lloyd, P., & Pavlidis, G. Th. (1983). The role of eye fixations in children's understanding and use of language. (Submitted for publication)

Lunzer, E. A. (1978). Short term memory and reading: Stage 1. In M. M. Gruneberg, P. E. Morris, & R. N. Sykes (Eds.), *Practical aspects of memory.* London: Academic Press.

Mackworth, N. H., & Bruner, J. (1970). How adults and children search and recognize pictures. *Human Development, 13,* 149–177.

Mattis, S., French, J. H., & Rapin, I. (1975). Dyslexia in children and young adults: Three independent neuropsychological syndromes. *Developmental Medicine and Child Neurology, 17,* 150.

McConkie, G. W., & Rayner, K. (1975). The span of the effective stimulus during a fixation in reading. *Perception & Psychophysics, 17,* 578–586.

Miles, T. R., & Ellis, N. C. (1981). A lexical encoding deficiency: Clinical observations. In G. Th. Pavlidis & T. R. Miles (Eds.), *Dyslexia research and its applications to education.* London: J. Wiley & Sons.

Morgan, W. P. (1896). A case of congenital word blindness. *British Medical Journal, 2,* 1378.

Mosse, H. L., & Daniels, C. R. (1959). Linear dyslexia. *American Journal of Psychotherapy, 13,* 826–841.

Naidoo, S. (1971). Symposium on reading disability. *Brit. J. Educ. Psychol., 41,* 19–22.

Naidoo, S. (1972). *Specific dyslexia.* London: Pitman.

Ojemann, G., & Mateer, K. (1979). Human language cortex: Localization of memory, syntax, and sequential motor-phoneme identification systems. *Science, 205,* 1401–1403.

O'Regan, J. K. (1979). Moment to moment control of eye saccades as a function of textual parameters in reading. In P. A. Kolers, M. Wrolstad, & H. Bouma (Eds.), *Processing of visible language.* New York: Plenum Press.

Orton, S. T. (1925). Word-blindness in school children. *Archives of Neurology and Psychiatry, 14,* 581–616.

Orton, S. T. (1937). *Reading, writing and speech problems in children.* London: Chapman and Hall.

Owens, F. W. (1978). Dyslexia: Genetic aspects. In A. L. Benton & D. Pearl (Eds.), *Dyslexia: An appraisal of current knowledge.* New York: Oxford University Press.

Pavlidis, G. Th. (1978). The dyslexic's erratic eye movements: Case studies. *Dyslexia Review, 1,* 22–28.

Pavlidis, G. Th. (1979). How can dyslexia be objectively diagnosed? *Reading, 13,* 3–15.

Pavlidis, G. Th. (1981). Do eye movements hold the key to dyslexia? *Neuropsychologia, 19,* 57–64. (a)

Pavlidis, G. Th. (1981). Sequencing, eye movements and the early objective diagnosis of dyslexia. In G. Th. Pavlidis & T. R. Miles (Eds.), *Dyslexia research and its applications to education.* London: J. Wiley and Sons. (b)

Pavlidis, G. Th., & Miles, T. R. (Eds.). (1981). *Dyslexia research and its applications to education.* London: J. Wiley and Sons.

Pavlidis, G. Th. (1982). *Erratic eye movement and dyslexia: Cause or effect?* Paper presented at the New York Academy of Sciences Conferences on Reading and Reading Disability, New York, May 7–8. (a)

Pavlidis, G. Th. (1982). *What can automated sequencing and erratic eye movements tell us about dyslexia.*

Paper presented at the 33rd Annual Conference of the Orton Dyslexia Society's Symposium on Disorders of Eye Movement in Dyslexia and their Significance, Baltimore, November 3–7. (b)

Pavlidis, G. Th. (1983). The objective diagnosis of dyslexia by erratic eye movements: A replication. (Submitted for publication)

Piaget, J., & Vinh–Bang, I. (1961). L'enregistrement des mouvements oculaires en jeu chez l'adulte dans la comparaison de verticules, horizontales ou obliques et dans les perceptions de la figure en equerre. *Arch. Psychol.* (Geneva), 38, 167–200.

Pirozzolo, F. J., & Rayner, K. (1978). The neural control of EMs in acquired and developmental reading disorder. In H. Avakian-Whitaker & H. A. Whitaker (Eds.), *Advances in Neurolinguistics and Psycholinguistics.* New York: Academic Press.

Rayner, K. (1978). Eye movements in reading and information processing. *Psychological Bulletin,* 85, 618–660.

Rubino, C. A., & Minden, H. A. (1973). An analysis of eye-movements in children with a reading disability. *Cortex,* 9, 217–220.

Rudel, R. G. (1980). Learning disability: Diagnosis by exclusion and discrepancy. *Journal of the American Academy of Child Psychiatry,* 53, 547–569.

Rutter, M., & Yule, W. (1975). The concept of specific reading retardation. *Journal of Child Psychology and Psychiatry,* 16, 181–197.

Spragins, A. B., Lefton, L. A., & Fisher, D. F. (1976). Eye movements while reading spatially transformed text: A developmental study. *Memory Cognition 4,* 36–42.

Stockwell, C. W., Sherard, E. S., & Schuler, J. V. (1976). EOG findings in dyslexic children. *Transactions of the American Academy of Ophthalmology and Otolol.,* 82, 239–243.

Symmes, J.S., & Rapoport, J. L. (1972). Unexpected Reading Failure. *American Journal of Orthopsychiatry,* 42, 82–91.

Taylor, S. E., Franckenpohl, H., & Pette, J. L. (1960). *Grade level norms for components of the fundamental reading skill* (EDL. Information Research Bulletin 3). Huntington, New York: Educ. Devel. Labs.

Tinker, M. A. (1958). Recent studies of eye movements in reading. *Psychological Bulletin,* 55, 215–231.

Vellutino, F. R. (1977). Alternative conceptualizations of dyslexia: Evidence in support of a verbal deficit hypothesis. *Harvard Educational Review,* 47, 334–354.

Vernon, M. D. (1971). *Reading and its difficulties.* Cambridge: Cambridge University Press.

Vernon, M. D. (1977). Varieties in deficiency in the reading process. *Harvard Educational Review,* 47, 396–410.

Vernon, M. D. (1979). Variability in reading retardation. *British Journal of Psychology,* 70, 7–16.

Vurpillot, C. (1976). *The visual world of the child.* London: George, Allen and Unwin.

Welchman, M. (1980). *Social and education implications of dyslexia.* Paper presented at International Symposium on Dyslexia research and its educational applications. Manchester, February 20–22.

Zangwill, O. L. (1981). Foreword in G. Th. Pavlidis & T. R. Miles (Eds.), *Dyslexia research and its applications to education.* London: J. Wiley & Sons.

Zangwill, O. L., & Blakemore, C. (1972). Dyslexia: Reversal of EM during reading. *Neuropsychologia,* 10, 371–373.

Zaporozhets, A. V. (1965). The development of perception in the preschool child. In P. H. Mussen (Ed.), European research in child development. *Monograph of Society for Research in Child Development,* 30, 82–101.

Zurif, E. B., & Carson, G. (1970). Dyslexia in relation to cerebral dominance and temporal analysis. *Neuropsychologia,* 8, 351–361.

Richard K. Olson, Reinhold Kliegl, and Brian J. Davidson

# 26

# Eye Movements in Reading Disability[1]

## I.   Introduction

The relation between eye movements and reading skill has intrigued psychologists and educators for nearly a century. The traditional experimental approach has been to compare group means for good and disabled readers on general eye movement parameters such as duration and number of fixations, frequency of regressions, and saccade length. The common result has been longer duration and higher fixation frequency, more regressions, and shorter saccades for average disabled readers when reading the same material as the average good reader (Tinker, 1965). Our research on these general parameters differs from the earlier studies in two important aspects. The reading materials are adjusted for each reader's word recognition skill, and our major focus is on individual differences in eye movements in relation to other reading and cognitive processes within the reading disabled group.

Recent neurologically oriented case studies of disabled readers have shown that acquired and congenital brain defects result in distinct subtypes of eye movement abnormalities (see Pirozzolo & Rayner, 1978a, for a review). A case reported by Pirozzolo and Rayner (1978b) showed an abnormal tendency to fixate from right to left along a line of text. They speculated that this was probably associated with a

[1]This research was supported by USPHS program project grant HDMH 11681-01A1. In the program project, subjects were first tested with several psychometric measures in Dr. DeFries's laboratory at the Institute for Behavior Genetics. The present report uses the WISC-R I.Q. and PIAT reading tests from this session.

congenital parietal lobe dysfunction. In contrast, a second case reported by Pirozzolo and Rayner displayed normal eye movements when reading very easy text,
but showed the frequently reported increase in fixations and regressions of disabled readers when he read text above his level of skill.

Other neurological case studies also indicate substantial individual differences
in word coding processes, with brain injury giving rise to distinct patterns of
reading disorders (e.g., Coltheart, 1981; Marshall & Newcombe, 1973). Several
investigators have suggested that these reading disorder subtypes can be related to
the selective impairment of visual and phonological word coding systems (Saffran
& Marin, 1977; Shallice & Warrington, 1980). Coltheart (1981) has argued that
similar differences in coding skills may exist within the general reading disabled
population. In fact, these individual differences have been observed by several
investigators (see Satz & Morris, 1981, for a review).

This chapter specifically addresses the relationship between individual differences in word coding processes and eye movements in reading disability. Our
broader goal is to understand the nature of individual differences in reading
disability through a convergent perspective on several different reading process
parameters.

Our reading disabled subjects participated in a project dealing with differential
diagnosis in reading disability through the University of Colorado Institute for
Behavior Genetics. They were first tested with several standard psychometric
measures such as the WISC-R IQ test and the Peabody Individual Achievement
Test (PIAT). Subjects who met the selection criteria, to be described, were tested
in our laboratory for word coding processes and eye movements.

The definition of specific reading disability in the project includes a WISC
verbal or performance IQ of at least 90, no obvious neurological or emotional
problems, normal socioeconomic and educational background, and reading skill at
approximately half of expected grade level. Forty-four reading disabled subjects
(34 males and 10 females) and 42 normal subjects (35 males and 7 females) were
included in the present analyses. Age in both groups ranged from 13–17 years.
Mean age, WISC full-scale IQ, and PIAT grade-equivalent subscores for word
recognition, spelling, and comprehension are presented in Table 26.1. The subjects were drawn from the Boulder, Colorado, area where socioeconomic levels
and quality of schools are above average for the country. The normal group is also
above the national norms in reading skill. However, the reading disabled group is
substantially below average despite their normal intelligence and their above average socioeconomic level and educational background. Thus, their reading failure
cannot be attributed to general intelligence or environmental deficits.


# II.   Word Coding Processes

## A.   Word Recognition

Three tasks considered in this chapter were part of a series designed to assess
various word coding processes. The first tested word recognition skill by present-

ing lists of 20 words across several grade levels from the Camp and McCabe (1977) reading and spelling test. The words were presented singly, in lowercase, three characters per degree of visual angle, on a television monitor placed 36 in. from the subject. Vocalization latency was monitored by a voice key. The first list presented was at least two grade levels below the subject's PIAT reading recognition score. Successively higher grade level lists were presented until the subject failed to recognize at least 50% of the words within the 2-sec time limit. The grade level list that was closest to 50% errors determined the subject's word recognition grade level.

## B.  Orthographic Coding

Orthographic and phonological coding tasks were adapted from a study of normal adult individual differences by Baron and Strawson (1976), (see Davidson, Kliegl, & Olson, 1981, for further details). In the orthographic coding task, subjects were presented 8 practice and 40 test trials containing two letter strings displayed side by side. One letter string was a word (e.g., *rain*), whereas the other was a phonologically identical nonword (e.g., *rane*). The subject's task was to press one of two buttons indicating whether the string to the left or to the right was a word. They were told to respond as quickly as possible but to try to avoid errors. Error and latency feedback were presented on the television monitor screen between trials.

## C.  Phonological Coding

Phonological coding skill has been identified by many researchers as the most substantial and fundamental difference between groups of good and disabled readers (see Rozin & Gleitman, 1977, for a review). Our test of individual differences in this skill was identical in structure to the orthographic task, except that neither of the letter strings was a word (e.g., *kake* and *dake*). However, one of these nonwords sounded like a word (e.g., *kake*). The target and distractor items were orthographically similar to each other and to the real word (e.g., *cake*) from which they were derived. As in the orthographic task, subjects pushed a button on the side of the perceived correct response and then received error and latency feedback. Again, the total stimulus series consisted of 8 practice and 40 test trials.

Recall that orthographic-task pairs were similar in phonology and, therefore, had to be discriminated primarily on the basis of orthographic differences. Phonology-task pairs presented no orthographic basis for lexical access but could be discriminated on the basis of phonology.

## III.   Eye Monitor and Reading Task

Following the word coding tasks, stories were presented for oral and silent reading while the subject's eye movements were recorded. Eye fixations were monitored with a Gulf & Western Applied Sciences Model 1996. This system uses infrared light to monitor pupil and corneal-reflection positions related to eye fixations. Fixation location was sampled at the rate of 60 Hz and the data were transfered to a PDP 11/03 computer for later analyses (Davidson, 1981).

During calibration and reading, subjects leaned forward into a goggles frame to stabilize head position. Calibration consisted of fixating each of nine points in a rectangular grid. Calibrated output of the eye monitor was later mapped to text locations with programs described in Kliegl and Olson (1981) and Kliegl (1981). Accuracy of the system was within one character position on 90% of the fixations. These programs also reduced the 60 Hz eye position data to fixations and moves yielding the fixation duration, regression, and saccade length measures used in the following analyses.

The stories were adapted from the Spache (1963) Diagnostic Reading Scales and were selected for grade level difficulty based on the subject's score in the earlier word recognition test. The stories ranged from one to two screens of text, 11 lines per screen, and about 60 character spaces wide (20° of visual angle). Following the eye movement calibration the subject was told to read the first story aloud and to remember it for a test of eight questions at the end of the story. After the first test, eye position was recalibrated and the second story was presented for silent reading, followed by an eight question test. We will begin the presentation and discussion of results with the group data and then proceed to our main concern: individual differences within the disabled reader group.

## IV.  Group Differences

Group data for word recognition grade level, orthographic reaction time, orthographic errors, phonological reaction time, and phonological errors are presented in Table 26.1. The results confirm that there are substantial group differences in word recognition and related coding skills.

Eye fixation measures presented in Table 26.2 include fixation duration, saccade length, Regressive Fixation Index (RFI), percentage of regressions, and reading rate in words per minute (wpm). Sample sizes are given in parentheses. The N's were different for reading aloud and silent because adequate data were not available for all subjects in both conditions.

The percentage of regression was computed by dividing the number of regressive fixations by the total number of fixations. These values are comparable to other studies (Tinker, 1965). For the individual difference analyses, a RFI was calculated by dividing the number of regressive fixations by the number of fixations that were preceded and succeeded by a right going saccade. Thus, fixations at the beginning and end of a line and fixations preceding a regressive fixation were not included. The RFI measure was thought to be a purer measure of regression tendencies than percentage of regressions, but in fact the correlation between the two measures was .97. Saccade length was computed by including only those forward saccades that were preceded and succeeded by a right going saccade. Saccades following a regression were excluded because subjects tend to

## TABLE 26.1
### Standardized Test and Word Coding Scores

| | Age | WISC | PIAT | | | Orthographic | | Phonological | | Word recognition |
|---|---|---|---|---|---|---|---|---|---|---|
| | | | Recognition | Spelling | Comprehension | Latency | Errors | Latency | Errors | |
| **Normal (n=42)** | | | | | | | | | | |
| $\bar{x}^a$ | 15.9 | 112 | 10.7 | 9.3 | 10.6 | 801 | 8.4 | 1318 | 17.4 | 11.9 |
| $(s)^b$ | (1.5) | (8) | (2.1) | (2.4) | (2.0) | (129) | (5.9) | (354) | (12.4) | (1.2) |
| **Disabled (n=44)** | | | | | | | | | | |
| $\bar{x}$ | 15.7 | 104 | 6.2 | 5.2 | 7.0 | 1054 | 13.3 | 2058 | 30.7 | 6.4 |
| $(s)$ | (1.4) | (10) | (2.1) | (1.6) | (2.4) | (311) | (6.0) | (909) | (13.8) | (2.5) |

[a] $\bar{x}$ is the mean group score.
[b] (s) is the standard deviation.

TABLE 26.2
Group and Condition Means (Standard Deviations) for Eye Movement Parameters

| | | Regression index | Regressions % | Fixation duration | Saccade length | Words per minute |
|---|---|---|---|---|---|---|
| Normal | | | | | | |
| Aloud | $x^a$ | 40.4 | 18.0 | 300 | 6.0 | 148 |
| ($n$=30) | (s)[b] | (17.9) | (5.1) | (30) | (.8) | (23) |
| Silent | $x$ | 44.0 | 19.2 | 283 | 7.1 | 158 |
| ($n$=32) | (s) | (18.8) | (6.8) | (33) | (1.0) | (45) |
| Disabled | | | | | | |
| Aloud | $x$ | 52.7 | 22.8 | 355 | 5.4 | 98 |
| ($n$=33) | (s) | (18.2) | (4.4) | (57) | (.7) | (26) |
| Silent | $x$ | 53.8 | 25.5 | 333 | 5.9 | 111 |
| ($n$=26) | (s) | (19.6) | (6.0) | (58) | (.8) | (32) |

[a] $x$ is the mean group score.
[b] (s) is the standard deviation.

skip over fixation locations that precede the regression, and this would artificially inflate the relation between RFI and saccade length.

All of the eye fixation group differences were significant, except for saccade length in the aloud condition. Although the differences were not as large as in previous studies because text difficulty was adjusted for word recognition skill, they follow the typical pattern of longer fixation duration, shorter saccades, and a higher percentage of regressive movements in disabled readers. The absence of a significant difference for saccade length in the aloud condition suggests that the good readers were restricted in their eye movements by the vocalization task. Saccade length increased significantly for good readers in the silent condition but not for the disabled readers.

## V.    Dimensions of Individual Differences

In this section we will discuss the separate relationships of word recognition, IQ, saccade length, and relative phonological skill to the RFI for disabled readers in the aloud condition. The subsequent section will combine these variables in multiple regression analyses for reader groups and conditions.

The standard deviations in Tables 26.1 and 26.2 indicate that there are substantial individual differences in IQ, word coding skills, and eye movement variables within the reading disabled group. The first question we asked was how these variables correlated with each other. The second step was to analyze selected variables in a series of theoretically motivated multiple-regression models.

Table 26.3 shows that RFI was significantly correlated with IQ, saccade length, and phonological latency. RFI was chosen as the criterion variable in the following models based on previous research and our initial hypotheses about how

TABLE 26.3
Correlations for Disabled Readers Reading Aloud

|  | Regressive fixation index | Word recognition | WISC | Saccade length | Phonological latency | Orthographic latency | Fixation duration |
|---|---|---|---|---|---|---|---|
| Word recognition | −.18 | | | | | | |
| WISC | .32 | .38 | | | | | |
| Saccade length | .56 | .44 | .48 | | | | |
| Phonological latency | .36 | −.51 | .07 | .10 | | | |
| Orthographic latency | −.14 | −.38 | .02 | .03 | .61 | | |
| Fixation duration | .05 | −.44 | −.30 | −.22 | .11 | .03 | |
| Words per minute | −.22 | .74 | .42 | .42 | −.41 | −.13 | −.63 |

the distribution of visual attention would relate to the other parameters. These hypotheses are described with the presentation of each of the following analyses.

## A.  Regressive Fixation Index and Word Recognition

The usual interpretation of a proportional increase in regressions with poor word recognition skill is that unknown words in the text elicit regressive saccades within words and to previous words for contextual support. We would expect this to be the case in the present study, if the adjustment of text difficulty for word recognition skill was not completely successful. Analyses of the oral reading errors showed that slightly more word recognition errors were made by subjects reading the lower-grade-level material. However, word recognition skill was not significantly related to RFI. Since RFI is a proportional score, its independence from word recognition does not imply that the low-grade-level material would be read with the same number of regressions; only the proportional increase is independent.

Although not significantly correlated with RFI, word recognition was correlated with the other variables that we use to predict RFI in the following three models. Since our main interest is in the influence of these variables, we use word recognition as a suppressor variable which removes variance in the predictors which is not related to RFI.

## B.  Regressive Fixation Index and IQ

IQ predicted 21% of RFI variance; the higher the IQ the higher the RFI. The predicted variance was 31% with one additional subject included in the initial analysis. This subject was not included in the final analysis because she was two standard deviations from the regression line. However, further consideration of her performance suggested a possible explanation for the relationship between IQ and RFI. Her word recognition, orthographic, and phonological skills were relatively good, but she had the lowest IQ (91) and the lowest RFI in the disabled reader group. She also had the lowest comprehension score. This general description fits the "word caller" syndrome (Goodman, 1968; Huttenlocher & Huttenlocher, 1973).

It may be characteristic of low IQ disabled readers that they do not monitor their understanding of the text and do not regress when comprehension breaks down. Disabled readers with high intelligence may more carefully monitor their understanding and would regress when necessary to integrate earlier with later text for comprehension. Although this seems to be a reasonable explanation of the IQ effect, other interpretations are possible. IQ is also correlated with saccade length ($r = .48$), and the following analysis will show that saccade length is the most powerful single predictor for RFI. When the complete regression model with all variables is evaluated, it will be shown that most of the variance shared between IQ and RFI is based on saccade length. This raises another possible explanation for the interrelation between IQ, RFI, and saccade length. Eyes of the more intelligent readers may take larger steps through the text. Sometimes this may result in overshooting the preferred center of a word, causing a short corrective regression within the word (O'Regan, 1980; Kliegl, Olson, & Davidson, Chapter 19 of this volume). This type of regression may combine with the comprehension and context related regressions described earlier to produce the effect of IQ on RFI. More research is needed to evaluate the various interpretations. This will involve the examination of the component scores in the WISC and the relation of eye fixations to specific text locations.

## C.  Regressive Fixation Index and Saccade Length

Saccade length predicted a substantial 53% of the variance in RFI. Subjects who made longer saccades also made relatively more regressions. There are several possible reasons for this result. At the perceptual level discussed earlier, long saccades could result in more frequent overshooting of the optimal position for fixating a word. At the cognitive level, long saccades could produce more frequent regressions if the subjects' gathering of visual information sometimes raced too far ahead of processes such as phonological coding, and syntactic and semantic analysis. A third hypothesis is that long saccades reflect a general processing strategy that depends on contextual support in the decoding of words. This strategy could be related to higher demands for comprehension among disabled readers with high IQ as well as the need to compensate for weak orthographic or phonological coding skills. The relationship of these skills to the RFI will be shown next.

## D.  Regressive Fixation Index and Relative Phonological Skill

Relative phonological skill is defined as the difference between the weighted logarithm of phonological latency and the weighted logarithm of orthographic latency. The weights were chosen to maximize the correlation of the difference with RFI. The model accounted for 34% of the variance in RFI. (Adding a similar calculation for the error rates resulted in a nonsignificant increase to 38%.)

Recall that these two tasks were considered to be tests of independent word coding skills (Baron & Strawson, 1976). However, orthographic latency was not significantly correlated with RFI. Because the two tasks are so similar in experimental procedure, subtracting orthographic latency reduces variance in phonological latency that is not associated with phonological skill. This extraneous variance could include subjects' general adaptation to the experimental situation and speed–accuracy criteria. In addition to the above view of the orthographic task as a control for extraneous variance, the adjusted phonological score is not independent of the orthographic score. In other words, what we call relative phonological skill is phonological skill relative to the subject's orthographic skill.

The finding that relatively poor phonological skill was associated with a relatively higher frequency of regressions was predicted. Our hypothesis was that stronger phonological codes would be associated with a more sequential left-to-right scanning strategy as graphemes were decoded to phonemes. Relatively weak phonological codes would be associated with less sequential processing within words and more frequent regressions to previous words to reinstate contextual support for decoding unfamiliar words. Weak phonological memory codes may also cause rapid forgetting of preceding text, resulting in a greater need for regressive fixations (Mark, Shankweiler, Liberman, & Fowler, 1977). Further discussion of the reasons for the relationship between RFI and relative phonological skill will be presented after the results from the silent reading condition.

## VI.  Multiple Regression Models of Individual Differences

### A.  Disabled Readers in the Aloud Condition

We have introduced three variables that alone or by interaction were significantly related to RFI during reading aloud. These variables were IQ, saccade length, and relative phonological latency. Word recognition skill served as a suppressor variable in all of the previous analyses. However, note that RFI variance related to word recognition (3%), IQ (21%), saccade length (53%), and phonological skill (34%) totals to 111%. Obviously there is some overlap in the variance these variables share with RFI. Composite Model 1 in Table 26.4 presents a hierarchical regression wherein the variables are entered in the order of word recognition, IQ, saccade length, and relative phonological latency. The $R$-squares show that for this sequence we always obtain significant increments. Relative phonological skill, entered on the final step, accounted for an additional 22% of the variance, compared with 31% when it was entered without IQ or saccade length. This regression model accounts for 78% of the RFI variance. To assess the

TABLE 26.4
Complete Models for Groups and Conditions

Disabled readers (aloud):

| | | | | | | |
|---|---|---|---|---|---|---|
| RFI = | −4.41WR + | 0.20IQ + | 19.60SL + | (32.55PL − | 101.26OL) + | 129.69 |
| SE: | .92 | .10 | 3.08 | 13.45 | 19.25 | 52.74 |
| R-square change: | .03 | .21 | .56 | | .78 | |

Disabled readers (silent):

| | | | | | | |
|---|---|---|---|---|---|---|
| RFI = | −4.91WR + | 0.36IQ + | 13.53SL + | (11.96PL − | 36.43OL) + | 3.55 |
| SE: | 1.97 | .19 | 4.18 | 27.63 | 43.32 | 115.09 |
| R-square change: | .02 | .22 | .49 | | .51 | |

Normal readers (aloud):

| | | | | | | |
|---|---|---|---|---|---|---|
| RFI = | −4.21WR + | 0.06IQ + | 14.09SL − | (18.21PL − | 55.08OL) − | 112.10 |
| SE: | 3.08 | .20 | 4.37 | 38.66 | 64.22 | 193.34 |
| R-square change: | .03 | .08 | .36 | | .38 | |

Normal readers (silent):

| | | | | | | |
|---|---|---|---|---|---|---|
| RFI = | −4.75WR − | 0.14IQ + | 7.29SL + | (19.32PL + | 4.82OL) + | 7.89 |
| SE: | 3.93 | .23 | 3.86 | 47.50 | 72.61 | 196.32 |
| R-square change: | .06 | .06 | .16 | | .18 | |

RFI: Regressive fixation index
WR: Word recognition
IQ: WISC
SL: Saccade length
PL: Phonology latency
OL: Orthographic latency
SE: Standard errors of regression coefficients

independent contribution of the variables in the model they were excluded one at a time and the decrement of the $R$-square was tested for significance. It can be seen in Table 26.4 that excluding phonological skill caused a drop to 56% of the variance. Additional analyses showed that the exclusion of word recognition left 60%, dropping IQ left 75%, and dropping saccade length left 46%. IQ was the only variable that did not make a significant difference in the variance accounted for. Most of its variance is shared with the other variables, particularly saccade length.

## B. Disabled Readers in the Silent Condition

The second model in Table 26.4 presents the results for the disabled readers in the silent condition. A significant difference between the aloud and silent models is the absence of an independent phonological skill effect in the silent condition. A possible reason for this difference is that the vocalization task presented an additional processing burden that may have been magnified for those who were weak in phonological skill, leading to greater word recognition, comprehension, and memory problems, and more associated regressions in the aloud condition. A related explanation would be that those who are slow in the generation of phonological codes would often find their eyes too far ahead of their voice in the aloud condition. In the silent condition, lexical access could be achieved visually and the slow generation of implicit phonological codes (postlexical access) would not require regressive fixations.

Our initial working hypothesis was that poor phonological skill would lead to more frequent regressions as the subject used contextual and visual information to aid in decoding unfamiliar words and focused less on the sequential phonemic decoding of letter patterns within words. We expected this hypothesized relation between eye movements and phonological skill to be valid for both aloud and silent reading conditions. Its absence in the silent condition suggests that the deployment of visual attention, indicated by RFI with these reading materials, is not systematically affected by phonological coding skill. Other eye movement parameters are being evaluated for their relation to relative phonological skill, and additional subjects are being tested with more difficult reading material. The materials in the present study were relatively easy, and the presence of more unfamiliar words may generate relationships between phonological skill and RFI in silent reading.

### C.  Normal Readers in Silent and Aloud Conditions

The only significant effect for normal readers was the $R$-square change of .08 to .36 when saccade length was entered in the aloud condition. A nonsignificant change of 10% was associated with saccade length in the silent condition. Thus, the only consistent effect across good and disabled readers was the relation between saccade length and the RFI. The absence of phonological effects for the good readers may be due to the fact that the good readers were generally high in phonological skill with much less variance. Also, the most difficult text, which all of the good readers read, was at the eighth-grade difficulty level. The relatively easy text and lack of word recognition problems may also have limited the effects of IQ.

## VII.  Conclusions

Our perspective on eye movements and reading disability is quite different from most previous research. The major focus is on individual differences *within* the reading disabled group, and several eye movement, reading process, and cognitive variables are explored simultaneously. What have we learned from this approach? First, it is clear that there were substantial individual differences between disabled readers that were independent of general reading skill. They varied widely in their relative frequency of regressive eye movements, length of saccades, IQ, and visual and phonological coding skills. Second, there was a strong relationship across individuals between different eye movement parameters. Those subjects who made longer saccades also tended to make relatively more regressive fixations. Third, there was a significant relationship between IQ, the RFI, and saccade length. Disabled readers with higher IQ tended to make longer saccades and have a higher RFI. Fourth, subjects who were weak in relative phonological skill tended to have a higher RFI, but only when reading aloud. Finally, all of the above relations were at least partially independent of word recognition skill. In establishing the existence of the above relations, we have raised new questions about their basis. Several hypotheses were offered to explain each of the relations. Additional analyses and research are needed to decide between them.

A general eye movement sequencing deficit in disabled readers has recently been proposed by Pavlidis (1981; Chapter 25 of this volume). He found that his reading disabled subjects had fixation problems in tracking a light that changed positions along a horizontal line. We have not observed this type of problem in our subjects while calibrating them, and the complex relations found between our variables do not seem explainable by a general eye movement deficit. Also, we did not confirm previous case study reports of some disabled readers' "irrepressible tendency" to scan text in a right to left direction (Ciuffreda, Bahill, Kenyon, & Stark, 1976; Gruber, 1962; Pirozzolo and Rayner, 1978b; Zangwill & Blakemore, 1972). These cases must be rare in our reading disabled population. Some disabled readers in our sample made more regressions than others, but these regressions were closely associated with word coding and higher cognitive processes.

# References

Baron, J., & Strawson, C. (1976). Orthographic and word-specific mechanisms in reading words. *Journal of Experimental Psychology: Human Perception & Performance, 2,* 386–393.

Camp, B., & McCabe, L. (1977). *Denver Reading and Spelling Test.* Denver, Colorado.

Ciuffreda, K. J., Bahill, A. T., Kenyon, R. V., & Stark, L. (1976). Eye movements during reading: Case reports. *American Journal of Optometry and Physiological Optics, 53,* 389–395.

Coltheart, M. (1981). Disorders of reading and their implications for models of normal reading. *Visible Language, 15,* 245–286.

Davidson, B. J. (1981). A rotating buffer system for on-line collection of eye monitor data. *Behavior Research Methods & Instrumentation, 13,* 112–114.

Davidson, B. J., Kliegl, R., & Olson, R. K. (1981). *Individual differences in reading disorders.* Paper presented at the meeting of the Midwestern Psychological Association, Detroit, April.

Goodman, K. S. (1968). The psycholinguistic nature of the reading process. In K. S. Goodman (Ed.), *The psycholinguistic nature of the reading process.* Detroit: Wayne State University Press.

Gruber, E. (1962). Reading ability, binocular coordination and the ophtalmograph. *Archives of Ophthalmology, 67,* 183–190.

Huttenlocher, P. R., & Huttenlocher, J. A. (1973). A study of children with hyperlexia. *Neurology, 23,* 1107–1116.

Kliegl, R. (1981). Automated and interactive analysis of eye-fixation data in reading. *Behavior Research Methods and Instrumentation, 13,* 115–120.

Kliegl, R., & Olson, R. K. (1981). Reduction and calibration of eye-monitor data. *Behavior Research Methods and Instrumentation, 13,* 107–111.

Mark, L. S., Shankweiler, D., Liberman, I. Y., & Fowler, C. A. (1977). Phonetic recoding and reading difficulty in beginning readers. *Memory & Cognition, 5,* 623–629.

Marshall, J. C., & Newcombe, F. (1973). Patterns of paralexia: A psycholinguistic approach. *Journal of Psycholinguistic Research, 2,* 175–199.

O'Regan, J. K. (1980). The control of saccade size and fixation duration in reading: The limits of linguistic control. *Perception & Psychophysics, 28,* 112–117.

Pavlidis, G. Th. (1981). Do eye movements hold the key to dyslexia? *Neuropsychologia, 19,* 57–64.

Pirozzolo, F. J., & Rayner, K. (1978). Disorders of oculomotor scanning and graphic orientation in developmental Gerstmann syndrome. *Brain & Language, 5,* 119–126. (a)

Pirozzolo, F. J., & Rayner, K. (1978). The neural control of eye movements in acquired and developmental reading disorders. In H. Avakian–Whitaker & H. A. Whitaker (Eds.), *Advances in neurolinguistics and psycholinguistics.* New York: Academic Press. (b)

Rozin, P., & Gleitman, L. (1977). The reading process and the acquisition of the alphabetic principle. In A. S. Reber & D. Scarborough (Eds.), *Toward a psychology of reading.* New Jersey: Erlbaum.

Saffran, E. M., & Marin, O. S. M. (1977). Reading without phonology: Evidence from aphasia. *Quarterly Journal of Experimental Psychology, 29,* 515–525.

Satz, P., & Morris, R. (1981). Learning disability subtypes: A review. In F. J. Pirozzolo & M. C. Wittrock (Eds.), *Neuropsychological and cognitive processes in reading.* New York: Academic Press.

Shallice, T., & Warrington, E. K. (1980). Single and multiple component central dyslexia syndromes. In M. Coltheart, K. Patterson, & J. C. Marshall (Eds.), *Deep dyslexia.* London: Routledge and Kegan Paul.

Spache, G. D. (1963). *Diagnostic reading scales.* Monterey, New York: McGraw-Hill.

Tinker, M. A. (1965). *Bases for effective reading.* Minneapolis: University of Minnesota Press.

Zangwill, O., & Blakemore, C. (1972). Dyslexia: Reversal of eye movements during reading. *Neuropsychologia, 10,* 371–373.

# 27

# Abnormal Patterns of Normal Eye Movements in Specific Dyslexia[1]

## I.  Introduction

In this chapter, we have surveyed three issues of interest concerning eye movement pattern diagnostic specificity in the dyslexias. The first issue addressed is the occurrence of the reverse staircase reading eye movement pattern and whether or not it is a pathognomonic sign of specific dyslexia. Early reports often associated it with a faulty return sweep ability in certain readers. However, the general impression in the recent literature is that the reverse staircase is a reading pattern unique to, but relatively uncommon in, specific dyslexia (Cuiffreda, Bahill, Kenyon, & Stark, 1976; Elterman, Abel, Daroff, Dell'Osso, & Bornstein, 1980). These successive, regressive saccades in the reading pattern also have been associated with the notion that there is a tendency for certain dyslexics to read in an opposite direction (Zangwill & Blakemore, 1972; Pirozzolo & Rayner, 1978a). Our findings argue not only for a broader prevalence of the pattern, but also for more than one cause in support of its employment.

The second issue involves the search for a nonverbal test that could provide the positive objective diagnostic for specific dyslexia. We limited the scope of our inquiry to the parameters of the following question: Can the nonverbal eye movement task of tracking a regularly and sequentially shifting target be used to delineate dyslexia? Recent findings in the literature (Pavlidis, 1981) suggested that such a delineation could be made. Nevertheless, the normal tracking re-

[1]This study received support from the NCC 2-86 cooperative agreement, NASA-AMES Research Center while Jones was a University of California Chancellor's Fellow.

481

sponse of the eye movement system to a regularly moving stimulus is subject to a complex prediction effect, and this variable is not widely understood.

The third and final issue is that of the interpretation of an abnormal reading eye movement record when all other information is excluded. Hartje (1972) demonstrated that it was difficult to use the standard reading eye movement task recording to either assess the contribution of an oculomotor disorder to reading difficulty or detect the presence of a reading disability. However, geometrically transformed text (Kolers, 1968) was used by Pirrozzolo and Rayner (1978a) to increase the diagnostic value of the reading eye movement record in a case of developmental Gerstmann syndrome. We have applied a similar reading test with some success in a case of congenital nystagmus.

Our address to these issues was based upon a correlative review of pertinent findings in the literature. In this preliminary investigation, we have presented illustrative short case reports that helped us to a positive appreciation of the complexity of the issues undertaken here.

## A.  The Reverse Staircase Reading Pattern

Successive backward eye movements that occurred during reading were first recorded early in this century. The terms *reverse stairway* (Gruber, 1962) and *reverse staircase* (Cuiffreda *et al.*, 1976) are, of course, analagous and were coined to denote the phenomenon because it opposed the characteristic, consistently forward staircase type of pattern common in normal reading eye movement recordings. This reverse reading pattern may also be described as a series or set of successive regressions and fixation pauses. It may be complete, that is, extending across the entire horizontal extent of text line width, or incomplete. We found that the phenomenon, when it was presented in the literature in the complete form, was usually associated with some form of reading difficulty or disability.

### 1.  HISTORICAL ASSOCIATION WITH RETURN SWEEP ABNORMALITY

The first published recording of a reverse staircase type of reading eye movement was made by Schmidt (1917), who reported: "In certain cases the return sweep is interrupted rather than continuous . . . ," and "this [return sweep abnormality] . . . is characteristic of only a few individuals, but where it does occur it tends to persist line after line." Several months later, Gray (1917) also reported on the reverse reading pattern, which he noted in the eye movement recordings of an experienced reader. Gray (1917) attributed this finding to a shift in attention on the part of the reader to an earlier point in the text for purposes of comprehension. Buswell (1922) noted that one of the subjects in his study lacked the "habit" of making a normal return sweep. He reported: "The subject [at the end of a line of print] . . . dropped down to the line below and then moved in a backward direction to the beginning of the next line." Buswell (1922) noted finding this reverse pattern in nearly half of the lines of print that the subject read and hypothesized that the reverse pattern represented a response to confusion.

Based upon the results of his reading eye movement studies, Anderson (1937) concluded that the reverse pattern denoted an inadequate return sweep and that it was employed by the reader to locate the beginning of the next line.

*Linear dyslexia* was a term ascribed by Wertham (1954) to children who demonstrated a reading impairment when attempting to read lines of print in succession. Wertham (1954) also believed the abnormality to be related to poor reading habits that could be reinforced by the excessive reading of comic books. Mosse and Daniels (1959) found that children with linear dyslexia at times also reversed the sequence of words when reading, and they concluded that the condition "occurs most frequently as a result of faulty reading habits acquired at an early age." Recordings by Taylor (1959) showed complete reverse staircases in two grade school students who, he believed, had not developed a proper "directional attack" on lines of print. Taylor (1959) also reported that children were often found who kept place while reading by retracing over a completed line with eye movement and who would then drop down to the beginning of the next line of print. Gruber (1962) attributed the "reverse stairway" pattern to readers who lacked control in executing the return sweep when reading, and who compensated for this deficiency by reversing fixation over the line just read. A classic example of the reverse pattern was clearly presented in one segmental reading record (Gruber, 1962); further information on the subject's reading performance or ability was not provided. However, we noted that the forward staircases shown immediately before and after the reverse sequence, in that instance, were very regular and only presented characteristics commonly associated with dyslexics' eye movements.

## 2. HISTORICAL ASSOCIATION WITH READING DISABILITY OR DIFFICULTY

Buswell (1922) examined the order of fixation eye movements of a first-grade student with less mature reading habits than her peers. He found that this subject read slowly with frequent use of short backward movements and commented: "Such eye movements indicate that the mental processes of the reader are chiefly concerned with a detailed analysis of words." Several instances of incomplete reverse staircases that occurred within lines of print were shown in the representative reading eye movement records of Buswell (1937), and we noted they were made by "poor" readers exclusively. Instances of incomplete reverse staircases were noted to be present in the recordings by Taylor (1959) of two 14-year-old boys before, but not after, they completed a remedial reading program of instruction for their poor reading ability. Upon close inspection, we noted two complete reverse staircases in the recordings by Hallpike (in Critchley, 1970) of a 31-year-old dyslexic reading elementary text. The reverse patterns occurred at the end sentences, apparently in place of return sweeps.

Zangwill and Blakemore (1972) found many right-to-left saccades in the reading eye movement record of a young adult dyslexic. Finding a normal oculomotor response and tachistoscopic word recognition in their subject, they hypothesized that the successive regressions were due to an "irrepressible tendency" for the dyslexic to read to the left. Ciuffreda *et al.* (1976) reported on the case of an adult dyslexic who exhibited at times incomplete "reverse staircase" patterns during reading. They (Cuiffreda *et al.*, 1976) argued that the incomplete reverse patterns in their dyslexic patient, which occurred within the lateral text boundaries and in the presence of normal return sweeps, did not support the hypothesis of an underlying return sweep abnormality as a cause. Pirrozolo and Rayner (1978a) recorded the reading eye movements of a 23-year-old patient with developmental Gerstmann syndrome and found instances of reverse staircases during the reading of standard text. They found that opposed staircases were eliminated and that reading performance was improved when this patient read text that was oriented upside-down. They concluded that the demonstrated tendency on the part this subject to read in a right-to-left direction reflected a spatial disorder, which was also supported by neuropsychological test results. Pavlidis (1978) reported that the regressions of dyslexics sometimes appeared in clusters of two or more in their reading records. Several incomplete reverse staircases are shown in the recordings (Pavlidis, 1981) of a dyslexic subject, in addition to incomplete reverse staircases made by a slow reader. In Adler's (1976) recordings, we noted several complete reverse staircases that were used by a specific dyslexic child who read a test paragraph above his measured grade level. Elterman *et al.* (1980) showed records of reverse staircases used by one dyslexic child reading above-grade-level text, used by another in lieu of a return sweep, and used by a third during dot symbol simulated reading but not during actual reading.

### 3. HISTORICAL ASSOCIATION WITH VISUAL SYSTEM ABNORMALITY

Remond, Leserve, and Gabersek (1957) found an abnormal number of regressive movements in the "scopogramme" of a patient with Broca's aphasia. Critchley (1953), without direct reference to fragmented return sweeps, noted that one reading problem individuals with a left homonymous hemianopia could have was that of locating the beginning of the next line of print. In a patient with a right hemianopia, Remond *et al.* (1957) found the amplitude of the progressions to be small. When the amplitude of the progression was of normal amplitude, a regression or "verification" often resulted. In contrast to that case, they found the reading eye movements of a patient with a left hemianopia to be fairly normal (although we noted one incomplete reverse staircase in the scopogram) with the exception of constant overshoot on the return sweep that necessitated a large rightward saccade to the beginning of the next line of print. "Overstepping" at the end of a return sweep was later noted by Gruber (1962) who attributed it to a "lack of lateral control of the eyes." Gassel and Williams (1963) reported that 12 of 18 patients with a left homonymous hemianopia had fragmented return sweeps in their reading eye movement patterns. Taylor's (1959) recordings showed reverse staircases in individual cases of Duane's syndrome, exotropia, hyperphoria, and monocular amblyopia. It was interesting to note an absence of the reverse patterns in Taylor's (1959) recordings of other subjects with the same or similar ocular abnormalities.

### 4.  HISTORIC ASSOCIATION WITH THE NORMAL READER

Presentation of the complete reverse staircase in the reading records of normal subjects was limited to Gray's (1917) finding of one such occurrence in an adult reading poetry for comprehension and Taylor's (1937) recordings of a young speed reader. The literature did, however, reveal numerous instances of incomplete reverse staircases in the reading records of normals as follows: Bayle (1942), Remond *et al.* (1957), Taylor (1959), Leserve (1968), recordings by Hallpike in Critchley (1970), Hartje (1972), Adler (1976), and Pavlidis (1981).

## B.  Methods

Horizontal eye movements were recorded using the infrared oculographic technique (Stark, Bahill, Cuiffreda, & Phillips, 1977). The reading stimuli consisted of test paragraph cards graded for reading ability (Educational Development Laboratories, Inc.).

Our clinical cases of specific dyslexia were diagnosed with exclusion criteria. The intelligence scores (WISC-R) of this group were above 90. The reading scores for this group (WRAT) showed at least a one grade-level deficit. Individuals with uncorrected refractive error, strabismus, amblyopia, severe emotional disturbance, inadequate opportunity to learn, or gross neurological deficit were excluded from the specific dyslexic category. Six children, ranging from 10 to 12 years of age, qualified as specific dyslexics for purposes of this study.

## C.  Results

### 1.  REVERSE STAIRCASES IN SPECIFIC DYSLEXICS

Reverse staircases occurred in the reading eye movements of all six specific dyslexics. Incomplete reverse occurred on the average of 1 out of every 3 lines read, whereas the complete pattern occurred approximately once for every 20 lines. The hypothesis that the mean duration of fixation pauses were less than the mean duration of midline fixation pauses was investigated with the Wilcoxon test. The test statistic showed the reverse staircase to be composed of significantly

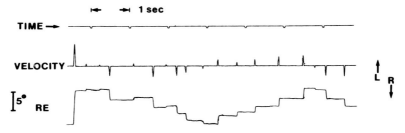

**FIGURE 27.1.** *The reading eye movement of a young specific dyslexic showing an occurrence of a complete reverse staircase. Note the prolonged fixation pauses within the reverse pattern.*

shorter fixation durations at the .05 level. In Case 1, an 11-year-old girl with specific dyslexia, used a complete reverse staircase composed of uncharacteristically long fixation durations, once while reading a paragraph of 10 lines (Figure 27.1). In all other complete reverse staircase occurrences in this case, the fixation durations were considerably less.

## 2. REVERSE STAIRCASES IN THE ABSENCE OF DYSLEXIA

In Case 2, a normal 19-year-old university student employed a reverse staircase while she read a test paragraph containing technical information. Interestingly, reverse staircases were not found in further extensive eye movement recording of this subject while she read nontechnical, standardized test paragraphs.

Individuals with spontaneous superior oblique palsies often complain of sudden diplopia and reading difficulty (Glaser, 1978). In Case 3, a 35-year old clinical psychologist complained of intermittent double vision and of lines of print often "running together" when reading. It was found that his complaint was due to a binocular misalignment caused by a right superior oblique paresis of unknown origin. During reading, he would occasionally close one eye, which resolved the reading disturbance, but later denied a knowledge of doing so for that reason. In contrast to monocular reading conditions that were normal, his binocular reading eye movement record was often replete with reverse staircases (Figure 27.2).

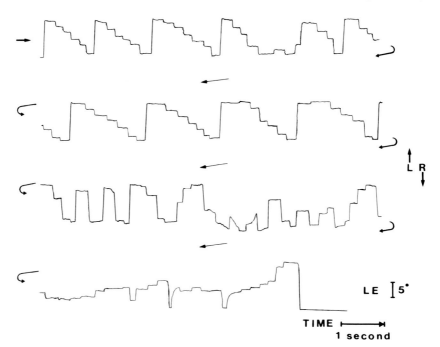

**FIGURE 27.2.** *This is the reading record of an adult patient with a right superior oblique paresis. The record begins at the upper left corner and should be read from left-to-right. Note the progressive breakdown the forward staircase pattern to reverse staircases, blink artifacts, and finally eye lid closure.*

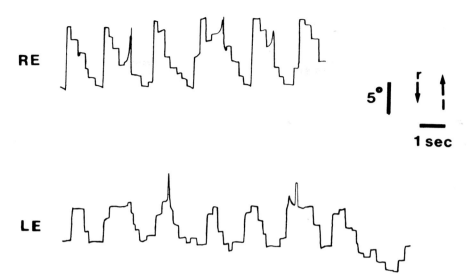

**FIGURE 27.3.** *The eye movement record of a patient with a demyelinating disease who read text with the normal eye (upper tracing) and who later attempted to read with the left eye and a central scotoma while the seeing eye was occluded (bottom tracing). Note the staircase fragments and the to-and-fro searching movements during attempted reading in the bottom tracing.*

In Case 4, a 21-year-old woman had been recently diagnosed as having optic neuritis and demyelenating disease. A deep central scotoma was found to be present in the visual field of the left eye in contrast to normal central field findings in the right eye. Oculomotor responses to random target tracking and reading tasks were normal under binocular conditions. When presented with standard text and with the normal (right) eye occluded, she reported seeing peripherally what she knew to be reading material, but could not read it. When directed to attempt reading despite all, she used searching eye movements including "reverse staircase" fragments during the futile exercise (Figure 27.3).

In Case 5, a 55-year-old man with a right homonymous hemianopia with macular sparing, was found to have a reading eye pattern characterized by episodes of reverse staircases, habitual undershoot of the return sweep, reduced overall reading performance (approximately 140 words per min with comprehension), and an overall regression rate of approximately 30%.

## D. Discussion

Our findings with regard to the reverse staircase pattern were in keeping with its previous historical associations. The reverse staircase reading eye movement pattern is not pathognomic of specific dyslexia, but we found it to be prevalent in that group's reading records. We hoped that some clue as to the basic nature the pattern could be obtained from its temporal characteristics. Reverse staircase fixation durations for the dyslexics were found to be shorter than the fixation durations following mid-line progressions. This suggested a "Zuber effect" (Cuiffreda *et al.*, 1976), that is, less verbal processing occurred during the reverse staircases, and the component fixation pauses were more closely related to the geometrically based saccadic eye movement latency or refractory period (Abrams & Zuber, 1972). This temporal effect in the reverse staircase was also informally noted in the segmental reading records shown in studies by Gruber (1962), Zangwill and Blakemore (1972), Cuiffreda *et al.* (1976), and Adler (1976). The long reverse fixation pauses noted in Case 1 (Figure 27.1) suggested a rare instance of actual reverse reading.

The stair-step eye movement pattern may be a fundamental type of visual search strategy. Aslin and Salapatek (1975) found that staircases were the normal pattern of infant eye movements, that is, the infants did not make large saccades directly to the target stimulus and similarly did not respond with smooth pursuit eye movements during ramp tracking.

The reverse staircase may be related to picture eye movement strategies. Akira Watanabe (personal communication and film of eye movement) used an electronic feedback device that imposed artificial tunnel vision upon a reading subject. Under such conditions, the subject made reverse staircases that disappeared when normal viewing conditions were returned. The subject made similar eye movement responses when he viewed pictures under the same visual conditions. When the central visual field was artificially masked, the reader responded with primarily horizontal to-and-fro searching movements that appeared to be guided by peripheral viewing; we noted similar searching patterns during attempted reading in the analogous neurophysiologically disrupted visual condition in Case 4 (Figure 27.3).

Hemianopic visual field defect may also contribute to reverse staircase use during reading. Meienberg, Zangemeister, Rosenberg, Hoyt, and Stark (1981) found that hemianopic patients often omitted head movement and made searching "stairstep" sequences of saccades into the blind hemifield in response to lateral target movement. Gassel and Williams (1963) noted a similarity between the pattern of the fragmented return sweep during reading and the pattern of eye movements when retracing a line to the left in patients with left homonymous hemianopia. In three patients with a right homonymous hemianopia and "pure" dyslexia, Gassel and Williams (1963) noted that their return sweep eye movements were normal, but "in these cases movements to the right were infrequent and irregular, and there were many uncorrected errors." In Case 5, a patient with a right blind hemifield, the habitual return sweep undershoot and reverse staircases that we noted in his recording were difficult to explain based upon the visual field status alone. Progressions to the right were smaller, but an abnormal number of regressions occurred in only half the lines he read. The patient might have inadvertently lost his place while reading, which would account for the concentration of reverse staircases at certain times in the recording; unfortunately, we had no way to be certain of this without a vertical eye movement record (Elterman *et al.*, 1980).

The visual confusion during reading caused by diplopic images was not resolved with the use of reverse staircases by Case 3. It was noteworthy to us that the reverse movements were resorted to before the closure of one eye and that the patient preferred to read with two eyes despite the resulting difficulty.

The instance of a reverse staircase in a normal reader (Case 2) drew our immediate attention during the recording session. It appeared to us, upon the reader's subjective report that she had rechecked the details of a certain statement in a technically oriented paragraph, to be related to comprehension effort. The amount of reading effort required to comprehend text and the complexity of the text may in some way account for the rarity of reports or presentation of complete reverse staircases in normals in the literature.

It is our impression, from all of the foregoing, that the reverse staircase reading pattern is employed or resorted to by the reader as a response to confusion. It is composed of normal eye movements. Its occurrence during reading may represent use of a fundamental, primarily geometrical eye movement search strategy that is secondary to a difficulty encountered with certain aspects of the physical reading process or comprehension effort. We thus find ourselves in agreement with the early conclusions of Gray (1917) and Buswell (1922) on this subject.

## II.  Eye Movement Response to Regularity in Sequential Target Patterns

The consensus in the literature supports the presence of a primary oculomotor deficit in at least some types of dyslexia. We will only mention several studies that support such a conclusion, since a thorough review of the literature concerning recorded eye movement task performance and dyslexia is available elsewhere (Pavlidis, 1981).

Gilbert (1953) was the first to associate abnormal simulated reading performance with poor reading ability. Leserve (1968) found that the eye movements of specific dyslexic children during successive fixations of fixed symbols was abnormal and presented a true ocular dyspraxia in contrast to her control group. She concluded that there was a maturation of eye movement performance independent of reading that depended upon spatial function. Elterman et al. (1980) reported abnormal successive fixation eye movement in two of five dyslexic children when they responded to a symbol-simulation reading stimulus and concluded that this finding supported the hypothesis of a primary oculomotor deficit in certain cases of developmental dyslexia.

A study by Pavlidis (1981) found that dyslexics as a group were unable to accurately follow sequential target movement within normal limits. The inaccuracies were attributed to "oculomotor control problems and/or sequential order deficit or faulty feedback between the two." The nature of normal predictive eye movement control and its role in producing inaccuracies under such test circumstances was not made clear.

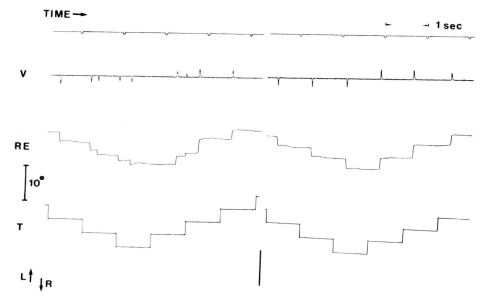

**FIGURE 27.4.** *An episode of inaccurate tracking eye movements (left record) and of accurate tracking (right record) in a young specific dyslexic girl as she attempted to follow the sequential target displacements illustrated at the bottom of each record.*

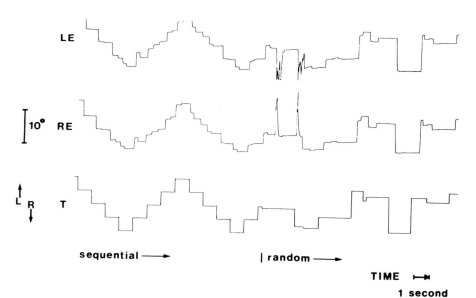

**FIGURE 27.5.** *The eye movement record of a young specific dyslexic boy who tracked sequential target displacements followed 2 sec later by a random tracking task. Prediction is evidenced by short, zero, or positive saccadic latencies that dominate sequential tracking record. A short episode of accurate sequential can be noted at the beginning of the record.*

## A.    Methods

Eye movement was measured as described previously. The task consisted of tracking a small spot target generated on an oscilloscope. Computer controlled target movement patterns were either random or regularly sequential in amplitude and frequency. Instructions for the task were: "Keep your eyes on the spot of light."

## B.    Results

Case 1, an 11-year-old girl with specific dyslexia (previously presented), was able to track a regular sequential target, at times with episodes of inaccuracy (Figure 27.4).

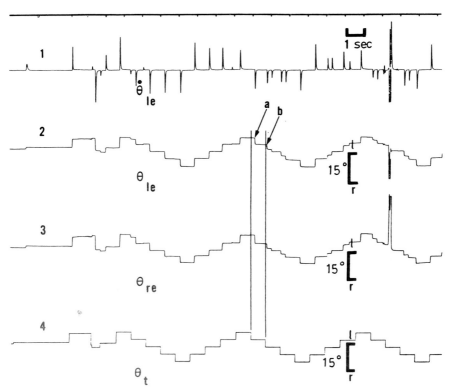

**FIGURE 27.6.**  *This is the eye movement recording of a normal young woman who followed a random target movement pattern followed by the first sequential tracking task of the session. Tracing 1 is the velocity of the left. Tracings 2,3, and 4 are horizontal records of the left eye, right eye, and target movement respectively. Arrow "a" indexes the normal delay of the eyes response to the target displacement (horizontal line), which in this instance is approximately 200 msec. Arrow "b" indexes a response delay of approximately 50 msec, which is short enough to indicate that the subject was preparing to make a saccade without waiting for the future target displacement.*

In Case 6, a 10-year-old boy with specific dyslexia, we found irregular eye tracking of the sequential target, possibly due to normal predictive guessing errors (Figure 27.5). Random target tracking, on the other hand, showed eye movement response latencies consistent with nonpredictive response.

Case 7, a normal 19-year-old university student, first tracked a randomly displaced horizontal stimulus spot followed by a sequential eye tracking task. She tracked the random target without difficulty, and this was also the case for the first left to right cycle of the sequential target. On the second and subsequent sequential cycles, tracking errors predominated. Inaccuracies desisted upon return to the random target mode but recurred within the first sequential cycle following this (Figure 27.6).

## C.    Discussion

Stark, Vossius, and Young (1962) found that apparent inaccuracies in the eye movements of normals as they tracked repetitive target displacements were due to varying amounts of over or under prediction. Random target displacements, on the other hand, usually elicited the standard delay in eye movement response. In Case 7, a normal adult, we noted nonpredictive error-free tracking eye movements during the first sequential cycle; the repetitive nature of the pattern had apparently not yet been recognized by the subject. We found that the dyslexics in our group showed small static refixation errors in sequential tracking and in random target tracking (Figures 27.4 and 27.5). Large amplitude saccadic errors, possibly due to anticipation, occurred occasionally during tracking of the predictable pattern but only after the first several jumps of the sequential target. In a recording by Pavlidis (1981) of a representative dyslexic subject tracking sequential lights, we noted that several saccadic errors were made when the target was stationary at the lateral extremes of the target displacement. Two examples of this occurred prior to the presumed first target movement in the task. These errors suggested to us a predictive response; the errors were in the appropriate direction and approximate amplitude for a future target displacement.

A target pattern need not be sequential for prediction to manifest itself. Meienberg et al. (1981) found that once an alternating pattern of target movement into and out of the blind hemifield of hemianopic patients was established, these patients would, if the target were extinguished while in the seeing field, make an eye movement into the blind field where the target was then expected to be. Eye movement abnormalities can be reflected in the sequential tracking pattern. Unfortunately, it is very difficult to assess the contribution of prediction, guessing, or abnormality to such a task without addition of a random task as a control.

Dyslexia is often associated with oculomotor disorders (Pavlidis, 1981). In investigations that distinguish specific from secondary dyslexia, eye movement abnormality in the latter category is more often found. In a study by Precht and Stemmer (1962) (cited in Critchley, 1970) of 50 school children with choreiform movements, they found 90% to have severe reading difficulties. In all of these cases, there were disturbances of conjugate eye movement and difficulty in fixation. Children with other obvious neurological signs were excluded from their study. Critchley (1970) pointed out that the group under study (Prechtl & Stemmer, 1962) was not related to the problem of specific dyslexia. The two dyslexic children who were reported by Elterman et al. (1980) to exhibit eye movement abnormalities during symbol simulated reading were also reported to have a history of seizure. We disagree that findings in such cases of secondary dyslexia support a primary oculomotor contribution to the reading disability characteristic of specific or developmental dyslexia. It is noteworthy, however, that the specific dyslexics were so delineated and we agree with Elterman et al. (1980) that "an ocularmotor disturbance should manifest an impairment even in a symbol simulation situation."

The unrelating nature of the reading disorder that is characteristic of specific dyslexia is reflected in this population's consistently abnormal reading eye movement patterns. The constancy of a given specific dyslexic's reading pattern abnormality stood in contrast, however, to the episodic nature of inaccuracies we found in their nonverbal sequential tracking tasks.

Assuming, for sake of argument, that a primary oculomotor deficit is the cause of the reading difficulty in specific dyslexia, then two hypotheses deserve consideration: First, if the oculomotor abnormality is intermittent or conditional, then one should expect episodes in the eye movement recordings and supportive testing corresponding to normal oculomotor function and reading ability. Conversely, if the oculomotor abnormality is constant and not conditional, then neither episodes corresponding to normal oculomotor function nor of normal reading ability should be evidenced in the eye movement recordings or supportive tests. Our experience, limited to a small group of specific dyslexics, has been that gross oculomotor abnormalities are not present, that tracking inaccuracies in response to predictable target displacements are episodic, and that the reading disability is unrelenting.

## III. Oculomotor Disorders and Reading

When nystagmus, a repetitive type of eye movement, is present in an individual, identification of fixation pauses, progressions, and regressions is difficult. Recordings of reading eye movements by Taylor (1959) showed the nystagmus superimposed upon the reading pattern of several subjects. He also noted an "unusual type" of nystagmus with an intermittent pattern that appears to be not nystagmus but saccadic intrusions. Nystagmoid head movements concurrent with ocular nystagmus may be compensatory and contribute to visual efficiency but act to further complicate the reading pattern (Metz, Jampolsky, & O'Meara, 1972; Gresty, Halmaygi, & Leech, 1976). Cuiffreda et al. (1976) presented the reading eye movement record of a 12-year-old girl with severe developmental complications and congenital jerk nystagmus with the fast phase to the right. Their (Cuiffreda et *al.*, 1976) reading recording of that case showed a nystagmoid pattern superimposed upon an extended forward staircase reading pattern. Hartje (1972), in a reading pattern comparison of normal subjects to aphasic patients, demonstrated the difficulty of deciding whether observed reading pattern abnormalities represented a verbal recognition disturbance or an oculomotor abnormality. However, using interpatient reading record comparisons Remond *et al.* (1957) were able to make a tentative distinction between the contribution of a right hemianopia and aphasia to reading difficulty based upon certain temporal characteristics of the hemianopic patient's reading eye movements.

## A.   Methods

A spot target ramp pattern provided a smooth pursuit stimulus for the subject to track. For comparison of results during reading of normally oriented material, a paragraph of text was geometrically transformed so that reading would proceed from right-to-left and from bottom-to-top of the test paragraph, for example "left the to this Read."

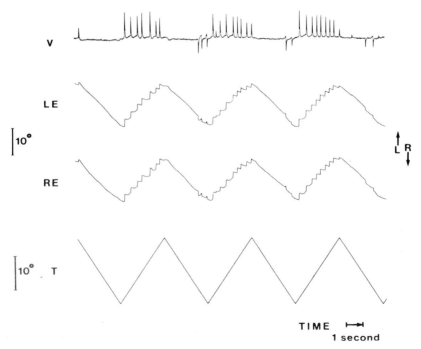

FIGURE 27.7. *The smooth pursuit eye movement record of a patient with congenital nystagmus tracking a ramp target pattern. When tracking the target to the right, the fast or jerk phase of the nystagmus was not exhibited.*

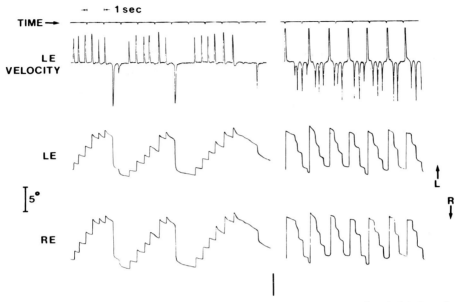

**FIGURE 27.8.** *The reading records of a patient with congenital nystagmus. The record on the left shows the response to reading geometrically transformed text characterized by superimposition of the nystagmus on the "forward" staircase and reduced reading performance. The right record, showing the response to reading normally oriented text, consisted of glissadic progressions and no regressions, which corresponded to very good reading performance.*

## B. Results

In Case 8, a 23-year-old student with a congenital left jerk nystagmus had complained of eye strain while studying for prolonged periods of time. His eye movement recordings showed suppression of the fast phase or jerk phase of the disorder when tracking ramp pattern target movement to the right (Figure 27.7). He read text rapidly to the right (approximately 500 words per min with comprehension), with regular glissadic saccades in the forward staircase and without regression (Figure 27.8). The overall eye movement pattern during reading was, in fact, very similar to that characteristic of a right dual jerk nystagmus (Daroff, R.B., Troost, A.B., & Dell'Osso, L.F., 1978). We also used transformed text (Kolers, 1968) as a diagnostic reading test (Finucci, Guthrie, Childs, Abbey, & Childs, 1976; Pirrozzolo & Rayner, 1978a) to study possible directional effects in this nystagmic patient. When the print was transformed (without letter reversal) such that reading now proceeded from right to the left along the horizontal lines of print, there was a marked slowing of the patient's reading rate (from 500 words to 200 words per min) with both phases of the nystagmus superimposed upon the "forward" staircases. He later reported that the print of the transformed text appeared "more blurred" and was therefore more difficult to read. A normal control demonstrated an overall reading performance mark of 360 words per min for the normal text and 279 words per min for the transformed text. When reading the transformed text, the nystagmus patient experienced twice the reduction from his basic reading performance compared to the normal control.

## C.  Discussion

The results in Case 8 clearly showed that this specific type of oculomotor disorder was reflected in the reading eye movement recording. The performance comparison with the normal control provides, perhaps, a rough guess regarding the specific contribution of this patient's nystagmus to reading under certain conditions, that is, the directional effect in the nystagmus during reading of transformed text demonstrated a hypothetical negative contribution if the patient were required by convention to read in right-to-left direction. Whether or not an opposite result would be found in a patient with the same form of nystagmus, but with a fast phase component to right, is not known. The abnormal appearance of the records remarkably belied the patient's actual performance in both cases. Gassel and Williams (1963) in their study on patients with right and left hemianopia reported: "Although normal reading records were associated with efficient reading considerably disturbed records were still compatible with good performance." The finding that good reading performance could be compatible with abnormal reading eye movement records was also demonstrated by Hartje (1972).

We found individual cases reported in literature to be of great value in helping to clarify our understanding of the various observations in normal and abnormal reading performance that we have made. Pirrozzolo and Rayner (1978b) presented several comprehensively documented cases of various types of aquired and developmental dyslexia with and without eye movement abnormalities and concluded that the nature of the patient's disorder was most often reflected in the reading eye movement pattern and that one cause alone, such as an underlying oculomotor deficit, could not explain the range of reading eye movement abnormality. Identification of isolation of those causes will undoubtedly continue to be the focus of much research effort, and we believe that as more knowledge of the adverse visual system conditions under which good reading performance is possible, it will permit a more accurate assessment of reading disability when it is coexistent with those conditions.

ACKNOWLEDGMENTS

We thank Emily Holden and Shirley Arao for help in the preparation of the manuscript.

# References

Abrams, S. G. & Zuber, B. L. (1972). Some temporal characteristics of information processing during reading. *Reading Research Quarterly, 8,* 40–51.

Adler, D. (1976). *Eye movements, scanpaths, and dyslexia*. Unpublished doctoral dissertation, University of California at Berkeley.

Adler-Grindberg, D., & Stark, L. (1978). Eye movements, scanpaths, and dyslexia. *American Journal of Optometry and Physiological Optics, 63,* 557–570.

Anderson, I. H. (1937). Studies of eye movements of good and poor readers. *Psychological Monographs, 48,* 1–35.

Aslin, R. N. & Salapatek, P. (1975). Saccadic localization of visual targets by the very young human infant. *Perception & Psychophysics, 17,* 293–302.

Bayle, E. (1942). The nature and causes of regressive movements in reading. *Journal of Experimental Education, 11*(1), 16–36.

Buswell, G. T. (1922). The fundamental reading habits: A study of their development. *Supplementary Educational Monographs*, 2, 1–150.

Critchley, M. (1953). *The parietal lobes*. London: Arnold.

Critchley, M. (1970). *The dyslexic child*. London: Heinemann.

Cuiffreda, K. J., Bahill, A. T., Kenyon, R. V., & Stark, L. (1976). Eye movements during reading: Case reports. *American Journal of Optometry and Physiological Optics, 53,* 389–395.

Daroff, R. B., Troost, B. T., & Dell'Osso, L. F. (1978). Nystagmus and related ocular oscillations. In T. D. Duane (Ed.), *Clinical Ophthalmology, 2*(11), 4.

Elterman, R. D., Abel, L. A., Daroff, R. B., Dell'Osso, L. F., & Bornstein, J. L. (1980). Eye movement patterns in dyslexic children. *Journal of Learning Disabilities, 13*(1), 16–21.

Finucci, J. M., Guthrie, J. T., Childs, A. L., Abbey, H., & Childs, B. (1976). The genetics of specific reading disability. *Annals of Human Genetics, 40*(1), 1–21.

Gassel, M. M., & Williams, D. (1963). Visual Function in patients with homonymous hemianopia, Part II, Oculomotor mechanisms. *Brain, 86*(1), 19–23.

Gilbert, L. C. (1953). Functional motor efficiency of eyes and its relation to reading. University of California Publications in Education, Vol. 2(3), 159–232.

Glaser, J. S. (1978). Infranuclear disorders of eye movements. In *Clinical Ophthalmology*, Vol. 2, T. D. Duane (Ed.), Maryland: Harper & Row.

Gray, C. T. (1917). Types of reading ability as exhibited through tests and laboratory experiments. *Supplementary Educational Monographs, 1*(5), 1–191.

Gresty, M., Halmaygi, G. M., & Leech, J. (1978). The relationship between head and eye movement in congenital nystagmus with head shaking: Objective recordings of a single case. *British Journal of Ophthalmology, 62,* 533–535.

Gruber, E. (1962). Reading ability, binocular coordination, and the ophthalmograph. *Archives of Ophthalmology, 67*(3), 280–288.

Hartje, W. (1972). Reading disturbances in the presence of oculomotor disorders. *European Neurology, 7,* 249–264.

Kolers, P. A. (1968). The recognition of geometrically transformed text. *Perception & Psychophysics, 3,* 57–64.

Leserve, N. (1968). L'Organisation du regard chez des enfants d'age scolaire, lecteurs normaux et dyslexiques. *Revue de Neuropsychiatrie Infantile, 16,* 323–349.

Leserve, N. (1976). Les mouvements oculaires d'exploration et lecture. *Bulletin D'Audiophonologie, 2,* 93.

Meienberg, O., Zangemeister, W. H., Rosenberg, M., Hoyt, W. F., & Stark, L. (1981). Saccadic eye movement strategies in patients with homonymous hemianopia. *Annals of Neurology, 9,* 537–544.

Metz, H. S., Jampolsky, A., & O'Meara, D. M. (1972). Congenital ocular nystagmus and nystagmoid head movements. *Americal Journal of Ophthalmology, 74*(6), 1131–1133.

Mosse, H. L., & Daniels, C. R. (1959). Linear dyslexia. *American Journal of Psychotherapy, 13,* 826–841.

Pavlidis, G. Th. (1978). The dyslexic's erratic eye movements; case studies, *Dyslexia Review, 1,* 22–28.

Pavlidis, G. Th. (1981). Sequencing, eye movements and the early objective diagnosis of dyslexia. In

G. Th. Pavlidis & T. R. Miles (Eds.), *Dyslexia research and its applications to education*. Chichester: John Wiley & Sons.

Pirozzolo, F. J., & Rayner, K. (1978). Disorders of oculomotor scanning and graphic orientation in developmental Gerstmann syndrome. *Brain & Language*, 5, 119–126. (a)

Pirozzolo, F. J., & Rayner, K. (1978). The neural control of eye movements in acquired and developmental reading disorders. In H. Avakian-Whitaker & H. A. Whitaker (Eds.), *Advances in neurolinguistics and psycholinguistics*. New York: Academic Press. (b)

Prechtl, H. F. R., & Stemmer, C. J. (1962). The coreiform syndrome in children. *Developmental Medicine & Child Neurology*, 4, 119–127.

Remond, A., Lesevre, N., & Gabersek, V. (1957). Approche d'une semeiologie electrographique du regard. *Revue Neurologie*, 96, 536–547.

Schmidt, W. A. (1917). An experimental study in the psychology of reading. *Supplementary Educational Monographs*, 1(2), 1–123.

Stark, L., Vossius, G., & Young, L. R. (1962). Predictive control of eye tracking movements. *I.R.E. Transactions on Human Factors in Electronics*, HFFE-3, 52–57.

Stark, L., Bahill, A. T., Cuiffreda, K. J., & Phillips, S. (1977). Neuro-Optometry: An evolving specialty clinic, *American Journal of Optometry & Physilogical Optics*, 54, 85–96.

Taylor, E. A. (1937). *Controlled reading*. Chicago: University of Chicago Press.

Taylor, E. A. (1959). *Eyes, visual anomalies and the fundamental reading skill*. New York: Reading and Study Skills Center.

Watanabe, A. *Personal communication and film study of reading eye movement and scanpaths*.

Wertham, F. (1954). *Seduction of the innocent*. New York: Rinehart.

Zangwill, O. L., & Blakemore, C. (1972). Dyslexia: Reversal of eye movements during reading. *Neuropsychologia*, 10, 371–373.

Francis J. Pirozzolo

# 28

# Eye Movements and Reading Disability

## I.   Introduction

This chapter addresses the question what can be learned about reading disability from eye movement behavior. Recent studies of normal readers have begun to provide a background against which we can judge the eye movement and reading behavior of normal and disabled readers. These studies, reviewed throughout this book, tell us above all that during reading the brain is constantly fed bits of perceptual and linguistic information about which rapid judgments must be made in order for the eye to be guided to places in the text that will most likely provide answers to the linguistic questions that are imposed by the text. Early research in this century on developmental reading disability showed some association between eye movement and visual perceptual disorders and reading failure, but closer scrutiny of the relationship between faulty eye movements and reading disability has shown that there is no causal association. Although a small percentage of disabled readers do show eye movement abnormalities, it has been suggested that the causal information processing may be visual–spatial disorientation and that faulty eye movements do not "cause" dyslexia (Pirozzolo & Rayner, 1978b).

The causal neurological problem in developmental reading disability has not been elucidated. Most disabled readers show no hard evidence of neuropathology (Pirozzolo & Hansch, 1982), although most have one or more of the "soft signs," including EEG abnormalities, speech difficulties, finger agnosia, directional disorientation, etc. There are now several studies that strongly suggest a structural abnormality underlying reading disorders. This work owes a debt to recent investi-

499

EYE MOVEMENTS IN READING:
PERCEPTUAL AND LANGUAGE PROCESSES

gations that point to an association between hemispheric specialization of language function and correlative anatomical asymmetries. Although it has been known for over 100 years that in most people the left cerebral hemisphere is specially endowed to carry out language functions, only recently have anatomical asymmetries been thought to account for this phenomenon. Geschwind and Levitsky (1968) studied 100 adult brains and found that 65% had wider left than right planum temporale, with 11% having a wider right planum and 24% having equal planum surface areas. The left planum temporale is roughly equivalent to the receptive language zone of the left hemisphere. This important finding, when combined with the demonstration by Witelson and Pallie (1973) that these asymmetries are present at birth, suggested that the additional neural tissue in the left hemisphere provides a more favorable anatomical site for language functions. Researchers agree that there is probably a strong association between anatomical and functional asymmetries, although several problems with this line of research still exist, the most important of which is determining why only 65 out of 100 brains have this left over right asymmetry, yet evidence from clinical studies suggests that 98% of right-handers and 60–70% of left-handers have left hemisphere language representation.

Autopsy data (Galaburda & Kemper, 1979) and data from a study of cerebral asymmetries revealed on computerized tomography (CT) (Hier, Perlo, Rosenberger, & LeMay, 1978) have shown that dyslexic subjects may, in fact, suffer from a reversal of the normal pattern of structural cerebral asymmetries. Galaburda and Kemper (1979) reported the results of a neuropathological examination of the brain of a 20-year-old disabled reader. Although the left hemisphere was consistently wider than the right along the anterior to posterior plane, there was no difference in size between the right and left planum temporale. The presumed language zones of the left hemisphere were not of normal appearance. There was evidence of atypical gyral pattern (polymicrogyria) and atypical cell-layer characteristics (cortical dysplasia). In addition to the limitations of a single case study, conclusions made on the basis of this report were cautious since the subject was also an epileptic. Additional suggestive evidence, however, comes from a study of the width of the parieto-occipital region on CT scan in learning disabled subjects (Hier, Perlo, Rosenberger, & LeMay, 1978). In this study, there was a strong relationship between so-called reversed cerebral asymmetry and developmental problems in speech and reading. If these and other related studies are supported by additional evidence of a subtle alteration in the cellular or biochemical structure of the language zones of the brain then some of the mystery of developmental reading disability will have been solved. Promising new methods that will undoubtedly be employed in the near future to attempt to measure in vivo differences between normal and disabled readers include positron emission tomography (PET) and nuclear magnetic resonance (NMR). PET scanning is a method that enables researchers to study the in vivo biochemistry of the brain. Early work has shown that cognitive activity can be mapped through the PET's assessment of cerebral glucose metabolism. Similarly, NMR is another imaging technique that employs low-energy radio waves to track the magnetic fields of polarized atomic nuclei. These methods can portray the activity of the brain by "lighting up" the pathways involved in certain cognitive tasks (Whitaker, 1979).

In the sections to follow, the importance of examining the eye's complex behavior will be demonstrated from a clinical perspective. A brief review will be provided of what can be learned about the brain from looking at the eye. The relationships between eye movements and brain function will be examined and a review of the role of eye movement disorders as a basis for developmental reading disability will follow.

## II. The Eye and the Brain

Examination of the behavior of the eye is one of the most accurate methods for determining the status of the human central nervous system (CNS). Clinicians can assess the conditions "behind the eye" in the brain by examining the eye's appearance and evaluating its movement. Brain disease can be signaled by increased intracranial pressure, which is manifested by papilledema, the lateral swelling and anterior elevation of the optic disc. From the appearance of the papilledema, it is even possible to determine how acute this process is through the examination of venous pulsations, distentions, hemorrhages, and the like. Evaluation of visual acuity and identification tells us the status of the retina, optic pathway, and the areas of the brain that govern discriminative vision and object recognition. Thorough examination of eye movements provides clues to the function of many CNS structures. The status of the six extraocular muscles that move the eye as well as the three cranial nerves that innervate these muscles can be determined by tests that require the subject to move the eyes in all directions. Problems at these lower levels are manifested in diplopia, gaze palsy, and nystagmus. An important part of the neurologic exam in coma is the assessment of the "doll's head" eye movement phenomenon, which gives evidence of the functioning of the very important deep brain structures. The eye movement exam also provides the clinician with a measure of the functioning of the cerebral cortex. Unilateral brain disease affecting the portions of the motor cortex and pre-motor cortex that program and launch saccadic eye movements prohibits eye movements to the contralateral side of space. It is even possible to determine whether the brain lesion affecting the patient is irritative (e.g., epilepsy) or destructive (e.g., stroke) by noting the direction of fixed gaze. In irritative lesions the gaze is fixed away from the side of the lesion and in destructive lesions the gaze is fixed toward the side of the lesion.

The examination of pursuit eye movements is important in the evaluation of diffuse disease processes, as well as in the assessment of certain psychiatric disorders. Careful testing of saccadic eye movements is known to provide useful data on the neurologic functioning of patients with a wide variety of brain disorders (see Pirozzolo, 1979). Furthermore, the tracking and recording of eye movements while subjects perform certain perceptual and cognitive tasks has provided a wealth of new information on the operating characteristics of the normal human brain. The objective of this chapter is to show how these studies contribute to knowledge about the normal reading eye movement process and to show how disordered eye movements may affect reading in children who have developmental reading disability.

## III.  Eye Movements Reflect Cognitive Processes

Some features of eye movement behavior reflect the brain's cognitive processing. This is a fact of neuropsychology that has received abundant documentation (see Rayner, 1978a, for review). Cognitive factors can affect saccadic latency and accuracy, but not saccadic velocity. In addition, cognitive factors can affect fixation duration, frequency, and density. Numerous studies (reviewed elsewhere in this book) provide the basic principles supporting these conclusions. These studies, carried out largely with normal subjects, point to relationships between cognitive behavior and movements of the eyes. In our laboratory we have used a variety of brain damaged and learning disabled subjects to confirm these findings.

Before the eye is launched into its ballistic flight to a predetermined region of visual space, computations about the location of an object to be fixated must be made. These computations are poorly understood, but probably involve subcortical brain mechanisms when the object is displaced by more than 10–15° from fixation (Frost & Poppel, 1976; Pirozzolo & Rayner, 1980) and cortical mechanisms when the object is nearer the fovea. This sensory information must be transmitted to brain mechanisms that perform motor execution. A decision is reached to launch a saccade to a specific region and the eye movement is initiated. Visual feedback occurs at some point at or near the end of the saccade and corrections to the motor program are made through corrective saccades. The initiation of a saccade, therefore, is under the control of a complex neural network that is heavily influenced by visual–spatial cognitive operations. Patients with Alzheimer's disease, a degenerative disease causing progressive intellectual deterioration (dementia), have profound impairments in saccadic latency (Pirozzolo & Hansch, 1981). Although normal elderly people are only slightly slower in initiating saccades than normal young people, dementia patients have eye movement reaction times of 350–500 msec, with a highly significant correlation between saccadic latency and dementia. These results, with others to be discussed in the section on developmental reading disability, show a strong cognitive component for what may appear to be a very basic, automated motor act. Increased latencies have been found with nearly all patients who have dementia (e.g., Pirozzolo, 1978; Pirozzolo & Rayner, 1978b). In addition, these patients have difficulty in saccadic accuracy and in exploratory eye movements when viewing thematic pictures (Hutton, Johnston, Shapiro, & Pirozzolo, 1979). In a study of eye movement strategies during a verbal problem solving task, Johnston and Pirozzolo (1981) showed that normal subjects' fixation durations, fixation densities, and sequential scan patterns were a function of cognitive operations. Aphasic subjects who have moderate auditory comprehension deficits have psycho-oculomotor strategies that differ from those of normals (Pirozzolo, Rubens, & Johnston, in preparation) and these differences are thought to reflect limitations in response selection (output) as well as linguistic problem solving ability. Aphasic patients' eye movements during reading (Pirozzolo & Rayner, 1978b) are not "normal," the pattern being one that reflects a linguistic problem solving disability rather than a visual–spatial or oculomotor deficit, much like that of the auditory–linguistic dyslexic to be discussed later.

## IV.   Eye Movement Disorders in Developmental Reading Disability

Disturbed reading eye movements have been suggested as a possible etiology of reading disability (e.g., see Zangwill & Blakemore, 1972). Although 60 years of research fails to support such a conclusion, some researchers continue to argue that faulty eye movements cause dyslexia (Levinson, 1981; Pavlidis, 1981). Methods that have been developed to train disabled readers to make smooth, regular "staircase" movements have been dramatically unsuccessful in remediating reading problems. Nevertheless, the reading eye movements of dyslexic children do differ from those of fluent readers in many respects (Tinker, 1958). These differences include increased numbers of fixations per line of text, increased numbers of regressions, longer fixation durations, and increased incidence of within-word short regressions and forward movements (see Pirozzolo, 1979, for review). These reading eye movement phenomena are clearly not evidence of any eye movement abnormality but suggest instead that a heavy linguistic demand is being placed upon the reader (e.g., grapheme to phoneme translation). These eye movement patterns are seen in normal younger children who are not fluent readers and in normal adults who are reading unfamiliar text (e.g., foreign language grammar text). Furthermore, as will be demonstrated in the following section, when the linguistic load is reduced (by having the subject read simple text) the reading eye movement pattern returns to normal.

The remaining features of eye movement behavior seen in disabled readers that suggest a faulty oculomotor system pertain to the reader's ability to make appropriately successive rightward eye movements that bring regions of unprocessed text onto the forea and to make accurate return sweeps. Some dyslexics have been observed to have a "irrepressible tendency" to scan text in a right-to-left manner (Zangwill & Blakemore, 1972). In the following section, evidence from a series of studies from our laboratory will suggest that this visual–spatial disorder does play a role in reading disability. It is probably not the case, however, that this phenomenon is an eye movement disorder per se. Rather, it can be best viewed as a spatial disorder. Children with these problems represent only a small proportion of disabled readers. They have great difficulty with a variety of visual–spatial functions and it can be suggested that because of the clustering of the visual–spatial symptomatology that this represents a specific form of dyslexia syndrome. In summary, the former group of eye movement "disorders" (increased fixations, regressions, and fixation durations) do not cause dyslexia. Instead, it can be argued that dyslexia causes these eye movement abnormalities. The latter symptom of poor eye guidance is infrequently seen in disabled readers (Pirozzolo & Rayner, 1978b). This eye movement disorder is probably not the cause of dyslexia. Instead, the faulty spatial mechanism, which guides the eye (rather than the oculomotor mechanism itself), is probably responsible for both reading and eye guidance problems.

# V.  Forms of Developmental Reading Impairment

Research on developmental dyslexia has suffered from the previously universal assumption that reading disability is a single neuropsychological entity caused by a brain dysfunction that is common to all dyslexics. Recent research strongly suggests that this assumption is probably false (Boder, 1973; Kinsbourne & Warrington, 1963; Mattis, French, & Rapin, 1975; Pirozzolo, 1979). These and other studies (see Denckla, 1980, for review) show that "syndromes" of developmental reading disability may exist, and that relatively discrete patterns of neuropsychological performance characterize each syndrome. Although agreement has not been reached on the exact subtypes that can be isolated from large clinical groups of developmental dyslexics (cf. Mattis, 1981; Satz & Morris, 1981), it has been suggested that at least two specific subtypes are found in all studies undertaking such analysis (Pirozzolo, 1979; Pirozzolo, 1981). These groups, called auditory–linguistic dyslexics and visual–spatial dyslexics (Pirozzolo, 1977), are separable on the basis of neuropsychological test performance, as well as reading, spelling, and writing performance. Table 28.1 provides a brief description of the features of these disorders.

Auditory–linguistic dyslexics represent the most common subtype of developmental reading disability, outnumbering visual–spatial dyslexics by perhaps as much as four to one (Boder, 1973; Mattis et al., 1975; Pirozzolo, 1979). Previous studies in our laboratory (Pirozzolo, 1979; Pirozzolo & Rayner, 1978a; Pirozzolo & Rayner, 1978b; Pirozzolo & Rayner, 1979; Pirozzolo, Rayner, & Whitaker, 1977) have used these two clinical groups to carefully study the problem of eye movement disorders in developmental reading disability. Prior to entry into our studies, children were given neurological, neuropsychological, and educational evaluations. Subjects were assigned to one of two groups on the basis of these test results. Although not all children from our clinic could be correctly assigned to a group (Pirozzolo & Hess, 1976), the groups can be considered neuropsychologically homogenous. Studies were designed to test subjects' abilities to

TABLE 28.1
Subtypes of Dyslexia

| Subgroup type | |
|---|---|
| Auditory–linguistic dyslexia | Visual–spatial dyslexia |
| Average to above average performance IQ | Average to above average verbal IQ |
| Low verbal IQ (relative to performance IQ) | Low performance IQ (relative to verbal IQ) |
| Developmentally delayed language onset | Right–left disorientation |
| Expressive speech defects | Early evidence of preference for mirror or inverted writing |
| Anomia, object naming, or color-naming defects | Finger agnosia |
| Agrammatism | Spatial dysgraphia (poor handwriting, poor use of space) |
| Reading errors mainly involving the phonological aspects of language | Reading errors involving visual aspects of text |
| Spelling errors characteristic of poor phoneme to grapheme correspondence | Spelling errors characteristic of letter and word reversals, omissions, etc. |
| Letter by letter decoding strategy | Use of phonetic decoding strategy |
| Normal eye movements | Faulty eye movements during reading |
| Relatively intact visual–spatial abilities | Oral language abilities relatively normal |

perform pursuit tasks, to launch saccades to verbal and nonverbal stimuli in the right and left visual fields, and to perform smooth, normal reading eye movements. A brief review of these studies will show that auditory–linguistic dyslexics do not show eye movement abnormalities and that visual–spatial dyslexics show faulty visual–spatial organization that probably disrupts the accurate placement of saccades during reading.

An evaluation of the reading eye movements of a case of auditory–linguistic dyslexia in a high-school educated adult was carried out and was the subject of a previous case study (Pirozzolo et al., 1977). The young man had average range intellectual abilities with an early developmental history of language disability (late language onset). His reading ability was approximately at the fifth-grade level, with slightly higher spelling and mathematical abilities. When this subject's reading eye movements were tracked and recorded while he read linguistically simple (third-grade level) text, a normal "staircase" pattern with few regressions was observed. When the subject was required to read more difficult text, fixation frequency and regression frequency greatly increased. The text difficulty factor, as shall be seen later, is an important control for determining whether eye movement abnormalities are secondary to linguistic difficulties.

Conversely, a case report illustrating the more dramatic eye movement and visual–spatial disorders that can occur in visual–spatial dyslexia was reported by Pirozzolo and Rayner (1978a). The female subject was a third year undergraduate who had a positive developmental history for visual–spatial disorders. She was apparently reading at age level until the third grade when the following incident occurred. At age 8 years her preferred reading and writing style was upside down and right-to-left. Her teacher at that time demanded that she return her book to the normal orientation because, as she explained, that was the only proper way to read. From that time, the subject read in the normal orientation, but continued to write beginning at the bottom of the page writing right-to-left and up the page. When this woman's eye movements were recorded while reading normally oriented text, she showed poor comprehension (fifth-grade level) and many instances of inappropriate right-to-left scanning and return sweep inaccuracies. When reading upside down text, her comprehension improved dramatically, much as if this strategy allowed her to make use of some prewired preference that effectively reduced the amount of time required to carry out the cognitive and perceptual tasks of reading. In addition, her reading eye movements were of the "normal" "staircase" variety, also supporting the aforementioned conclusion. The text difficulty factor did not significantly alter the reading eye movement pattern in the normal orientation, suggesting that the abnormalities observed were below that of the level of language processing (i.e., visual–spatial and–or oculomotor).

Subsequently, a larger study of saccadic latency and reading eye movements was designed to determine whether, in fact, the pattern of eye movement behavior differs between auditory–linguistic and visual–spatial dyslexics (Pirozzolo, 1979). Previous research had shown that normal adults show shorter saccadic latencies for rightward than for leftward saccades (Rayner, 1978b) when identifying words in the left and right visual field. It has been argued that this asymmetry reflects a hemispheric specialization factor since right-handers exhibit this tendency and left-handers do not (Pirozzolo & Rayner, 1979). Normal readers and auditory–linguistic dyslexics were both found to have shorter latencies for rightward saccades. Visual–spatial dyslexics had shorter latencies for leftward saccades. These findings were in agreement with other neuropsychological observations in suggesting that visual–spatial dyslexics have difficulty in executing tasks that require visual–spatial perception and a visual–motor response.

When the eye movements during reading were recorded and analyzed, the two groups of dyslexic readers could again be differentiated on the basis of their performance. Two conditions were used in this study. Subjects were asked to read relatively easy text in the first condition and more difficult text in the second condition. Measures employed were mean number of fixations per line of print, mean fixation duration, mean number of return sweep inaccuracies, and mean percentage of regressions. While reading easy text normal readers made approximately six fixations per line of text (text visual angle = 12°), fixation durations of 250 msec, and 15% regressions with very few return sweep inaccuracies. Difficult text increased the number of fixations and regressions but not fixation durations or return sweep inaccuracies. Thus, the increased linguistic processing load influenced the number of fixations but it did not influence the spatial–oculomotor task of returning the eye to the next line of print. Auditory–linguistic dyslexics had the same pattern of performance with respect to the text difficulty factor as normal readers. Text difficulty increased fixations and regressions but did not influence the return sweep or fixation duration. Auditory–linguistic dyslexics' baseline performance while reading easy text differed from normals' in that fixation durations averaged approximately 275 msec. Visual–spatial dyslexics also had fixation durations in the range of 275 msec for both conditions. Increased text difficulty, however, did not influence the number of regressions for this group. The hallmark characteristic of oculomotor performance by these disabled readers was the presence of significant numbers of return sweep inaccuracies, which were present in both conditions to the same degree. This finding again suggests that the visual–spatial problem of dysmetric return sweeps is independent of the linguistic nature of the reading task. Visual–spatial dyslexics did show evidence of frequent right-to-left scanning, the "irrepressible tendency" to scan text from right-to-left. A further observation supported the claim of a spatial disorientation factor being responsible for the poor scanning strategy. When audiotapes were compared with eye movement records, a somewhat frequent anomaly was discovered—the completion of one line of text followed by a return sweep that landed more than one line of text below the previous line. Similarly, in the saccadic latency task described above, visual–spatial dyslexics made more frequent eye movements into the incorrect visual field.

## VI. Conclusion

One hundred years of research on developmental reading disability has not elucidated the etiologic factors that underlie this cognitive disorder. Cytoarchitectonic, radiologic, neurophysiologic, and neuropsychologic research, however, is beginning to show a possible causal association between atypical neural structure of the language zones of the left hemisphere and reading disorders. Just as there are varieties of acquired reading disability caused by lesions in different areas of the brain (Benson, 1981), there are varieties of developmental reading deficits. One basic scheme for differentiating the forms of reading problems in children is through the clinical inferential method. At least two subgroups can be characterized through this neuropsychological assessment technique: auditory–linguistic dyslexia and visual–spatial dyslexia. There is substantial agreement among researchers that these two forms exist and good agreement that other forms probably exist (cf., Denckla, 1979). Disabled readers with oral language deficits greatly outnumber those with symptoms of visual–spatial perceptual deficits. Auditory–linguistic dyslexics show no evidence of eye movement disorders, either during reading or while performing other nonreading tasks. Visual–spatial dyslexics do show a number of eye movement abnormalties (such as faulty oculomotor scanning strategies during reading), but these abnormalities probably result from poor visual–spatial programming of saccadic eye movements rather than from impairments in the motor mechanisms that trigger ocular movement.

# References

Benson, D. F. (1981). Alexia and the neuroanatomical basis of reading. In F. J. Pirozzolo & M. C. Wittrock (Eds.), *Neuropsychological and cognitive processes in reading.* New York: Academic Press.

Boder, E. (1973). Developmental dyslexia: A diagnostic approach based on three atypical reading–spelling patterns. *Developmental Medicine and Child Neurology, 15,* 663–687.

Denckla, M. B. (1979). Childhood learning disabilities. In K. Heilman & E. Valenstein (Eds.), *Clinical neuropsychology.* New York: Oxford University Press.

Frost, D., & Poppel, E. (1976). Different programming modes of human saccadic eye movements as a function of stimulus eccentricity. *Biological Cybernetics, 23,* 39–48.

Galaburda, A., & Kemper, T. L. (1979). Cytoarchitectonic abnormalities in developmental dyslexia: A case study. *Annals of Neurology, 6,* 94–100.

Geschwind, N., & Levitsky, W. (1968). Human brain: Left–right asymmetries in temporal speech region. *Science, 161,* 186–188.

Hier, D. B., LeMay, M., Rosenberger, P., & Perlo, V. P. (1978). Developmental dyslexia. *Archives of Neurology, 35,* 90–92.

Hutton, J. T., Johnston, C., Shapiro, I., & Pirozzolo, F. J. (1979). Oculomotor programming disturbances in the dementia syndrome. *Perceptual and Motor Skills, 49,* 312–314.

Johnston, C., & Pirozzolo, F. J. (1981). Eye movements and cognitive strategies. *Perceptual and Motor Skills, 53,* 623–632.

Kinsbourne, M., & Warrington, E. K. (1963). Developmental factors in reading and writing backwardness. *British Journal of Psychology, 54,* 145–156.

Levinson, F. (1981). *Dyslexia: A solution to the riddle.* New York: Springer–Verlag.

Mattis, S. (1981). Dyslexia syndromes in children: Toward the development of syndrome-specific treatment programs. In F. J. Pirozzolo & M. C. Wittrock (Eds.), *Neuropsychological and cognitive processes in reading.* New York: Academic Press.

Mattis, S., French, J., & Rapin, I. (1975). Dyslexia in children and young adults: Three independent neuropsychological syndromes. *Developmental Medicine and Child Neurology, 17,* 150–163.

Pavlidis, G. (1981). Do eye movements hold the key to dyslexia? *Neuropsychologia, 19,* 57–64.

Pirozzolo, F. J. (1977). *Visual–spatial and oculomotor deficits in developmental dyslexia: Evidence for two neurobehavioral syndromes of reading disability.* Unpublished doctoral dissertation, University of Rochester, 1977.

Pirozzolo, F. J. (1978). Slow saccades. *Archives of Neurology, 35,* 618.

Pirozzolo, F. J. (1979). *The neuropsychology of developmental reading disorders.* New York: Praeger.

Pirozzolo, F. J. (1981). Language and brain: Neuropsychological aspects of developmental reading disability. *School Psychology Review, 10,* 350–355.

Pirozzolo, F. J., & Hansch, E. C. (1981). Oculomotor reaction time reflects degree of diffuse cerebral dysfunction. *Science, 213.*

Pirozzolo, F. J., & Hansch, E. C. (1981). The neurobiology of developmental reading disorders. In R. N. Malatesha & P. G. Aaron (Eds.), *Neuropsychological and neurolinguistic aspects of reading disorders.* New York: Academic Press.

Pirozzolo, F. J., & Hess, D. W. (1976). *A neuropsychological analysis of the ITPA.* Paper presented at the annual convention of the New York State Orton Society, Rochester.

Pirozzolo, F. J., & Rayner, K. (1978). Disorders of oculomotor scanning and graphic orientation in developmental Gerstmann Syndrome. *Brain and Language, 5,* 119–126. (a)

Pirozzolo, F. J., & Rayner, K. (1978). The neural control of eye movements in acquired and developmental reading disorders. In H. A. Whitaker & H. A. Whitaker (Eds.), *Studies in neurolinguistics* (Vol. 4). New York: Academic Press. (b)

Pirozzolo, F. J., & Rayner, K. (1979). Cerebral organization and reading disability. *Neuropsychologia, 17,* 485–489.

Pirozzolo, F. J., & Rayner, K. (1980). Handedness, hemispheric specialization, and saccadic eye movement latencies. *Neuropsychologia, 18,* 225–229.

Pirozzolo, F. J., Rayner, K., & Whitaker, H. A. (1977). *Left hemisphere mechanisms in dyslexia.* Paper presented at the annual convention of the International Neuropsychological Society, Sante Fe.

Pirozzolo, F. J., Rubens, A. B., & Johnston, C. (1982). *Eye movements in aphasia.* Manuscript in preparation.

Rayner, K. (1978). Eye movements in reading and information processing. *Psychological Bulletin, 85,* 618–660. (a)

Rayner, K. (1978). Saccadic latencies for parafoveally presented words. *Bulletin of the Psychonomic Society, 11,* 13–16. (b)

Satz, P., & Morris, R. (1981). Learning disability subtypes: A review. In F. J. Pirozzolo & M. C. Wittrock (Eds.), *Neuropsychological and cognitive processes in reading.* New York: Academic Press.

Tinker, M. A. (1958). Recent studies of eye movements in reading. *Psychological Bulletin, 55,* 215–231.

Whitaker, H. A. (1979). Preface. In F. J. Pirozzolo, *The neuropsychology of developmental reading disorders.* New York: Praeger.

Witelson, S., & Pallie, W. (1973). Left hemisphere specialization for language in the newborn: Neuroanatomical evidence of asymmetry. *Brain, 96,* 641–646.

Zangwill, O., & Blakemore, C. (1972). Dyslexia: Reversal of eye movements during reading. *Neuropsychologia, 10,* 371–373.

# 29

# What Can Eye Movements
# Tell Us about Dyslexia?

## I.   Introduction

I shall start out by backing up a bit from my title and making a few general comments about dyslexia research. This seems necessary since dyslexia appears to be (from my outsider's perspective, at least) a field where there are many contradictory claims, and often it is difficult to know where truth lies.

The natural place to start would appear to be to define dyslexia. There appears to be wide agreement that the definition is one of exclusion: a dyslexic is someone who has a severe reading problem that is not explainable by a list of factors. Pavlidis's list seems to be representative: "intelligence, motivation, emotional stability, physical health, socio-economic background, educational opportunities, language spoken at home, parent education, teacher quality, culture." Later on, he also makes clear that he excludes children with vision problems. Although there appears to be much hand-wringing in some quarters about such a definition by exclusion (e.g., Satz & Morris, 1981), there is no serious problem with it as long as it is remembered that *dyslexia* refers to a fascinating unsolved problem for the researcher rather than to a disease that is well understood. Although a definition in terms of known causal agents would be better, it appears premature given the current status of the research.

In dyslexia, there is also the dichotomy between developmental dyslexia (i.e., people with reading problems from the beginning of their reading history) and acquired dyslexia (i.e., people who once could read normally but now have trouble due to brain injury or disease). The four chapters in this part of the book and this review concern themselves almost exclusively with developmental dyslexia.

EYE MOVEMENTS IN READING:
PERCEPTUAL AND LANGUAGE PROCESSES

Despite the complaints made by many authors about the nonuniformity of the operational definition of dyslexia, my impression on reading through the literature was that, in the recent literature at least, there was surprising agreement. While there appear to be minor differences in the criteria used, most people seem to agree that some criterion is needed to exclude people with minor reading retardation. The usual criterion for a severe reading problem appears to be something like excluding people who are less than 1.5–2 years below the norm in reading grade level. This exclusion of children with mild reading problems seems necessary if one is to make significant progress in uncovering the basic causes of reading problems. If a child is only a bit below the norm in reading, it is unlikely that there will be a clear difference between such a child and normal readers on any instrument devised to diagnose the basic problem. Unfortunately, what sometimes happens is that some measure is claimed as an index of dyslexia. Then a study is done comparing good readers to poor readers (e.g., the bottom half or bottom third of the distribution of readers in a particular population) that finds no clear differences between good and poor readers. Some reviewers will then use this weak null result as evidence that this index is unimportant in diagnosing dyslexia.

Although variations in the criterion of severity of the reading deficit should only create small problems in comparing studies, variations in the definition of the other exclusionary criteria can cause more serious problems, especially for studies in which a case is being made that the sample studied is representative of dyslexics in general (e.g., Pavlidis, Chapter 25 in this volume; Olson, Kliegl, & Davidson, Chapter 26 in this volume). Looking ahead briefly, the problem is that the reading difficulties of dyslexics must be caused by something: an oculomotor, perceptual, language, and/or cognitive deficit. The exclusionary definition of dyslexia (sometimes termed "specific dyslexia"), if taken literally, implies that the deficit or deficits are manifest only during reading. Since it is quite implausible that whatever constellation of deficits the dyslexic has will in fact only appear in reading, the spirit of the exclusionary definition is that whatever the deficits are that are observed in other tasks, they are mild enough so that they cause little difficulty elsewhere. This leads to a problem in the dyslexia literature, since people could have somewhat different criteria about the severity of the perceptual deficit, language deficit, IQ deficit, and the like that is used to discriminate between "perceptually disabled," "language disabled," "retarded," and dyslexic. Another problem in defining the population of dyslexics is that we are not really sure what kind of prescreening goes on before the experimenter applies his or her exclusionary criteria. What tests does the school system administer to children in order to diagnose them as dyslexic or as having a reading problem? Are certain labs known for their treatment of certain kinds of reading problems and thus do they get an unrepresentative sample of dyslexics? For example, Pavlidis has been written up in national newspapers in Great Britain and has appeared on television. These reports have emphasized his expertise in diagnosing eye movement problems. Thus, people with severe reading retardation who appear to have no language or cognitive deficits and/or have reason to believe that they have eye control problems would tend to seek him out. On the other hand, since the current popular view in the United States appears to be that dyslexia is mainly a language problem, a different prescreening may be happening in most American studies.

To summarize, there appears to be a reasonable consensus that there is a population of people, called dyslexics, that have severe reading problems, but who are not socioeconomically disadvantaged, have no motivation problems, and appear to have cognitive, language, and/or perceptual–motor problems that are subtle enough that the person performs at least acceptably in all other important real-world tasks. That is not to say that people with more general learning problems might not also have the same specific problems as these "dyslexics," but the consensus is that studying purer dyslexics should be first on the agenda if we are to understand the kind of problems that are relatively specific to reading.

Two related methodological points are worth raising. Although obvious, they appear to be rarely stated in the dyslexia literature. First is the problem of regression toward the mean. Since the dyslexics studied are those poor readers who score about average or above in IQ tests and other standardized instruments, they are clearly well above average in the population of retarded readers on these measures. Since these instruments are less than perfectly reliable, one has reason to believe that if the dyslexics were retested, they would score lower on these standard measures (i.e., regressing to the mean of the population of poor readers from which they were drawn). Although this problem is unavoidable, the situation could be improved if researchers reported the mean and standard deviation of the test scores for the population of poor readers from which the dyslexics were drawn as well as a measure of the reliability of the test. With that information, one could make some estimate of how much the actual test scores of the dyslexics are likely to exceed their "true scores."

Another point that is rarely commented on is the logic of matching dyslexics and control subjects. If dyslexics and control subjects are truly matched on standard intelligence tests and the like despite the demonstrated reading problem of the dyslexics, then the presumption must be that the dyslexics are supranormal on at least some skills in order to compensate both for the underlying deficits that cause the reading problem, and for the additional handicap of a reading problem (especially after they have entered school). This point does not invalidate the research commonly reported, but I feel that part of the diagnosis of dyslexia as defined earlier will have to be the identification of those supranormal skills that do not seem to be of much help in compensating for their deficits in the reading situation, but appear to compensate for them in IQ and other standardized tests.

## II.   Approaches to Dyslexia

Most research on dyslexia appears to have as a major objective the understanding of the basic types of dyslexia. There are two interlocking motives that underlie this goal: (*a*) to be able to diagnose individuals with reading problems so as to be able to give the best remediation possible; (*b*) to be able to get greater insight into how the process of reading works. Although most researchers hope that their research serves both ends, they are often not clear, in written reports, about the relevance of their research to either of these objectives.

I shall refer to the two major approaches in developmental dyslexia as the clinical method and the representative sample method. In the clinical method, a few people are studied in great detail, and often the people studied are not selected because they are representative of dyslexics, but because their deficit is particularly clear and, it is hoped, illustrative of a basic deficit in dyslexia. In the representative sample method, of necessity a large sample of dyslexics is chosen, and as a usual result, each subject is studied in less detail than in the clinical method.

Obviously, both methods have their merits. The clinical method is needed to diagnose individual patients and to recommend remediation. It is also much better suited to achieving detailed characterizations of an individual's reading problem. On the other hand, the representative sample method is needed to answer questions about the population of dyslexics in general. Probably, the best approach is to use both methods in combination, possibly following up some of the most interesting subjects from a representative sample in much greater detail using the clinical method.

## III.   The Role of Eye Movements

### A.   The Basic Issues

Although most researchers appear to agree that the basic focus of dyslexia research at this point is to identify the basic types or dimensions of dyslexia and to characterize these types as carefully as possible, there is less agreement than one would have hoped after several decades of research in dyslexia about what the basic types are. However, a rough consensus may be emerging. The dominant position appears to be that there are at least two types of dyslexia, at least in clinical populations (e.g., Boder, 1973; Mattis, 1981; Pirozzolo, Chapter 28 in this volume). The list of candidates put forward for basic types includes the following: visual–spatial perceptual disorders, language disorders, oculomotor disorders, and sequencing disorders. Several authors distinguish subtypes within those basic categories as well. However, there still appears to be considerable controversy about the prevalence of the basic types and even whether there is more than one basic type (e.g., Pavlidis, Chapter 25 in this volume; Velluntino, 1979). Moreover, there is often a great deal of vagueness about what is meant by a particular type.

In the articles in this volume, the focus is on a single indicator of reading: the eye movement record. Although this record has been shown to be an invaluable tool for understanding the process of reading, it is not a panacea in dyslexia research. In fact, the more limited goals that the research appears to be addressing itself to are: (*a*) Are oculomotor problems a common cause of dyslexia? (*b*) How can we characterize these oculomotor problems? (*c*) If there are other problems, how can the eye movement record help in analyzing them?

## B.   Are Eye Movements the Cause of Dyslexia?

The major problem confounding a simple answer to this question is that poor readers' eye records will look abnormal compared to good readers regardless of whether eye movement control is the problem. If they are having difficulty understanding the text, they will tend to fixate longer, make smaller saccades, and have more regressions. Thus, for example, one can not use the percentage of eye movements in reading that are regressions by itself as a measure of oculomotor problems. The approaches taken, or at least suggested, in the preceding chapters appear to fall in three categories: (*a*) to determine whether there are oculomotor problems in nonlinguistic tasks as well; (*b*) to determine whether the oculomotor indices change if nonperceptual variables are manipulated (e.g., text difficulty); (*c*) to devise a measure that differentiates the *pattern* of eye movements of the person with eye control problems from the pattern of eye movements of the person with other problems. The chapters in Part VII all employ at least one of these methods.

The question about whether there are dyslexics who have oculomotor problems and those who do not appears to be fairly clearly answered in the clinical literature, most notably in Pirozzolo and Rayner (1978), discussed in Pirozzolo's chapter. One of their major diagnostic devices was to manipulate text difficulty. They reasoned that if the problem was basically one of faulty eye control, then the manipulation of text difficulty should make little difference in the abnormality of the eye movement record, whereas if the difficulty was more linguistic or cognitive then the abnormality of the eye record would decrease as the text was made appropriately easy for the subject. They found a clear differentiation along those lines in the subjects they studied, and furthermore, other details corroborated their classification. The subjects with oculomotor difficulties had problems making return sweeps in reading, and, in fact, one of the subjects read much more easily when the text was upside down, something extremely difficult to explain if the problem were linguistic or cognitive. Classifying the subjects may have been easy partly because the clinical method was used, and thus relatively extreme cases were studied.

Thus, it appears to be relatively safe to say that there are at least two types of dyslexics: those whose problems involve eye control and those whose problems do not. The issue, about which there still seems to be considerable controversy, is what percentage of dyslexics have eye control problems and what percentage do not.

The two studies that use the representative sample approach in Section VII

(Olson *et al.*; Pavlidis) come to opposing conclusions: Olson *et al.* conclude that there appear to be few people in their sample who have serious eye control problems; Pavlidis concludes that such eye control problems are the sole cause of the reading problems found in his dyslexic sample. Unfortunately, given the data at hand, it is hard to come to any definitive conclusion about who is right (if either). A major problem, discussed earlier, is that there may be biases beyond the experimenter's control about what subjects are referred to them. The following is an attempt to compare the two studies as carefully as possible.

First of all, there appear to be some differences in the procedures stated for diagnosing the dyslexics. Pavlidis appears to exclude subjects with either performance or verbal WISC scores below 90; Olson *et al.* exclude people with full-scale scores below 90. If many dyslexics score lower on the verbal than on the performance part of the test, Pavlidis's criterion may be significantly stricter in excluding people with language difficulties. He does not state how many of his "poor readers" were people who were originally sent to him diagnosed as dyslexics but were put in this group because of low verbal IQ scores. Pavlidis's other criterion of excluding subjects because of "inadequate motivation to read" sounds dangerously subjective, and may further exclude other people standardly diagnosed as dyslexics.

Despite the above, the data from the two studies, where they can be compared, are not that different. Pavlidis reports that his dyslexic group makes 30% regressions as compared to 21% for the normal control group, whereas Olson *et al.* report values of 26% and 19%, respectively. There are minor differences in procedure (Pavlidis used text a little easier than that at the appropriate reading level; Olson *et al.* used text at the appropriate reading level). In addition, Pavlidis's subjects' mean age was about 10 years (Pavlidis, 1981) and Olson *et al.*'s subjects' mean age was about 15, so that the relatively small differences in level of performance seem reconcilable. Pavlidis argues that since his dyslexic group was worse than his poor reader group, there is a qualitative difference between them, since the groups were both reading text adjusted for their reading level. This argument has merit, but I see two problems. First, it would have been better to use Pirozzolo and Rayner's manipulation and also study the eye movement pattern with more difficult text, since the most conclusive evidence for a qualitative difference would have been if the percentage of regressions was little affected by text difficulty for the dyslexic group but strongly affected by text difficulty in the poor reader group. As it is, a skeptic could explain Pavlidis's observed difference by saying that the dyslexic group was just a little more reading disabled than the poor reader group. Second, Pavlidis's claims for nonoverlapping distributions for the groups seem a bit overblown. If the percentage of eye movements that are regressions are approximately normally distributed in each of Pavlidis's groups, then I estimate that about 30–35% of the dyslexics have regression scores within one standard deviation of the mean of the normal or poor reader group. Thus, it would appear unlikely that all of the dyslexic group have severe oculomotor difficulties.

Neither study, unfortunately, attempts to give a measure that would be evidence for a different *pattern* of regressions in the reading task that would suggest oculomotor difficulties. From clinical descriptions of people with such difficulties, it would seem that the average number of fixations needed to execute a return sweep or a measure of repetitive regressions (controlled for absolute number of regressions) could help to measure the frequency of regressions due to oculomotor difficulties with the text. Pavlidis presents reading eye movement records of dyslexics and poor readers and argues for qualitative differences. I find the qualitative difference in pattern hard to see.

The best evidence for a qualitative difference between the dyslexic group and the poor reader group is the "lights test," in which subjects are supposed to execute a simple sequential tracking of a light with their eyes. Since the task has no linguistic component, differences on the task would appear to be diagnostic of eye control difficulties. The differences between groups that Pavlidis reports are impressive, although again he exaggerates the separation a bit. If the groups are normally distributed, about 15% of the dyslexic group would be within one standard deviation of the mean of the poor readers on the lights test. Olson *et al.* did not carefully test for eye control problems (since this was not the major focus of their study). They do report that the poor readers had little problem with tracking during the calibration procedure, which is a sequential tracking task. However, the lights task may be faster and more demanding, and thus more diagnostic of eye control problems.

However, Olson *et al.* report data that imply that many of their dyslexics have language and/or cognitive deficits. Their dyslexics have a mean word recognition score that is about half of grade level, and their latency in making phonetic judgments is about 50% longer than the controls. It seems implausible that these major deficits are caused by the relatively minor deficit in eye control indexed by percentage regressions (26% vs. 19% for the normal readers). Thus oculomotor problems are unlikely to be the sole cause of the reading problems for Olson *et al.*'s subjects, and the severity of the deficits in the word attack skills suggest that linguistic and/or cognitive deficits may explain most of the reading problems.

What is one to conclude? Given the data from Pavlidis's lights test, it appears that many of his subjects have serious eye control problems, and given Olson *et al.*'s other data, it appears that most of their subjects have serious language problems. Yet, the two groups did not look that different in the one task where they could be compared. It is unfortunate that Olson *et al.* did not conduct the lights test and that Pavlidis did not report data on word attack skills. The latter should measure linguistic difficulties and be relatively unaffected by eye control problems.

Which group is representative of dyslexics? Most researchers appear to agree with Pirozzolo, who claims that only a minority of dyslexics have eye control problems. It is worth noting in this regard that a recent study by Stanley, Smith, and Howell (1982) has employed the lights test and has gotten results different from Pavlidis. Their data showed only one subject in the group of dyslexics who appeared to have any difficulty with the lights test.

## C.  Toward Diagnosing Eye Control Problems

Although neither of the representative sampling studies were as complete as one would have wished in measuring the dyslexics, the four chapters in Part VII point the way to procedures that could be used to diagnose eye control problems. First, a simple nonlinguistic test such as the lights test would seem to be easy to use and should diagnose serious eye control problems. However, converging operations are needed as well, especially in the case of less severe eye control problems. First, more qualitative measures should be used to assess the eye movement pattern. Clinical studies of people with clear eye movement control problems seem invaluable in this regard so that one can assess what is qualitatively different about the pattern of eye movements in such subjects. Second, it would seem necessary to study the pattern of eye movements at several levels of text difficulty. Presumably, if a subject had a mild eye control problem, he or she would only make a few more regressions than the norm, but the deficit should be small and consistent across various levels of text difficulties.

Jones and Stark (Chapter 27 in this volume) make it clear that I have probably oversimplified the task ahead in that there is probably more than one type of eye control problem. They identify at least two: one a problem with involuntary movement of the eye (nystagmus) that Pavlidis has apparently excluded from his sample, and a sequencing problem as described by Pavlidis. It would be better if there were quantitative indices that would allow us to differentiate the subject populations, as well as help to diagnose milder forms of the problems.

One technique that could be used to distinguish among eye control problems is to assess whether the reading difficulty is much less when the requirement to move the eyes is removed. Normal subjects can read text presented rapidly and sequentially word by word in a single location (e.g., Potter, Kroll, & Harris, 1980). It would be interesting to see whether dyslexics with oculomotor problems could also read well using this rapid serial visual presentation (RSVP) technique. If so, it would suggest that their problem is one of eye movement guidance as opposed to a problem in maintaining fixation. Such a technique might also be of some value as an aid to such dyslexics.

## D.  Use of Eye Movements to
## Diagnose Linguistic Difficulties

Recently, there has been an explosion of research using the eye movement record to investigate the reading process in skilled readers. Notable gains, as discussed elsewhere in this book, have been made in analyzing both perceptual and linguistic stages in reading. It thus seems reasonable to use eye movements to study the difficulties dyslexics are having when they read. The Olson *et al.*

chapter is the only one of the four that reports in any detail the relationship of linguistic difficulties to the eye movement record. In particular, they attempt to use measures from both the eye movement record and other independently obtained measures to predict the "regression fixation index" (RFI), which is highly correlated with the percentage of eye movements that are regressions.

Unfortunately, the research seems to lack theoretical focus. The authors investigate several models using the technique of stepwise multiple regression to try to predict the RFI. However, they do not make very clear what general conclusions follow from their models or how their data fit in with other studies in the literature. I draw several conclusions from their chapter. First, the percentage of regressions appears to covary with the size of the saccade. Thus, on the face of it, the percentage of regressions that an individual reader makes may be somewhat a matter of strategy: Some readers may be bolder and move forward ahead farther and then have to make more regressions; others move forward more cautiously and make fewer regressions. This result provides another reason for not using percentage regressions as an important diagnostic tool. Second, neither the word recognition score ($r = -.18$) nor the phonological latency score ($r = .36$) accounted for a particularly impressive percentage of the variance of the RFI within the reading disabled group when reading aloud. (It would be nice to have the data from silent reading.)

Since these measures have been thought to be reliable indices of reading difficulty, the results seem disappointing and suggest these measures may only tell a small part of the story in dyslexia. However, that conclusion may be premature. First of all, since the correlations are within the group of dyslexic readers and a fairly strict criterion of severity of reading impairment has been set, the range of scores on these measures within the group may be restricted (especially for word recognition) and thus low correlations may be misleading. Second, the problem may not be in the use of these measures of word attack skills or grapheme to phoneme correspondence to predict dyslexia, but in the use of global measures such as the RFI, average saccade length, or average fixation duration to reflect qualitative differences in the reading process. As Part III indicates, the use of the eye movement record is likely to be especially useful for studying the linguistic processes underlying reading when the text is manipulated and specific places of special interest in the text are studied (e.g., Inhoff, Chapter 10 in this volume; K. Ehrlich, Chapter 15 in this volume). In the case of phonological skills, for example, one might compare fixation durations for orthographically "regular" and "irregular" words (e.g., "won" vs. "one"), since one might expect that readers with poor phonological skills would show little difference in their ability to process the two types, whereas dyslexics who had relatively intact phonological skills but impaired "direct" visual skills would show large differences between regular and irregular words.

It is certainly an open question whether such well-defined subtypes of linguistic deficits exist in the population of developmental dyslexics. However, since it appears reasonably certain that they exist in the population of acquired dyslexics (e.g., Coltheart, 1981), it seems like a reasonable hypothesis to investigate. Unfortunately, it strikes me that the correlational method employed by Olson *et al.* is a bit premature. They appear to be simultaneously trying to understand their instruments and their subjects. A first step would appear to be to find striking cases of developmental dyslexia that appeared to be prototypical of one kind of problem or another and then to see what in the eye movement record appeared to be the best indicator of this reading problem. Only then, it seems to me, would there be much chance of uncovering basic dimensions of dyslexia in the eye movement records of a representative sample. The same comment applies as well to other indices that one might want to use to diagnose dyslexia, such as word attack skills.

## E.   Dyslexia and Models of Reading

The preceding discussion and the four other chapters in Part VII concern themselves almost entirely with a characterization of types of developmental dyslexia, and say little about the implications of the research for understanding the reading process. This is in marked distinction to the largely clinical work in acquired dyslexia, where modeling the reading process is a major concern (e.g., Coltheart, 1981). In fact, the work in acquired dyslexia seems to provide the strongest evidence for the theory hinted at earlier that there are at least two independent routes to the lexicon, a "direct" visual route, and one involving a system of grapheme–phoneme translation (e.g., Marshall & Newcombe, 1966, 1973).

What are the syndromes of developmental dyslexia likely to tell about the reading process (assuming such distinct types in fact exist)? First, let us consider the type with oculomotor problems. If a subject has difficulty maintaining fixation, then it is likely that the resultant blurring and so forth would interfere with the reading process, but such a syndrome would tell us little of interest about reading. However, if the problem is more subtle than that, for example, being restricted to eye *movement* control, such eye movement problems might help us to understand reading better. What is most intriguing in this regard is a comment by Jones and Stark that there are normal readers who show the same abnormal patterns of eye fixations as the dyslexic readers with eye control problems. They do not make clear, however, what the frequency of these abnormal patterns are in such readers. If one can find subjects who have relatively intact reading skills while displaying relatively severe disruptions in their eye movements, such subjects would be extremely interesting to study. The existence of such subjects would somewhat call into question that the abnormal eye movement pattern of the dyslexics was the sole cause of the reading difficulty, and would suggest that there is a deeper problem as well, such as the sequencing problem suggested by Pavlidis. However, my feeling is that if an underlying problem in dyslexia is one of sequencing as suggested by Pavlidis and others (e.g., Bakker, 1972), the construct must be sharpened considerably. The problem cannot be as general as Pavlidis presents it, since virtually all human behavior involves sequencing, yet these subjects appear to have a relatively specific problem with reading.

Although there may be subtle and deep aspects to the reading problems of dyslexics with eye control problems, dyslexics who have linguistic and/or cognitive difficulties would seem to be a more promising group to study to get basic insights into the reading processes. In particular, it would be valuable to identify those skills, which if severely impaired, make reading close to impossible, yet which allow oral language comprehension to be relatively intact. In this regard, two tasks that appear to signal severe reading problems are naming deficits (e.g., long latencies to name line drawings of objects, colors) and difficulty in abstracting the phonetic code in spoken language. It would clearly be of value to know whether these deficits are invariably accompanied by reading problems, since in some theories of fluent reading phonetic codes are not involved at all (e.g., Smith, 1973). For people with these "verbal deficits" who have severe reading problems, tasks with individual words are likely to be more diagnostic than analyzing their grossly nonfluent reading of text. However, if fairly severe deficits on these dimensions are accompanied by less severe problems, then the eye movement record might be particularly valuable in uncovering how these deficits disrupt the reading process. In addition, studying how people with severe deficits in one skill carry on relatively normally with the reading process might provide some important clues in programs of remediation.

# References

Bakker, J. F. (1972). *Temporal order in disturbed reading-developmental and neuropsychological aspects in normal and reading-retarded children.* Rotterdam: Rotterdam University Press.

Boder, E. (1973). Developmental dyslexia: Prevailing diagnostic concepts and a new diagnostic approach. *Bulletin of the Orton Society, 23,* 106–118.

Coltheart, M. (1981). Disorders of reading and their implications for models of normal reading. *Visible Language, 15,* 245–286.

Marshall, J. C., & Newcombe, F. (1966). Syntactic and semantic errors in paralexia. *Neuropsychologia, 4,* 169–176.

Marshall, J. C., & Newcombe, F. (1973). Patterns of paralexia: A psycholinguistic approach. *Journal of Psycholinguistic Research, 2,* 175–199.

Mattis, S. (1981). Dyslexia syndromes in children: Toward the development of syndrome-specific treatment programs. In F. Pirozzolo & M. Wittrock (Eds.), *Neuropsychological and cognitive processes in reading.* New York: Academic Press.

Pavlidis, G. Th. (1981). Sequencing eye movements and the early objective diagnosis of dyslexia. In G. Th. Pavlidis & T. R. Miles (Eds.), *Dyslexia research and its applications to education.* London: J. Wiley.

Pirozzolo, F. J., & Rayner, K. (1978). The neural control of eye movements in acquired and developmental reading disorders. In H. Whitaker & H. A. Whitaker (Eds.), *Studies in neurolinguistics, Vol. 4.* New York: Academic Press.

Potter, M., Kroll, J. F., & Harris, C. (1980). Comprehension and memory in rapid sequential reading. In R. S. Nickerson (Ed.), *Attention and Performance* (Vol. 8). Hillsdale, New Jersey: Erlbaum.

Satz, P., & Morris, R. (1981). Learning disability subtypes: A review. In F. Pirozzolo & M. Wittrock (Eds.), *Neuropsychological and cognitive processes in reading.* New York: Academic Press.

Smith, F. (1973). *Understanding reading.* New York: Holt, Rinehart, & Winston.

Stanley, G., Smith, G. A., & Howell, E. A. (1982). Eye movements and sequential tracking in dyslexic and control children. *British Journal of Psychology,* in press.

Velluntino, F. R. (1979). *Dyslexia: Theory and research.* Cambridge, Massachusetts: MIT Press.

# Index

PERSPECTIVES IN
NEUROLINGUISTICS, NEUROPSYCHOLOGY, AND
PSYCHOLINGUISTICS: A Series of Monographs and Treatises

R. W. RIEBER (Ed.). Language Development and Aphasia in Children: New Essays and a Translation of "Kindersprache und Aphasie" by Emil Fröschels

GRACE H. YENI-KOMSHIAN, JAMES F. KAVANAGH, and CHARLES A. FERGUSON (Eds.). Child Phonology, Volume 1: Production and Volume 2: Perception

FRANCIS J. PIROZZOLO and MERLIN C. WITTROCK (Eds.). Neuropsychological and Cognitive Processes in Reading

JASON W. BROWN (Ed.). Jargonaphasia

DONALD G. DOEHRING, RONALD L. TRITES, P. G. PATEL, and CHRISTINA A. M. FIEDOROWICZ. Reading Disabilities: The Interaction of Reading, Language, and Neuropsychological Deficits

MICHAEL A. ARBIB, DAVID CAPLAN, and JOHN C. MARSHALL (Eds.). Neural Models of Language Processes

R. N. MALATESHA and P. G. AARON (Eds.). Reading Disorders: Varieties and Treatments

MICHAEL L. GEIS. The Language of Television Advertising

LORAINE OBLER and LISE MENN (Eds.). Exceptional Language and Linguistics

M. P. BRYDEN. Laterality: Functional Asymmetry in the Intact Brain

KEITH RAYNER (Ed.). Eye Movements in Reading: Perceptual and Language Processes

*In Preparation:*

S. J. SEGALOWITZ (Ed.). Language Functions and Brain Organization